Communications
in Computer and Information Science

3009

Series Editors

Gang Li, *School of Information Technology, Deakin University, Burwood, VIC, Australia*

Joaquim Filipe, *Polytechnic Institute of Setúbal, Setúbal, Portugal*

Zhiwei Xu, *Chinese Academy of Sciences, Beijing, China*

Rationale

The CCIS series is devoted to the publication of proceedings of computer science conferences. Its aim is to efficiently disseminate original research results in informatics in printed and electronic form. While the focus is on publication of peer-reviewed full papers presenting mature work, inclusion of reviewed short papers reporting on work in progress is welcome, too. Besides globally relevant meetings with internationally representative program committees guaranteeing a strict peer-reviewing and paper selection process, conferences run by societies or of high regional or national relevance are also considered for publication.

Topics

The topical scope of CCIS spans the entire spectrum of informatics ranging from foundational topics in the theory of computing to information and communications science and technology and a broad variety of interdisciplinary application fields.

Information for Volume Editors and Authors

Publication in CCIS is free of charge. No royalties are paid, however, we offer registered conference participants temporary free access to the online version of the conference proceedings on SpringerLink (http://link.springer.com) by means of an http referrer from the conference website and/or a number of complimentary printed copies, as specified in the official acceptance email of the event.

CCIS proceedings can be published in time for distribution at conferences or as postproceedings, and delivered in the form of printed books and/or electronically as USBs and/or e-content licenses for accessing proceedings at SpringerLink. Furthermore, CCIS proceedings are included in the CCIS electronic book series hosted in the SpringerLink digital library at http://link.springer.com/bookseries/7899. Conferences publishing in CCIS are allowed to use our online conference service (Meteor) for managing the whole proceedings lifecycle (from submission and reviewing to preparing for publication) free of charge.

Publication process

The language of publication is exclusively English. Authors publishing in CCIS have to sign the Springer CCIS copyright transfer form, however, they are free to use their material published in CCIS for substantially changed, more elaborate subsequent publications elsewhere. For the preparation of the camera-ready papers/files, authors have to strictly adhere to the Springer CCIS Authors' Instructions and are strongly encouraged to use the CCIS LaTeX style files or templates.

Abstracting/Indexing

CCIS is abstracted/indexed in DBLP, Google Scholar, EI-Compendex, Mathematical Reviews, SCImago, Scopus. CCIS volumes are also submitted for the inclusion in ISI Proceedings.

How to start

To start the evaluation of your proposal for inclusion in the CCIS series, please send an e-mail to ccis@springer.com

Mariella Särestöniemi · Daljeet Singh ·
Erika Jarva · Jarmo Reponen
Editors

Digital Health and Wireless Solutions: Towards Trustworthy and Person-Centric Digital Health

Second Nordic Conference, NCDHWS 2026
Oulu, Finland, June 16–17, 2026
Proceedings, Part I

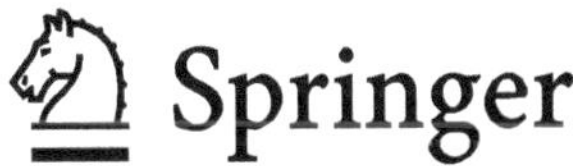 Springer

Editors
Mariella Särestöniemi
University of Oulu
Oulu, Finland

Daljeet Singh
University of Oulu
Oulu, Finland

Erika Jarva
University of Oulu
Oulu, Finland

Jarmo Reponen
University of Oulu
Oulu, Finland

ISSN 1865-0929   ISSN 1865-0937 (electronic)
Communications in Computer and Information Science
ISBN 978-3-032-28811-0   ISBN 978-3-032-28812-7 (eBook)
https://doi.org/10.1007/978-3-032-28812-7

Foreword

Digital health functions as an umbrella concept encompassing a wide range of technology-enabled approaches to healthcare. It includes electronic health services traditionally referred to as eHealth, telemedicine, electronic health counselling, and the active involvement of citizens and patients in promoting their own health through the use of digital technologies. In recent years, this umbrella has expanded to include advanced computational methods, such as artificial intelligence-based analytics, and more recently, generative artificial intelligence and large language models. When combined with genomic data, large-scale health datasets, and sensor-based measurements of citizens' health status, these technologies enable the generation of precise and actionable information. Such information can be leveraged both to improve the overall quality of healthcare systems and to enhance the care of individual patients.

Digital transformation in healthcare aims to make healthcare processes more efficient through the systematic use of digital tools. Wireless technologies, in particular, enable the collection of relevant health data outside traditional clinical environments, while mobile devices allow citizens to actively participate in their own care. Together, these developments contribute to making healthcare services increasingly independent of time and place, whenever physical encounters are not strictly necessary.

The Nordic countries are at the forefront of this digital transformation of healthcare and consistently rank among the top performers in the European Union's Digital Economy and Society Index (DESI). Finland provides a prominent example: all public healthcare patient record systems have been fully electronic since 2007. National health information infrastructure components—including a nationwide electronic health record archive, electronic prescriptions, and a Health Information Exchange (HIE) connecting different healthcare service providers—have been in place since 2010. Citizen engagement is also substantial: on a monthly basis, approximately one fifth of the population regularly accesses their personal health data through the My Kanta Pages patient portal linked to the HIE. Comparable patient portals are in use across the other Nordic countries as well.

As a field of research, digital health is of particular relevance in Finland, not least due to the major administrative reform implemented in 2023. This reform merged public healthcare service providers, social welfare services, and rescue services into large regional entities known as Wellbeing Services Counties. Beyond changes in governance and financing, the reform involves extensive integration of information systems and the adoption of a "Digital First" principle in service delivery. The guiding objective is to provide services digitally and independently of location whenever face-to-face contact is not required.

At the European level, future developments and research opportunities are influenced by initiatives such as the European Health Data Space (EHDS), which aims to harmonize health data used both for primary purposes in patient care and for secondary purposes in research and innovation. At the same time, regulatory frameworks such as the EU

Artificial Intelligence Act and the EU Medical Device Regulation define the boundaries within which artificial intelligence can be deployed responsibly in healthcare. Efforts are also underway to strengthen methods for evaluating the effectiveness of digital health applications and, through Health Technology Assessment (HTA), to establish frameworks for the reimbursement of software-based health solutions. It is hoped that these regulatory developments will support, rather than constrain, Europe's ability to advance as a leading source of health innovations.

The Second Nordic Conference on Digital Health and Wireless Solutions (NCD-HWS 2026) was organized by the University of Oulu's *6G Enabled Sustainable Solutions* (6GESS) and *Digital Health* (DigiHealth) research programs, in collaboration with the Profi6-Fibrobesity, Profi8-Health Dimensions, and Oulu Brain & Mind research programs. Our regional partners included Oulu University of Applied Sciences, Oulu University Hospital, the Wellbeing Services County of North Ostrobothnia (Pohde), and Business Oulu. Together, these initiatives brought multidisciplinary expertise spanning medical and health sciences, biosciences, health economics, information technology, sensor technologies, and wireless communications. Once again, we hosted an international multidisciplinary conference that provided an excellent forum for professionals, researchers, and industry leaders from diverse fields to exchange insights and discuss the latest advances in digital health and related technologies.

The conference host city of Oulu has long been at the forefront of research and development in digital health and wireless communications. Electronic health records, telemedicine, and mobile health services have been developed and deployed here for nearly three decades. Active research initiatives continue in areas such as artificial intelligence, novel sensor technologies, and edge computing. At the same time, strong emphasis is placed on the scientific evaluation of the impact of these innovations, as well as on addressing the associated educational needs.

The organization of a multidisciplinary conference of this scale—bringing together diverse academic, clinical, industrial, and societal perspectives—would not have been possible without the dedicated efforts of numerous colleagues and experts. I would like to thank the multidisciplinary Organizing Committee, my co-chair Simo Saarakkala, and our two coordinators, Chao Ding and Tuire Salonurmi, for their highly constructive collaboration. I would further like to express my special appreciation to the Chair of the Scientific Program Committee and Publication Chair, Mariella Särestöniemi, who, together with the committee members and International Reviewers, ensured the high scientific quality of the conference content.

I am also grateful to our distinguished international invited speakers for sharing their expertise in digital health and related technologies, and to the members of the International Advisory Committee for their valuable guidance. My sincere thanks go to Elina Laukka for leading the Student Volunteer Committee, and to all student volunteers whose invaluable support ensured smooth conference operations. I would also like to thank our media team, Katja Longhurst and Sallamaari Syrjä, for their excellent work in maintaining the conference's digital presence. My gratitude further extends to Minna Komu for her efforts in engaging industry partners, as well as to Oulu University Hospital and the Wellbeing Services County of North Ostrobothnia for their support in conference arrangements and for providing a rich and unique research environment.

Finally, I would like to thank all those who contributed to the success of NCDHWS 2026—whether as organizers, contributors, or participants.

June 2026   Jarmo Reponen

Preface

The Nordic Conference on Digital Health and Wireless Solutions (NCDHWS) is an international, multidisciplinary conference that brings together experts and professionals from engineering, medicine, and health sciences working at the intersection of digital health and wireless technologies. Following the successful inaugural conference in 2024, NCDHWS was organized for the second time, continuing its mission to foster interdisciplinary collaboration and advance innovative, impactful digital health solutions.

The organization of NCDHWS relies on close cooperation among multidisciplinary committees and a shared effort to harmonize the diverse scientific cultures and evaluation practices of different research fields. Consequently, the program committee chairs, organizing committee, program committee, and international advisory committee included representatives from a wide range of disciplines as well as from 32 different countries, reflecting the international and interdisciplinary nature of the conference.

The conference proceedings are published in a Springer CCIS Open Access book with three thematically organized volumes: *Volume I: Towards Trustworthy and Person-Centric Digital Health*, *Volume II: Integrating AI, LLMs and Multimodal Health Data for Next-Generation Decision Support*, and *Volume III: Connected Digital Health: Digital Twins, Wearables, Wireless Systems, and Secure Architectures.*

This Volume I focuses on the foundations of trustworthy and person centric digital health. The contributions address digital health transformation and innovation with an emphasis on personalization, ethics, usability, and real-world impact within healthcare and social care systems. Topics include personalized digital health solutions ranging from omics to telemedicine and eRehabilitation, health technology assessment and impact evaluation, user experience and adoption of health information systems, as well as organizational, policy, and governance perspectives that shape implementation in practice. Additionally, digital health education is a recurring theme, with studies addressing skills development and innovative educational approaches, including the use of emerging technologies such as AI, XR, and simulation in the training of healthcare professionals. Together, these works provide a human-centred and system-level perspective on digital health, highlighting how technological innovation is translated into meaningful, sustainable, and responsible practice.

Reflecting varied publication practices across disciplines, the conference accepted three types of submissions: full papers (10–30 pages), short papers (5–9 pages), and abstracts (1–4 pages). Full and short papers are published in the main body of the Springer book and indexed, while abstracts appear in the back matter. In total, 159 submissions were received, including 90 full papers, 32 short papers, and 37 abstracts.

All submissions underwent a rigorous double-blind peer-review process involving approximately 190 international reviewers. Each full and short paper was evaluated by three to five reviewers with appropriate scientific expertise, while abstracts were reviewed by two to three reviewers. The EDAS platform was used for submission and review management, ensuring confidentiality and the automated handling of conflicts of interest. Reviewers assessed submissions using a five-point scoring scale, provided confidence levels, and offered detailed, constructive feedback. Final acceptance decisions were based on weighted average scores that incorporated reviewer confidence. Submissions with a rounded weighted average score of at least 3 ("marginally accept") were accepted, contingent upon authors revising their work in accordance with reviewers' comments. This revision requirement applied to all accepted papers. Plagiarism checks were conducted using the plagiarism detection tools integrated into EDAS, and authors were asked to take corrective action when similarity scores exceeded acceptable thresholds. EDAS also ensured confidentiality by preventing program committee chairs from accessing reviews of their own papers or from viewing reviewer identities. In total, 137 papers were accepted for publication, comprising 107 full and short papers and 30 abstracts.

We gratefully acknowledge the support of the Springer Nature team for their guidance and assistance throughout all practical aspects of the book publication process. We also extend our sincere thanks to all members of the conference committees, including the organizing committee, program committee, and international advisory committee, whose collective efforts made the organization of this multidisciplinary conference possible.

We would further like to thank the City of Oulu, European Capital of Culture 2026, for supporting the conference and for providing the opportunity to organize a get-together event at the Oulu City Hall, which greatly enriched the conference experience and facilitated informal networking and interaction among participants.

In addition, we express our deep appreciation to the keynote and invited speakers, who took time from their busy schedules to travel to Oulu and deliver inspiring presentations on their research. Finally, we sincerely thank all authors for choosing NCDHWS 2026 as a forum to present their research. Through the combination of high-quality contributed papers and excellent invited talks, this multidisciplinary gathering proved to be both productive and successful, fostering meaningful discussions and new opportunities for collaboration.

June 2026

Mariella Särestöniemi
Daljeet Singh
Erika Jarva
Jarmo Reponen

Organization

General Chairs (Conference President and Vice-president)

Jarmo Reponen	University of Oulu, Finland
Simo Saarakkala	University of Oulu, Finland

Program Committee Chairs

Mariella Särestöniemi (Chair)	University of Oulu, Finland
Daljeet Singh	University of Oulu, Finland
Erkki Harjula	University of Oulu, Finland
Minna Isomursu	University of Oulu, Finland
Miia Jansson	University of Oulu, Finland
Erika Jarva	University of Oulu, Finland
Mark van Gils	University of Tampere, Finland
Jarmo Reponen	University of Oulu, Finland
Johanna Uusimaa	University of Oulu, Finland
Johannes Kettunen	University of Oulu, Finland
Mika Martikainen	University of Oulu, Finland
Janne Hukkanen	University of Oulu, Finland
Ali Mobasheri	University of Oulu, Finland

Publication Chairs

Mariella Särestöniemi	University of Oulu, Finland
Daljeet Singh	University of Oulu, Finland
Erika Jarva	University of Oulu, Finland
Jarmo Reponen	University of Oulu, Finland

Organization Committee

Jarmo Reponen (Chair)	University of Oulu, Finland
Simo Saarakkala (Vice-chair)	University of Oulu, Finland
Chao Ding	University of Oulu, Finland

Tuire Salonurmi	University of Oulu, Finland
Mariella Särestöniemi	University of Oulu, Finland
Erkki Harjula	University of Oulu, Finland
Matti Hämäläinen	University of Oulu, Finland
Minna Isomursu	University of Oulu, Finland
Johanna Uusimaa	University of Oulu, Oulu University Hospital, Finland
Miia Jansson	University of Oulu, Finland
Salla Kangas	University of Oulu, Finland
Ritva Saastamoinen	University of Oulu, Finland
Essi Erkkilä	University of Oulu, Finland
Minna Komu	OuluHealth/BusinessOulu, Finland
Teija Kekonen	Oulu University Hospital, Finland
Elina Laukka	Oulu University of Applied Sciences, Finland
Mark van Gils	University of Tampere, Finland

Program Committee

Chew Han Shi (Jocelyn)	National University of Singapore, Singapore
Tam Wai San (Wilson)	National University of Singapore, Singapore
Raja Omman Zafar	Dalarna University, Sweden
Sarthak Acharya	University of Oulu, Finland
Ijaz Ahmad	VTT Technical Research Centre of Finland, Finland
Roni Ahola	University of Tampere, Finland
Outi Ahonen	Laurea University of Applied Sciences, Finland
Mika Alhonkoski	University of Turku, Finland
Slawomir Ambroziak	Gdańsk University of Technology, Poland
Ulla Ashorn	University of Turku, Finland
Aslak Aslaksen	Bergen University Hospital, Norway
Tunc Asuroglu	VTT Technical Research Centre of Finland, Finland
Himanshi Babbar	Chitkara University, India
Christian Becker	University of Stuttgart, Germany
Woubset Behutiye	University of Oulu, Finland
Gro Rosvold Berntsen	Norwegian Center for eHealth Research, Norway
Roberto Blanco	University of Turku, Finland
Mikael Brix	University of Oulu, Finland
Maria Bulgheroni	Ab.Acus srl, Italy
Stefano Caputo	University of Florence, Italy
Constantino Alvarez Casado	University of Oulu, Finland

Bhushan B. Chaudhari	SVKM's Institute of Technology, India
Wei Ling Chua	National University of Singapore, Singapore
Omedev Dahia	Galgotias University, India
Nils Dahlström	University of Linköping, Sweden
Livio Dalvia	Sapienza University of Rome, Italy
Aysen Degerli	VTT Technical Research Centre of Finland, Finland
Manish Deshwal	Chandigarh University, India
Satu Elo	Oulu University of Applied Sciences, Finland
Jeppe Eriksen	University of Aalborg, Denmark
Gökçe Banu Laleci Ertürkmen	Software Research & Development and Consultancy Corporation, Turkey
Shan Feng	University of Turku, Finland
Hany Ferdinando	University of Oulu, Finland
Dimitris Filos	Aristotle University of Thessaloniki, Greece
Huber Flores	University of Tartu, Estonia
Mark van Gils	University of Tampere, Finland
Heidi Gilstad	Norwegian University of Science and Technology, Norway
Guido Giunti	University of Oulu, Finland
Casandra Grundstrom	Norwegian University of Science and Technology, Norway
Ankur Gupta	Netaji Subhas University of Technology, India
Akhil Gupta	Symbiosis Institute of Technology, India
Sanaul Haque	LUT University, Lappeenranta, Finland
Erkki Harjula	University of Oulu, Finland
Nina Hautala	University of Oulu, Finland
Ying He	University of Technology Sydney, Australia
Tharaka Hewa	University of Oulu, Finland
Sari Huikko-Tarvainen	Medical Research Center Oulu, Finland
Krista Hylkilä	University of Oulu, Finland
Piia Hyvämäki	Oulu University of Applied Sciences, Finland
Matti Hämäläinen	University of Oulu, Finland
Minna Hökkä	Kajaani University of Applied Sciences, Finland
Iiris Hörhammer	Aalto University, Finland
Esa-Ville Immonen	University of Oulu, Finland
Milla Immonen	Lapland University of Applied Sciences, Finland
Antti Isosalo	University of Oulu, Finland
Erika Jarva	University of Oulu, Finland
Joel Jaskari	University of Tampere, Finland
Sara Jayousi	University of Florence, Italy
Vesa Jormanainen	University of Helsinki, Finland

Hem Dutt Joshi	Thapar Institute of Engineering & Technology, India
Emmi Kaivanto	University of Oulu, Finland
Janne Kananen	University of Oulu, Finland
Salla Kangas	University of Oulu, Finland
Mari Kangasniemi	University of Turku, Finland
Kimmo Kansanen	Norwegian University of Science and Technology, Norway
Outi Kanste	University of Oulu, Finland
Minna Karjalainen	University of Oulu, Finland
Pasi Karppinen	University of Oulu, Finland
Markus Karttunen	Oulu University of Applied Sciences, Finland
Jani Katisko	Oulu University Hospital, Finland
Haneda Katsuyaki	Aalto University, Finland
Tuija Keinänen	Oulu University Hospital, Finland
Heli Kerimaa	University of Oulu, Finland
Ali Khaleghi	Norwegian University of Science and Technology, Norway
Ulla-Mari Kinnunen	University of Eastern Finland, Finland
Chaïmaâ Kissi	Ibn Tofail University, Morocco
Pyry Kiviharju	Aalto University, Finland
Sivarama Krishna Akhil Koduri	University of the Cumberlands, USA
Laura Kohonen-Aho	University of Oulu, Finland
Jussi Koivunen	Oulu University Hospital, Finland
Jorma Komulainen	University of Eastern Finland, Finland
Juha Korpelainen	Oulu University Hospital, Finland
Hilkka Korpi	Oulu University of Applied Sciences, Finland
Pirkko Kouri	Finnish Society of Telemedicine and eHealth, Finland
Elizabeth Krupinski	Emory University School of Medicine, USA
Heli Kuivila	University of Oulu, Finland
Atul Kumar	Indian Institute of Technology, India
Rajeev Kumar	University of Chitkara, India
Sumit Kumar	Jain University, India
Tanesh Kumar	Aalto University, Finland
Timo Kumpuniemi	University of Oulu, Finland
Maria Kääriäinen	University of Oulu, Finland
Elina Laukka	Oulu University of Applied Sciences, Finland
Jay J. J. Lee	University of Hong Kong, China
Fedor Lehocki	Slovak University of Technology in Bratislava, Slovakia
Hilkka Liedes	VTT Technical Research Centre of Finland, Finland

Tarmo Lipping	University of Tampere, Finland
Tinja Lääveri	Aalto University, Finland
Bessie Malila	University of Johannesburg, South Africa
Andigoni Malousi	Aristotle University of Thessaloniki, Greece
Terence McSweeney	University of Oulu, Finland
Sharon Guardado Medina	University of Oulu, Finland
Heta Merikallio	University of Oulu, Finland
Nora Mickelson	University of Turku and Turku University Hospital, Finland
Kristina Mikkonen	University of Oulu, Finland
Ayan Mondal	Indian Institute of Technology Indore, India
Lorenzo Mucchi	University of Florence, Italy
Karla MunozEsquivel	Atlantic Technological University, Ireland
Joyce Mwangama	University of Cape Town, South Africa
Teemu Myllylä	University of Oulu, Finland
Vasiliki Mylonopoulou	University of Gothenburg, Sweden
Mariaana Mäki-Asiala	University of Oulu, Finland
Niko Männikkö	Oulu University of Applied Sciences, Finland
Tuija Männistö	University of Eastern Finland, Finland
My Nguyen	RMIT University, Australia
Marketta Niemelä	LAB University of Applied Sciences, Finland
Anne Oikarinen	University of Oulu, Finland
Diana Moya Osario	Linköping University, Sweden
Sofia Ouhbi	Uppsala University, Sweden
Hanna Paananen	University of Jyväskylä, Finland
Juha Pajari	University of Eastern Finland, Finland
Juha Pajula	VTT Technical Research Centre of Finland, Finland
Mika Paldanius	Oulu University of Applied Sciences, Finland
Ankur Pandley	Rajiv Gandhi Institute of Petroleum Technology, India
Egor Panfilov	University of Oulu, Finland
Lauri Parkkonen	Aalto University, Finland
Juha Partala	University of Oulu, Finland
Ella Peltonen	University of Oulu, Finland
Renu Popli	Chitkara University, India
Pawani Porambage	VTT Technical Research Centre of Finland, Finland
Tarja Pölkki	University of Oulu, Finland
Prabhat Ram	University of Oulu, Finland
Ahmad Rayani	King Saud University, Saudi Arabia
Jarmo Reponen	University of Oulu, Finland

Peeter Ross   Technical University of Tallinn, Estonia
Heidi Ruotsalainen   Oulu University of Applied Sciences, Finland
Rajkumar Saini   Luleå University of Technology, Sweden
Tuire Salonurmi   University of Oulu, Finland
Ama Samarasinghe   RMIT University, Australia
Pedro Moreno Sanchez   Tampere University, Finland
Laura Sandström   University of British Columbia, Canada
Daniel Pinto dos Santos   University Hospital of Cologne, Germany
Kaija Saranto   University of Eastern Finland, Finland
Kamran Sayrafian   National Institute of Standards and Technology,
                                  USA
Aleksi Schrey   University of Turku, Finland
Imran Shah   University of Oulu, Finland
Shallu Sharma   Bennett University, India
Stephan Sigg   Aalto University, Finland
Heidi Siira   University of Oulu, Finland
Pekka Siirtola   University of Oulu, Finland
Daljeet Singh   University of Oulu, Finland
Gurjinder Singh   Chitkara University, India
Eeva Sliz   University of Oulu, Finland
Anthony Smith   University of Queensland, Australia
Simone Soderi   IMT School for Advanced Studies Lucca, Italy
Jack Soh   University of Oulu, Finland
Mariella Särestöniemi   University of Oulu, Finland
Atthapongse Taparugssanagorn   Asian Institute of Technology, Thailand
Gianluigi Tiberi   London South Bank University, UK & UBT Srl,
                                  Italy
Jani Tikkanen   Kuura Health Ltd, Finland
Jussi-Pekka Tolonen   Oulu University Hospital, Finland
Paulus Torkki   University of Helsinki, Finland
Posco Tso   Loughborough University, UK
Annukka Tuomikoski   Northern Ostrobothnia Wellbeing Services
                                  County, Finland
Timo Tuovinen   University of Oulu, Finland
Delfin Tursin   University of Oulu, Finland
Shingo Ueki   Kyushu University, Japan
Johanna Uusimaa   University of Oulu, Finland
Minna Vanhanen   Oulu University of Applied Sciences, Finland
Sampsa Vanhatalo   University of Helsinki, Finland
Antti Vehkaoja   University of Tampere, Finland
Paula Veikkolainen   University of Oulu, Finland
Märt Vesinurm   Aalto University, Finland

Gillian Vesty	RMIT University, Australia
Johanna Viitanen	Aalto University, Finland
Sidsel Villumsen	University of Aalborg, Denmark
Mari Virtanen	Metropolia University of Applied Sciences, Finland
Anna-Leena Vuorinen	University of Tampere, Finland
Alpo Värri	University of Tampere, Finland
Fan Wang	University of Oulu, Finland
Zhou Wentao	National University of Singapore, Singapore
Brigitte Woo	National University of Singapore, Singapore
Xiaoting Wu	University of Oulu, Finland
Miyae Yamakawa	Osaka University, Japan
Rameem Zahra	Netaji Subhas University of Technology, India
Yingchun Zeng (Chloe)	National University of Singapore, Singapore
Aleksandra Zienkiewicz	University of Oulu, Finland
Ece Üreten	Delft University of Technology, Netherlands

International Advisory Committee

Najeeb Al-Shorbaji	eHealth Development Association, Jordan
Slawomir Ambroziak	Gdańsk University of Technology, Poland
D. K. Arvind	University of Edinburgh, UK
Rimma Axelsson	Karolinska Institutet, Sweden
Gro Rosvold Berntsen	Norwegian Centre for E-health Research, Norway
Paolo Bifulco	University Federico II of Naples, Italy
Paola Buedo	University of Munich, Germany
Filipe Cardonso	Polytechnic Institute of Setúbal, Portugal
Jessica Centracchio	University Federico II of Naples, Italy
Akshay Chaudhari	Stanford University, USA
Luis M. Correia	University of Lisbon, Portugal
Georg Dorffner	Medical University of Vienna, Austria
Sandra Dudley	London South Bank University, UK
Osama Elhassan	UAE Health Informatics Society, UAE
Flavio Esposito	Saint Louis University, USA
Simone Farah	UNIFASE/Petrópolis Faculty of Medicine, Brazil
Vahid Farrahi	TU Dortmund University, Germany
Michael Fuchsjäger	Medical University Graz, Austria
Mohammad Ghvami	London South Bank University, UK
Hassan Ghazal	Moroccan Society for Telemedicine and eHealth, Morocco

Michele Y. Griffith	International Society for Telemedicine and eHealth, USA
Ingfrid S. Haldorsen	Haukeland University Hospital, Norway
Clayton Hamilton	World Health Organization, Denmark
Manami Hori	Tokai University, Japan
Lars Hulbæk	MedCom, Denmark
Michael Inouye	University of Cambridge, UK
Vesa Jormanainen	Ministry of Social Affairs and Health, Finland
Dipak Kalra	European Institute for Innovation through Health Data, Belgium
Ulla-Mari Kinnunen	University of Eastern Finland, Finland
Hiroshi Kondoh	Tottori University, Japan
Ilkka Korhonen	University of Tampere, Finland
Elisabeth A. Krupinski	Emory University, USA
Line Helen Linstad	Norwegian Centre for E-health Research, Norway
Anthony Maeder	Flinders University, Australia
Janne Martikainen	University of Eastern Finland, Finland
Lorenzo Mucchi	University of Florence, Italy
Miika Nieminen	University of Oulu, Finland
Jérôme Noally	University of Pompeu Fabra, Spain
Aud Uhlen Obstfelder	Norwegian University of Science and Technology, Norway
Peter van Ooijen	University Medical Center Groningen, Netherlands
Kaija Saranto	University of Eastern Finland, Finland
Kamran Sayrafian	National Institute of Standards and Technology, USA
Päivi Sillanaukee	Ministry of Social Affairs and Health, Finland
Piotr H. Skarzynski	Institute of Physiology and Pathology of Hearing, Poland
Anthony Smith	University of Queensland, Australia
Attaphongse Taparugssanagorn	Asian Institute of Technology, Thailand
Rosanna Tarricone	Bocconi University, Italy
Gianluigi Tiberi	Umbria Bioengineering Technologies, Italy
Paulus Torkki	University of Helsinki, Finland
Yoshito Tsushima	Gunma University, Japan
Gillian Vesty	RMIT University, Australia
Johanna Viitanen	Aalto University, Finland
Anssi Ylimaula	OunasHealth, Finland

Contents

Health Technology Assessment and Impact Evaluation

User Experience, Acceptance and Adoption of Health Information Systems

Education in Digital Health

Abstracts

Digital Health Transformation, Innovations and Future Visions

Profiting from 6G System for the Smart Hospital of the Future

Fan Wang[1,2]($\boxtimes$) , Seppo Yrjölä[3] , Risto Jurva[3] , Timo Koivumäki[1] ,
Aigerim Dairabekova[1] , and Petri Ahokangas[1]

[1] Martti Ahtisaari Institute, Oulu Business School, University of Oulu, Oulu, Finland
`{fan.wang,timo.koivumaki,aigerim.dairabekova,`
`petri.ahokangas}@oulu.fi`
[2] Research Unit of Health Sciences and Technology, University of Oulu, Oulu, Finland
[3] Centre for Wireless Communications, University of Oulu, Oulu, Finland
`{Seppo.Yrjola,Risto.Jurva}@oulu.fi`

Abstract. Technologically enabled smart hospitals are emerging as a future trend in modern healthcare, yet their objectives and the role of advanced connectivity such as 6G remain unclear. This study explores the concept of smart hospitals and their aims for future patient care from technological, business, and regulatory perspectives, considering diverse stakeholder viewpoints. To address this, we propose a five-layered "C-service" business model for deploying 6G systems to support smart hospital objectives. The connectivity layer ensures ultra-reliable, low-latency communication for real-time monitoring and telemedicine. The computing layer enables distributed edge processing for rapid decision-making and immersive applications such as AR-assisted surgery. The content layer leverages integrated sensing and communication capabilities in 6G to facilitate secure transmission of medical data and imaging. The context layer interprets this data through AI-driven analytics and digital twinning, supporting personalized care and predictive diagnostics. Finally, the commerce layer integrates multi-layered communication and data platforms for efficient healthcare transactions, reducing administrative burdens and enabling new business models for value-based care. By minimizing hospital admissions through proactive health management, 6G-enabled smart hospitals empower patients and seamlessly integrate services across physical and virtual environments. This framework highlights how next-generation connectivity can transform healthcare delivery, improve operational efficiency, and create sustainable business models for future smart hospitals.

Keywords: Smart hospital · 6G · business model.

1 Introduction

The transformation of healthcare systems is increasingly shaped by the integration of advanced technologies, with the concept of the smart hospital emerging as a central focus of innovation. Among the most promising enablers of this transformation is the anticipated development of sixth-generation (6G) mobile communication networks, which are expected to drive a paradigm shift from volume-based service delivery toward value-based healthcare. In this context, patient outcomes become closely linked to operational efficiency and cost-effectiveness.

© The Author(s) 2026
M. Särestöniemi et al. (Eds.): NCDHWS 2026, CCIS 3009, pp. 3–18, 2026.
https://doi.org/10.1007/978-3-032-28812-7_1

The evolution of information and communication technologies (ICT) has accelerated data-driven innovation, fostering the convergence of physical and virtual environments. The availability of affordable technologies and the exponential growth of data have positioned digital transformation as a source of competitive advantage across all sectors, including healthcare. Recent academic discourse has highlighted emerging technologies such as artificial intelligence (AI), machine learning (ML), metaverse applications, terahertz (THz) spectrum-based radio access, edge computing, and private localized networks—all of which are expected to build upon the capabilities of 6G. Despite this growing interest, the current status and future trajectory of smart hospitals remain unclear.

The vision for 6G includes novel architecture and advanced technologies designed to address critical challenges faced by healthcare organizations, including aging populations, workforce shortages, and budget constraints. However, the term "smart hospital" lacks an accepted definition, and its practical implications, benefits, and implementation strategies are still evolving. This conceptual ambiguity poses challenges for researchers and practitioners seeking to advance in the field.

To address these gaps, this study adopts a workshop-based methodology to engage key stakeholders in a co-creative process. Thus, this study moves beyond descriptive accounts of smart hospitals by empirically identifying stakeholder-driven value creation mechanisms in 6G-enabled healthcare ecosystems.

The objective is to develop a shared understanding of what constitutes a smart hospital in contemporary healthcare settings and to identify strategic directions for its future development by leveraging the 6G system. This helps to explore how emerging connectivity infrastructures such as 6G may enable the evolution of smart hospitals, based on stakeholder perceptions of digital healthcare futures. Accordingly, the research question guiding this study is:

How do stakeholders envision value creation and capture in 6G-enabled smart hospitals?

2 Theoretical Approach

2.1 Business Models and 6G Ecosystems

A business model serves as a conceptual framework for understanding how organizations create, deliver, and capture value [1]. Traditionally, business models have been applied to analyze competitive advantage and strategic positioning, representing a firm's logic for delivering products and services to customers [2, 3]. With the rise of digitalization, this approach has been extended to e-business, where novel technologies and services enable new forms of value creation across private, public, and third-party sectors. In this context, business models are essential for translating technological potential into economic value [4–6].

The dominant lens for studying business models emphasizes three interrelated dimensions: value creation, value delivery, and value capture [7]. Amit and Zott [5] further conceptualize value creation through the content, structure, and governance of transactions, highlighting factors such as efficiency, novelty, and performance expectancy as critical drivers in digital business environments [4, 8]. However, focusing exclusively on internal technological processes and product innovation is insufficient for explaining value architecture, as it neglects the role of external actors, resources, and activities [9]. Consequently, the scope of business model research has expanded toward network-level interconnectedness and an ecosystemic perspective, emphasizing integrated and interdependent processes of value co-creation and co-capture [10].

This ecosystemic view aligns with Service-Dominant Logic (SDL), which frames value as co-created through collaborative activities and active stakeholder engagement rather than being embedded in products or services alone [11, 12]. SDL provides a process-oriented understanding of business models, highlighting dynamic interactions among actors in digital ecosystems.

Building on these foundations, Ahokangas et al. [14], Ahokangas et al. (2022) [13] extend business model theory to the context of mobile communication technologies, introducing a layered approach to connectivity-driven value creation. Connectivity is positioned as a fundamental enabler for user participation, digital content exchange, and platform-based business models, which leverage artificial intelligence and data-driven services. This perspective is operationalized through data platforms that integrate computing, content, context, and commerce, forming the backbone of emerging 6G ecosystems.

Further refinement is provided by Yrjölä [15], who proposes a 5C layered framework comprising five archetypical value propositions: connection, content, context, computing, and commerce. Each layer represents distinct yet interrelated sources of value and revenue models for profiting from 6G mobile communications. For instance, the connectivity layer enables data transmission and sensing; the computing layer provides distributed processing capabilities at the edge; the context layer interprets content through AI-driven analytics; and the commerce layer facilitates seamless transactions with minimal friction. These layers can generate and capture value individually, across multiple layers, or through their combined integration [16, 17]

The theoretical evolution of business models from firm-centric logic to ecosystemic and layered frameworks offers a foundation for analyzing how 6G-enabled smart hospital ecosystems can create, deliver, and capture value. This perspective emphasizes the importance of connectivity, data platforms, and stakeholder co-creation in shaping future healthcare services. Kumar et al. (2025) [49] argue that 6G will enable highly connected, data-driven smart hospitals that improve patient care and efficiency, but its adoption is constrained by infrastructure costs, interoperability challenges, and the need for robust governance frameworks.

2.2 Smart Hospitals in 6G Era

The concept of the smart hospital has emerged at the intersection of digital transformation, healthcare innovation, and advanced communication infrastructures. It is described by Kumar et al. (2025) [49] as a "digital or intelligent hospital " that is an example of how cutting-edge technologies, data-driven strategies, and patient-centered care have come together in the healthcare sector. Smart hospitals are increasingly seen as digitally integrated healthcare environments that leverage technologies such as the Internet of Medical Things (IoMT), artificial intelligence (AI), big data analytics, and advanced connectivity to enable real-time monitoring, predictive diagnostics, and personalized care [18, 19] with the aim of improving existing patient care methods at a minimal cost [20]

Unlike traditional hospitals, which are primarily organized around physical infrastructure and discrete care delivery, smart hospitals operate as continuous, data-driven ecosystems [21]. From an organizational perspective, smart hospitals can be conceptualized as ecosystems of interdependent actors that co-create value through digitally mediated interactions [22]. These ecosystems include healthcare providers, patients, technology firms, telecommunications operators, regulators, and data intermediaries. Value creation in such systems is not limited to organizational boundaries but emerges through coordination, data exchange, and platform-based interactions. Importantly, smart hospitals are increasingly characterized by the centrality of data as a strategic resource [20, 23]. Health data becomes the foundation for clinical decision-making, operational optimization, and new service development [24]. This shift aligns with broader transformations in digital ecosystems, where value is co-created through data flows and network effects rather than through isolated service provision [25]. Smart technologies, well-integrated with the help of sufficient connectivity, allow the right people to access the right information at the right time to offer better services [21].

However, the transformation toward smart hospitals also raises critical questions regarding governance, coordination, and legitimacy. As multiple actors participate in data-intensive healthcare ecosystems, issues related to trust, accountability, interoperability, and data ownership become central to the sustainability of these systems [23, 26]. Another essential prerequisite for developing a smart hospital is the creation and optimization of clinical and administrative processes, as well as the design and deployment of innovative technologies and equipment. These conditions cannot be met without interconnected assets [27].

With its ultra-high-speed connectivity, low latency, and massive device interconnection, 6G technology enables real-time data transmission and processing, allowing for the provision of advanced care solutions such as remote surgeries, AI-driven diagnostics, and enhanced telemedicine services [24]. The integrations of the 6G connectivity networks into smart hospitals offer transformative potential, offering data security features, seamless communication between various hospital departments, and enhancing operational efficiency. Nevertheless, this transformation requires significant infrastructure upgrades, high expenditures for implementation, as well as massive trainings for the health professionals [24].

3   Method

3.1   Research Design

A qualitative research design was employed to explore a comprehensive understanding of the phenomenon under investigation [28, 29].

3.2   Sample and Setting

A convenience sample of 19 participants was recruited from the health and technology research community, healthcare professionals (HCPs), and representatives of mobile network operators, all engaged in digital innovation for smart hospitals at the University of Oulu. No specific inclusion or exclusion criteria were applied.

3.3 Data Collection

Data were collected through a workshop held on the premises of the Oulu university hospital, utilizing the World Café method as a participatory approach. All discussions at the four thematic tables were audio-recorded and subsequently transcribed using Microsoft Teams. The transcripts were then refined and verified by the research team to ensure accuracy.

The workshop began with a brief introduction outlining its objectives. Participants were then presented with four key themes: (1) the hospital of the future, (2) stakeholder expectations and key actors in building smart hospitals, (3) digitalization and future directions, and (4) regulatory perspectives.

Following the principles of the World Café format [30], participants, each bringing diverse expertise from various organizations, were divided into small groups of 4 to 5 individuals. This structure facilitated dynamic, rotating discussions across all themes, encouraging collaborative reflection and knowledge exchange. At each table, one designated chairperson facilitated the discussions, guiding participants to share insights and explore digital technology and their expected benefits for future hospitals. After completing the rotation through all discussion tables, participants reconvened to engage in a plenary session, during which they reflected and synthesized their collective insights.

3.4 Data Analysis

The workshop data was transcribed by Microsoft Teams and later manually corrected by the first author, with verification by the research group. The unit of analysis (phrases) was defined prior to analysis, and hidden content (e.g., sighs, pitch changes, and pauses) was excluded from the data analysis. Thematic analysis was performed and categorized data through themes in the context of smart hospitals, and the results are presented based on the four key themes of round tables. Themes were validated through comparison across workshop groups and participant categories.

4 Results

4.1 The Hospital of the Future

The concept of "future hospitals," as discussed by participants, revolves around several key aims and visions for the transformation of healthcare delivery. Future hospitals are envisioned to focus on preventive care, aiming to reduce the need for patients to visit hospitals by promoting healthier lifestyles and enabling early interventions. The goal is to minimize hospital visits through proactive health management, supported by digital solutions, patient empowerment, and better integration of services.

Future hospitals are expected to leverage advanced technologies, such as portable diagnostic devices and telemedicine, to enhance patient care. A significant emphasis is placed on patient-centered care, where services are designed around the needs and experiences of patients. Effective care delivery depends on understanding the diverse backgrounds of patients and tailoring services to meet their specific needs. The integration of data across different healthcare systems to provide a holistic view of patient health can be seen as a key enabler. Meanwhile, improving communication and ensuring that patients have clear and accessible pathways to care remain essential.

Accessibility was another major theme. Participants emphasized the importance of making healthcare services available regardless of geographic location. This includes the use of remote monitoring and telehealth services to reach patients in rural or underserved areas. The need for remote monitoring and diagnostic devices or mobile health care constructions that can be used outside hospital settings was highlighted. Such technologies should enable continuous patient monitoring and early diagnosis, particularly for individuals living far from healthcare facilities.

Future hospitals also aim to optimize workflows and reduce administrative burdens on HCPs. Participants emphasized that using technology to automate processes and improve efficiency would allow providers to focus more on direct patient care. Accessing data from multiple sectors is essential for delivering holistic patient care that addresses not only medical needs but also social and psychological factors. Participants believe this can be achieved using personal data and data-driven decision-making to enhance patient outcomes. Real-time data sharing and monitoring will enhance the quality of care and support more personalized treatment strategies.

Overall, the discussions from the first theme of the workshop reflect a shared vision for future hospitals that prioritize preventive care, patient engagement, technological integration, and a holistic approach to health management.

4.2 The Key Players or Actors in Future Hospitals

The second key theme examines the stakeholder's perspective, focusing on the roles they are expected to assume in future healthcare systems and the tasks associated with smart hospitals and technological innovation. The stakeholders identified during the workshop discussions are presented in Table 1.

The analysis of stakeholders highlights the diverse roles and responsibilities required to enable the transition toward smart hospitals and technology-driven healthcare. Each stakeholder group contributes uniquely to the development, implementation, and sustainability of innovative solutions, emphasizing the need for collaborative approaches across sectors. The future of hospitals will rely on effective collaboration among diverse stakeholders to establish a more integrated, efficient, and patient-centered healthcare ecosystem.

4.3 Digitalization and Future Directions

The discussion highlighted considerable differences in the level of digitalization among hospitals. While some institutions have implemented advanced technologies, many continue to adopt a conservative approach to digital services. Participants emphasized the importance of intuitive design and clear, comprehensive instructions to ensure effective use of digital tools. The participants emphasized the necessity of creating user-friendly interfaces and providing clear guidance for both healthcare professionals and patients as end users. The importance of designing systems from the patient's perspective was strongly emphasized, particularly through the integration of proactive engagement strategies informed by individual health data. Consequently, there was a consensus that the

Table 1 Key stakeholders in the smart hospital and its relevance.

Stakeholder	Relevance
HCPs	Doctors, nurses, and other providers are central to future hospitals. Their engagement with new technologies and adaptability are crucial for implementation
Patients	Patients are key players. Their needs, preferences, and experiences should drive the design and delivery of healthcare services
Technology developers	Companies developing healthcare technologies (software, devices) play a major role in enhancing care and streamlining operations
Regulatory bodies	Agencies that set standards for healthcare practices, data sharing, and privacy. Their regulations shape technology adoption
Policymakers	Government officials influence healthcare policy and funding, affecting hospitals' ability to invest in digitalization
Insurance providers	Insurers determine coverage for new technologies and services, influencing patient access and hospital implementation
Community organizations	Local health and community groups promote health initiatives and ensure accessibility for diverse populations
Higher educational institutions	Universities and research centers contribute through innovation, research, and training of HCPs

continuous development of patient-centric digital services is essential to support and enhance access to health information and healthcare resources.

With regards to the utilization of health data, several challenges were identified in sharing patient information across different healthcare providers, primarily due to strict regulations governing data access and exchange. Participants discussed the potential for more seamless data integration across EU countries to improve patient care. The conversation also emphasized the need for secure and reliable technologies, particularly when handling sensitive patient data. Furthermore, participants stressed that data management systems must guarantee high levels of security to build trust among patients.

Technological innovations were a major focus, especially the potential of portable diagnostic devices and remote monitoring to support early diagnosis and treatment. These innovations align with the vision of smart hospitals and preventive healthcare. Participants expressed interest in the integration of AI and machine learning to enhance service delivery and patient outcomes. The transformative potential of AI in diagnostics, treatment planning, and personalized medicine was widely discussed, with future applications expected to be supported by 6G connectivity and private networks.

Several bottlenecks within the current healthcare system were identified, including inadequate communication among healthcare providers and fragmented data infrastructures. There is a pressing need for seamless integration of healthcare systems and devices to ensure interoperability across different manufacturers and platforms. Attention was also directed toward reducing patient waiting times and establishing clear pathways to care, which are closely linked to improving healthcare accessibility.

Regarding HCPs, participants recognized that while work organization can vary, inefficiencies persist in current systems. Technology should be designed to improve hospital workflows. Participants noted that existing workflows often lead to delays and inefficiencies, negatively impacting both patient care and HCPs' experiences. The need for more streamlined processes was emphasized, with suggestions for better planning and management tools to improve operational efficiency.

The discussions highlighted that HCPs frequently experience significant stress due to the demands of their roles, which can lead to burnout. This issue is exacerbated by inefficient workflows that require excessive time spent on administrative tasks rather than patient care. There was a strong call for solutions that allow professionals to focus more on patient interactions, which could help mitigate burnout. Integrating technology into healthcare workflows was discussed as a potential solution to reduce burnout. By automating routine tasks and improving data sharing, HCPs could dedicate more time to direct patient care. Participants emphasized the need for user-friendly systems that facilitate better communication and data management, helping to alleviate pressure on healthcare workers.

A forward-looking perspective on the healthcare workforce emerged, highlighting the need for ongoing training and support to adapt to new technologies and care models. Equipping HCPs to meet the demands of modern healthcare is essential for maintaining high-quality care. This effort also requires addressing conservatism and reluctance to adopt wireless and digital solutions. The cost of implementing new technologies was identified as a significant factor. While advanced technologies offer substantial benefits, they must also be cost-effective to ensure widespread adoption.

The effectiveness of healthcare services is closely tied to patient experience. If patients feel their needs are unmet, even the most efficient systems may be perceived as ineffective. The conversation highlights the need to balance operational efficiency with quality of care and patient satisfaction. The discussion reflected the challenges in measuring healthcare effectiveness, particularly in defining and applying appropriate metrics. While many metrics exist, participants noted a lack of focus on long-term effectiveness and the real impact on patient health. Although hospitals and healthcare systems commonly measure performance, there is a need for more refined indicators that accurately capture patient outcomes and service quality. The discussion emphasized shifting the focus from purely operational metrics to patient-centered outcomes, including assessing whether appropriate services are delivered and whether they effectively improve health.

The collective understanding of technological requirements for advancing healthcare delivery centered on key dimensions: security, usability, system integration, patient-centered design, and performance metrics.

4.4 Regulatory Perspectives and Key Actors in Building Smart Hospitals

The discussions regarding regulatory perspectives highlighted the complexities of data sharing and the implications of existing regulatory frameworks. There are strict regulations governing how patient data can be shared between healthcare providers, particularly across different countries within the European Union. Patient consent is often required before their data can be accessed by other HCPs. The Data Governance Act was mentioned, emphasizing that individuals have control over their data, including who can access it and how it can be used.

Participants expressed concerns that current regulations may create barriers to efficient healthcare delivery. For example, the requirement for patient consent and strict data access controls can slow down the process of sharing critical health information. While regulations are essential for protecting patient privacy, there was recognition that they can also hinder the integration of digital services and reduce the overall efficiency of healthcare systems.

The challenge of balancing regulatory requirements with the need for innovation in healthcare was a recurring theme. Participants noted that overly stringent regulations could stifle the development of new technologies and services that have the potential to benefit patients. There was a call for a regulatory framework that supports innovation while maintaining patient safety and data protection.

Differences in regulatory frameworks across countries were also discussed, as they complicate international collaboration in healthcare. Participants noted that varying regulations can pose challenges for data sharing and the implementation of cross-border healthcare services. There was an ongoing discussion about how regulations might evolve in response to technological advancements and changing healthcare needs. Participants expressed a desire for adaptable regulatory frameworks that can accommodate new developments in digital health.

5 Discussion

5.1 The Aim of Smart Hospitals

The thematic analysis of the workshops presents a vision for the future of healthcare that emphasizes holistic and integrated care models, where technology plays a central role in monitoring and managing patient health beyond traditional hospital settings [31]. This transformation is driven by technological advancements, regulatory changes, and the growing adoption of patient-centered care models, which emerged as dominant themes in discussions about future hospitals [32]. There is broad consensus that the current healthcare delivery model is insufficient to meet the evolving needs of modern patients. Participants highlighted the need to transition toward patient-centric services that prioritize accessibility, convenience, and proactive care. This shift reflects broader societal expectations for personalized and responsive healthcare systems. Therefore, the findings suggest that the transformation toward smart hospitals is not driven by specific technologies alone, but by infrastructural capabilities that are expected to be realized through 6G.

Empowering patients to actively participate in their healthcare journey was strongly emphasized [33]. This includes providing access to personal health data, ensuring transparent communication about care options, and offering digital tools for self-management. Patient engagement was viewed not only as an ethical imperative but also as a strategic approach to improving adherence, satisfaction, and health outcomes [34].

Future hospitals should prioritize accessibility by offering remote services [35, 36], particularly for patients unable to visit healthcare facilities in person. Digitalization plays a critical role in enabling healthcare services that can be accessed from home, including remote monitoring and virtual consultations. This approach is especially relevant given demographic trends indicating an increasing number of senior citizens who are likely to require more healthcare services. In the context of preventive care, the focus should shift toward well-being services that support everyday activities for elderly individuals living at home.

Accessibility also involves the ability to share patient data across different healthcare providers. Participants stressed that patients should have control over their data and have the ability to consent to its sharing, which is important for ensuring timely and appropriate care [37]. Effective inter-organizational collaboration and seamless data sharing were viewed as critical enablers of improved patient outcomes. The ability to exchange information across systems and providers enhances continuity of care, supports clinical decision-making, and fosters integrated care pathways.

Many patients present with multiple health issues requiring coordinated care across various specialties, yet the current system often struggles to address these complex needs effectively. Participants emphasized the need for better guidance and support systems to help patients navigate care pathways. Integration of services and collaboration among healthcare providers were seen as essential for improving accessibility and ensuring comprehensive care without unnecessary barriers.

The issue of HCPs burnout was prominently discussed. Optimizing workflows and reducing administrative burdens are vital to allow providers to focus on patient care rather than bureaucratic tasks. Addressing these challenges is critical for maintaining workforce motivation, retention, and overall system resilience.

5.2 6G-Enabled Smart Hospital Service Model Framework

Future hospitals and care systems must leverage digital tools, telemedicine, and data analytics to enhance clinical decision-making, streamline operational workflows, and reduce administrative burdens in order to achieve their objectives. Technology is not only a facilitator of efficiency but also a driver of innovation in care delivery. Technology integration is at the core of discussions surrounding the development of smart hospitals. As healthcare systems evolve, the ability to seamlessly connect devices, data, and processes in real time becomes critical for delivering efficient, patient-centered care.

While the study participants did not explicitly distinguish between 5G and 6G communication networks, their expectations reflect capabilities associated with next-generation infrastructures such as ultra-low latency, real-time analytics, and massive device connectivity. 6G, positioned as both a system and a general-purpose technology (GPT) platform, reflects this expectation [38–40]. This foundation supports diverse service models with distinct value propositions, such as real-time remote monitoring,

AI-driven diagnostics, and immersive telemedicine experiences [41–46]. By leveraging 6G's capabilities, smart hospitals can create integrated ecosystems that enhance operational efficiency, improve clinical outcomes, and deliver personalized healthcare services (Table 2).

Table 2　6G-enabled Smart Hospital Service (Business) Model Framework.

Service model	Technologies	Value proposition	Aim of the smart hospital
Connection model	Virtual and/or physical ubiquitous mobile communication network infrastructure	Resilient and secure access to personal health data, transparent communication about care options, and digital tools for self-management	Enable trustworthy connected and preventive and participatory care including remote and mobile healthcare
Computing model	Virtual and/or physical edge-core-cloud continuum computing infrastructure and related services for other layers	Enhanced secure and privacy clinical decision-making through real time AI and data analytics	Personalized care Improved diagnostic accuracy and efficiency
Content model	Smart devices and networks: Internet of things (IoT), location, Integrated Sensing and Communication (ISAC)	Provide the right data to the right user at the right time leveraging novel device and network capabilities for sensing and monitoring	Access to rich health data, reduce barriers, and ensure security
Context model	Sensor fusion and Digital twin (integration of data)	Integrate health data into digital twin for personalized and context-aware healthcare services	Integrate health data to improve patient experience and operational efficiency
Commerce model	Integrate 6G system into multi-layered smart hospital platform via Application Programming Interfaces (APIs)	Seamless access to data and analysis reduces in-person hospital visits by offering online consultations and other relevant medical services	Optimize resources while maintaining quality care

Regulatory discussions also raised concerns regarding data governance and interoperability standards. While regulatory frameworks are essential for ensuring data protection, patient safety, and ethical compliance, they must also be designed to foster innovation [47]. The key challenge is to find a balance where regulations do not hinder technological progress but instead enable the responsible and scalable adoption of new solutions. Achieving this balance requires adaptive policy-making and close collaboration among stakeholders [48].

A key limitation of this study is the composition of the dataset, which primarily reflects the perspectives of researchers actively engaged in smart hospital initiatives. As a result, the views of real patients and frontline healthcare professionals were largely absent from the discussions. Their actual needs and priorities may differ from those assumed by researchers, creating potential gaps in the applicability of the findings.

Future research should adopt a more inclusive approach by engaging a broader range of stakeholders, such as particularly patients and HCPs, to ensure that proposed solutions align with practical realities and user expectations. Methods such as interviews, surveys, and co-creation workshops can provide richer insights into diverse perspectives. In addition, conducting a comprehensive stakeholder analysis will be essential for identifying roles, responsibilities, and interdependence within the healthcare ecosystem. It will strengthen the relevance and impact of recommendations for digitalization and smart hospital development.

6 Conclusions

Based on the workshop data, this paper envisions the future direction of healthcare and outlines the trajectory toward which healthcare systems are evolving in the era of 6G. The study provides guidance for technology developers to understand the aims of future hospitals, which will leverage the five-layered 6G architecture, including connection, content, context, computing, and commerce models, to enable preventive care, reduce hospital visits, and promote healthier lifestyles through early interventions [15]. The goal is to minimize hospital admissions via proactive and extended health management supported by 6G-enabled digital solutions, patient empowerment, and seamless integration of services across physical and virtual environments.

The connectivity layer ensures ultra-reliable, low-latency communication for real-time monitoring and telemedicine [39]. The computing layer provides distributed processing at the local edge, enabling rapid decision-making and immersive applications such as AR-assisted surgery [40, 41]. The content layer leveraging integrated sensing and communication capabilities in 6G and facilitates secure transmission of medical data and imaging [25, 42]. The context layer interprets this data using AI-driven analytics and digital twinning to support personalized care and predictive diagnostics [43]. Finally, the commerce layer integrates multi-layered communication and data platforms for efficient healthcare transactions, reducing administrative burdens and enabling new business models for value-based care [44–46].

A critical aspect of this transformation involves addressing regulatory impacts on healthcare delivery, particularly the challenges posed by international regulatory differences in data governance and interoperability [47, 48]. A balanced approach is required, which means one that ensures patient data protection while remaining adaptable to the demands of modern, hyper-connected healthcare systems. This includes fostering innovation through 6G-driven technologies without compromising safety, privacy, or ethical standards.

This research reflects a comprehensive vision for the future of healthcare, prioritizing patient-centered approaches, technological integration, and a collaborative, data-driven ecosystem enabled by the 6G five-layered model. Addressing challenges such as regulatory complexity, professional burnout, and accessibility will be essential to realizing this vision. Furthermore, the study emphasizes the importance of interdisciplinary collaboration among HCPs, supported by 6G-enabled system for real-time communication, sensing, and data sharing. By working together across disciplines, service providers can deliver more comprehensive care and effectively respond to the multifaceted needs of patients in next-generation healthcare environments.

Acknowledgments. The authors thank all the participants for the workshop.

Disclosure of Interests

The authors declare that they have no known competing financial interests or personal relationships that could have appeared to influence the work reported in this paper.

References

1. Teece, D.J.: Profiting from innovation in the digital economy: enabling technologies, standards, and licensing models in the wireless world. Res. Policy. **47**, 1367–1387 (2018). https://doi.org/10.1016/j.respol.2017.01.015
2. Sánchez, P., Ricart, J.E.: Business model innovation and sources of value creation in low-income markets. Eur. Manag. Rev. **7**, 138–154 (2010). https://doi.org/10.1057/emr.2010.16
3. Spiegel, O., Abbassi, P., Zylka, M.P., Schlagwein, D., Fischbach, K., Schoder, D.: Business model development, founders' social capital and the success of early stage internet start-ups: a mixed-method study. Inf. Syst. J. **26**, 421–449 (2016). https://doi.org/10.1111/isj.12073
4. Amit, R., Han, X.: Value creation through novel resource configurations in a digitally enabled world. Strateg. Entrep. J. **11**, 228–242 (2017). https://doi.org/10.1002/SEJ.1256
5. Amit, R., Zott, C.: Value creation in e-business. Strateg. Manag. J. **22**, 493–520 (2001)
6. Chesbrough, H., Rosenbloom, R.S.: The role of the business model in capturing value from innovation: evidence from Xerox Corporation's technology spin-off companies. Ind. Corp. Chang. **11**, 529–555 (2002)
7. Teece, D.J., Linden, G.: Business models, value capture, and the digital enterprise. J. Organ. Des. **6**, 8 (2017). https://doi.org/10.1186/s41469 017 0018 x
8. Costa-Climent, R., Haftor, D.M., Staniewski, M.W.: Using machine learning to create and capture value in the business models of small and medium-sized enterprises. Int. J. Inf. Manag. **73**, 102637 (2023)
9. Jocevski, M., Arvidsson, N., Ghezzi, A.: Interconnected business models: present debates and future agenda. J. Bus. Ind. Marketing. **35**, 1051–1067 (2020). https://doi.org/10.1108/JBIM-06-2019-0292
10. Iivari, M.M., Ahokangas, P., Komi, M., Tihinen, M., Valtanen, K.: Toward Ecosystemic business models in the context of industrial internet. J. Bus. Model. Suppl. Special Issue: Sustainability And Scalability of B. **4**, 42–59 (2016)
11. Vargo, S.L., Lusch, R.F.: Service-dominant logic: what it is, what it is not, what it might be. In: The Service-Dominant Logic of Marketing, pp. 61–74. Routledge (2014)
12. Ranjan, K.R., Read, S.: Value co-creation: concept and measurement. J. Acad. Mark. Sci. **44**, 290–315 (2016)
13. Ahokangas, P., Matinmikko-Blue, M., Yrjölä, S.: Envisioning a future-proof global 6G from business, regulation, and technology perspectives. IEEE Commun. Mag. **61**, 72–78 (2022)

14. Ahokangas, P., Matinmikko-Blue, M., Yrjölä, S., Hämmäinen, H.: Platform configurations for local and private 5G networks in complex industrial multi-stakeholder ecosystems. Telecomm Policy. **45**, 102128 (2021)
15. Yrjölä, S.: Business Models and Profiting from Innovation in Future Mobile Communications (2024)
16. Moqaddamerad, S., Xu, Y., Iivari, M., Ahokangas, P.: Business models based on co-opetition in a hyper-connected era: the case of 5G-enabled smart grids. In: Collaboration in a Hyper-connected World: 17th IFIP WG 5.5 Working Conference on Virtual Enterprises, PRO-VE 2016, Porto, Portugal, October 3–5, 2016, Proceedings 17, pp. 559–568. Springer (2016)
17. Xu, Y., Ahokangas, P., Louis, J.-N., Pongrácz, E.: Electricity market empowered by artificial intelligence: a platform approach. Energies (Basel). **12**, 4128 (2019)
18. Polit, D., Beck, C.: Essentials of Nursing Research: Appraising Evidence for Nursing Practice. Lippincott Williams & Wilkins (2020)
19. Creswell, J.W., Poth, C.N., qualitative inquiry and research design: choosing among five approaches. Sage publications (2016)
20. Löhr, K., Weinhardt, M., Sieber, S.: The "world café" as a participatory method for collecting qualitative data. Int. J. Qual Methods. **19**, 1609406920916976 (2020)
21. Rajak, S., Summaq, A., Kumar, M.P., Ghosh, A., Elumalai, K., Chinnadurai, S.: Revolutionizing healthcare with 6G: a deep dive into smart, connected systems. IEEE Access. **12**, 194150–194170 (2024). https://doi.org/10.1109/ACCESS.2024.3519567
22. Jovy-Klein, F., Stead, S., Salge, T.O., Sander, J., Diehl, A., Antons, D.: Forecasting the future of smart hospitals: findings from a real-time delphi study. BMC Health Serv. Res. **24**, 1421 (2024). https://doi.org/10.1186/s12913-024-11895-z
23. Lavallee, D.C. et al.: mHealth and patient generated health data: stakeholder perspectives on opportunities and barriers for transforming healthcare. mHealth. mHealth. **6** (2019)
24. Tanniru, M.: Engagement leading to empowerment—digital innovation strategies for patient care continuity. J Hosp. Manag. Health Policy. **3** (2019)
25. Kim, Y., Lee, S.: Energy-efficient wireless hospital sensor networking for remote patient monitoring. Inf. Sci (N Y). **282**, 332–349 (2014). https://doi.org/10.1016/j.ins.2014.05.056
26. Nguyen, T.N., Piuri, V., Qi, L., Mumtaz, S., Lee, W.H.-C.: Guest editorial innovations in wearable, implantable, Mobile, & remote healthcare with IoT & Sensor Informatics and patient monitoring. IEEE J. Biomed. Health Inform. **27**, 2152–2154 (2023). https://doi.org/10.1109/JBHI.2023.3265411
27. Heart, T., Ben-Assuli, O., Shabtai, I.: A review of PHR, EMR and EHR integration: a more personalized healthcare and public health policy. Health Policy Technol. **6**, 20–25 (2017)
28. Ahad, A., Jiangbina, Z., Tahir, M., Shayea, I., Sheikh, M.A., Rasheed, F.: 6G and intelligent healthcare: taxonomy, technologies, open issues and future research directions. Internet Things. **25**, 101068 (2024). https://doi.org/10.1016/j.iot.2024.101068
29. de Alwis, C., Pham, Q.-V., Liyanage, M.: 6G for Healthcare (2023)
30. Nayak, S., Patgiri, R.: 6G communication technology: a vision on intelligent healthcare. Health Inform.: Comput. Perspect. Healthc, 1–18 (2021)
31. Srinivasu, P.N., Ijaz, M.F., Shafi, J., Woźniak, M., Sujatha, R.: 6G driven fast computational networking framework for healthcare applications. IEEE Access. **10**, 94235–94248 (2022). https://doi.org/10.1109/ACCESS.2022.3203061
32. Gupta, N., Gupta, S.K., Jain, V.: Machine learning in healthcare cybersecurity: role of human activity recognition and impact of 6G in smart healthcare. In: In: 6G-Enabled IoT and AI for Smart Healthcare, pp. 143–156. CRC Press (2023)
33. Dhaya, R., Kanthavel, R.: Role of machine learning in 6G technologies: healthcare and education sectors. In: Challenges and Risks Involved in Deploying 6G and Next Gen Networks, pp. 130–147. IGI Global (2022)

34. Wu, X., Yang, Y., Bilal, M., Qi, L., Xu, X.: 6G-enabled anomaly detection for Metaverse healthcare analytics in internet of things. IEEE J. Biomed. Health Inform. **1–10** (2023). https://doi.org/10.1109/JBHI.2023.3298092

35. Khan, I.A. et al.: Big data analytics model using artificial intelligence (AI) and 6G Technologies for Healthcare. IEEE Access. **12**, 97924–97937 (2024). https://doi.org/10.1109/ACCESS.2024.3427333

36. Wang, F., Jurva, R., Ahokangas, P., Yrjölä, S., Matinmikko-Blue, M.: Expert perspectives on future 6G-enabled hospital Metaverse. In: Särestöniemi, M., Keikhosrokiani, P., Singh, D., Harjula, E., Tiulpin, A., Jansson, M., Isomursu, M., van Gils, M., Saarakkala, S., Reponen, J. (eds.) Digital Health and Wireless Solutions, pp. 3–20. Springer Nature Switzerland, Cham (2024)

37. Batista, E., López-Aguilar, P., Solanas, A.: Smart health in the 6G era: bringing security to future smart health services. IEEE Commun. Mag. **62**, 74–80 (2024). https://doi.org/10.1109/MCOM.019.2300122

38. Gray, B., Purdy, J.: Collaborating for our Future: Multistakeholder Partnerships for Solving Complex Problems. Oxford University Press (2018)

39. Zeadally, S., Bello, O.: Harnessing the power of internet of things based connectivity to improve healthcare. Internet Things. **14**, 100074 (2021). https://doi.org/10.1016/j.iot.2019.100074

40. Sodhro, A.H., Zahid, N.: AI-enabled framework for fog computing driven e-healthcare applications. Sensors. **21**, 8039 (2021)

41. Attaran, M.: The impact of 5G on the evolution of intelligent automation and industry digitization. J. Ambient. Intell. Humaniz. Comput. **14**, 5977–5993 (2023). https://doi.org/10.1007/s12652-020-02521-x

42. Lv, Z., Kumar, N.: Software defined solutions for sensors in 6G/IoE. Comput. Commun. **153**, 42–47 (2020). https://doi.org/10.1016/J.COMCOM.2020.01.060

43. Guo, C.: Big data analytics in healthcare: data-driven methods for typical treatment pattern mining. J. Syst. Sci. Syst. Eng. **28**, 694–714 (2019). https://doi.org/10.1007/s11518-019-5437-5

44. Alexander, C.A.: Healthcare driven by big data analytics. Am. J. Eng. Appl. Sci. **11**, 1154–1163 (2018). https://doi.org/10.3844/ajeassp.2018.1154.1163

45. Ahmad, H.F., Rafique, W., Rasool, R.U., Alhumam, A., Anwar, Z., Qadir, J.: Leveraging 6G, extended reality, and IoT big data analytics for healthcare: a review. Comput. Sci. Rev. **48**, 100558 (2023). https://doi.org/10.1016/j.cosrev.2023.100558

46. Galetsi, P., Katsaliaki, K., Kumar, S.: Values, challenges and future directions of big data analytics in healthcare: a systematic review. Soc. Sci. Med. **241**, 112533 (2019). https://doi.org/10.1016/J.SOCSCIMED.2019.112533

47. Starkbaum, J., Felt, U.: Negotiating the reuse of health-data: research, big data, and the European general data protection regulation. Big Data Soc. **6**, 2053951719862594 (2019). https://doi.org/10.1177/2053951719862594

48. Hoeyer, K.: Datafication and accountability in public health: introduction to a special issue. Soc. Stud. Sci. **49**, 459–475 (2019). https://doi.org/10.1177/0306312719860202

49. Kumar, A., Masud, M., Alsharif, M.H., Gaur, N., Nanthaamornphong, A.: Integrating 6G technology in smart hospitals: challenges and opportunities for enhanced healthcare services. Front Med. (Lausanne) **12**, 1534551 (2025). https://doi.org/10.3389/fmed.2025.1534551. PMID: 40255587; PMCID: PMC12006048

Identifying Social Sustainability Drivers and Future Scenarios in Digital Healthcare Through a Stakeholder-Based Method

Sehrish Khan[1]([✉]) [iD], Petri Ahokangas[2] [iD], Johanna Annunen[3,4] [iD], Johanna Uusimaa[3,5] [iD], Jonna Komulainen-Ebrahim[3,6] [iD], and Minna Isomursu[1,7] [iD]

[1] M3S, Faculty of Information Technology and Electrical Engineering, University of Oulu, 90750 Oulu, Finland
`Sehrish.khan@oulu.fi`
[2] Martti Ahtisaari Institute, Oulu Business School, University of Oulu, 90570 Oulu, Finland
[3] Research Unit of Clinical Medicine and Medical Research Center Oulu, Oulu University Hospital and University of Oulu, 90014 Oulu, Finland
[4] Neurocenter, Oulu University Hospital, 90029 Oulu, Finland
[5] Medical Research Center Oulu, Oulu University Hospital, 90220 Oulu, Finland
[6] Department of Children and Adolescents, Division of Pediatric Neurology, Oulu University Hospital, Oulu, 90029 Oulu, Finland
[7] Faculty of Medicine, University of Oulu, 90014 Oulu, Finland

Abstract. In this paper, we present a scenario-based method for identifying stakeholders' insights for sustainable digital healthcare by leveraging future digital healthcare scenarios and changing social sustainability drivers. This study aims to propose a scenario-based stakeholder insight method to support the development of inclusive and socially sustainable digital healthcare futures. The first eleven change drivers associated with social sustainability were extracted from the digital healthcare literature and presented to various stakeholders to rank their impact and predictability regarding the social sustainability of digital healthcare. Moreover, the proposed method is also designed to extract insights from stakeholders regarding the implementation of different future scenarios, (i) the consequences of various future scenarios, (ii) the risks and challenges of achieving the future scenarios, and (iii) recommendations for policymakers. The study's stakeholders include medical doctors, digital healthcare researchers, developers, and digital health-related businesses. The results present the most decisive, impactful, and predictable scenario as "connected care for all," an inclusive digital healthcare system accessible to all without digital exclusion. Moreover, results show the most impactful and uncertain change driver, as rated by stakeholders. The proposed method can be used to understand stakeholders' social sustainability requirements, leading to a sustainable digital healthcare future.

Keywords: Digital healthcare · social sustainability · future healthcare scenarios · User-centered digital healthcare.

M. Särestöniemi et al. (Eds.): NCDHWS 2026, CCIS 3009, pp. 19–33, 2026.
https://doi.org/10.1007/978-3-032-28812-7_2

1 Introduction

1.1 Social Sustainability of Digital Healthcare

Social sustainability (SS) in digital healthcare is often discussed in general and value-oriented terms. Still, the core idea can be stated plainly: within software engineering for e-health, SS is the "support of current and future generations to have the same or greater access to social resources by pursuing social equity" [1]. That definition anchors the conversation, yet what counts as "access" in practice may vary by context—think rural clinics navigating unstable bandwidth versus urban hospitals worrying about trust and language. In more practice-oriented writing, SS in e-health is said to focus on ensuring equitable access to e-health technologies and addressing the digital divide, with specific attention to digital literacy, privacy, and data security. At the societal scale, scholars reviewing digital transformation suggest SS should show up as tangible gains in social cohesion, quality of life, equality, diversity, democracy, and governance; that's ambitious, and it may suggest that "doing digital" is necessary but not sufficient for real social progress [2]. Altogether, the literature points toward an evidence-based SS dimension that (i) pushes for equitable access to tools like telemedicine and e-health apps, (ii) supports social equity across generations, (iii) builds digital skills and narrows digital divides, and (iv) improves everyday quality of life and participation through digital systems; in practice, the weight on each element will likely depend on setting, and policy. Amid the technical and disciplinary complexity, the public health concept of health equity provides a clarifying lens. It is "the state in which everyone has a fair and just opportunity to attain their highest level of health," a reminder that digital projects succeed socially only when the people most likely to be left behind can actually benefit [3] (Centers for Disease Control and Prevention [CDC] 2024).

1.2 Why Future Scenarios

Future scenarios are essential to consider because they help stakeholders and policymakers think about uncertainty without pretending to predict everything. In a field like sustainable digital healthcare, where policy and people constantly push and pull on each other, imagining several plausible futures may be one of the few tools that actually helps. These scenarios can encourage policymakers and designers to make choices that seem better prepared for shifts in regulations, patient expectations, or even something as ordinary but disruptive as changes in reimbursement models. They also tend to bring different groups to the same table; clinicians, researchers, and developers often bring different perspectives, and scenario work gives them a structured way to compare them. It is worth admitting that scenarios don't guarantee perfect decisions; they offer a framework that appears to support clearer thinking about trade-offs and long-term consequences. Instead of relying on a single "ideal" future, the process encourages people to explore a range of possibilities and, hopefully, uncover needs and requirements that might otherwise remain hidden. Scenario-based methodology has been used in numerous studies [4–7]. These studies highlight that a scenario-based approach provides evidence-based knowledge and methodologically consistent research, helping policy and decision-makers design long-term goals for socially sustainable digital healthcare.

1.3　Change Drivers

Main factors like equity and inclusion, digital literacy, human-centred design, data privacy, ethical AI, collaboration, policy, sustainable infrastructure, patient empowerment, workforce well-being, and responsible digital transformation all shape whether digital healthcare becomes a trusted, accessible, and socially sustainable system. Research shows that equity and inclusion are essential for digital health to improve outcomes and quality of life, rather than widening gaps. Access, context, and inclusion determine who benefits [8, 9]. Digital literacy and usability, supported by human-centered design, play a significant role in making digital health accessible to everyone. Studies link patients' trust, comfort, and the fit of the design to their needs with their engagement [10, 11]. Privacy, security, and ethical AI are seen as necessary for public trust and long-term use. These are most effective when built into policy, procurement, and governance throughout the entire process [11, 12]. Working together across sectors and building strong infrastructure makes it possible to scale digital health solutions reasonably and meet real-world needs [11, 13]. Finally, focusing on healthcare professionals' well-being and the reality of digital transformation helps make sure technology reduces fragmentation and burden. These improvements are linked to lasting value and a better quality of life for the population [9, 12].

1.4　Objective

The primary objective of this study is to develop and apply a scenario-based method to identify stakeholders' insights and requirements for achieving socially sustainable digital healthcare futures by integrating future digital healthcare scenarios with changing social sustainability drivers.

2　Related Studies

Various methods have been reported in the literature to study stakeholder insights. Table 1 shows some of the studies. However, there is a gap in methods and research studies, as multiple future-scenario-based methods are rarely used to assess the social sustainability of digital healthcare, including primary healthcare stakeholders. The existing research on digital health sustainability uses methods such as Delphi panels, participatory design, critical system heuristics, and discrete-choice experiments. However, these approaches do not provide a structured mechanism for eliciting stakeholders' sustainability requirements in future digital-health contexts. Furthermore, prior studies do not systematically examine multiple types of future scenarios to address scenario-specific consequences, risks, policy implications, or stakeholder-level impacts. Consequently, literature lacks a comprehensive, scenario-based method for operationalizing social sustainability requirements in digital healthcare. Therefore, the proposed methodology addressed this gap by introducing a scenario-based stakeholder-elicitation method that identifies requirements for sustainable digital healthcare and incorporates multi-scenario evaluation and policy-relevant insights for long-term planning.

Table 1 Comparison of related studies based on aims, stakeholders, and scenario usage

Publication	Aim	Stakeholders	Scenario-based	References
Guise et al. (2021)	Develop and test a model for stakeholder involvement in resilient healthcare (protocol)	Patients, caregivers, providers, managers, regulators	Not explicitly reported	[14]
Godage et al. (2023)	Assess the sustainability requirements and gaps of the national HHIMS in Sri Lanka	Wide range of actors involved/affected by HHIMS[a] across large hospitals	Implicit boundary-reflection; no explicit future scenarios reported	[15]
Haig et al. (2023)	Develop a value framework for patient-facing digital health technologies	Patients, clinicians, industry, players/decision-makers, influencers across three countries	No	[16]
Savira et al. (2023)	Identify consumer preferences for telehealth vs. in-person care	General population (n = 1,025)	Yes, four clinical choice scenarios	[17]
De Guzman et al. (2024)	Quantify GP[b] preferences for telehealth service attributes	General practitioners (n = 60)	Yes, DCE[c] choice sets (described as choice sets rather than "scenarios")	[18]
Maaß et al. (2024)	Identify indicators for national digital public health maturity	International experts in public health, informatics, and policy	No	[19]
Vo et al. (2024)	Synthesise DCE-based preferences for virtual-care models	Mixed (patients, clinicians, others across included DCE studies)	Yes, DCE choice tasks	[20]
Austin et al. (2020)	Map definitions and factors influencing the sustainability of virtual care	Stakeholders represented via the included studies (n = 54)	No	[21]

(continued)

Table 1 (*continued*)

Publication	Aim	Stakeholders	Scenario-based	References
Giunti et al. (2025)	Examine power dynamics in participatory design of digital health solutions	Patients, healthcare professionals, and family members.	Not explicitly reported	[22]
Piera Jiménez et al. (2026)	Co-create principles for digital health equity in catalonia	Citizens/caregivers, clinicians, managers, digital-health experts	Yes, explicit future scenario	[23]

[a]HHIMS = Hospital Health Information Management System; [b] GP = General practitioners; [c] DCE = Discrete Choice Experiment.

3 Method

This study uses a step-by-step approach to understand the future of social sustainability in digital healthcare and to gather opinions from multiple stakeholders. The proposed method consists of four stages.

In the first stage, we thoroughly reviewed the literature to understand the concepts of change drivers of social sustainability in digital healthcare and their impact on the design of future scenarios. Seven change drivers were presented to the stakeholders to ask for the (i) Impact and (ii) Predictability on a five-point Likert scale. The Predictability factor also presents uncertainty.

After analyzing the questionnaire responses, we moved to the second stage: developing four distinct future scenarios. We used the quadrant method to develop four different scenarios that align with the axes of impact and predictability.

The third stage is creating different stakeholder groups as participants based on their expertise: (1) healthcare professionals, (2) developers and designers, (3) researchers, and (4) professionals from the information technology (IT) and healthcare industries.

The fourth stage is to frame questions for each scenario and to seek responses from each group during a workshop to gather stakeholders' opinions and insights (Fig. 1).

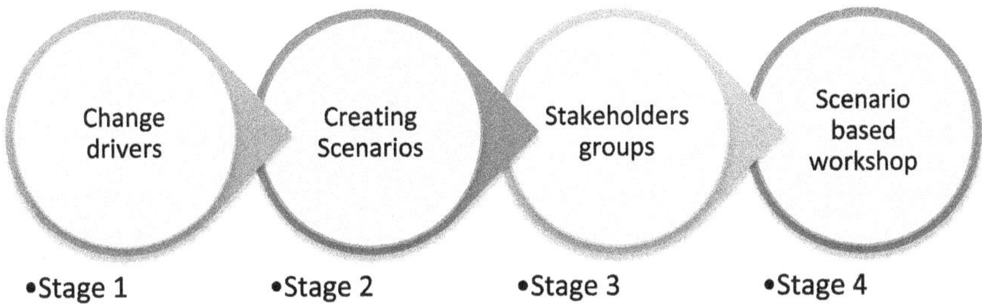

Fig. 1 Proposed methodology

3.1 Change Driving of SS in Digital Healthcare

Several change drivers were identified in the literature regarding social sustainability in digital healthcare. Table 2 describes these drivers. These drivers were also used to map the four future scenarios, based on participants' responses and reported in the results section.

Table 2 Change drivers reported in the literature

Publication	Change driver	Evidence (supported by)	References
Kim and Backonja (2025)	Equity and inclusion in healthcare access	Scoping reviews and frameworks consistently identify digital inclusion as foundational to equitable outcomes	[8]
Hameed et al. (2024)	Well-being of healthcare professionals (HCP)	System-level reviews and policy analyses link digital transformation, workload, and sustainability	[24]
Hameed et al. (2024)	Social policy and regulatory frameworks	Reviews and frameworks emphasize governance, procurement, privacy/security as enablers	[24]
Tung et al., (2025)	Digital literacy and education	Empirical "digital readiness" measures and frameworks show that literacy/trust drives adoption	[10]
Hameed et al. (2024)	Data privacy and ethical AI	Privacy/ethics repeatedly identified as prerequisites for trust and equitable uptake	[24]
World Economic Forum (2026)	Closer collaboration among stakeholders	Framework and policy analyses underline multi-stakeholder collaboration across the lifecycle	[13]
World Economic Forum (2026)	Human-cantered design	Frameworks and empirical work tie usability/co-design to equitable adoption.	[13]

(continued)

Table 2 (*continued*)

Publication	Change driver	Evidence (supported by)	References
Hameed et al. (2024)	Digital transformation and health-tech adoption	A comprehensive review and policy synthesis show the system-level benefits/risks for sustainability	[24]
Hameed et al. (2024)	Sustainable healthcare infrastructure	Reviews/policy analyses identify infrastructure as a prerequisite for resilient digital systems	[24]
Tung et al., (2025)	Empowered patients (wearables, personal data)	Empirical readiness and equity commentary show that engagement depends on literacy/trust	[10]
Kim and Backonja (2025)	Quality of life	Frameworks connect equity/digital inclusion to improved QoL and social sustainability	[8]

3.2 Scenario Selection

Four future scenarios are presented in Table 3 based on the factors (Impact and predictability) ranked by the stakeholders in the previous stage through a pre-workshop questionnaire.

Table 3 Scenario emergence and change drivers

Quadrant	Participant ratings reflecting	Scenarios emergence
High Impact AND High Predictability	Drivers matter a lot and are under control	Connected Care for All
High Impact AND Low Predictability	Drivers matter a lot, but the system is unstable or unclear	Chaotic Health scape
Low Impact AND Low Predictability	Social foundations are weak and unpredictable	Digital Divide Nightmare
Low Impact AND High Predictability	Tech works, but does not improve equity or inclusion	Tech-Driven Elitism

3.3 Participants/Stakeholders

Four groups were formed to explore and engage with the four future scenarios, each comprising four participants. Group 1 consisted of four (4) healthcare professionals:

three medical doctors and practitioners, each with more than 10 years of clinical and teaching experience, and one medical researcher with 15 years of research experience. Group 2 was based on "developers and designers," including mobile and web application developers for rehabilitation. Group 3 consists of four "researchers," each with more than 10 years of experience on various aspects of digital healthcare. Group 4 comprises professionals working in the Information technology (IT) and healthcare industries. Fig. 2 shows the groups and the total number of participants.

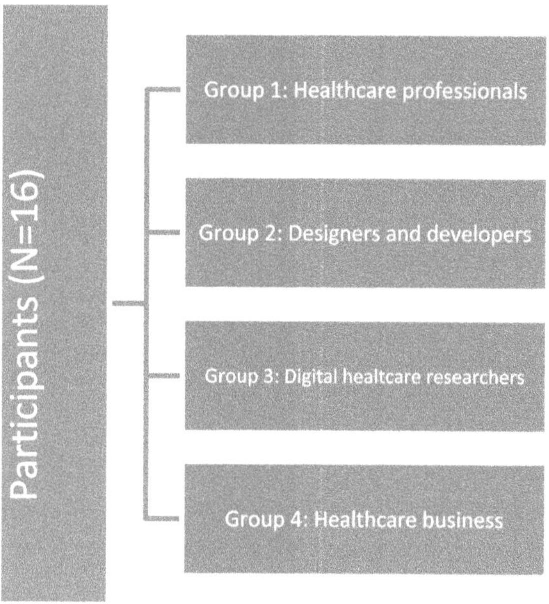

Fig. 2 Categorization of stakeholder groups participating in the workshop.

3.4 Workshop with Stakeholders (Data Collection)

Data collection was done in a scenario-based workshop, which aimed at scenario assessment and validation, particularly (1) to achieve a better understanding of social sustainability in digital healthcare for the future, and (2) to evaluate and validate the four alternative scenarios for the future through multidisciplinary discussion. The scenario assessment will help to understand the future scenarios at a practical level. The Miro software [21] was used to ask questions and collect insights from stakeholders. During the workshop, four activities were planned around four scenarios and presented to participants. These activities comprised asking stakeholders' perspectives, focusing on five different themes: (1) Impact on Stakeholders, (2) Achievability and Real-World Impact, (3) Challenges and Risks, (4) Steps to Ensure Success, and (5) Recommendations for policymakers. In addition to the above four activities, participants were also asked to rank the future scenarios as (1) Plausible, (2) preferable, and (3) probable (Table 4).

Table 4 Method to extract qualitative, detailed insights from stakeholders on future scenarios

Question Number	Common Theme of each question	Scenario 1: Connected Care for All (Inclusive Digital Healthcare)	Scenario 2: Chaotic Healthscape (Ethical AI in Healthcare)	Scenario 3: Digital Divide Nightmare (Monopolistic Tech in Healthcare)	Scenario 4: Tech-Driven Elitism (Digital Literacy and Digital Exclusion)
Q1	Impact on stakeholders	Digital healthcare's effect on research priorities	Exploitative AI compromising research integrity	Professionals coping with a lack of AI access	Digital exclusion's effects on rural populations
Q2	Achievability and Real-World Impact:	Failure of universal digital healthcare	Success of the exploitative AI scenario	Success of a profit-driven AI scenario	Success of the digital exclusion scenario
Q3	Challenges and Risks:	Unequal access to digital healthcare	Unethical AI use in healthcare	Profit-driven AI healthcare services	Lack of patient education on digital tools
Q4	Steps to Ensure Success:	Positive outcomes of universal digital healthcare	Negative outcomes of unregulated AI in healthcare	Negative outcomes of inaccessible healthcare systems	Strategies for low digital literacy groups
Q5	Policy and decision-making interventions	Ensure inclusive and equitable digital healthcare	Implement strict ethical AI regulations	Prevent monopolistic tech exploitation in healthcare	Ensure equitable digital healthcare access

4 Results

4.1 Change Drivers

The response on change drivers was collected through a Likert scale-based answer for each change driver against two factors: (i) Impact, and (2) predictability. Fig. 3 shows the stakeholders' responses to these change drivers. To calculate the mean and standard deviation (SD) of the five-stage Likert scale, which was converted to 1 to 5 points, with 1 being the lowest and 5 being the highest impact.

The SD for each response is lower, ranging from 0.6 to 1, indicating strong agreement among the stakeholders. There are a few responses with SD greater than 1 and less than 1.15, showing moderate to high agreement.

The highest-impact driver with the highest predictability (i.e., lower uncertainty) is "closer stakeholder collaboration" and "Social policy and regulatory frameworks." However, the lowest predictability (i.e., highest uncertainty) driver consists of "Empowered patients" (3.44 ± 1.09) and "Equity and inclusion in healthcare access." (3.50 ± 1.15), however, the responses of stakeholders for these two change drivers for predictability mentioned above have SD of more than 1, which reflects most of the stakeholders responded as moderate (Likert scale 3) to highest (Likert scale 5).

It is also important to note that most change drivers are expected to have a moderate to high impact on stakeholders, as shown in Fig. 3.

4.2 Scenario-Mapping Based on Stakeholder Rating

Alignment of change driver rating by stakeholders with future scenarios shows that the rating mostly aligns with the first scenario, which is "connected care for all", representing the most desirable future scenario (Table 5).

Table 5 Alignment of stakeholder rating with future scenarios

Scenario	Impact and predictability pattern	Results alignment
Connected care for all	Most drivers fall into high impact and medium to high predictability	Highly aligned, as most of the drivers fall here (Collaboration, Policy, Equity, Infrastructure, HCD[a], Privacy)
Chaotic healthscape	Drivers have high Impact but low predictability (i.e., uncertainty)	Partial alignment with stakeholders, rating as a few drivers show this pattern (Equity predictability low, HCD[a] predictability low)
Digital divide nightmare	Social foundation drivers (Equity, Literacy, Empowerment) show low to Medium Impact and low Predictability	Not aligned with stakeholders' ranking as the most social foundational drivers got a high impact rating (Equity mean = 4.12, Empowered mean = 4.00, Infrastructure mean = 4.12)
Tech-driven elitism	Tech drivers have High Impact, but social inclusion drivers have medium to low impact	Weak alignment because the technology-related drivers are high, but equity and inclusion are high as well, so the gap is small

[a] HCD = Human-centered design

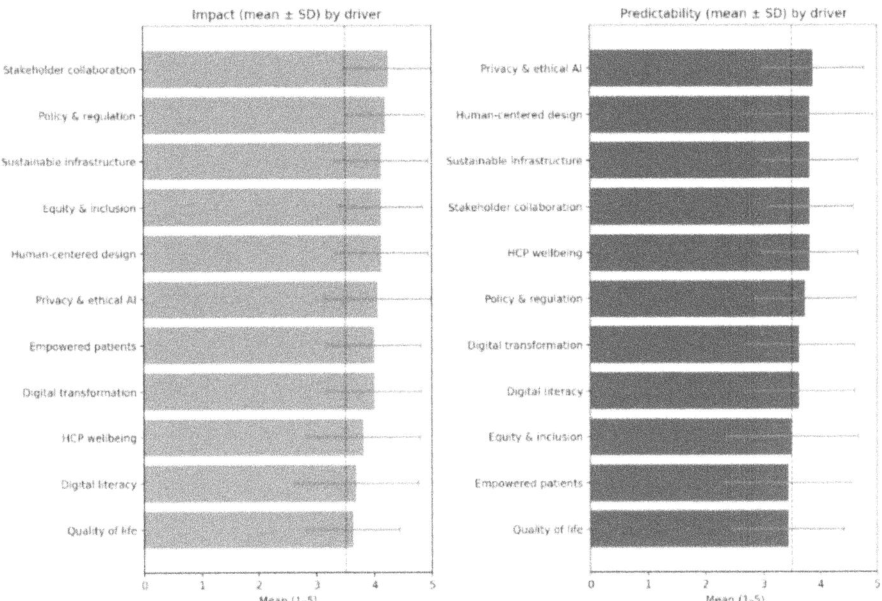

Fig. 3 Stakeholder response in terms of the impact and predictability of change drivers.

5 Discussion

These ratings identify (a) the drivers' stakeholders consider most critical for the social sustainability of digital healthcare and (b) the perceived foreseeability of the consequences associated with these drivers. The ratings can be mapped onto a two-axis framework: Impact (low to high) and Predictability (low to high), as illustrated in Fig. 4. This framework yields four distinct quadrants, each representing a contrasting future: (1) Connected Care for All (high impact and high predictability), where the system can scale inclusive, trusted digital care if many enablers are rated as both important and foreseeable; (2) Chaotic Healthscope (high impact and low predictability), where key levers are important but uncertain, leading to system fragmentation, variable quality, and diminished trust; (3) Digital Divide Nightmare (low impact and low predictability), where foundational social enablers such as equity, literacy, empowerment, and infrastructure are undervalued and uncertain, resulting in the exclusion of vulnerable groups; and (4) Tech-Driven Elitism (low social impact and high predictability for technology), where technology functions effectively but inclusion is not prioritized, concentrating benefits among a select few.

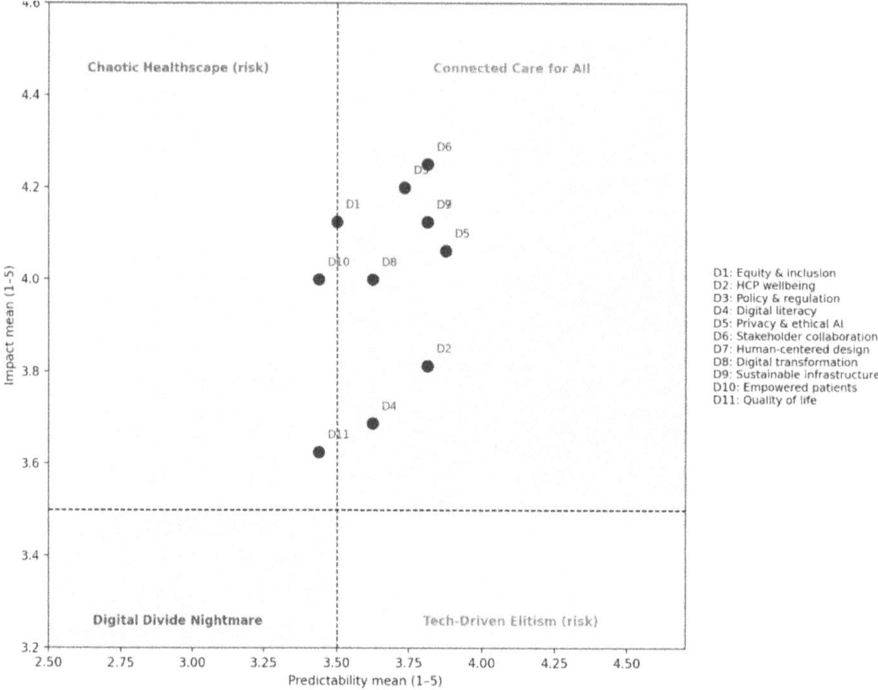

Fig. 4 Impact-predictability matrix with scenario quadrants

The ratings represent stakeholders' current assessments, while the scenarios facilitate exploration of potential future trajectories if these assessments persist or if circumstances evolve. Although the data strongly supports the first scenario, consideration of the alternative scenarios reveals potential risks, blind spots, and necessary safeguards, such as factors that could shift a high-impact driver into low predictability or groups that may remain excluded. Such a scenario-based approach is also adopted in the literature to get stakeholders' perspectives on sustainable healthcare [25].

Overall, these results, insights, and requirements will help policy and decision-makers work on digital healthcare scenarios amid changing social sustainability drivers. The results of this study will add value by providing empirical evidence on the effectiveness of the scenario-based methodology and by highlighting the opinions of different stakeholders on this topic.

In the future, stakeholders' qualitative insights elucidate the reasons behind specific driver scores, identify early warning signals, and inform practical actions such as building equity guardrails, investing in literacy, strengthening governance, and supporting workforce well-being. Overall, the four scenarios are derived from the ratings using the Impact–Predictability axes and are further refined through discussion to prioritize actions that advance the system toward the preferred future and mitigate undesirable outcomes. The work can also be extended by including three additional groups: a group representing healthcare users (patients), a group of healthcare policymakers, and a third group of sustainability researchers.

6 Conclusion

This study presented a scenario-based methodology to get stakeholders' perspectives on enhancing the social sustainability of digital healthcare. First, eleven change drivers were identified from the literature, which stakeholders subsequently ranked by perceived impact and predictability. Among the drivers, "closer stakeholder collaboration" emerged as the most influential, followed by "equity and inclusion," "policy and regulation," and "sustainable infrastructure." Furthermore, four future scenarios of social sustainability emerged, based on two factors: impact and predictability. When stakeholders responded to each change driver mapped onto the four scenarios, the result showed that the "connected care for all" scenario most closely aligned with their expectations. The future work includes a detailed analysis of four scenarios to identify the plausible, preferable, and probable scenarios, and the actions required to attain the most plausible scenarios, based on stakeholder insights.

Acknowledgments. The work has been supported by the University of Oulu & The Research Council of Finland Profi6 336449.

Disclosure of Interests The authors have no competing interests to declare that are relevant to the content of this article.

References

1. Grua, E.M., De Sanctis, M., Malavolta, I., Hoogendoorn, M., Lago, P.: Social sustainability in the e health domain via personalized and self adaptive mobile apps. In: Software Sustainability, pp. 301–328. Springer (2021)
2. Qadri, U.A., Abd Ghani, M.B., Abbas, U., Kashif, A.R.: Digital technologies and social sustainability in the digital transformation age: a systematic analysis and research agenda. Int. J. Ethics Systems. **41**, 142–169 (2025)
3. Control, C. for D., Prevention: About Health Equity (2024).
4. Peyroteo, M., Lapão, L.V.: Strategic scenarios for the digitalisation of chronic disease care management: a 10-year foresight case study in Lisbon's primary healthcare setting. Technol. Forecast. Soc. Change. **220**, 124290 (2025). https://doi.org/10.1016/j.techfore.2025.124290
5. Cordova-Pozo, K., Rouwette, E.A.J.A.: Types of scenario planning and their effectiveness: a review of reviews. Futures. **149**, 103153 (2023). https://doi.org/10.1016/j.futures.2023.103153
6. Mackiewicz, K., Freiheit, R.: Foresight for digital health 2030: scenarios, barriers, and enablers for a sustainable future. International Journal of Social Science and Human Research. **8**, 861–870 (2025) https://doi.org/10.47191/ijsshr/v8-i2-11
7. Ahokangas, P., Perälä-Heape, M., Jämsä, T.: Alternative futures for individualized connected health. In: Gurtner, S., Soyez, K. (eds.) Challenges and Opportunities in Health Care Management, pp. 61–74. Springer International Publishing, Cham (2015). https://doi.org/10.1007/978-3-319-12178-9_5
8. Kim, K.K., Backonja, U.: Digital health equity frameworks and key concepts: a scoping review. J. Am. Med. Inform. Assoc. **32**, 932–944 (2025). https://doi.org/10.1093/jamia/ocaf017
9. Pierce, R.: Digital health equity: crafting sustainable pathways. PLOS Digital Health. **4**, e0000703 (2025). https://doi.org/10.1371/journal.pdig.0000703

10. Tung, E.L., Press, V.G., Peek, M.E.: Digital health readiness and health equity. JAMA Netw. Open. **7** (2025)
11. Culli, L.: Bridging the Digital Divide in Health Care: a New Framework for Equity (Digital Health Care Equity Framework). https://publichealth.jhu.edu/2025/bridging-the-digital-div ide-in-health-care-a-new-framework-for-equity (2025).
12. Hammad, A.W.A.: A Bilevel multiobjective optimisation approach for solving the evacuation location assignment problem. Adv. Civ. Eng. **2019,** (2019). https://doi.org/10.1155/2019/605 2931
13. Forum, W.E.: How equitable healthcare means a healthier future., https://www.weforum.org/ stories/2026/01/healthcare-sustainable-equitable-ai/ (2026).
14. Guise, V., Aase, K., Chambers, M., Canfield, C., Wiig, S.: Patient and stakeholder involvement in resilient healthcare: an interactive research study protocol. BMJ Open. **11**, e049116 (2021). https://doi.org/10.1136/bmjopen-2021-049116
15. Godage, P., Siribaddana, P., Hewapathirana, R.: Sustaining digital health systems through key stakeholders' engagement: a critical systems heuristics perspective. Oxf. Open Digit. Health. **1**, oqad014 (2023). https://doi.org/10.1093/oodh/oqad014
16. Haig, M., Main, C., Chávez, D., Kanavos, P.: A value framework to assess patient facing digital health technologies that aim to improve chronic disease management: a Delphi approach. Value Health. **26**, 1474–1484 (2023). https://doi.org/10.1016/j.jval.2023.06.008
17. Savira, F. et al.: Consumer preferences for telehealth in Australia: a discrete choice experiment. PLoS One. **18**, e0283821 (2023). https://doi.org/10.1371/journal.pone.0283821
18. De Guzman, K.R., Smith, A.C., Snoswell, C.L.: General practitioner preferences for telehealth consultations in Australia: a pilot survey and discrete choice experiment. Prim. Health Care Res. Dev. **25**, e49 (2024). https://doi.org/10.1017/S1463423624000136
19. Maaß, L., Zeeb, H., Rothgang, H.: International perspectives on measuring national digital public health system maturity through a multidisciplinary Delphi study. NPJ Digit. Med. **7**, 92 (2024). https://doi.org/10.1038/s41746-024-01078-9
20. Vo, L.K. et al.: Stakeholders' preferences for the design and delivery of virtual care services: a systematic review of discrete choice experiments. Soc. Sci. Med. **340**, 116459 (2024). https:// doi.org/10.1016/j.socscimed.2023.116459
21. Austin, S.F., Jansen, J.E., Petersen, C.J., Jensen, R., Simonsen, E.: Mobile app integration into dialectical behavior therapy for persons with borderline personality disorder: qualitative and quantitative study. JMIR Ment. Health. **7** (2020). https://doi.org/10.2196/14913
22. Giunti, G., Mylonopoulou, V., Rivera Romero, O., Isomursu, M.: Power dynamics analysis of participatory design in digital health research: case study. In: Studies in Health Technology and Informatics, pp. 454–458. IOS Press (2025). https://doi.org/10.3233/SHTI250760
23. Piera Jiménez, J. et al.: Cocreating principles for digital health equity: cross sectional, qualitative study for participatory human centered design in Catalonia. J. Med. Internet Res. **28**, e84129 (2026)
24. Hameed, K., Naha, R., Hameed, F.: Digital transformation for sustainable health and Wellbeing: a review and future research directions. Discov. Sustain. **5**, 104 (2024). https://doi.org/ 10.1007/s43621-024-00273-8
25. Pereno, A., Eriksson, D.: A multi-stakeholder perspective on sustainable healthcare: from 2030 onwards. Futures. **122**, 102605 (2020). https://doi.org/10.1016/j.futures.2020.102605

Implementation of the Digital-First Policy in Finnish Well-Being Services Counties: A Cross-Sectional Survey

Maiju Kyytsönen[1,2(✉)] ⓘ, Arild Faxvaag[3] ⓘ, Rune Pedersen[4,5] ⓘ, Jeppe Eriksen[6] ⓘ, Ove Lintvedt[4] ⓘ, and Jarmo Reponen[7] ⓘ

[1] Finnish Institute for Health and Welfare, FI-00271 Helsinki, Finland
`maiju.kyytsonen@thl.fi`
[2] University of Eastern Finland, FI-70211 Kuopio, Finland
[3] Department of Neuromedicine and Movement Science, NTNU – Norwegian University of Science and Technology, NO-7491 Torgarden, Trondheim, Norway
[4] Norwegian Centre for E-health Research, N-9038 Tromsø, Norway
[5] NORD University, 8049 Bodø, Norway
[6] Aalborg University, Rendsburggade 14, 9000 Aalborg, Denmark
[7] Research Unit of Health Sciences and Technology, University of Oulu, FI-90014 Oulu, Finland

Abstract. Digital-first policies aim to prioritise digital channels in the delivery of social and health care services. In Finland, well-being services counties (WSCs) became responsible for organising public health and social services in 2023, alongside the release of a national digital-first policy. This study assesses the progress of digital-first policy implementation in WSCs and identifies socio-technical factors that enable or constrain this process. A cross-sectional survey was conducted among chief information officers, chief digital officers, and other information management specialists across Finnish WSCs. The survey examined digital infrastructure, resource availability, collaboration practices, and the perceived facilitators and barriers to increasing the use of digital services. All but one WSC reported having fully or partially adopted the digital-first policy. However, infrastructure and resources for digital service development were often perceived as insufficient, and key barriers were related to organisational practices and technical infrastructure rather than to clients or patients. Strategic prioritisation, targeted funding, and management support emerged as central facilitators. The findings highlight the importance of strategic alignment, workflow redesign, and cross-organisational collaboration in the effective implementation of digital-first policies in social and health care systems.

Keywords: Digital-first policy · Service system · Digital transformation · Policy analysis

© The Author(s) 2026
M. Särestöniemi et al. (Eds.): NCDHWS 2026, CCIS 3009, pp. 34–47, 2026.
https://doi.org/10.1007/978-3-032-28812-7_3

1 Introduction

Digital services are expected to enhance patients' and clients' access to services and improve the effectiveness and efficiency of the service system [1–5]. Wellbeing services counties (WSCs) are the responsible entities for organising public health and social services and rescue services in Finland. They have been operational since early 2023, replacing the previous structures of municipalities and hospital districts. Following the structural change, the digitalisation of social and healthcare services has advanced both in alignment with the new structure and independently, for example, due to the COVID-19 pandemic and AI projects. In 2023, Finland's Ministry of Social Affairs and Health set a national strategic goal stating that 'digital channels are the primary choice whenever appropriate or for customers that are able to use digital services' [6]. The new strategy marks a clear departure from the previous one, which focused on integrating digital services into the service portfolio and ensuring that clients had the option to use them [7]. However, at the beginning of the decade, patients' demand for digital services in the public sector appears to have exceeded the available supply [8], although the situation has begun to ease since 2024 [9]. Achieving a mature stage of digitalisation requires substantial investment and a strategically phased approach [1, 10, 11]. The process typically begins with data digitisation, followed by the application of next-generation technologies to leverage this data and the development of innovative service models. At full maturity, resource allocation can be aligned with outcomes rather than volume, enabling more efficient and value-driven operations [12]. In Finland, systematic efforts towards the digital transformation of service systems began three decades ago [13]. In recent years, efforts have been made to harmonise digital infrastructures, ranging from foundational information systems to client-facing digital services.

Consistent with socio-technical systems theory, policy implementation is influenced by the interdependence of technological systems and social arrangements [12, 13]. Although digitalisation in Finland has advanced well, it has mainly concentrated on converting existing communication channels and data pathways into digital formats [14, 15]. For instance, Kanta Services serves as a solution for data sharing across organisations and between social and health care sectors and provides a patient portal for individuals to access their data. Studies show that Kanta Services has improved the situation but has not managed to solve all obstacles to data exchange between professionals from different organisations [14, 15].

Digital transformation entails profound changes, such as redesigning workflows, integrating predictive analytics into decision-making processes, and restructuring care pathways [1], to enable a proactive, data-driven, and integrated service delivery model. In this effort, adequate infrastructure is crucial for realising the advantages of digitalisation [16, 17]. The extent to which Finland has progressed toward deeper transformation remains uncertain, as although digitalisation is relatively mature, evidence of systematic, socio-technical transformation is still emerging.

Other Nordic countries also pursue strategies closely aligned with Finland's approach to digitalisation and information management in health and social care, with a shared policy focus on empowering citizens and promoting prevention and digital-first principles [16]. For example, in Norway, the current policy emphasises interoperability and the European Health Data Space to enable seamless data sharing across care sectors, representing a sociotechnical shift aimed at improving system sustainability by reducing clinician burden and enhancing patient safety [17]. Technology adoption is framed as essential to addressing workforce shortages, as in Finland [6, 18]. Centralised services such as Helsenorge, where citizens can access their health data, support the multisector "digital by default" approach [19], illustrating how organisational change and digital tools are combined to strengthen long-term care.

Comparable policy developments are also evident in Denmark, where current recommendations reinforce "digital and technological first" principles, promote faster scaling of labour-saving technologies, and strengthen the digital competencies of health professionals [20]. In 2024, a large-scale health reform began, which outlined the establishment of Digital Health Denmark (from 2027) to accelerate the national deployment of digital solutions. A key element of the reform is the "digital front door," which grants citizens the right to connect with healthcare providers through digital channels whenever possible and appropriate [21]. Taken together, Nordic policy directions consistently prioritise digital-first service models, but differ in how they operationalise data management, patient activation, and service system reforms.

Barriers to the utilisation of digital health services have predominantly been examined from the patient perspective. A recent review identified five common barriers: (1) limited digital skills, (2) lack of interest, (3) restricted access to technology, (4) concerns regarding quality of care, and (5) technical problems and usability issues [22]. Technology adoption among patients can be understood as a staged diffusion process, wherein individual uptake occurs at varying rates and is mediated by enabling and hindering conditions such as social support and psychological factors [23]. User satisfaction is a critical determinant of successful health technology adoption [24].

Digital health services can be leveraged to provide timely and appropriate care that aligns with patients' needs. Achieving this, however, requires competence at all levels of the health system, including clients, front-line professionals, administrators, and decision-makers [25]. When a digitally literate patient seeks help for a health concern, a digital front door can help in directing them to a healthcare professional with the appropriate competence profile, supporting efficient navigation and reducing unnecessary service use. Therefore, harnessing digital data to inform clinical and organisational decision-making can enhance care outcomes and support more efficient allocation of resources across the system [12].

The implementation of the digital-first policy is the responsibility of the WSCs, as their service provision is largely funded by the state through a budget that does not specify how services should be delivered [26]. A recent review identified a research gap in studies addressing the management implications of digitalisation across diverse stakeholder groups [27]. Therefore, this study adopts an evaluation approach to assess the progress of digital-first policy implementation in WSCs and to identify socio-technical factors that enable or constrain this process [28, 29]. Drawing on data from chief information officers (CIOs) and information management specialists, the study focuses on digital infrastructure, resource availability, collaboration, and perceived facilitators and barriers to implementation.

2 Materials and Methods

A Digital Service System Survey for WSCs was developed by two researchers specialising in the digitalisation of social and healthcare services. Feedback and ideas from 21 experts were utilised during the development process. In addition, one CIO of a WSC piloted the survey using a think-aloud protocol in an online meeting, providing valuable insights for further refinement. The survey was initially distributed to the CIOs or chief digital officers of each WSC in September 2025 and remained open for one month. The contact information of CIOs was obtained via the WSCs' websites or switchboards. Before the structural reform of the social and health care sectors, it was common for each hospital district to have its own CIO. In many WSCs, however, there was no CIO; instead, information management responsibilities were carried out by a person holding another professional title. Nevertheless, each respondent can be regarded as an information management specialist with substantial experience in the field. In total, ten CIOs completed the survey; additional respondents included chief digital officers and ICT managers representing their organisation's information management or digital services units. The accompanying instructions encouraged respondents to complete the survey collaboratively with other specialists. Overall, the mentioned respondents held 16 distinct professional titles. Ethical approval was not required before data collection for this cross-sectional study, as participants represented their organisations, and no sensitive personal information was gathered. Participation was voluntary, which was stated in the cover letter.

Research themes of the questionnaire are presented in Table 1. The data was analysed using descriptive statistics in IBM SPSS Statistics Version 29.0.2.0. A Fisher's exact test with Monte Carlo simulation (10,000 samples) was performed to examine the association between digital-first policy and infrastructure, as well as digital-first policy and resources. Figure 1 shows a boxplot illustrating the distribution of the variable, including the median (vertical line), first quartile, third quartile, and the upper and lower whiskers representing the maximum and minimum non-outlier values, along with outliers (circles).

Table 1. Research themes in the questionnaire.

Theme	Question	Reclassification
Digital-first policy	Is your wellbeing services county currently following the strategic objective for the digitalisation and information management of social and health care: 'digital channels are the primary choice whenever appropriate or for customers that are able to use digital services'?" Answer options: Yes, Partly, No	
Infrastructure	How adequate is the digital service infrastructure in your wellbeing services county in relation to the strategic goal: 'digital channels are the primary choice whenever appropriate or for customers that are able to use digital services'? In this context, infrastructure refers to the underlying digital structures and basic prerequisites of social and healthcare services, such as information systems and skilled personnel. Scale: 1 = Completely inadequate, 2 = Inadequate, 3 = Somewhat inadequate, 4 = Somewhat adequate, 5 = Adequate, 6 = Completely adequate	1 + 2 + 3 = Inadequate 4 = Somewhat adequate 5 + 6 = Adequate
Resources	"How sufficient are the resources in your wellbeing services county for developing the infrastructure of digital services?" Scale: 1 = Completely insufficient, 2 = Insufficient, 3 = Somewhat insufficient, 4 = Somewhat sufficient, 5 = Sufficient, 6 = Completely sufficient	1 + 2 + 3 = Inadequate 4 = Somewhat adequate 5 + 6 = Adequate
Collaboration	How important is collaboration with the following parties for the development of the digital service system on a scale of 1 to 5? 1 = Not at all important, 2 = Not very important, 3 = Neutral, 4 = Fairly important, 5 = Very important	

(continued)

Table 1. (*continued*)

Theme	Question	Reclassification
Barriers	Select the three most significant barriers to increasing the use of digital services offered to clients/patients. Discoverability of available services Inadequate communication Deficiencies in management Limited range of digital services Lack of suitable digital services Usability issues Under-resourcing of services relative to demand Lack of development resources Need for changes in professionals' work processes Skills gaps among professionals Lack of IT support for professionals Clients/patients prefer in-person or telephone services Clients'/patients' insufficient digital skills Technology is unsuitable for the client base Lack of language versions Lack of integration, e.g., between digital services and social and health centres Other, please specify	Statements selected by at least three respondents are presented in Fig. 1. One response originally categorised as "Other, please specify" was reclassified under "Lack of integration".
Support	Select the three most important factors that have supported the increase in the use of digital services offered to clients/patients: Discoverability of the services offered Communication Support from management Comprehensive range of digital services High quality of services Good usability of services Longer opening hours compared to other service channels Shorter waiting times compared to other service channels Prioritisation of digital service system development within the wellbeing services county Targeted additional funding for development Outsourcing digital service provision to specialised providers Changes in professionals' work processes Training for professionals IT support for professionals Professionals' enthusiasm for digital working Involvement of professionals in development Involvement of clients/patients in development Provision of digital support for clients/patients Provision of language versions Integration, e.g., between digital services and social and health centres Other, please specify	Statements selected by at least three respondents are presented in Fig. 2.

3   Results

In total, representatives from 21 of the 23 WSCs responded to the survey. The WSCs largely adhered to the digital-first policy (Table 2). Only one WSC had not implemented the policy, whereas 42.9% (n = 9/21) fully complied and 52.4% (n = 11/21) partially complied. Table 2 presents the adequacy of infrastructure and resources in relation to compliance with the digital-first policy. The associations between adherence to the digital-first policy and infrastructure (p = 0.059) or resources (p = 0.087) were not statistically significant.

Table 2. CIOs' assessment of the adequacy of infrastructure and resources according to compliance with the digital-first policy (n = 21).

	Digital-first policy		
	Yes	Partly	No
Infrastructure			
Inadequate	2	6	0
Somewhat adequate	6	4	0
Adequate	1	1	1
Resources			
Inadequate	2	8	0
Somewhat adequate	6	3	1
Adequate	1	0	0

Respondents viewed private companies and other WSCs in the same collaborative area as the most important parties for developing the digital service system (See Fig. 1). In-house companies, which are legally separate entities owned and controlled by a WSC, were also viewed as important partners. WSCs outside the WSC's own collaborative area and government institutions were viewed as neutral or fairly important partners. Non-profit organisations and DigiFinland Ltd., which is co-owned by the state and WSCs with a mission to develop public digital services, were placed in the middle of the scale. Universities and universities of applied sciences were viewed as neutral or not very important parties for collaboration.

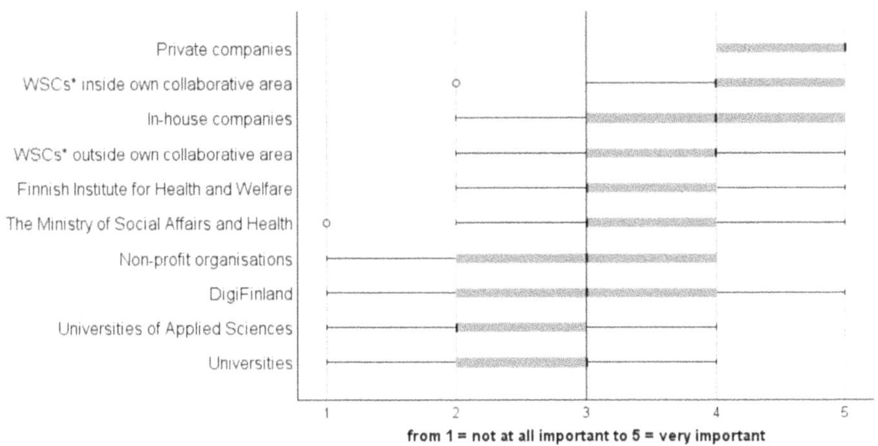

Fig. 1. Boxplot of the CIOs' assessment of the importance of collaboration for the development of the digital service system (n = 21).

The main barrier to increasing the use of digital services was the need for change in professionals' work processes (76%) (Fig. 2). This barrier was most often accompanied by a lack of development resources (33%, n = 7/21) and deficiencies in management (29%, n = 6/21). In addition to these barriers being repeated in the responses of the same respondents, they were also the most frequently selected barriers. Lack of integration and the view that many clients and patients prefer in-person or phone calls were chosen as the key barriers by 29%, and a limited range of digital services by 24%.

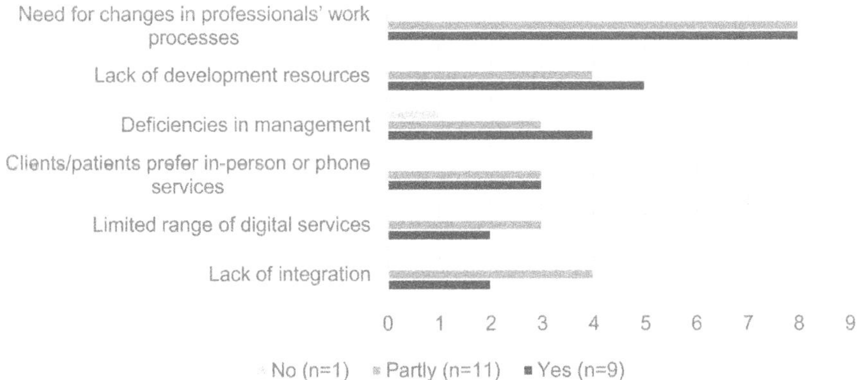

Fig. 2. The main barriers to increasing the use of digital services by adherence to the digital-first policy (n = 21).

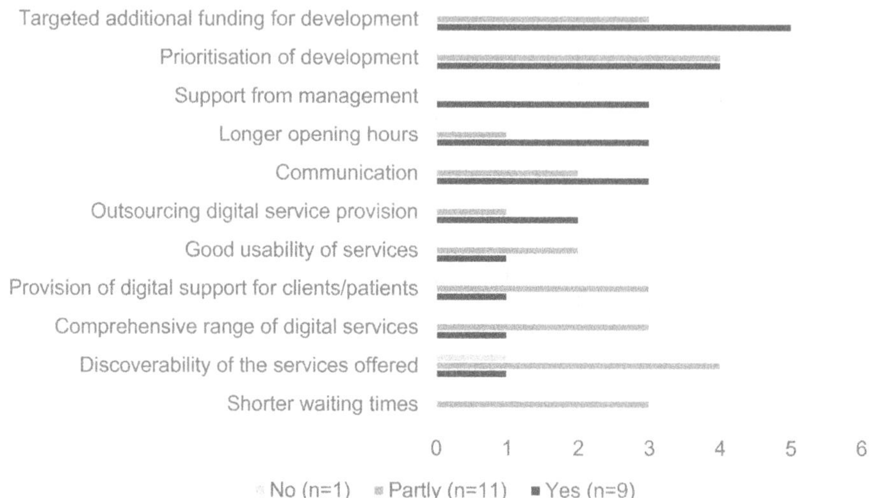

Fig. 3. The main facilitators to increasing the use of digital services by adherence to the digital-first policy (n = 21).

Perceptions of factors supporting the increased use of digital services for clients and patients varied considerably (see Fig. 3). The most frequently identified facilitators were targeted additional funding for development and prioritisation of digital service system development (38%). Other commonly cited factors were the discoverability of services (29%) and communication (24%).

4   Discussion

This study aimed to assess the extent to which WSCs have advanced in implementing the digital-first policy by analysing digital infrastructure, resource availability, collaboration, and the facilitators and barriers reported by CIOs and other specialists responsible for information management within WSCs. Respondents indicated that the digital-first policy had either been adopted or was in the process of adoption. The perceived adequacy of infrastructure and the resources allocated for its development did not demonstrate statistical significance in the analysis, a finding likely attributable to the limited sample size. Private companies and other WSCs within the same collaborative area were identified as the most critical partners for advancing the digital service system. Key barriers and facilitators to expanding the use of digital services were related to resources and organisational practices.

The digital infrastructure, which we defined as the underlying digital structures and fundamental prerequisites of social and healthcare services, such as information systems and skilled personnel, was adequate at three WSCs. Resources for developing this infrastructure were adequate at one WSC. Previous research has shown that policymakers often identify the lack of additional resources as a barrier to implementing health technology interventions [30], while simultaneously suggesting that improving financial incentives could increase the use of digital health services [31]. In any case, investments in digital infrastructure appear to be unavoidable in WSCs.

Attitudes towards collaboration emerged as another critical factor. An earlier study emphasised greater cooperation within the healthcare ecosystem as essential for accelerating digital transformation [12]. Our findings indicate that private companies, in-house providers, and other WSCs within the same collaborative area are valued as key partners in developing digital service systems. Additionally, WSCs outside their own collaborative area were appreciated, possibly due to benchmarking purposes and cross-border services, such as Health Village. Conversely, universities and universities of applied sciences were not perceived as important partners, which is a concern from the perspective of evidence-based social and health care. Addressing these gaps requires clarifying roles, building coordination mechanisms, and creating paths for communication across organisational boundaries to enable meaningful collaboration.

The capacity of integrated care systems to realise the benefits of digital technologies is contingent upon sustained strategic investments. These investments serve as foundational enablers, ensuring that technological adoption translates into systemic efficiency and measurable value rather than isolated digital initiatives [1, 30, 31]. Respondents consistently agreed that professionals' workflows must be redesigned to increase the use of digital services offered to clients and patients. Workflows were also central in all Nordic countries' digital strategies in the context of supporting health operations [16]. Our result suggests that many digital initiatives have been implemented without adequately adapting professionals' workflows and providing the necessary resources [1, 32–34]. Strengthening collaboration, particularly at the interfaces between stakeholders such as information management units and front-line staff, appears essential. This kind of collaboration can be facilitated by managers, which furthermore strengthens the strategic approach.

Other commonly reported barriers included insufficient development resources and deficiencies in management. These were complemented by facilitators selected by respondents whose WSC adhered to the digital-first policy: targeted additional funding for development, prioritisation of digital service system development, and management support. Together, these factors underline the importance of aligning the service system at the strategic level towards a shared trajectory, supported by active management engagement in change processes [1, 35].

When planning new interventions, it is crucial to allocate resources for training, human capital development, and IT integration [35]. In our study, only one WSC identified deficiencies in professionals' skills as a key barrier to increasing the use of digital services, which is supported by another study concluding that nurses' informatics competency is good [36]. Instead, the lack of system integration was highlighted as a major barrier by just six WSCs in a situation where many WSCs depend on digital services provided by private providers, for example, in gatekeeping functions that determine access to further services. If these services are not adequately integrated into the WSCs' information systems, it can hamper the development of patient-and client-centred workflows and care pathways.

A prior review found that half of the included studies identified an individual-level barrier related to patients' lack of interest in digital health services, often linked to a preference for in-person care [22]. In our study, only six respondents considered this a major barrier. Patient and client perspectives were reflected in the responses in other ways; factors such as effective communication, convenient opening hours, and good usability were perceived as encouraging greater adoption of digital services, all of which contribute to delivering a service that is both attractive and valuable to clients and patients. These views align with the Finnish atmosphere, where, despite the national digital-first policy, the use of digital services is voluntary for clients and patients, which ensures equal possibilities of service use for everyone [6]. Another facilitator highlighted in earlier research, which was not considered central by our respondents, was the involvement of front-line staff and patients in development [1, 33, 35], which may help align service production with real patient needs.

Overall, only one WSC adhered to the digital-first policy in circumstances where it had sufficient resources and infrastructure to support its implementation. If we accept that the ability to align resources with intended outcomes reflects the maturity of digitalisation [12], it appears that the WSCs still have considerable progress to make. The envisioned end state could be one in which patients are guided through the service system via the digital front door in a meaningful and as seamless a manner as possible, supported by the data generated throughout their journey and by service pathways that enable professionals to use their expertise to its full value.

The study has several limitations. First, two WSCs did not respond to the survey, which prevented us from obtaining a complete sample. Nevertheless, the response rate of 91.3% can be considered satisfactory. Second, the research was conducted by the Finnish Institute for Health and Welfare, which has a national steering role in the field of information management. However, the researchers involved in this study do not participate in these steering activities, and participants were informed that the survey was conducted for scientific purposes and was voluntary. These conditions likely provided respondents with greater freedom to answer freely compared with mandatory national data collections used for steering. Lastly, two survey questions included long option lists from which respondents were asked to select the three most suitable choices. Before data collection, a survey expert was consulted regarding the length of these lists, after which the original format was retained. After data collection, the researchers confirmed that no order bias appeared to be present.

5   Conclusions

The digital-first policy has been adopted in all WSCs except one. Implementing a digital-first approach requires a complex digital transformation, which presents significant challenges at various organisational levels. Our results showed that CIOs and other specialists responsible for information management within a WSC identified modifying professionals' workflows as a key challenge to expanding digital services. While resources were generally seen as insufficient, our results indicate that prioritising the development of the digital service system is crucial to increasing digital service usage. Collaboration with frontline staff, patients, clients, and academic institutions remains underutilised. In the coming years, monitoring the implementation of the digital-first policy will be essential for understanding how the situation evolves and which aspects of the change process are viewed as significant within WSCs. The WSCs could also benefit from a scientific roadmap that integrates the perspectives of different stakeholders, such as CIOs, patients and front-line staff, to support and accelerate a meaningful digital-first policy adoption process. At this stage, based on the findings, we recommend:

- ensuring that the digital-first policy is strategically led;
- strategic objectives are aligned with adequate resource allocation;
- collaboration is strengthened at different interfaces of stakeholders; and
- workflow design is placed at the centre of implementation processes.

Acknowledgments. We thank all representatives of the well-being services counties who participated in the Digital Service System Survey, as well as all experts who contributed to the design of the survey. We also extend our thanks to the three anonymous reviewers for their valuable insights on the manuscript.

Disclosure of Interests The authors have no competing interests to declare that are relevant to the content of this article.

References

1. Ebo, T.O., Clement David-Olawade, A., Ebo, D.M., et al.: Transforming healthcare delivery: a comprehensive review of digital integration, challenges, and best practices in integrated care systems. Digit. Eng. **6** (2025). https://doi.org/10.1016/j.dte.2025.100056
2. Böckerman, P., Kortelainen, M., Laine, L.T., et al.: Information technology, improved access, and use of prescription drugs. J. Eur. Econ. Assoc. **23**, 396–430 (2025). https://doi.org/10.1093/jeea/jvae034
3. Dahlberg, A., Jukarainen, S., Kaartinen, T., Orre, P.: Cost minimization analysis of digital-first healthcare pathways in primary care. Npj. Digit. Med. **8**, 546 (2025). https://doi.org/10.1038/s41746-025-01937-z
4. Vainio, H., Eklund, A., Soininen, L., et al.: Evaluation of the performance of telephone triage service. Scand. J. Trauma Resusc. Emerg. Med. **33**, 172 (2025). https://doi.org/10.1186/s13049-025-01462-8
5. Laukka, E., Jansson, M., Suonnansalo, P., et al.: Effectiveness of interactive digital health services in non-communicable diseases: an umbrella review and evidence synthesis from 26 meta-analyses. Int. J. Nurs. Stud. **174**, 105277 (2025). https://doi.org/10.1016/j.ijnurstu.2025.105277
6. Ministry of Social Affairs and Health: Strategy for digitalisation and information management in healthcare and social welfare (2024)
7. Ministry of Social Affairs and Health: Information to Support Well-being and Service Renewal: eHealth and eSocial Strategy 2020. Ministry of Social Affairs and Health| (2015)
8. Kyytsönen, M., Aalto, A.-M., Virtanen, L., et al.: Patients' perceived access to healthcare: comparison of in person, phone call, and telehealth appointments. Finnish Institute for Health and Welfare (2024)
9. Haaga, T., Mauno, V., Saxell, T., et al.: Digital clinics are reshaping public primary health care. In: SoteDataLab. https://sotedatalab.fi/en/uutinen/digiklinikka-muuttamassa-julkista-perust erveydenhuoltoa/ (2024). Accessed 19 Mar 2026
10. Kruse, C.S., Williams, K., Bohls, J., Shamsi, W.: Telemedicine and health policy: a systematic review. Health Policy Technol. **10**, 209–229 (2021). https://doi.org/10.1016/j.hlpt.2020.10.006

11. Rodler, S., Schütz, J.M., Styn, A., et al.: Mapping telemedicine in German private practice urological care: implications for transitioning beyond the COVID-19 pandemic. Urol. Int. **105**, 650–656 (2021). https://doi.org/10.1159/000515982
12. Gopal, G., Suter-Crazzolara, C., Toldo, L., Eberhardt, W.: Digital transformation in healthcare—architectures of present and future information technologies. Clin. Chem. Lab. Med. CCLM. **57**, 328–335 (2019). https://doi.org/10.1515/cclm-2018-0658
13. Ministry of Social Affairs and Health: Sosiaali- ja terveydenhuollon tietoteknologian hyödyntämisstrategia (1995)
14. Vehko, T., Ikonen, J., Kyytsönen, M., et al.: Tietojärjestelmät lähihoitajien työn tukena eri toimintaympäristöissä: kokemuksia tuotemerkeittäin 2022. Finn. J. EHealth EWelfare. **15**, 199–218 (2023). https://doi.org/10.23996/fjhw.125395
15. Lääveri, T., Reponen, J., Vehko, T., Viitanen, J.: Physicians' experiences of health information exchange in Finland after ten years of national patient data repository services. In: Intelligent Health Systems—from Technology to Data and Knowledge, pp. 637–641. IOS Press (2025)
16. Faxvaag, A., Reponen, J., Hardardottir, G.A., et al.: Towards accountable E-health policies in the Nordic countries. Stud. Health Technol. Inform. **316**, 339–343 (2024). https://doi.org/10.3233/SHTI240413
17. Directorate of e-Health: National e-health strategy for the health and care sector [Nasjonal e-helsestrategi for helse- og omsorgssektoren] (2023)
18. Official Norwegian Reports: Time for action: Personnel in a sustainable health and care service [Tid for handling—Personellet i en bærekraftig helse- og omsorgstjeneste]. regjeringen.no (2023)
19. Norwegian Ministry of Local Government and Modernisation: Digital agenda for Norway in brief [Regjeringens digitaliseringsprogram i kortversjon]. Government of Norway (2016)
20. Danish Ministry of the Interior and Health: The Danish Resilience Commission: Summary report (2023)
21. Sundhedsreformen: Ministry of Interior and Health Denmark, India. https://www.ism.dk/temaer/sundhedsreformen-2024 (2024). Accessed 12 Jan 2026
22. Kemp, M., Rising, K.L., Laynor, G., et al.: Barriers to telehealth uptake and use: a scoping review. JAMIA Open. **8**, ooaf019 (2025). https://doi.org/10.1093/jamiaopen/ooaf019
23. Turja, T., Jylhä, V., Rosenlund, M., Kuusisto, H.: Beyond early and late adopters: reimagining health technology readiness through health-related circumstances. Sustain. Futur. **10**, 101003 (2025). https://doi.org/10.1016/j.sftr.2025.101003
24. Thabet, Z., Albashtawi, S., Ansari, H., et al.: Exploring the factors affecting telemedicine adoption by integrating UTAUT2 and IS success model: a hybrid SEM-ANN approach. IEEE Trans. Eng. Manag. **71**, 8938–8950 (2024). https://doi.org/10.1109/TEM.2023.3296132
25. Malmivaara, A.: Vision and strategy for healthcare: competence is a necessity. J. Rehabil. Med. **52**, jrm00061 (2020). https://doi.org/10.2340/16501977-2684
26. Finland: Laki hyvinvointialueiden rahoituksesta [Act on the Financing of Wellbeing Services Counties] (2021)
27. Stoumpos, A.I., Kitsios, F., Talias, M.A.: Digital transformation in healthcare: technology acceptance and its applications. Int. J. Environ. Res. Public Health. **20**, 3407 (2023). https://doi.org/10.3390/ijerph20043407
28. Pawson, R., Tilley, N.: Realistic Evaluation. SAGE Publishing Ltd, India. https://uk.sagepub.com/en-gb/eur/realistic-evaluation/book205276 (1997). Accessed 5 Dec 2025
29. Scriven, M.: Evaluation Thesaurus. SAGE Publishing Inc., India (1991) https://us.sagepub.com/en-us/nam/evaluation-thesaurus/book3562. Accessed 5 Dec 2025
30. Neher, M., Nygårdh, A., Broström, A., et al.: Perspectives of policy makers and service users concerning the implementation of eHealth in Sweden: interview study. J. Med. Internet Res. **24**, e28870 (2022). https://doi.org/10.2196/28870

31. Assing Hvidt, E., Atherton, H., Keuper, J., et al.: Low adoption of video consultations in post–COVID-19 general practice in northern Europe: barriers to use and potential action points. J. Med. Internet Res. **25**, e47173 (2023). https://doi.org/10.2196/47173

32. Marwaha, J.S., Landman, A.B., Brat, G.A., et al.: Deploying digital health tools within large, complex health systems: key considerations for adoption and implementation. Npj Digit. Med. **5** (2022). https://doi.org/10.1038/s41746-022-00557-1

33. Nadav, J., Kaihlanen, A.-M., Kujala, S., et al.: How to implement digital Services in a way that they integrate into routine work: qualitative interview study among health and social care professionals. J. Med. Internet Res. **23**, e31668 (2021). https://doi.org/10.2196/31668

34. Saukkonen, P., Elovainio, M., Salovaara, S., et al.: Perceived effects of digitalization on social work in Finland: a network analysis approach. Int. Soc. Work. **67**, 1464–1481 (2024). https://doi.org/10.1177/00208728241265015

35. Schiffhauer, B., Seelmeyer, U.: Responsible digital transformation of social welfare organizations. In: Ifenthaler, D., Hofhues, S., Egloffstein, M., Helbig, C. (eds.) Digital Transformation of Learning Organizations, pp. 131–144. Springer International Publishing, Cham (2021)

36. Kinnunen, U.-M., Kuusisto, A., Koponen, S., et al.: Nurses' informatics competency assessment of health information system usage: a cross-sectional survey. Comput. Inform. Nurs. CIN. **41**, 869–876 (2023). https://doi.org/10.1097/CIN.0000000000001026

Electronic Health Record System Market Concentration in Finland, 2007–2028

Timo Tuovinen[1,2(✉)] , Petra Kuikka[1,2] , Paula Veikkolainen[1,2] ,
Niina S. Keränen[1,2] , Virpi Ekholm[3], Vesa Jormanainen[4] ,
and Jarmo Reponen[1,2]

[1] FinnTelemedicum, Research Unit of Health Sciences and Technology, University of Oulu,
Oulu, Finland
`timo.tuovinen@oulu.fi`
[2] Medical Research Center Oulu, Oulu University Hospital and University of Oulu, Oulu,
Finland
[3] Viestintä Virpi Ekholm, Nokia, Finland
[4] Department of Public Health, Doctoral School of Health Sciences, Doctoral Programme in
Population Health, University of Helsinki, Helsinki, Finland

Abstract. The market for electronic health record (EHR) systems is notably concentrated, with a small number of vendors dominating the landscape. In this study, we analyze market concentration in Finland's public healthcare EHR system between 2007 and 2020 using data from the Use of Information and Communication Technology in Finnish Healthcare surveys (2007, 2011, 2014, 2017, and 2020). To capture recent developments and upcoming changes, data on the current status and future EHR system plans of the wellbeing services counties were collected through a separate survey, extending the monitoring period to 2028. The results show that the Finnish public healthcare EHR market was highly concentrated throughout 2007–2020, and that market concentration is expected to increase further by 2028.

Keywords: Electronic health records · Brand · Market share ·
Herfindahl-hirschman index · Finland

1 Introduction

Since the pioneering implementations in the 1980–1990s, electronic health record (EHR) systems have evolved into a central tool in modern healthcare not only for the secure and readily accessible storage of patient data, but also holds promise for standardizing care, supporting quality and efficiency reporting, guiding operational management, and enabling data-driven clinical decision-making and interoperability. EHRs are real-time digital systems that typically store patients' medical histories, diagnoses, treatment, medications, allergies, immunizations, referrals, radiology images, and laboratory results [1]

M. Särestöniemi et al. (Eds.): NCDHWS 2026, CCIS 3009, pp. 48–60, 2026.
https://doi.org/10.1007/978-3-032-28812-7_4

Healthcare service systems and their digital solutions typically differ substantially across countries, for example in regulation, structure, and processes. As a result, requirements and approaches to EHR systems' implementation vary. Top-down models establish a national EHR under central authority, while bottom-up approaches rely on regional or local EHR systems. National health information exchange (HIE) platforms, such as Kanta Services in Finland, can link regional systems through a middle-out approach [1, 2]

While only every tenth hospital in USA used EHR systems as late as in 2010 [3, 4], public healthcare EHR coverage in Finland had almost reached 100% already by 2007 [5]. However, after the passage of the Health Information Technology for Economic and Clinical Health (HITECH) act of 2009 in the USA, hospitals have rapidly adopted EHRs [4, 6]. In the Nordic countries, high digital maturity, public trust, and integrated digital infrastructures have driven early and sustained adoption, albeit not without challenges in fragmentation, usability and workflow integration. For example, by January 2001, 53 of the 72 hospitals in Norway had purchased a license for an electronic medical records system, covering 77% of hospital beds [7]. The WHO Global Observatory for eHealth reported differences in the implementation of EHRs across countries in 2015 [8]. By 2021, the use of EHRs had increased globally similarly to USA [9].

The global health informatics market has been projected to reach $123 billion, by 2025 [10], and the global EHR market is currently valued at approximately $30–50 billion. The market for EHR systems is becoming notably concentrated, with a few major vendors dominating the landscape from global perspective. This concentration is evident in both the USA and international markets. In the USA six major vendors cover approximately 90% of the market share for EHR systems [4]. This high level of market concentration suggests limited competition, potential barriers for new entrants, and in some cases slow development activities. Concentration is high in the USA hospital sector, where the Herfindahl-Hirschman Index (HHI) surpassed 3000 by 2021, primarily driven by the dominance of Epic Systems and Oracle Health (Cerner). Over the past decade, Epic-based systems have also been adopted in the Nordic countries, with installations in Finland, Denmark, and Norway [11].

A previous Finnish study from 2019 investigated the market shares of EHR systems used in public primary healthcare (health centers) and hospital districts in 2017 demonstrating that EHR system markets were already highly concentrated (HHI = 3300) [12].

While previous studies have examined EHR market concentration at specific time points, evidence on its long-term development remains limited. Longitudinal monitoring is necessary to assess structural persistence, as sustained high concentration may indicate vendor lock-in and barriers to competition, with implications for healthcare system organization, interoperability, and policy.

In this research study, we describe the EHR systems market and measure market concentration trends over time in Finland in 2007–2028.

2 Materials and Methods

2.1 Organization of Healthcare in Finland

Until 2023, public primary healthcare was organized by 309 municipalities, while specialized hospitals' medical care was provided by twenty hospital districts jointly owned by the municipalities in each region – and by the county of Åland [13]. Some municipalities also formed joint municipal authorities over the years responsible for primary healthcare. Within the hospital districts, five university hospitals provided tertiary care. The private sector accounted for one-third of outpatient physician visits, although with a narrower range of services; half of these visits occurred within occupational healthcare [14].

Since January 1, 2023, responsibility for public healthcare and social welfare services in Finland has been transferred to 21 Wellbeing Services Counties, the City of Helsinki, and the Autonomous Region of Åland, forming a total of 23 administrative entities (compared with 195 separate municipal and joint arrangements and 22 rescue service providers in 2022) [15]. Each wellbeing services county integrates primary and specialized healthcare, social welfare, and rescue services under a single administrative structure funded primarily by the government through tax revenue.

2.2 Data Used in this Study

Longitudinal survey on the availability and extent of use of information systems in Finnish healthcare (2007–2020). This study used longitudinal survey data from the 'Use of Information and Communication Technology in Finnish Healthcare' surveys conducted in 2007, 2011, 2014, 2017, and 2020. The dataset constitutes long-term monitoring data, with the most recent measurement conducted after the full implementation of the national Kanta Services HIE system. This study only examined public healthcare providers because private sector data were not available comprehensive enough to assess market shares.

The survey was conducted among public healthcare providers in Finland and a sample of private medical service providers. The target population of public healthcare providers included all 21 hospital districts responsible for specialized healthcare (specialized hospitals) and all primary healthcare organizations. Primary healthcare organizations were defined as independent municipalities or cooperation areas organized as municipal consortia or responsibility models. Responses were collected using web-based questionnaires (Webropol). The questions were kept comparable with those used in earlier surveys and were updated to reflect developments in health information and communication technology. The questionnaires were distributed by email to medical directors and chief information officers in specialized hospitals and to chief physicians in primary healthcare. For private healthcare providers, the questionnaires were addressed to chief executive officers or other designated contact persons. The functionality of the questionnaires was tested prior to distribution to the participating organizations.

Responses were compiled at the organizational level. In hospital districts where specialized healthcare providers were also responsible for primary healthcare services for municipalities, only the specialized healthcare questionnaire was administered. In these cases, responses from specialized healthcare providers were transferred to the primary healthcare survey. At the end of the official response period, non-responding organizations were reminded by email and telephone. Submitted questionnaires were reviewed, and incomplete responses were supplemented through follow-up by telephone or email with organizational representatives.

The study included all 21 hospital districts in 2007, 2011, 2014, 2017, and 2020. For primary healthcare organizations, response rates (number of organizations) were 100% (229/229, to the most important question; 87–96% to the rest of the questions) in 2007, 86% (139/161) in 2011, 88% (135/153) in 2014, 86% (121/141) in 2017, and 96% (130/136) in 2020, corresponding to population coverages of 91%, 95%, 95%, and 99%, respectively. Response rates among private healthcare providers were 62% (28/45) in 2007, 31% (30/97) in 2011, 45% (24/46) in 2014, 57% (26/46) in 2017, and 44% (12/28) in 2020, including organizations operating as corporate groups. Variations in the number of participating primary and private healthcare organizations across survey years reflected changes in municipal healthcare organizational arrangements and mergers among private healthcare providers, respectively.

Additional data sources (2025–2028). A separate survey was conducted among chief digital and information officers in the wellbeing services counties within mainland Finland to assess future patient information systems in these areas [16]. The survey was distributed to the target group on November 20, 2025, and the final responses were received on December 7, 2025. Survey included four questions: 1. What EHR systems are currently in use in your wellbeing services county? 2. If the area has already switched to a common EHR system, when were the last implementations? 3. If the transition to a common system is just beginning, what is the timetable for this? Which patient information system has been selected for the wellbeing services county? 4. Anything else you would like to say about the topic? Responses were obtained from all wellbeing services counties. Raw data from the survey was made available to researchers for this study.

In this study, Helsinki University Hospital (HUS) and Åland were analysed together with the wellbeing areas. Information about city of Helsinki and the HUS Group was publicly available [17]. In addition, publicly available information indicated that a new EHR system (Cosmic), supplied by the Swedish company Cambio, was introduced in the Åland healthcare in fall of 2025 [18, 19].

Table 1 shows EHR vendors and brands in Finnish wellbeing services counties in 2025.

Verification data. For 2013, the available verification data consisted of a publication by the Finnish Institute for Health and Welfare that examined EHR systems in public primary healthcare units [20]. No significant differences were observed between the findings of that publication and the results of our survey X^2 (1, N $= 286$) $= 0.3925$, p $= 0.98$.

2.3 Data Analysis

The data were analyzed by means of descriptive methods, and we present results by using graphs.

Market concentration. The Herfindahl–Hirschman Index (HHI) is a standard metric used to quantify market concentration and competitiveness. It is calculated by squaring the market share of each firm competing in a market and summing these values:

$$HHI = \sum_{i=1}^{n} s_i^2 \tag{1}$$

where s_i is the market share of firm as a whole percentage and n is the number of firms in the market.

According to established interpretations, markets are considered competitive and unconcentrated when the HHI is below 1500, moderately concentrated when the HHI ranges from 1500 to 2500, and highly concentrated when the HHI exceeds 2500, indicating oligopolistic or monopolistic market structures with significant barriers to entry [11].

In contrast to the previous study by Jormanainen et al. [12], which examined EHR market concentration in 2017, the present study calculated the HHI based on customer organizations, except for the most recent data on wellbeing services counties, city of Helsinki, and Åland for which population-based market shares were also calculated.

3 Results

3.1 Development of EHR System Market Shares Between 2007–2020

The market shares of the EHR brands have remained relatively stable both in the primary healthcare as well as in specialized hospitals (hospital districts) (Fig. 1). Among smaller trademarks, some have exited the market (HealthNet and Musti). The Epic-based Apotti EHR system was introduced at HUS in stages in 2018–2021, and today it covers all HUS hospitals as well as primary healthcare in the city of Helsinki and wellbeing services county of Vantaa and Kerava. In addition, branding changes have occurred, with Effica becoming Lifecare and Pegasos, Miranda, and Uranus later merging to form Omni360.

Table 1. EHR vendors and brands in Finnish wellbeing services counties in 2025.

Vendor	EHR system brand	Comments
Apotti	Apotti (Epic)	Built on the core software of the US-based Epic Systems.
Cambio	Cosmic	The leading EHR vendor in Sweden; currently implemented in the Åland region.
CGI	Omni360	Successor to legacy systems including Miranda, Uranus, and Pegasos.
Esko Systems	Esko	An in-house company, primarily owned by the Northern Ostrobothnia and Lapland wellbeing services counties.
TietoEvry	LifeCare	Successor to the Effica system.

A Market shares of EHR systems in public primary care

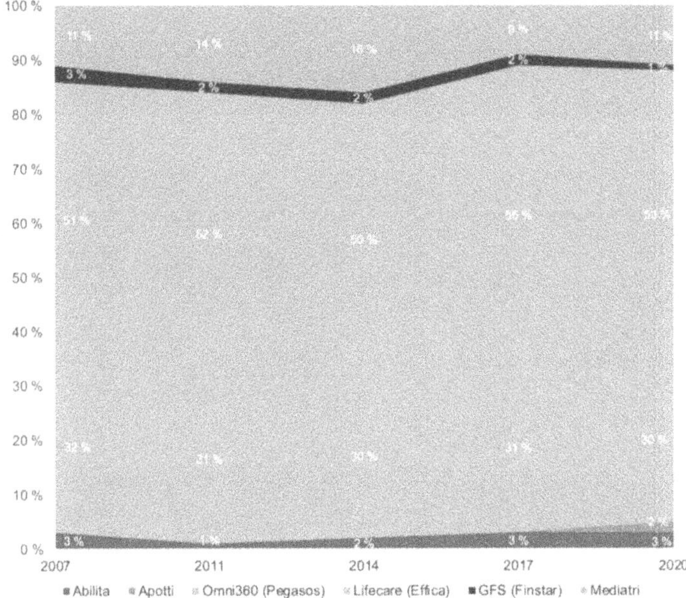

B Market shares of EHR systems in hospital districts (specialized hospitals)

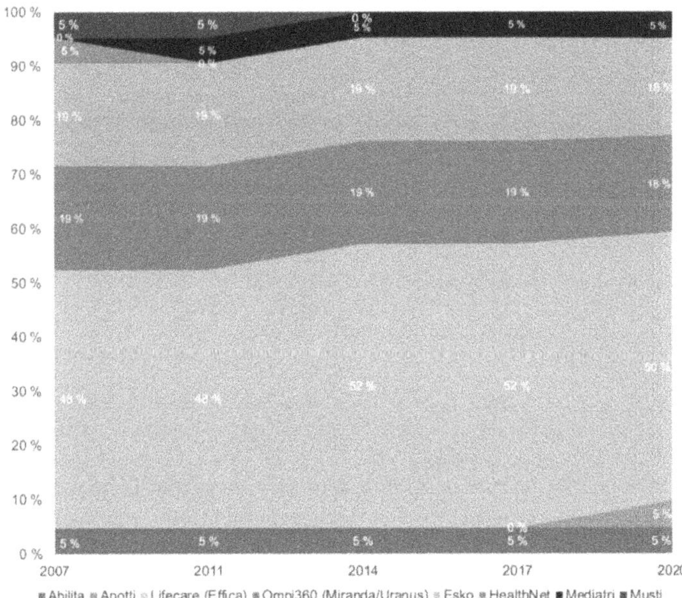

Fig. 1. Development of market shares of EHR systems in Finland in public primary health-care (panel A) and specialized hospital care within hospital districts (panel B), measured by the number of customer organizations. For comparability, earlier EHR product brands and product families were grouped according to current naming conventions, with Effica becoming Lifecare and Pegasos, Miranda, and Uranus later merging to form Omni360.

3.2 Status of EHR Implementation in Wellbeing Services Counties in Finland (2025–2028)

All wellbeing services counties reported that they have already chosen their future EHR system to cover the entire county (both primary healthcare and specialized hospitals' medical care).

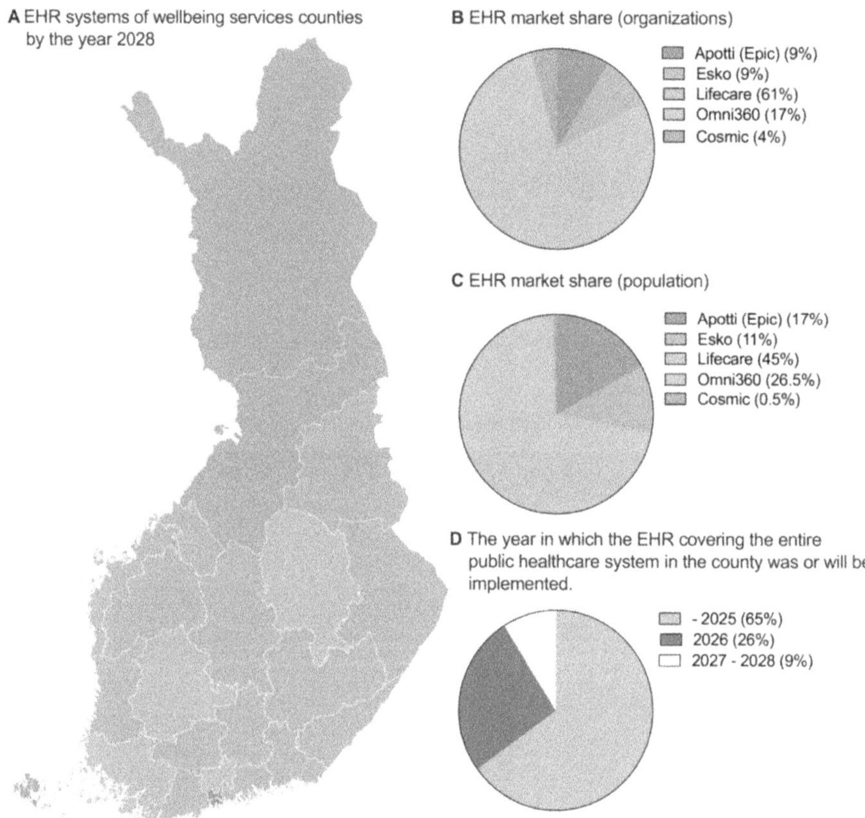

Fig. 2. EHR market by 2028. Panel A shows the EHR systems reported by wellbeing services counties, either currently in use or already decided upon. Panel B presents the market shares of EHR vendors measured by the number of customer organizations. Panel C presents market shares measured by the population covered by welfare regions. Panel D shows the reported timing of full implementation of an EHR system covering the entire welfare region.

In the future, the Finnish public healthcare market is expected to be concentrated among five EHR system trademarks (Fig. 2). The most commonly selected system is Lifecare (formerly Effica), which has also previously dominated the Finnish public healthcare EHR market (Fig. 1). The second most common system chosen by wellbeing services counties is Omni365 (formerly Pegasos, Uranus and Miranda). Esko and Apotti (Epic) are similar in terms of customer organization shares. The Cosmic system, introduced in Åland in 2025, has the smallest market share, both in terms of the number of organizations and the population served.

Two thirds (65%) of respondents reported that the implementation of wellbeing services county wide EHR system had already been completed, either in their previous organizations or at the welfare services county level (c.f. Fig. 2D). In addition, one out of four (26%) of the respondents indicated that implementation was at an advanced stage and expected that an EHR system covering the entire wellbeing services county would be in use during 2026. Two respondents (9%) reported that the transition to a single EHR system at the wellbeing services county level would occur during 2027–2028.

3.3   Trends in EHR System Market Concentration in Finland

Throughout the study period, the Finnish EHR market was highly concentrated, as indicated by the HHI, largely due to two vendors holding more than 80% of the market share (Fig. 1). In public primary healthcare, the greater market concentration was higher (average HHI = 3813) than in specialized hospitals in hospital districts (average HHI = 3275). The reform from municipality-based healthcare organization to welfare services counties, city of Helsinki and HUS Group appears to have further increased market concentration (HHI = 4178) (Fig. 3).

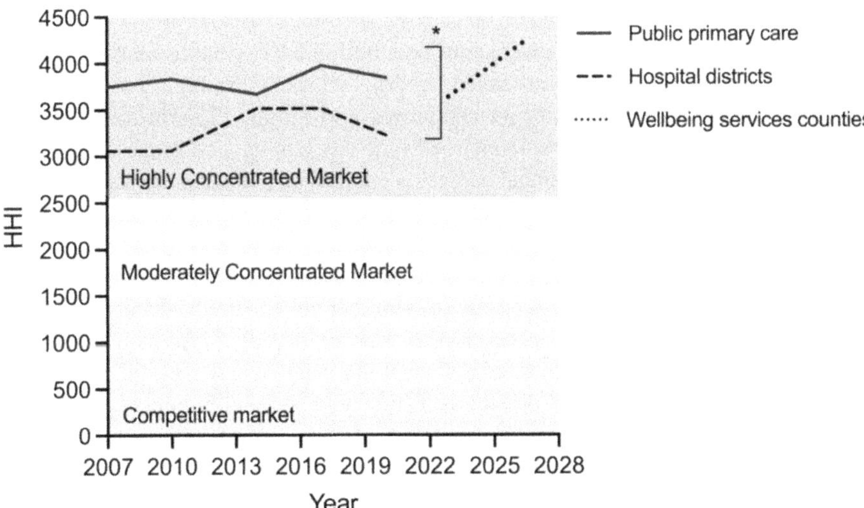

Fig. 3. Herfindahl–Hirschman Index (HHI) for public healthcare in Finland, 2007–2028. Observed values (2007–2020) are based on survey data; projected values (dotted line) incorporate planned EHR system choices of wellbeing services counties and reflect increased concentration driven by organizational consolidation. * Social and healthcare reform on 1 January 2023 forming wellbeing services counties.

4 Discussion

Our research shows that the Finnish EHR market has been highly concentrated throughout measured history in 2007–2020, and this development, to become even more concentrated by 2028, has continued with the social welfare and healthcare reform that formed wellbeing services counties, city of Helsinki and the HUS Group. To the best of our knowledge, this is the longest longitudinal monitoring series of the EHR market development in any country.

Similar developments has been reported in several other countries. For example, the hospital EHR vendor market in the USA changed substantially in 2012–2021 [6]. During this period, two vendors (Epic and Cerner) increased their market shares noticeably, and the market shifted from being considered competitive to highly concentrated, since these two vendors covering 72% of hospital beds. Further based on bed numbers, the HHI for USA hospital EHRs has been estimated at 1452 in 2012 increasing to >3000 in 2021.

In our data, a very similar development trend will happen in Finland by 2028, with Lifecare and Omni360 accounting for 78% of customer organizations and 71% of the wellbeing services counties' population base. In terms of exhibited substantial market concentration, the situation appears to be even more pronounced for the United Kingdom general practitioners where it has exhibited marked market concentration, with two vendors (TPP and EMIS) holding a combined market share of 73% in 2011, increasing to 99% by 2024. HHI for English general practice EHRs has increased from 4608 in 2017 to 5120 in 2024 [21]

Our study shows that only few changes occurred in EHR systems market shares in 2007–2020. This may relate to so-called vendor lock-in. Transitions from one EHR system to another involve significant challenges and pitfalls [22]. In addition, such transitions are labor-intensive, personnel-and time-consuming, and remarkably expensive. Key challenges include financial burdens, demands on personnel resources, patient safety risks due to limited access to legacy records, data integrity during migration, cybersecurity concerns, and issues related to semantic interoperability [22].

The high market concentration can lead to several challenges, including high maintenance costs and difficulties in keeping up with technological advancements such as telemedicine and artificial intelligence [23]. Consolidation also creates cybersecurity risks such as single-point-of-failure tail risk meaning that single successful attack could expose even millions of patients' private data and could potentially impact clinical care and other healthcare functions across thousands of sites [24]. Additionally, interoperability issues are prevalent, as vendors may be reluctant to dilute their market share by enhancing compatibility with other systems [25, 26].

On the other hand, other perspectives have been presented in the literature. Although an increase in the number of vendors in the EHR market may enhance competition, reduce costs, and improve quality, it may also raise the risk of interoperability challenges, since EHR systems do not always communicate effectively with one another [11]. Additionally, staff usually becomes accustomed to specific systems, and job mobility is easier when the same system is used across organizations. Fewer systems also simplify national architecture planning. However, similar benefits could be achieved through standardization. This could include not only standardization of underlying technical solutions and data formats, but also standardization of user interface components. This can be compared to the automotive industry, where basic use is standardized, yet manufacturers compete through differences in user experience. Another benefit of extended standardization is decreased vendor dependance.

All the wellbeing services counties in Finland reported that they will implement a single EHR system for both primary healthcare and specialized hospitals by 2028, which will significantly affect healthcare operations. On the other hand, occupational healthcare and private healthcare sector sustain the need for interoperability and national HIE. In addition, cooperation between wellbeing services counties requiring specialized expertise and division of labor will continue to require interoperability between different systems.

Large-scale EHR systems are increasingly adopted in European healthcare and are often framed as platform-based ecosystems that enable third-party integration and innovation. In line with this trend, Norwegian health authorities initiated the Akson program in 2018 to procure a common EHR system for most Norwegian municipalities. The system was intended to replace existing EHR solutions across municipal health services, with implementation planned for 2025–2030. While the program represents a major long-term investment, it generated considerable debate among stakeholders regarding its scope, design, and strategic direction [27] leading to ending the project in 2020–2021 [28, 29].

Regulatory initiatives such as the European Health Data Space (EHDS) and Regulation (EU) 2025/327 are expected to promote increased standardization and cross-border interoperability of health data. For example, the EHDS promotes interoperability by standardizing a common data transfer format. These developments may require substantial modifications to external interfaces of electronic health records or other patient information systems and pharmacy data systems to enable compliant data exchange. However, the practical implications of EHDS for healthcare organizations remain partially uncertain, and the national implementation approaches are still evolving [30]. It is also not yet clear how responsibilities will be distributed across national infrastructures, including the future role of Kanta Services within this framework even though the Kanta Services will remain the national HIE in Finland.

Looking forward, it remains uncertain whether these regulatory changes will lead to significant shifts in market structure. While existing systems are currently well established, the extent to which new entrants may emerge is unclear. Future research could systematically monitor these developments and examine EHDS-related impacts at European or Nordic levels, providing comparative insights into regulatory implementation and interoperability outcomes.

5 Conclusions

This study provides a rare longitudinal analysis of EHR market concentration, demonstrating that the Finnish market has remained persistently highly concentrated over time and is to become even more concentrated following the reform of social welfare, healthcare and rescue services and the establishment of wellbeing services counties, the City of Helsinki, and the HUS Group. Rather than representing a lack of change, this structural stability aligns with current eHealth literature, which identifies vendor lock-in, high switching costs, and consolidation as defining features of mature digital health infrastructures. Notably, the formation of wellbeing services counties represents a rare large-scale organizational reform, and its effects on EHR market structure have not previously been empirically documented.

Comparable trends observed internationally suggest that increasing concentration is a common feature of contemporary EHR markets. While concentration may offer certain operational and architectural advantages, it also raises concerns related to competition, costs, innovation, and interoperability. In the context of ongoing regulatory initiatives such as the EHDS, understanding baseline market structures and their persistence is essential, as their impact on market dynamics remains uncertain. Continued longitudinal and comparative monitoring is therefore needed to assess how regulatory, organizational, and technological developments influence market structure, interoperability, and healthcare system performance – and perhaps patient outcomes.

Acknowledgments. The study was part of the national "Monitoring and Evaluation of Social and Healthcare Information System Services" (STEPS 3.0) research project. STEPS 3.0 was co-funded by Ministry of Social Affairs and Health (STM) and participants and coordinated by the National Institute for Health and Welfare (THL). This work was also supported by the University of Oulu and the Research Council of Finland, Profi6 336449.

Disclosure of Interests Timo Tuovinen works for the Finnish Medical Association, and has been involved in the STEPS project, conducting surveys used in this study. Jarmo Reponen has led a survey for healthcare organizations in the STEPS project, which examined the availability and extent of use of information systems. Vesa Jormanainen is currently Medical Counsellor at the Ministry of Social Affairs and Health of Finland.

References

1. Tornero Costa, R. et al.: Electronic health records and data exchange in the WHO European region: a subregional analysis of achievements, challenges, and prospects. Int. J. Med. Inform. **194**, 105687 (2025)
2. Coiera, E.: Building a National Health IT system from the middle out. J. Am. Med. Inform. Assoc. **16**(3), 271–273 (2009)
3. Jha, A.K. et al.: Use of electronic health Records in U.S. hospitals. N. Engl. J. Medicine. **360**(16), 1628–1638 (2009)
4. Jiang, J. (Xuefeng), Qi, K., Bai, G., Schulman, K.: Pre-pandemic assessment: a decade of progress in electronic health record adoption among U.S. hospitals. Health Aff. Scholar. (2023) 1(5).
5. Winblad, I., Reponen, J.: Terveyskeskusten ja sairaanhoitopiirien sähköisten potilaskerto-musjärjestelmien tuotemerkit vuosina 2002–2010. Finn. J. Ehealth Ewelfare. **2**(4), 162–169 (2010) https://journal.fi/finjehew/article/view/3865
6. Holmgren, A.J., Apathy, N.C.: Trends in US Hospital electronic health record vendor market concentration, 2012–2021. J. Gen. Intern. Med. **38**(7), 1765–1767 (2023)
7. Lærum, H., Ellingsen, G., Faxvaag, A.: Doctors' use of electronic medical records systems in hospitals: cross sectional survey. BMJ. **323**(7325), 1344–1348 (2001)
8. Global diffusion of eHealth: making universal health coverage achievable: report of the third global survey on eHealth: World Health Organization (2016) 154

9. Slawomirski, L., et al.: Progress on implementing and using electronic health record systems: developments in OECD countries as of 2021 (2023). Report No. 160

10. Machado, A.C., Martins, M., Cordeiro, B., Au-Yong-Oliveira, M.: Where is the health informatics market going? In: World Conference on Information Systems and Technologies, pp. 584–595 (2020)

11. Sorace, J. et al.: Quantifying the competitiveness of the electronic health record market and its implications for interoperability. Int. J. Med. Inform. **136**, 104037 (2020)

12. Jormanainen, V., Parhiala, K., Reponen, J.: Terveyskeskusten ja erikoissairaanhoidon sairaaloiden sähköisten potilaskertomusten markkinat olivat erittäin keskittyneet vuonna 2017—onko syytä olla huolissaan? Finn. J. Ehealth eWelfare. **11**(1–2), 109–124 (2019)

13. Keskimäki, I.: Development of primary health care in Finland. Report No. 9 (2022). https://www.lshtm.ac.uk/media/62361

14. Vehko, T. et al.. E-health and e-welfare of Finland Check Point 2022 (2023). https://urn.fi/URN:ISBN:978-952-343-891-0

15. OECD/European Observatory on Health Systems and Policies: Country Health Profile 2025: Finland. State of Health in the EU (2025). https://eurohealthobservatory.who.int/publications/m/finland-country-health-profile-2025

16. Ekholm, V.: Valtaosa alueista valitsi Lifecaren. Suomen Lääkärilehti (2025) [cited 2026 Jan 31]. www.laakarilehti.fi/e46664

17. Oy Apotti Ab: n omistuspohja muuttuu. Apotti webpage (2024) [cited 2026 Jan 31]. https://www.apotti.fi/apotin-omistuspohja-muuttuu/

18. Ruotsin käytetyin potilastietojärjestelmä otettiin käyttöön Ahvenanmaalla—Atostek mahdollisti integraatiot Suomen kansallisiin palveluihin: Atostek webpage (2025) [cited 2026 Jan 31]. https://atostek.com/ruotsin-kaytetyin-potilastietojarjestelma-otettiin-kayttoon-ahvenanmaalla-atostek-mahdollisti-integraatiot-suomen-kansallisiin-palveluihin/

19. Ekholm, V.: Ahvenanmaalla ratkotaan uuden potilastietojärjestelmän haasteita. Suomen Lääkärilehti (2026) 13 [cited 2026 Jan 31]. www.laakarilehti.fi/e46912

20. Rintanen, H., Puromäki, H., Heinämäki, L.: Terveyskeskuksen avosairaanhoidon järjestelyt Suomessa—Kysely terveyskeskuksille keväällä 2013 (2014) [cited 2026 Jan 31]. Report No. 18. https://urn.fi/URN:ISBN:978-952-302-216-4

21. Bradley, S.H.: We need to create a competitive market for electronic health record systems. Br. J. Gen. Practice. **75**(760), 497–499 (2025)

22. Huang, C., Koppel, R., McGreevey, J.D., Craven, C.K., Schreiber, R.: Transitions from one electronic health record to another: challenges, pitfalls, and recommendations. Appl. Clin. Inform. **11**(5), 742–754 (2020)

23. Berger, S.M.: Communication and documentation in the electronic health record. In: Practical Problems and Approaches in Genetic Counseling, pp. 51–56. CRC Press, Boca Raton (2025)

24. Holmgren, A.J., Apathy, N.C., Kanter, G.P.: Electronic health record market consolidation and implications for cybersecurity. Health Aff. Scholar. **3**(8) (2025)

25. Eden, K.B. et al.: Barriers and facilitators to exchanging health information: a systematic review. Int. J. Med. Inform. **88**, 44–51 (2016)

26. Ünver, M.B.: What cloud interoperability connotates for EU policy making: recurrence of old problems or new ones looming on the horizon? Telecomm Policy. **43**(2), 154–170 (2019)

27. Ellingsen, G., Christensen, B., Wynn, R.: A common electronic health record for Norwegian municipalities. Stud. Health Technol. Inform. (2022) https://ebooks.iospress.nl/doi/10.3233/SHTI220288

28. Haraldsen, A.: Akson—et monument over en feilslått helsepolitikk. Digi Daglig. (2022) [cited 2026 Jan 31]. https://www.digi.no/artikler/kommentar-akson-et-monument-over-en-feilslatt-helsepolitikk/518860

29. Ekroll, H.C., Torset, N.S.: Staten har brukt en halv milliard på omstridt IT-prosjekt. Nå setter regjeringen foten ned. Aftenposten (2022) 11 [cited 2026 Jan 31]. https://www.aftenposten.no/norge/i/gE6MgL/staten-har-brukt-en-halv-milliard-paa-omstridt-it-prosjekt-naa-setter-regjeringen-foten-ned
30. Cervera de la Cruz, P., Lalova-Spinks, T., Shabani, M.: Implementation of the European health data space: a qualitative study on expectations of health data experts from 23 countries. Health Policy. **161**, 105428 (2025)

Digital Health: From Policy to Reality in the Nordic Countries

Arild Faxvaag[1]([✉]) [iD], Jarmo Reponen[2] [iD], Guðrún Auður Harðardóttir[3] [iD],
Tuulikki Vehko[4] [iD], Johanna Viitanen[5] [iD], Jeppe Eriksen[6] [iD], Rune Pedersen[7] [iD],
Sabine Koch[8] [iD], Christian Nöhr[6] [iD], and Vivian Vimarlund[9] [iD]

[1] Department of Neuromedicine and Movement Science, NTNU, Trondheim, Norway
arild.faxvaag@ntnu.no
[2] Research Unit of Health Sciences and Technology, University of Oulu, Oulu, Finland
[3] Ministry of Health, Reykjavik, Iceland
[4] Finnish Institute for Health and Welfare, Helsinki, Finland
[5] Department of Computer Science, Aalto University, Espoo, Finland
[6] Department of Sustainability and Planning, Aalborg University, Aalborg, Denmark
[7] Department of Learning, Informatics, Management and Ethics, Health Informatics Centre,
Karolinska Institutet, Stockholm, Sweden
[8] Norwegian Centre for e-Health research, Tromsø, Norway
[9] Department of Computer and Information Science, Linköping University, Linköping, Sweden

Abstract. The Nordic countries are done with implementing a first generation
of digital tools in their healthcare systems. This means that the primary tool for
documenting clinical work, laboratory analyses and work within medical imaging
is a healthcare information system. Also, patient portals now allow clinicians to
reach out to patients and vice versa through a digital channel. A third category
of tools are health registries that support a wide range of administrative, quality
improvement and research workflows. In a few years, EHDS will lead to a single
market for health data EHR-systems and wellness applications in Europe. This
development takes place at the same time as generic information technologies (e.g.
machine learning, AI and digital twins) threaten to upend any sector. A healthcare
information system tool may come out of a design and have an intended value,
but in the end, it is the actual, real-life value that matters. What is there to learn
from the pioneering work within digital health that has been carried out in the
Nordic countries? What are the implications for the forthcoming EHDS-related
work? This paper presents the outline of a review of evaluation studies from the
Nordic countries.

Keywords: EHR-systems · e-Health · Digital health · Digital health policy ·
Evaluation research

1 Introduction

The healthcare systems in the Nordic countries are largely funded and owned by the public. Ever since the advent of information technology tools, Nordic health authorities have
recognized the potential that lies within adapting such tools to the workflows and needs

© The Author(s) 2026
M. Särestöniemi et al. (Eds.): NCDHWS 2026, CCIS 3009, pp. 61–65, 2026.
https://doi.org/10.1007/978-3-032-28812-7_5

in their healthcare sectors and have invested heavily in developing digital infrastructures and in implementing EHRs and other information system tools (Hyppönen et al. 2013). As of today, personnel from all parts of the sector now use a healthcare information system as their primary tool for work (Nordic council of ministers 2024). Likewise, patient portals now allow for a digital interface to the healthcare system for patients. A third category of tools are the national health registries that allow for accounting, reimbursement, quality improvement and research.

As the information systems have found their places in the healthcare system, they have turned into an infrastructure that is critical both for the institutions and for the clinician users. The institutions and clinician user may have had an influence on the design of a new information system, but in the end, once implemented, the healthcare information systems also tend to shape their users. As clinicians adapt to a digital health information environment, the manners in which the information system ease their work quickly leads to a dependency on having access to the system (Lium et al. 2008). Many other aspects are problematic. To mention a few: EHR-systems serve as a portal into health and healthcare data that are specific to the individual patient, meant to support clinicians in making decisions that are to benefit the very same patient. Yet, the patient-specific data are fragmented: Information about an important healthcare event in one institution does not automatically flow to the next institution that is to provide care to the patient. Digital health is widely considered an important tool for health policy-making. However, expressing health policy directly in the information systems face the risk that the information system gets outdated once the policy it builds on is replaced by a newer. The current generation of healthcare information systems are information silos that does not take into account the need for interaction with institutions that surround our healthcare sectors, namely the institutions responsible for developing biomedical knowledge and tools (i.e. research institutions) and the institutions that feed healthcare systems with qualified personnel (i.e. the educational institutions).

Understanding the true impacts of healthcare information systems and infrastructures are important, not only for digital health policy makers but also for product owners, for institutions and people involved in HTA, procurement processes, investment decision-making, benefit management and for society as a whole. The EHDS regulations aim to establish a single market for health data, EHR-systems and wellness applications in Europe. This translates into opportunities for local EHR system product owners, policy-makers, researchers, citizens, patients and numerous other stakeholders. At the same time, generic information technology tools such as machine learning, AI and digital twins are positioned to transform our sector.

In general, all healthcare information system solutions are a result of design and engineering. All information system solutions relate to the problems they intend to solve, and herein lies the potential value of the solutions. But in the end, it is the actual, real-life value of the solutions that matters to the payers and the stakeholders that are to benefit from taking the solutions into use. The Nordic countries are one of the very few places in the world where the real-life value of implemented healthcare information systems can be studied. What is there to learn from the pioneering work within digital health that has been carried out in the Nordic countries? What are the implications for the forthcoming EHDS-related work? This paper presents the outline of a review of evaluation studies from the Nordic countries. We aim to explore which stakeholders and perspectives are taken into account in studies that assess effects and impacts of EHR-system implementations.

2 Methods

This investigation is to be carried out as a literature review using PubMed[1] and the literature databases available at Engineering village.[2] See Table 1 for a preliminary concept table.

Table 1. Concept table.

Evaluation of EHR-systems	Evaluation method	Norway, Sweden, Denmark, Iceland, Finland
PubMed:		
"Medical Records Systems, Computerized/statistics and numerical data"[Mesh] OR "Medical Records Systems, Computerized/trends"[Mesh] OR "Hospital Information Systems/statistics and numerical data"[Mesh]	Operations Research [MeSH] OR Qualitative Research [MeSH] OR Surveys and Questionnaires [MeSH] OR "Task Performance and Analysis"[MeSH] OR "Quality improvement"[Mesh]	"Norway"[MeSH] OR "Sweden"[MeSH] OR "Denmark"[MeSH] OR "Finland"[MeSH] OR "Iceland"[MeSH]
Engineering village:		
"Health record systems" OR "Electronic health record" OR "eHealth"	"Operations research" OR Qualitative research" OR "Survey" OR "Questionnaire" OR "Evaluation study"	Norway OR Sweden OR Finland OR Iceland OR Denmark

Inclusion criteria: Full text available in English or in one of the Nordic Languages. Published in a peer reviewed journal. Study assessing the effects and/or side effects, utility and values of EHR-systems or other information systems used in healthcare. Qualitative or quantitative design. Data sampled from healthcare information systems or users (clinician or non-clinician) of such systems.

Properties to be extracted from each included publication (preliminary description): Publication year, Study design, Population sampled, stakeholders identified.

---

[1] Pubmed, available at https://pubmed.ncbi.nlm.nih.gov/?otool=inoubitlib

[2] Engineering Village: provided by Springer Verlag, available at https://www.engineeringvillage. com/app/search/quick/

3   Results

A search using the preliminary concepts developed and presented in Table 1 was carried out on January 31 2026. The PubMed search resulted in 76 records; The Engineering village search yielded 31 records. All records were downloaded in the Endnote format and imported to the Zotero[3] reference management system for further analysis. After removing of duplicates, non-nordic studies and studies not evaluating the implementation of an EHR-system or another healthcare information system, 74 papers remained (Figure 1).

4   Discussion

The discussion will hopefully enable us to theorize over the insights developed through the analysis of the existing literature. We will hopefully be able to show how the insights relates to policy makers working with the implementation of the EHDS-regulations and to developers and owners of EHR- and wellness systems.

Acknowledgments. This study is funded by the institutions that employ the authors of the publication and by the Nordic Council of Ministers (NCM) e-health group.

Disclosure of Interests   The authors have no competing interests to declare that are relevant to the content of this article.

References

Hyppönen, H., Faxvaag, A., Gilstad, H., Audur Hardardottir, G., Jerlvall, L., Kangas, M., et al.: Nordic eHealth Indicators: Organisation of research, first results and the plan for the future. Nordic Council of Ministers (2013) https://urn.kb.se/resolve?urn=urn:nbn:se:norden:org:div a-675

Lium, J.T., Tjora, A., Faxvaag, A.: No paper, but the same routines: a qualitative exploration of experiences in two Norwegian hospitals deprived of the paper based medical record. BMC Med. Inform. Decis. Mak. **8**(1), 2 (2008)

The Nordic Council of ministers: THE NORDICS—a sustainable and integrated region? Baseline report for Our Vision 2030 2024. https://www.norden.org/en/publication/nordics-sustainable-and-integrated-region-baseline-report-our-vision-2030

---

[3] Zotero, available from https://www.zotero.org

Personalised Digital Health – From Omics to Interventions, Telemedicine and eRehabilitation

Dynamic Digital Precision Nutrition for Cardiometabolic Prevention in Cancer Survivorship

Maryam Gholamalizadeh[1] , Saeid Doaei[1,2(✉)] , and Raul Zamora-Ros[1]

[1] Unit of Nutrition and Cancer, Cancer Epidemiology Research Program, Catalan Institute of Oncology, Bellvitge Biomedical Research Institute (IDIBELL), L'Hospitalet deLlobregat, Barcelona, Spain
Sdoaei@idibell.cat

[2] Faculty of Nutrition and Food Technology, National Nutrition and Food Technology Research Institute, Shahid Beheshti University of Medical Sciences, Tehran, Iran

Abstract. Cancer survivorship has improved substantially in recent decades, yet long-term health remains strongly influenced by cardiometabolic complications such as obesity, insulin resistance, dyslipidaemia, hypertension, and cardiovascular disease. These conditions arise from a complex interaction of treatment-related toxicities, pre-existing metabolic vulnerabilities, lifestyle disruptions, and genomic susceptibility. Personalised dietary strategies have the potential to mitigate these risks, but conventional approaches rely on population-level guidelines that overlook the profound interindividual variability in metabolic responses observed among cancer survivors. Integrating digital nutrition-related biomarkers with genomic, dietary, and lifestyle data enables a more dynamic and responsive model of care. Continuous measures of postprandial physiology, body composition, eating behaviour, physical activity, sleep, and food-environment exposure provide real-time insight into how each individual's metabolism and behaviour evolve during survivorship. When combined with multi-omics risk profiling, these data support a Dynamic Digital Precision Nutrition (DDPN) approach in which dietary recommendations are continuously adapted to the survivor's physiological state, behavioural patterns, and environmental context. This framework offers a pathway toward more precise, adaptive, and clinically actionable nutrition interventions aimed at reducing cardiometabolic complications and improving long-term health outcomes in cancer survivors.

Keywords: Cancer survivorship · Digital biomarkers · Personalised nutrition

1 Introduction

Cancer survivorship, as individuals who have completed primary treatment and have no active disease [1], has expanded rapidly over recent decades due to advances in early detection, targeted therapies, and supportive care [2]. As more individuals live several years or decades beyond their diagnosis, the long-term health challenges they

© The Author(s) 2026
M. Särestöniemi et al. (Eds.): NCDHWS 2026, CCIS 3009, pp. 69–80, 2026.
https://doi.org/10.1007/978-3-032-28812-7_6

face have become increasingly important determinants of overall survival and quality of life. Among these challenges, cardiometabolic complications, including obesity, insulin resistance, dyslipidaemia, hypertension, and cardiovascular disease, represent a major and growing burden. These conditions arise from a multifaceted interplay of treatment-related toxicities, systemic inflammation, endocrine disruption, pre-existing metabolic vulnerabilities, lifestyle changes, and underlying genomic susceptibility [3]. Their cumulative impact places cancer survivors at substantially elevated risk of premature morbidity and mortality compared with the general population.

Despite the scale and complexity of this problem, current prevention strategies remain largely rooted in population-based dietary and lifestyle guidelines. Such generalized recommendations fail to account for the profound interindividual variability in metabolic responses to food, physical activity, sleep patterns, and environmental exposures, a variability that is further amplified by cancer treatments and survivorship trajectories. As a result, many survivors receive guidance that is insufficiently tailored to their physiological state, behavioural patterns, or treatment-specific risks, limiting the effectiveness of traditional prevention approaches.

Cancer survivorship is highly heterogeneous, with substantial variation in treatment exposures, symptom trajectories, and metabolic disturbances across tumour types [4]. While the cardiometabolic mechanisms that drive long-term risk, such as insulin resistance, visceral adiposity, autonomic imbalance, and circadian disruption, are shared across many cancers, the magnitude and pattern of these disturbances differ between survivor groups. This heterogeneity underscores the need for a flexible framework that can be applied broadly yet validated in a phased manner [5]. Survivors of breast, colorectal, prostate, and hematologic cancers, who often exhibit pronounced and well-characterized metabolic dysfunction, represent strong candidates for initial implementation and refinement before expanding to a wider range of cancer types [6].

Digital nutrition assessment in cancer survivorship has traditionally relied on self-reported dietary intake, sporadic clinic-based measurements, and broad lifestyle recommendations. These approaches provide only fragmented snapshots of behaviour and physiology, making it difficult to detect early metabolic deviations or understand how survivors respond to dietary exposures in real-world settings. Given the substantial heterogeneity in treatment effects, metabolic vulnerability, and behavioural patterns across survivor groups, there is a growing need for continuous, high-resolution data streams that can capture how eating patterns, postprandial responses, and body-composition dynamics evolve over time.

Recent advances in digital nutrition-related biomarkers offer a pathway to meet this need. Technologies such as continuous glucose monitoring, smartphone-based meal-timing and eating- pattern tracking, wearable-enabled postprandial physiology, and digital body-composition assessment provide a multidimensional, real-time view of how dietary behaviours interact with metabolic function. When integrated with genomic, lifestyle, clinical, and contextual information, these data enable the development of Dynamic Digital Precision Nutrition (DDPN)—a model in which dietary recommendations are continuously adapted to an individual's physiological responses and behavioural patterns rather than delivered as static, population-level guidance.

This adaptive, feedback-driven approach has the potential to more effectively mitigate cardiometabolic risk and enhance long-term survivorship care (Fig. 1).

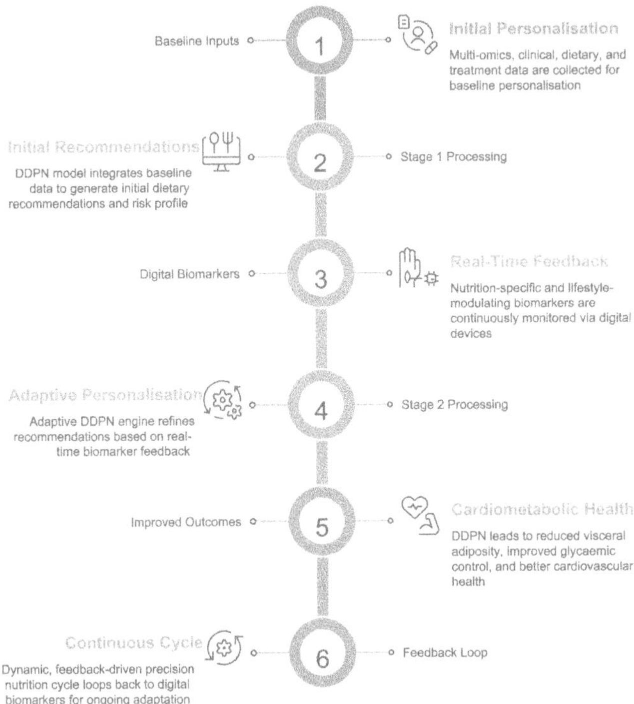

Fig. 1. Dynamic digital precision nutrition (DDPN) workflow for cardiometabolic prevention.

2 Digital Nutrition Related Biomarkers Relevant to Cardiovascular Risk

Digital nutrition-related biomarkers encompass a diverse set of physiological, behavioural, and environmental indicators that collectively provide a multidimensional view of how individuals interact with food and how these interactions shape cardiometabolic risk [7, 8]. In cancer survivors—where treatment effects, metabolic instability, and lifestyle disruptions amplify interindividual variability—these biomarkers offer a powerful means of capturing real-world dietary behaviours, postprandial physiological responses, energy-balance patterns, body-composition dynamics, and food-environment exposures. By enabling continuous, objective, and context-specific monitoring, they form the foundation of a Dynamic Digital Precision Nutrition (DDPN) approach, in which dietary recommendations can be tailored and adaptively refined based on each survivor's evolving metabolic profile and lived environment. The following sections outline the major categories of digital nutrition-related biomarkers most relevant to cardiovascular risk.

While several of these biomarker categories capture nutrition-specific processes (e.g., meal timing, eating- pattern dynamics, postprandial responses, and digital body-composition measures), others influence nutrition more indirectly, including sleep-wake patterns that modulate glycaemic control and physical-activity rhythms that shape energy balance and metabolic flexibility

2.1 Eating Pattern Digital Biomarkers

Eating pattern biomarkers capture habitual patterns of food intake that influence cardiometabolic health, including meal timing, eating-window duration, eating rate, bite count, chewing patterns, snacking frequency, and night-time eating [9]. These patterns are strongly associated with obesity, insulin resistance, circadian misalignment, and elevated cardiometabolic risk. Recent advances in digital health have enabled objective, continuous monitoring of these patterns using multimodal sensing technologies [10]. Acoustic wearables and neck-mounted microphones detect chewing and swallowing events with high temporal resolution, while wrist-worn accelerometers identify micromovements associated with hand-to-mouth gestures [11]. Computer-vision systems embedded in smartphones or smart glasses automatically recognize foods and estimate bite count and eating rate. AI-enhanced food-logging applications further support passive or semi-passive dietary capture. Together, these technologies provide a granular, real-world assessment of eating patterns that surpasses traditional self-report methods, although the technology is still evolving and current systems have notable limitations.

2.2 Postprandial Physiological Response Biomarkers

Postprandial physiological responses represent some of the most robust digital biomarkers linking dietary exposures to cardiovascular risk. Key indicators include postprandial glucose excursions, glycaemic variability, time in range, postprandial heart rate and heart rate variability (HRV), skin temperature fluctuations, and autonomic responses to food intake [12]. These biomarkers reflect metabolic flexibility, inflammatory burden, and endothelial stress—mechanisms central to the development of atherosclerosis and cardiometabolic disease. Continuous glucose monitoring (CGM) systems provide minute by minute glucose profiles, enabling precise quantification of glycaemic responses to meals. Wearable photoplethysmography (PPG) sensors integrated into smartwatches measure HRV and heart rate dynamics, while skin temperature sensors capture thermoregulatory responses associated with metabolic load [13]. Emerging sweat biosensors quantify metabolites such as lactate and electrolytes, offering additional insight into metabolic stress [14]. These technologies collectively allow real-time, ecologically valid assessment of physiological responses to dietary intake, although an important practical consideration is that some sensors, such as CGM, are minimally invasive and therefore less acceptable for routine use in individuals without diabetes.

2.3 Energy Balance and Lifestyle Biomarkers

Energy balance and lifestyle biomarkers encompass physical activity patterns, sedentary time, energy expenditure, sleep duration and quality, and circadian rhythm stability [15].

These factors modulate cardiometabolic risk by influencing adiposity, insulin sensitivity, lipid metabolism, and systemic inflammation. Modern wearable devices equipped with triaxial accelerometers quantify activity intensity and sedentary behaviour with high precision, while optical heart rate sensors estimate energy expenditure [16]. Actigraphy based sleep monitors assess sleep duration, fragmentation, and efficiency, and integrated temperature and light sensors provide information on circadian alignment [17]. Novel metabolic tracking devices estimate substrate utilization (fat vs. carbohydrate oxidation) through breath analysis or wearable gas exchange sensors [18]. These multimodal data streams offer a comprehensive view of lifestyle patterns that interact with dietary behaviours to shape cardiovascular risk trajectories.

2.4 Digital Body Composition Biomarkers

Digital body composition biomarkers include percent body fat, visceral adiposity, lean mass distribution, total body water, and digitally-derived waist circumference [19]. These indicators are among the strongest predictors of cardiometabolic and cardiovascular disease, particularly visceral fat, which is closely linked to insulin resistance, dyslipidaemia, and systemic inflammation. Smart scales using bioelectrical impedance analysis (BIA) provide accessible, repeated measurements of body composition, while smartphone-based 3D imaging algorithms estimate waist circumference and abdominal adiposity with increasing accuracy [20]. Infrared body scanners and wearable impedance sensors enable more continuous or context-specific monitoring of body composition changes. These digital tools enhance the precision and frequency of body composition assessment, supporting early identification of cardiometabolic risk [21].

2.5 Digital Food Environment Biomarkers

Digital food environment biomarkers capture the external influences shaping dietary behaviour, including grocery purchase patterns, online food ordering behaviour, exposure to digital food marketing, and geospatial access to healthy or unhealthy food outlets [22]. These environmental factors strongly influence dietary quality and, consequently, cardiovascular risk. Measurement approaches increasingly rely on large scale digital traces: loyalty card purchase data reveal habitual food acquisition patterns; food delivery platforms provide detailed logs of ordering behaviour; and social media analytics quantify exposure to unhealthy food advertising [23]. Geolocation data from smartphones enable mapping of an individual's food environment, while AI-based neighbourhood food environment models integrate multiple data sources to characterize environmental risk. These digital indicators offer a powerful lens for understanding how external contexts interact with individual behaviours to shape cardiometabolic outcomes.

3 Applying Digital Nutrition Related Biomarkers to Cardiovascular Disease Prevention in Cancer Survivors

Integrating digital nutrition related biomarkers into cardiovascular disease (CVD) prevention strategies for cancer survivors requires careful consideration of the unique metabolic, physiological, and behavioural challenges imposed by cancer and its treatments. Among the five major categories of digital biomarkers, postprandial physiological response biomarkers and energy balance and lifestyle biomarkers hold the highest priority. Cancer therapies (e.g., chemotherapy, radiotherapy, endocrine therapy, and corticosteroids) frequently induce hyperglycaemia, insulin resistance, autonomic dysfunction, and circadian disruption, all of which substantially elevate cardiometabolic risk [24]. Continuous glucose monitoring (CGM), glycaemic variability metrics, and postprandial heart rate and HRV responses therefore provide critical, real-time insights into metabolic instability and should form the core of early risk stratification and dietary personalization efforts. These biomarkers enable detection of exaggerated glycaemic excursions, impaired metabolic flexibility, and autonomic imbalance, which are common in survivors and strongly predictive of future CVD [25].

Energy balance and lifestyle biomarkers represent the second major priority. Cancer survivors often experience profound fatigue, reduced physical activity, prolonged sedentary time, sleep disturbances, and circadian misalignment [26]. These factors accelerate visceral adiposity, impair glucose regulation, and exacerbate systemic inflammation [27]. Wearable-derived measures of activity intensity, sedentary behaviour, sleep duration and quality, and circadian rhythm stability provide a comprehensive picture of lifestyle related cardiometabolic stress. Their integration into survivorship care allows clinicians to identify high risk behavioural patterns and tailor interventions such as gradual activity progression, sleep stabilization strategies, and time restricted eating aligned with circadian physiology.

Digital body composition biomarkers constitute the third priority, particularly in the context of sarcopenic obesity, a phenotype highly prevalent among cancer survivors and strongly associated with CVD [28]. Smart BIA devices, 3D smartphone imaging, and wearable impedance sensors can detect early shifts in visceral fat, lean mass, and waist circumference—changes that may not be reflected in body weight alone. These measurements are essential for guiding protein intake, exercise prescriptions, and metabolic risk monitoring.

Eating pattern biomarkers, including meal timing, eating rate, snacking patterns, and night-time eating, provide valuable behavioural context but should be interpreted alongside physiological data. Cancer related symptoms such as nausea, appetite loss, emotional distress, and treatment induced taste alterations can significantly modify eating patterns [29]. Therefore, these biomarkers are most effective when used to refine personalized dietary strategies (e.g., optimizing meal timing to improve glycaemic control or reducing rapid eating to mitigate postprandial spikes).

Digital food environment biomarkers offer additional contextual insight into survivors' access to healthy foods, reliance on online food delivery, and exposure to unhealthy food marketing. While these indicators are less directly linked to physiological risk, they are important for designing sustainable, equity focused interventions, particularly for survivors facing socioeconomic or functional limitations [30].

Tool burden should be considered when interpreting the digital biomarkers and their measurement methods. In this context, burden refers to the level of intrusiveness, patient effort, and day-to-day usability required by each measurement tool, allowing methods to be classified as low-, moderate-, or high-burden based on their practicality in survivorship care. The following Table 1 provides a concise overview of the key digital nutrition related biomarkers relevant to cancer survivorship, summarizing their clinical priority in cancer survivors and the burden categorized measurement methods used to capture them.

Table 1. Integrated digital nutrition related biomarkers, measurement methods, and priority levels for cardiometabolic risk stratification and personalized nutrition in cancer survivors.

Category	Digital nutrition-related biomarkers (Shortened)	Measurement methods (Burden-Categorized)	Priority	Key considerations (Shortened)
Postprandial physiological response	Glucose peaks; GV; TIR; postprandial HR/HRV; skin-temp response; autonomic response	**Low-burden**: Smartwatch PPG/ECG; HR/HRV; skin-temp wearables **Moderate**: Short-term CGM **High**: None	Very High	Detects therapy-induced metabolic and autonomic instability; guides timing and glycaemic-load adjustments
Energy balance and lifestyle	Activity intensity; sedentary time; energy expenditure; sleep duration/quality; circadian stability	**Low-burden**: Accelerometers; optical HR; actigraphy; PPG sleep; light sensors **Moderate**: Chest-strap HR; multi-sensor wearables **High**: None	Very High	Identifies behavioural drivers of fatigue, circadian disruption, and cardiometabolic stress
Digital body composition	Body fat%; visceral fat; lean mass; total body water; digital waist	**Low-burden**: Smart BIA; smartphone 3D scan **Moderate**: Multi-frequency BIA; infrared scanners **High**: DEXA (if used)	High	Detects sarcopenic obesity and visceral fat gain; informs nutrition/exercise tailoring
Eating pattern	Meal timing; eating window; eating rate; bite count; chewing; snacking; night eating	**Low-burden**: Food logging; wrist-motion sensors; actigraphy timestamps **Moderate**: Acoustic chewing sensors; computer-vision bites **High**: Neck-mounted swallowing sensors	Moderate–High	Helps refine practical dietary strategies; requires contextual interpretation
Digital food environment	Purchase patterns; online ordering; marketing exposure; food-outlet access	**Low-burden**: Loyalty cards; receipts; delivery logs; GPS **Moderate**: GIS + AI geolocation **High**: None	Moderate	Supports long-term adherence; secondary to physiological and lifestyle markers

4 Implementation Challenges for Dynamic Digital Precision Nutrition (DDPN)

Integrating DDPN into survivorship care requires structured pathways that translate digital biomarker data into clinically actionable decisions while balancing measurement priority and patient burden. Very high-priority biomarkers—such as postprandial glycaemic dynamics, heart-rate and HRV responses, sleep quality, circadian stability, and physical activity—can be monitored using low-burden tools including smartwatch-based PPG/ECG sensing, actigraphy-grade activity and sleep tracking, and short-window CGM assessments. These data streams enable clinicians to identify metabolic vulnerability during routine survivorship visits through DDPN dashboards that summarise glucose trends, autonomic responses, sleep–wake patterns, and early shifts in body composition. Remote-monitoring models extend this capability by continuously collecting data from wearables, CGM devices, and dietary applications, with adaptive algorithms updating recommendations as physiology evolves.

Higher-priority digital body-composition biomarkers—such as visceral fat, lean mass, and digital waist indices—are incorporated periodically using low-burden smart BIA or smartphone-based 3D scanning, allowing detection of sarcopenic obesity and treatment-related metabolic decline. Moderate- to high-priority eating-pattern biomarkers and moderate-priority food-environment indicators are introduced selectively for survivors whose behavioural or contextual barriers impede cardiometabolic control, using tools such as smartphone food logging, wrist-motion sensors, or digital purchase-pattern data. This tiered, burden-aligned approach ensures that DDPN begins with a minimal viable digital panel and expands only when additional complexity is likely to yield meaningful clinical benefit.

Sustained patient engagement is supported through personalised goals, brief motivational prompts, and simplified feedback loops that accommodate varying levels of digital literacy, symptom burden, and functional capacity. Clinicians likewise require concise training on interpreting CGM metrics, HRV patterns, sleep indicators, and digital body-composition outputs, supported by standardised response protocols that minimise additional workload. Finally, continuous digital monitoring introduces essential considerations related to privacy, data security, and patient autonomy; transparent consent processes, secure data-storage practices, and clear governance frameworks are critical for maintaining trust, particularly when AI-generated insights influence clinical decisions. Addressing these methodological, technological, behavioural, and ethical dimensions collectively will be key to enabling scalable, responsible, and clinically meaningful deployment of DDPN in cancer survivorship.

5 Future Research Directions

Advancing DDPN from a conceptual framework to evidence-based clinical strategy requires a staged research agenda that reflects both the heterogeneity of cancer survivorship and the complexity of digital biomarker integration. Early feasibility studies should evaluate the usability, acceptability, and data completeness of a DDPN-enabled digital platform that integrates wearables, continuous glucose monitoring, dietary assessment tools, and environmental sensors. These studies can clarify patient engagement patterns, identify barriers to sustained monitoring, and refine the adaptive algorithms that generate personalised dietary recommendations.

Observational cohort studies across diverse cancer types can then be used to characterise digital biomarker trajectories, quantify interindividual variability, and determine how treatment exposures, symptom burden, and behavioural patterns shape metabolic risk. Such studies will help identify which survivor groups exhibit the strongest and most actionable digital signatures, informing prioritisation for subsequent intervention trials.

Randomised or adaptive clinical trials represent the next step, testing whether DDPN-guided nutrition improves glycaemic control, reduces visceral adiposity, enhances metabolic flexibility, and improves quality of life compared with standard survivorship care. These trials may initially focus on high-risk groups (e.g., survivors of breast, colorectal, prostate, or hematologic cancers) before expanding to broader populations. Longitudinal follow-up will be essential to determine whether improvements in digital biomarkers translate into reductions in long-term cardiometabolic morbidity and mortality.

Finally, implementation science approaches will be needed to evaluate scalability, integration into survivorship clinics, cost-effectiveness, and equity of access. These studies will help ensure that DDPN can be deployed in real-world settings and benefit diverse survivor populations.

6 Conclusion

Dynamic Digital Precision Nutrition (DDPN) offers a next-generation framework for tailoring dietary guidance in cancer survivorship by integrating digital nutrition-related biomarkers into a continuously adaptive system. These biomarkers capture real-time variation in postprandial physiology, eating behaviour, body-composition dynamics, and contextual food-environment exposures, dimensions that conventional assessments cannot adequately reflect. By linking dietary recommendations to an individual's evolving metabolic responses, behavioural patterns, and environmental constraints, DDPN transforms nutrition care from static, population-based advice into a dynamic, feedback-driven process. This approach has the potential to more effectively mitigate cardiometabolic risk, enhance long-term survivorship care, and support sustainable, personalised nutrition strategies for a growing population of cancer survivors.

A natural next step is determining how these biomarker domains should be weighted within the DDPN framework to optimise cardiometabolic prevention for your specific survivor population.

Acknowledgments. The authors acknowledge the support of their institutional affiliations, including the Bellvitge Biomedical Research Institute (IDIBELL) and the Catalan Institute of Oncology (ICO), for providing an intellectually stimulating research environment and facilitating interdisciplinary collaboration. AI-based tools were used solely for language editing and clarity enhancement under full human oversight. All scientific content, conceptual development, and interpretation were entirely generated by the authors.

IDIBELL acknowledges support from the Generalitat de Catalunya through the CERCA Program. MGh was supported by the Sara Borrell program (CD24/00222) from the Instituto de Salud Carlos III (Co-funded by European Social Fund (ESF) investing in your future).

Disclosure of Interests The authors have no competing interests to declare that are relevant to the content of this article.

References

1. Fitch, M.I.: Take care when you use the word survivor. Can. Oncol. Nurs. J. **29**, 218 (2019)
2. Wagle, N.S. et al.: Cancer treatment and survivorship statistics, 2025. CA Cancer J. Clin. **75**, 308–340 (2025). https://doi.org/10.3322/caac.70011
3. Albulushi, A., Balushi, A.A., Shahzad, M., Bulushi, I.A., Lawati, H.A.: Navigating the crossroads: cardiometabolic risks in cancer survivorship—a comprehensive review. Cardio-Oncol. **10**, 36 (2024). https://doi.org/10.1186/s40959-024-00240-2
4. Rituraj, Pal, R.S., Wahlang, J., Pal, Y., Chaitanya, M., Saxena, S.: Precision oncology: transforming cancer care through personalized medicine. Med. Oncol. **42**, 246 (2025). https://doi.org/10.1007/s12032-025-02817-y
5. Natto, H.A., Sahoo, D., Muneera, N.: Benefits of personalized diet, nutrition, and exercise programs for cancer survivors. Int. J. Trends Onco Science., 12–22 (2024)
6. Kc, M. et al.: Relative burden of cancer and noncancer mortality among long-term survivors of breast, prostate, and colorectal cancer in the US. JAMA Netw. Open. **6**, e2323115 (2023). https://doi.org/10.1001/jamanetworkopen.2023.23115
7. Van Den Brink, W.J., Van Den Broek, T.J., Palmisano, S., Wopereis, S., De Hoogh, I.M.: Digital biomarkers for personalized nutrition: predicting meal moments and interstitial glucose with non-invasive, wearable technologies. Nutrients. **14**, 4465 (2022). https://doi.org/10.3390/nu14214465
8. Blendea, L. et al.: From traditional medical patterns to artificial intelligence: the applicability of digital biomarkers in reinventing personalised nutrition. BRAIN Broad Res. Artif. Intell. Neurosci. **16**, 179–192 (2025)
9. Hiraguchi, H., Perone, P., Toet, A., Camps, G., Brouwer, A.-M.: Technology to automatically record eating behavior in real life: a systematic review. Sensors. **23**, 7757 (2023). https://doi.org/10.3390/s23187757
10. Hiraguchi, H., Perone, P., Toet, A., Camps, G., Brouwer, A.-M.: Technology to automatically record eating behavior in real life: a systematic review. Sensors. **23** (2023). https://doi.org/10.3390/s23187757
11. Zhou, J., Cai, M., Shi, M.: Wearable sensing in eating episode monitoring: an updated systematic review protocol. BMJ Open. **15**, e092175 (2025). https://doi.org/10.1136/bmjopen-2024-092175
12. Berry, S.E. et al.: Human postprandial responses to food and potential for precision nutrition. Nat. Med. **26**, 964–973 (2020). https://doi.org/10.1038/s41591-020-0934-0
13. Stan, I.E., D'Auria, D., Napoletano, P.: A systematic literature review of innovations, challenges, and future directions in telemonitoring and wearable health technologies. IEEE J. Biomed. Health Inform. **30**, 2630–2645 (2026). https://doi.org/10.1109/JBHI.2025.3598056
14. Qiao, Y., Qiao, L., Chen, Z., Liu, B., Gao, L., Zhang, L.: Wearable sensor for continuous sweat biomarker monitoring. Chem. **10**, 273 (2022). https://doi.org/10.3390/chemosensors10070273
15. Ruiz-González, D., Hidalgo-Migueles, J., Ramos-Maqueda, J., Vargas-Hitos, J.A., Jiménez-Jáimez, J., Soriano-Maldonado, A.: Device-Measured Physical Activity, Sedentary Time, and Sleep in Patients with Arrhythmogenic Cardiomyopathy: Descriptive Values and Stability over 30 Measurement Days. medRxiv (2022)

16. Hodkinson, A. et al.: Interventions using wearable physical activity trackers among adults with cardiometabolic conditions: a systematic review and meta-analysis. JAMA Netw. Open. **4**, e2116382 (2021). https://doi.org/10.1001/jamanetworkopen.2021.16382
17. Van Den Brink, W.J. et al.: Sleep as a window of cardiometabolic health: the potential of digital sleep and circadian biomarkers. Digit. Health. **11**, 20552076241288724 (2025). https://doi.org/10.1177/20552076241288724
18. Heng, W., Yin, S., Chen, Y., Gao, W.: Exhaled breath analysis: from laboratory test to wearable sensing. IEEE Rev. Biomed. Eng. **18**, 50–73 (2025). https://doi.org/10.1109/RBME.2024.3481360
19. Heymsfield, S., Bell, J.D., Heber, D.: Phenotyping, body composition, and precision nutrition. In: Precision Nutrition, pp. 143–152. Elsevier (2024). https://doi.org/10.1016/B978-0-443-15315-0.00008-0
20. Thomas, D.M., Crofford, I., Scudder, J., Oletti, B., Deb, A., Heymsfield, S.B.: Updates on methods for body composition analysis: implications for clinical practice. Curr. Obes. Rep. **14**, 8 (2025). https://doi.org/10.1007/s13679-024-00593-w
21. Carrier, B. et al.: Wearables for health monitoring: body composition estimates of commercial smartwatch and clinical bioelectrical impedance device. Front. Sports Act. Living. **7**, 1644082 (2025). https://doi.org/10.3389/fspor.2025.1644082
22. Granheim, S.I., Løvhaug, A.L., Terragni, L., Torheim, L.E., Thurston, M.: Mapping the digital food environment: a systematic scoping review. Obes. Rev. **23**, e13356 (2022). https://doi.org/10.1111/obr.13356
23. Hetz, K. et al.: The development and potential of a digital out of home food environment monitoring platform. Nutrients. **15**, 3887 (2023). https://doi.org/10.3390/nu15183887
24. Sharma, R. et al.: Cardio-oncology: managing cardiovascular complications of cancer therapies. Cureus. **15** (2023)
25. Cleary, S., Rosen, S.D., Gilbert, D.C., Langley, R.E.: Cardiovascular health: an important component of cancer survivorship. BMJ Oncol. **2**, e000090 (2023). https://doi.org/10.1136/bmjonc-2023-000090
26. Cao, C., Patel, A.V., Liu, R., Cao, Y., Friedenreich, C.M., Yang, L.: Trends and cancer-specific patterns of physical activity, sleep duration, and daily sitting time among US cancer survivors, 1997–2018. JNCI J. Natl. Cancer Inst. **115**, 1563–1575 (2023). https://doi.org/10.1093/jnci/djad146
27. Bou Matar, D. et al.: Adipose tissue dysfunction disrupts metabolic homeostasis: mechanisms linking fat dysregulation to disease. Front. Endocrinol. **16**, 1592683 (2025). https://doi.org/10.3389/fendo.2025.1592683
28. Liu, C. et al.: Sarcopenic obesity and outcomes for patients with cancer. JAMA Netw. Open. **7**, e2417115 (2024). https://doi.org/10.1001/jamanetworkopen.2024.17115
29. Aldossari, A., Sremanakova, J., Sowerbutts, A.M., Jones, D., Hann, M., Burden, S.T.: Do people change their eating habits after a diagnosis of cancer? A systematic review. J. Hum. Nutr. Diet. **36**, 566–579 (2023). https://doi.org/10.1111/jhn.13001
30. Chavan, P.P., Kedia, S.K., Yu, X.: Physical and functional limitations in US older cancer survivors. J. Palliat. Care Med. **7**, 1–8 (2017)

Feasibility Evaluation of a Multidisciplinary Digital Rehabilitation Delivered by Community Health Workers for Mild Stroke in Indonesia

Eeva Aartolahti[1(✉)], Suci Muqodimatul Jannah[2], Opifia Dian Wahyono[3],
Dela Fariha Fuadi[4], Andrew Wijaya Saputra[4], Nesi[4],
Moh Rendy Herdiansyah[3], Michael Oduor[1], Kari-Pekka Murtonen[1],
Muhammad Irfan[2,3], Katariina Korniloff[1], and Hilmi Zadah Faidullah[2]

[1] Institute of Rehabilitation, Jamk University of Applied Sciences, Jyväskylä, Finland
eeva.aartolahti@jamk.fi
[2] Department of Physiotherapy, Faculty of Health Sciences, Universitas Aisyiyah Yogyakarta,
Yogyakarta, Indonesia
[3] Indonesia Physiotherapy Association, Jakarta, Indonesia
[4] Physiotherapy Study Program, Institut Kesehatan Hermina, Jakarta, Indonesia

Abstract. Access to post-stroke rehabilitation remains limited in many low- and middle-income countries, particularly in primary healthcare and community settings. Digital rehabilitation solutions supported by community health workers (CHWs) may offer a feasible strategy for expanding access to stroke rehabilitation in resource-constrained contexts. This study evaluated the feasibility of a multidisciplinary digital rehabilitation intervention delivered by CHWs to individuals with mild chronic stroke in Indonesia. Additionally, we explored the participant-reported change in functioning.

A four-week pilot feasibility study was conducted in a primary care area in Jakarta without access to rehabilitation services. Seventeen individuals with mild chronic stroke and five CHWs participated in the study. The intervention comprised app-based physiotherapy, occupational therapy, and speech therapy exercises delivered to participants' homes with CHW support. Feasibility outcomes included adherence to home-based exercises and usability, which were assessed using the System Usability Scale (SUS). Preliminary indications of change were evaluated using the Global Rating of Change (GRC).

Adherence to the therapeutic exercises was generally high. Most participants (76.5%) reported meaningful improvements in their functioning (GRC $\geq +3$). Usability was rated as good to excellent by the CHWs (median SUS: 77.5) and acceptable to good by individuals with stroke (median SUS: 69.4). Informal assistance from family members was frequently required; 64% needed help with opening the app or understanding and performing exercises.

In conclusion, CHW-facilitated multidisciplinary digital rehabilitation appears feasible and shows promising preliminary benefits for people with mild stroke in low-resource community settings. These results highlight the importance of family involvement in supporting digital rehabilitation in community settings.

Keywords: Stroke rehabilitation · Telerehabilitation · Mobile applications · Community health workers · Caregivers · Feasibility studies

© The Author(s) 2026

M. Särestöniemi et al. (Eds.): NCDHWS 2026, CCIS 3009, pp. 81–89, 2026.
https://doi.org/10.1007/978-3-032-28812-7_7

1 Introduction

Globally, stroke is a major cause of long-term functional disability and remains the third most common cause of death and disability, as measured by disability-adjusted life years (DALYs) [1]. Nearly 94 million people are currently living after a stroke, many with persistent impairments affecting mobility, upper limb function, communication, cognition, and independence in activities of daily living. The global burden of stroke-related disability is concentrated in low- and lower-middle-income countries (LMICs), which account for approximately 89% of stroke-related DALYs [1]. In these settings, access to post-acute and long-term rehabilitation services remains limited, particularly in rural and underserved urban areas [2]. In Indonesia, rehabilitation professionals are scarce at the primary healthcare level, and many people with stroke receive little or no structured rehabilitation following hospital discharge, contributing to prolonged functional limitations and restricted participation in daily lives.

Digital health interventions have been proposed to address inequities in rehabilitation access in resource-constrained contexts. Digital rehabilitation has demonstrated effectiveness in improving functional outcomes after stroke, with several interventions delivered remotely showing outcomes comparable to conventional face-to-face care [3]. However, the evidence base remains limited for multidisciplinary digital rehabilitation models [4], particularly those integrating physiotherapy, occupational therapy, and speech therapy, and delivered within community settings through non-specialist health workers.

Evaluating feasibility is essential when implementing digital rehabilitation solutions, as it reflects how practical, acceptable, and workable an intervention is in real-world conditions [5] and can be evaluated through engagement and usability. System usability refers to the extent to which users can effectively, efficiently, and satisfactorily interact with a system [6, 7] and is considered a core requirement for the design and evaluation of digital rehabilitation systems [7]. In low-resource settings, limited digital literacy and variable access to technology further heighten the importance of feasibility assessments for successful implementation [8]. The World Health Organization (WHO) highlights rehabilitation as an essential component of high-quality health systems [9] and a key strategy for improving long-term outcomes after stroke. Rehabilitation is defined as interventions that optimize functioning and reduce disability in interactions with a person's environment, emphasizing a person-centered and goal-oriented approach [10]. Rehabilitation task shifting to community health workers (CHWs) supported by digital tools is aligned with this framework and the principles of community-based rehabilitation [11], offering a way to expand access in low-resource settings. Our previous work using a digital rehabilitation solution in primary healthcare demonstrated that CHW-supported physiotherapy-focused digital rehabilitation is both acceptable and feasible [12], providing a foundation for assessing the feasibility of the present multidisciplinary stroke rehabilitation model in the present study.

The aim of this feasibility study was to evaluate the use of a multidisciplinary digital rehabilitation solution (Inclusion App) delivered by CHWs to people with mild chronic stroke in home settings in Indonesia. Specifically, this study assessed feasibility in terms of adherence and usability, as well as preliminary indications of change based on self-reported changes in functioning.

2   Materials and Methods

2.1   Study Design

A multi-method 4-week pilot feasibility study was conducted in August-September 2025 to analyze the usability, user engagement, and CHW resource requirements of the Inclusion App for multidisciplinary home-based therapeutic exercises delivered with the help of CHWs.

2.2   Setting and Participants

The setting was a densely populated primary healthcare catchment area located in Central Jakarta, which predominantly serves low-income households and is characterized by the absence of rehabilitation professionals.

The study involved two participant groups: individuals using home-based rehabilitation through the Inclusion App and CHWs supporting the intervention. Seventeen individuals with a history of stroke participated in this feasibility study (Table 1). The mean age of the participants was 63 years (SD 9.0), and 10 (58.8%) were women. Most participants lived with family members and had access to a mobile phone, whereas access to the home Internet varied. Baseline functional status was characterized using the 12-item World Health Organization Disability Assessment Schedule (WHODAS 2.0). Participants reported mild to moderate functional challenges across all domains of functioning, with many experiencing difficulties in cognitive tasks, physically demanding activities, everyday self-care, social interactions, household or work-related roles, and community participation. An unmet need for rehabilitation services was evident, as 15 of the 17 participants stated that they currently had no access to such services.

Table 1. Rehabilitation user characteristics and functional status (N = 17).

	Value
Age, years, median (range)	64 (45–80)
Female, n (%)	10 (59)
Male, n (%)	7 (41)
Education ≥ secondary, n (%)	12 (71)
Lives with family, n (%)	16 (94)
Has a smart phone in family, n (%)	16 (94)
Has consistent internet access at home, n (%)	7 (41)
Prior experience with using technologies, n (%)	5 (29)
WHODAS 2.0 total score, median (range)	23 (0–75)
Any WHODAS difficulty, n (%)	16 (94)
Access to rehabilitation services, n (%)	2 (12)

In addition, five female CHWs with a mean age of 52 (SD 6.5) years participated in the study. All the CHWs had prior experience in community-based health or social care roles. CHWs reported moderate to high prior experience with digital technologies, supporting the feasibility of a CHW-facilitated digital rehabilitation approach in this study.

2.3 Intervention

In this pilot study, the Inclusion App incorporated guided exercises in physiotherapy, occupational therapy, and speech therapy for individuals with stroke. The speech therapy intervention involved oral exercises consisting of five distinct movements, each performed for 15 repetitions across five sets of exercises. Occupational therapy included seven upper limb exercises, including passive stretching, stereognosis exercises, range of motion exercises, and sensory exercises, each performed for 10 repetitions in a single set. Physiotherapy comprised seven movements focused on lower limb stretching, each performed for three repetitions in one set. All exercises were available in video format with written instructions, and users had the option to download the exercises in PDF format. CHWs were responsible for introducing the Inclusion App, supporting people with stroke in its use, and providing guidance on home-based rehabilitation exercises.

In-person group training sessions were conducted to enable CHWs to effectively support stroke rehabilitation using the Inclusion App and to assist with recruitment and data collection. These sessions were held twice, each lasting 2–3 h, and were delivered by physiotherapists, speech therapists and occupational therapists. The training covered core exercise principles, correct exercise execution, and safety precautions, including how to respond if the patients experienced symptoms during exercise.

2.4 Measures

Primary Outcome: Feasibility. Feasibility was evaluated through (1) self-reported adherence to digital rehabilitation, quantified by the weekly frequency of use, that is, performing different therapeutic exercises; (2) perceived usability of the Inclusion App using the System Usability Scale (SUS) [13] together with the standard seven-point adjective usability rating scale (worst imaginable to best imaginable) for both CHWs and stroke survivors; and (3) resource requirements of CHWs. Additionally, CHW experiences in delivering rehabilitation and using the app were explored through a focus group discussion. The discussion addressed the practical use of the app, perceptions of its usefulness and limitations, and views on training needs and future applicability of the app. Notes were taken to capture key feedback, as the session was not audio-recorded.

Secondary outcome: Participant-reported changes. Changes in functioning were evaluated using the Global Rating of Change (GRC) scale [14]. The person was asked, "Please rate the overall change in your condition from the time that you began the exercise program until now (choose only one)." The seven negative response options varied from -7 (very great deal worse) through -1 (a tiny bit worse (almost the same)) and positive response options from $+1$ (a tiny bit better (almost the same)) to $+7$ (a very great deal better). The research team translated the surveys and reviewed them for semantic equivalence.

Background information. A questionnaire was included to collect socio-demographic information on participants' age, gender, education, technology use, smartphone ownership, and Internet availability. Functional limitations of the participants with stroke were measured using the 12-item World Health Organization Disability Assessment Scale (WHODAS 2.0) [15], a standardized instrument for measuring disability across various health conditions and cultural contexts. WHODAS 2.0 results were analyzed and reported in accordance with WHO guidance; for the 12-item version, only total scores were calculated, and domain level reporting was not performed.

2.5 Data Analysis

Descriptive statistics were used to summarize the participants' characteristics, feasibility, and perceived changes in functioning, with analyses conducted using Microsoft Excel (Microsoft 365). Owing to the small sample size typical of pilot studies, the results were reported descriptively without inferential testing. The focus group discussion was examined using a descriptive qualitative approach, and the findings are presented narratively to highlight the key issues raised by the participants.

2.6 Ethical Considerations

This study was reviewed and approved by the Health Research Ethics Committee of Universitas 'Aisyiyah Yogyakarta in December 2024 (Ref. no. 4082/KEP-UNISA/XII/2024) and conducted in accordance with the Declaration of Helsinki. Written informed consent was obtained from all participants prior to their enrollment.

3 Results

3.1 Feasibility

Adherence to therapeutic exercise was highest in speech therapy, followed by physiotherapy and occupational therapy (Fig. 1). Overall, most participants reported exercising at least 2–3 times per week across all rehabilitation domains, with daily practice being the most commonly observed in speech therapy. While seven participants (35%) reported that they did not need any help in exercising or using the application, 10 (59%) reported that they needed help either to open the application (n = 5) or to explain, monitor, and guide performance (n = 6).

Among individuals with mild chronic stroke (N = 17), the median SUS score was 69.4 (range 50.0–77.8), corresponding to acceptable to good perceived usability. Adjective usability ratings were predominantly positive but more moderate than those of the CHWs. Ten individuals with stroke selected "Good", four selected "Excellent," and two selected "OK." None of the participants selected any negative categories. Among the CHWs (N = 5), the median SUS score was 77.5 (range 77.5–90.0), indicating good to excellent perceived usability. Consistent with these scores, adjective usability ratings

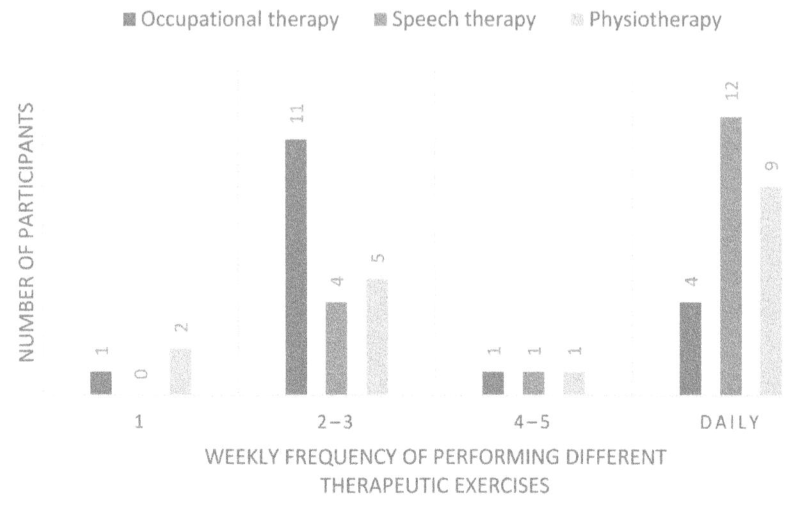

Fig. 1. Weekly adherence to therapeutic home exercise among participants (n = 17) with mild stroke. Rehabilitation delivered by CHWs and a mobile application.

were clustered at the highest end of the scale: three CHWs selected "Best imaginable" and two selected "Excellent."

Community health workers (CHWs) unanimously regarded the Inclusion App as advantageous, user-friendly, and applicable to various conditions, including limb stiffness, tingling sensations, and facial paralysis. Home visit frequencies varied from daily to weekly, with durations ranging from 30 min to 1 h. The app content was deemed relevant and appropriate. CHWs utilized all available programs and recommended the inclusion of hand exercises using a ball to enhance the app's functionality.

3.2 Participant Reported Changes in Functioning

As shown in Table 1, the participants with stroke demonstrated low-to-moderate functional limitations at baseline. They predominantly reported a positive perceived change on the GRC scale (Table 2). Using an a priori responder definition, 13 of 17 individuals (76.5%) were classified as improved (GRC $\geq$ + 3), including 8 individuals (47.1%) who reported substantial improvement (GRC $\geq$ + 5). Two participants reported worsening (GRC $\leq$ − 1), whereas the remaining participants reported small improvement (GRC + 1 to + 2). These findings suggest an overall favorable self-reported- change in this feasibility sample.

Table 2. Global rating of change (GRC) distribution (N = 17)

GRC category	n (%)
− 3 Somewhat worse	2 (11.8)
+ 1 A tiny bit better	1 (5.9)
+ 2 A little bit better	1 (5.9)
+ 3 Somewhat better	5 (29.4)
+ 5 Quite a bit better	6 (35.3)
+ 6 A great deal better	1 (5.9)
+ 7 A very great deal better	1 (5.9)

GRC scale: − 7 = A very great deal worse, 0 = no change, + 7 = A very great deal better

4 Discussion

This feasibility study demonstrated that a multidisciplinary CHW-supported digital rehabilitation solution was both acceptable and feasible for people with mild stroke living in a low-resource community. Participants generally reported mild to moderate functional challenges and positive perceived change in functioning, and both CHWs and users perceived the Inclusion App as usable, although CHWs rated it higher.

The adherence level, with most participants exercising at least two to three times weekly, was likely sufficient to support meaningful functional improvement, as reflected in the positive GRC responses. In this study, adherence was assessed through self-report because the application does not process personal data and, therefore, does not allow individual-level usage monitoring. Although objective adherence measures could offer a more accurate picture of exercise implementation, their use is challenging. For example, many exercises are too stationary for activity sensors and offline use, or merely opening the application without exercising may distort usage of log interpretations. Nonetheless, when technically and ethically feasible, incorporating complementary adherence monitoring methods in future research could help strengthen the assessment of user engagement.

These findings are consistent with prior telerehabilitation studies showing that remote or technology-supported rehabilitation can be feasible and yield functional benefits after stroke, although prior research has been highly limited to high-resource settings [3]. The differences between our findings and those from higher-resource settings may be partly explained by limited digital literacy, variable Internet access, and the substantial role of CHWs and family members in facilitating app use and exercise performance. These contextual factors likely enhanced adherence and usability but also mean that our results may reflect a supported model rather than independent digital rehabilitation, highlighting that CHW and caregiver involvement is a key consideration for future implementation.

Nevertheless, the study provides important practical implications: CHW-facilitated digital rehabilitation appears to align well with WHO recommendations for extending rehabilitation capacity through task sharing [11] and demonstrates the potential for scaling services in underserved communities and primary health care, where rehabilitation professionals are scarce [9]. From an implementation perspective, further work is needed to understand the time and resource demands of CHW-supported home rehabilitation, as well as practical models for supervision and quality assurance to maintain fidelity. Broader cost and resource implications should also be examined to determine long-term sustainability and scalable deployment. As a small, shorter study relying on self-reported outcomes, generalization is limited; however, the findings offer promising early evidence, inform future product development, and provide a foundation for larger, more rigorous effectiveness trials and implementation research.

5 Conclusion

Task-shifting rehabilitation delivery to community health workers, supported by digital technologies, represents a promising strategy for expanding access to post-stroke rehabilitation in resource-constrained settings. Future digital rehabilitation programs in low-resource contexts may benefit from explicitly acknowledging and supporting the role of family members or informal caregivers, alongside task-shifted rehabilitation delivery models.

Acknowledgments. The authors gratefully acknowledge the Indonesian Speech Therapy Association and Indonesian Occupational Therapy Association for their expert contributions to the development of the rehabilitation content and design of the study protocol. This study is part of the NextStep to Scale: Advancing Digital Rehabilitation in East Africa and Southeast Asia project, coordinated by Jamk University of Applied Sciences in collaboration with Physiotools Ltd. And GoodLife Technology Ltd. This project is financed by the Ministry for Foreign Affairs of Finland/Finnpartnership.

Author roles Conceptualization and Protocol Development: (EA, HZF, SMJ, ODW, DFF, MRH, MI, KPM); Methodological and Technical Input (EA, HZF, SMJ, DFF, AWS, N, MO); Data analyses and interpretation (EA, HZF, SMJ, ODW, DFF, MRH, MI); Funding acquisition (EA, KK, KPM); Writing – original draft (EA); Critical review and final approval (All authors).

Disclosure of Interests Authors SMJ and ODW were employed by Physitrack, the company responsible for the Inclusion App. Author ODW was involved in training the CHWs who participated in the study. Author SMJ contributed to data management, under the supervision of HZF. The company had no involvement in data interpretation or manuscript preparation. The authors declare no other potential conflicts of interest regarding the research, authorship, or publication of this article.

The AI tool Microsoft Copilot and the AI-assisted Paperpal solution were used for essential language editing, with key suggestions for correcting grammar and improving readability.

References

1. Feigin, V.L., Brainin, M., Norrving, B., et al.: World stroke organization: global stroke fact sheet 2025. Int. J. Stroke **20**, 132–144 (2025)

2. Kayola, G., Mataa, M.M., Asukile, M., et al.: Stroke rehabilitation in low- and middle-income countries: challenges and opportunities. Am. J. Phys. Med. Rehabil. **102**, S24 (2023)
3. Najafabadi, M.G., Shariat, A., Ingle, L., et al.: The clinical effectiveness of tele-rehabilitation interventions on balance and activities of daily living in post-stroke survivors: an umbrella review of systematic reviews. Disabil. Rehabil. **47**, 5718–5724 (2025)
4. Raymond, M.J., et al.: Delivery of allied health interventions using telehealth modalities: a rapid systematic review of randomized controlled trials. Healthcare **12**, 1217 (2024)
5. Støme, L.N., Wilhelmsen, C.R., Kværner, K.J.: Enabling guidelines for the adoption of eHealth solutions: scoping review. JMIR Form Res **5**(4), e21357 (2021)
6. Price, M., et. al.: Evaluation of eHealth system usability and safety. In: Lau, F., Kuziemsky, G. (eds.) Handbook of eHealth Evaluation, pp. 337–350 (2017)
7. Ghaben, S.J., Mat Ludin, A.F., Mohamad Ali, N., Beng Gan, K., Singh, D.K.A. A framework for design and usability testing of telerehabilitation system for adults with chronic diseases: A panoramic scoping review. Digital Health, 9 (2023)
8. Njoroge, M., Zurovac, D., Ogara, E.A., Chuma, J., Kirigia, D.: Assessing the feasibility of eHealth and mHealth: a systematic review and analysis of initiatives implemented in Kenya. BMC. Res. Notes **10**(1), 90 (2017)
9. Gimigliano, F., Negrini, S.: The world health organization "Rehabilitation 2030: a call for action." Eur. J. Phys. Rehabil. Med. **53**, 155–168 (2017)
10. World Health Organization: Rehabilitation. https://www.who.int/news-room/fact-sheets/det ail/rehabilitation. Accessed 30 Jan 2026
11. World Health Organization: Community-based rehabilitation: CBR guidelines. https://www. who.int/publications/i/item/9789241548052. Accessed 30 Jan 2026
12. Oduor, M. & Aartolahti, E.: Community health workers and service users' experiences of a community-based digital rehabilitation application. Jamk Arena Public. (2024)
13. Brooke, J.: SUS—a quick and dirty usability scale. In: Jordan, P.W., et. al. (eds.) Usability Evaluation in Industry, pp. 189–194 (1996)
14. Kamper, S.J., Maher, C.G., Mackay, G.: Global rating of change scales: a review of strengths and weaknesses and considerations for design. J. Man. Manip. Ther. **17**, 163–170 (2009)
15. World Health Organization: Measuring health and disability: manual for WHO disability assessment schedule (WHODAS 2.0). In: Üstün, T., Kostanjsek, N., Chatterji, S., Rehm, J. (eds.). World Health Organization, Geneva (2010)

Hybrid Teleophthalmology Pilot for Ophthalmologist Appointments

Anniina Häyrynen and Joonas Wirkkala[✉] [iD]

Silmäasema Eye Hospital, Helsinki, Finland
`joonas.wirkkala@silmaasema.fi`

Abstract. Purpose: To evaluate the feasibility, diagnostic performance and clinical outcomes of a hybrid teleophthalmology model combining on-site optometrist examinations with synchronous live video ophthalmologist appointment in a private clinic setting.

Methods: This pilot study included adult participants who underwent hybrid teleophthalmology assessments at two optical stores in Finland. Participants underwent standardized examinations performed by a pretrained optometrist, including refraction, anterior segment video microscopy, fundus photography and optical coherence tomography (OCT). The data collected were reviewed in real time during the live video ophthalmologist appointment.

Results: A total of 105 participants (210 eyes; mean age 69.2±9.8 years; 65% female) were included. Of all participants, 13% had no prior ophthalmologist visits. All hybrid teleophthalmology appointments were completed, with no cancellations due to technical issues. Complete anterior segment video microscopy and OCT imaging were achieved in 99% and 94% of participants, respectively, while complete fundus photography was obtained in 79%, with 69% being of full diagnostic quality. Clinically relevant ocular pathology was frequently detected, most commonly dry eye syndrome (26%), cataract (27%), macular degeneration (18%) and glaucoma suspicion (7%). Treatment was initiated in 30% of participants while 19% required referral to hospital eye care, most often for cataract surgery.

Conclusion: This pilot demonstrates the feasibility and scalability of a hybrid teleophthalmology model for delivering comprehensive eye care. It enables accurate diagnosis, treatment initiation and targeted referrals while improving access to specialist ophthalmological care.

Keywords: Teleophthalmology · Telemedicine · Digital health

1 Introduction

Access to timely and comprehensive ophthalmological care remains a challenge, particularly in rural areas, where specialist services are scarce. The demand for ophthalmology services is increasing due to population aging and the high prevalence of chronic eye diseases such as cataract, glaucoma, age-related macular degeneration (AMD) and diabetic retinopathy, yet the supply of ophthalmologists is limited and unevenly distributed geographically [1–3]. Teleophthalmology has emerged as a promising approach to delivering accessible eye care with diverse imaging and examination modalities [3, 4].

M. Särestöniemi et al. (Eds.): NCDHWS 2026, CCIS 3009, pp. 90–102, 2026.
https://doi.org/10.1007/978-3-032-28812-7_8

This is particularly relevant in Finland, where, according to the Finnish Medical Association, a substantial proportion of ophthalmologists practice in the private sector: 45% work exclusively in private practice and a further 40% practice in both private and public sectors. Therefore, strong private networks such as Silmäasema, which provide a broad network of optical stores and eye hospitals offering both optometrist and ophthalmology appointments, play a central role in routine eye care delivery, while public ophthalmology services are less accessible in many non-urban regions. Moreover, in Finland, diabetic retinopathy screening is currently the only organized ophthalmic screening program [5], and public screening pathways do not routinely provide a comprehensive diagnostic evaluation.

Teleophthalmology applications have traditionally focused on disease-specific screening or asynchronous referral pathways and virtual clinics, most commonly for diabetic retinopathy, glaucoma or AMD [6, 7]. While these approaches can reduce the number of face-to-face visits, their diagnostic scope is usually limited [4, 8] and community-based screening studies suggest that up to 14% of individuals may have more than one ophthalmological condition [8].

In this study, we present a novel and, to our knowledge, one of the most comprehensive and multidisciplinary hybrid models for teleophthalmology eye examination within a private clinic setting. The model combines standardized on-site clinical assessments performed by trained optometrists at local optical stores with synchronous evaluation and live video ophthalmologist appointment. The aim of this pilot study was to evaluate the feasibility, diagnostic yield and clinical outcomes of this teleophthalmology model, in providing comprehensive eye care to underserved populations without compromising diagnostic accuracy or continuity of care.

2 Materials and Methods

This retrospective analysis of a pilot study includes teleophthalmology-based ophthalmologist appointments for consecutive participants in private ophthalmologist practice in Silmäasema optical stores. According to Finnish regulations and guidance for evidence-based management, formal ethical approval was not required. All procedures adhered to the principles outlined in the Declaration of Helsinki and only anonymized, non-identifiable participant data was used in the analysis.

Participants were recruited via local optical stores when planning a visit to an ophthalmologist by front desk staff and optometrists. Participants were considered eligible if they were aged 18 years or older and able to participate in a non-urgent eye examination without acute symptoms. Exclusion criteria included sudden visual loss, recent onset of floaters or flashes, history of retinal detachment, visual field loss, diplopia, severe eye pain or other signs requiring immediate in-person assessment. Furthermore, to ensure eligibility for a hybrid teleophthalmology model, participants were required to be independently mobile and have a normal cognitive function, including adequate speech recognition and comprehension. As visual field testing could not be performed, participants requiring a medical certificate for driver's license renewal were also excluded and referred for an in-person examination.

Two local Silmäasema optical stores were included in this pilot due to their limited availability of ophthalmologist services. Optical stores were located in the City of Ylivieska (population 15 000) and the City of Kokkola (population 48 000). Furthermore, these stores had necessary facilities and optometrist resources for this hybrid teleophthalmology model. All participants underwent a standardized examination conducted by local licensed optometrists. The protocol is illustrated in Fig. 1. In brief, the optometrist performed the initial workup with the participant at a local optical store. Before the pilot started, seven optometrists were trained to acquire all examinations and performance was validated by an ophthalmologist (AH). For technical issues, constant remote support was available for optometrists. The comprehensive ophthalmological evaluation included measurement of best-corrected visual acuity (BCVA), refraction with prescription for eyeglasses, IOP (iCare) and examinations for the anterior segment (Topcon DC-4 Digital Camera), fundus imaging (Canon CR-2 AF or CX-1) and OCT (Optopol Revo 60). From one eye, a total of five images were taken, one image with macula and optic disc centered, and further temporal, inferior and superior fields. Fundus photography was considered complete if a total of 10 images were obtained (five per eye). All collected data were transferred to electronic health records and Topcon Harmony in real time, where they were reviewed by an experienced ophthalmologist.

Following completion of the on-site optometric examination and real-time data transfer, the care pathway immediately proceeded to a live video ophthalmologist appointment conducted via Microsoft Teams. During this appointment, the ophthalmologist reviewed the examination findings, completed the electronic health record, issued eyeglass prescriptions or electronic medication prescriptions when indicated and established the diagnosis and treatment plan, which were discussed with the participant. When required, participants were referred either to an on-site ophthalmologist or to a hospital eye clinic for further care.

Primary outcomes included the completion rate of remote examinations, technical feasibility including data quality and the proportion of cases requiring referral to an on-site ophthalmologist or local hospital. Secondary outcomes included clinical findings or treatment plans. For the subgroup analysis, participants with no previous ophthalmology visits were compared to participants with previous visits.

Descriptive statistics were used to summarize demographic characteristics, examination completion rates, technical performance and clinical outcomes. Continuous variables were reported as means $\pm$ standard deviations (SD) and categorical variables as counts and percentages. Data analysis was conducted using SPSS. Statistical analyses included Pearson's chi-squared test and Student's t-test, with significance set at $p < 0.05$.

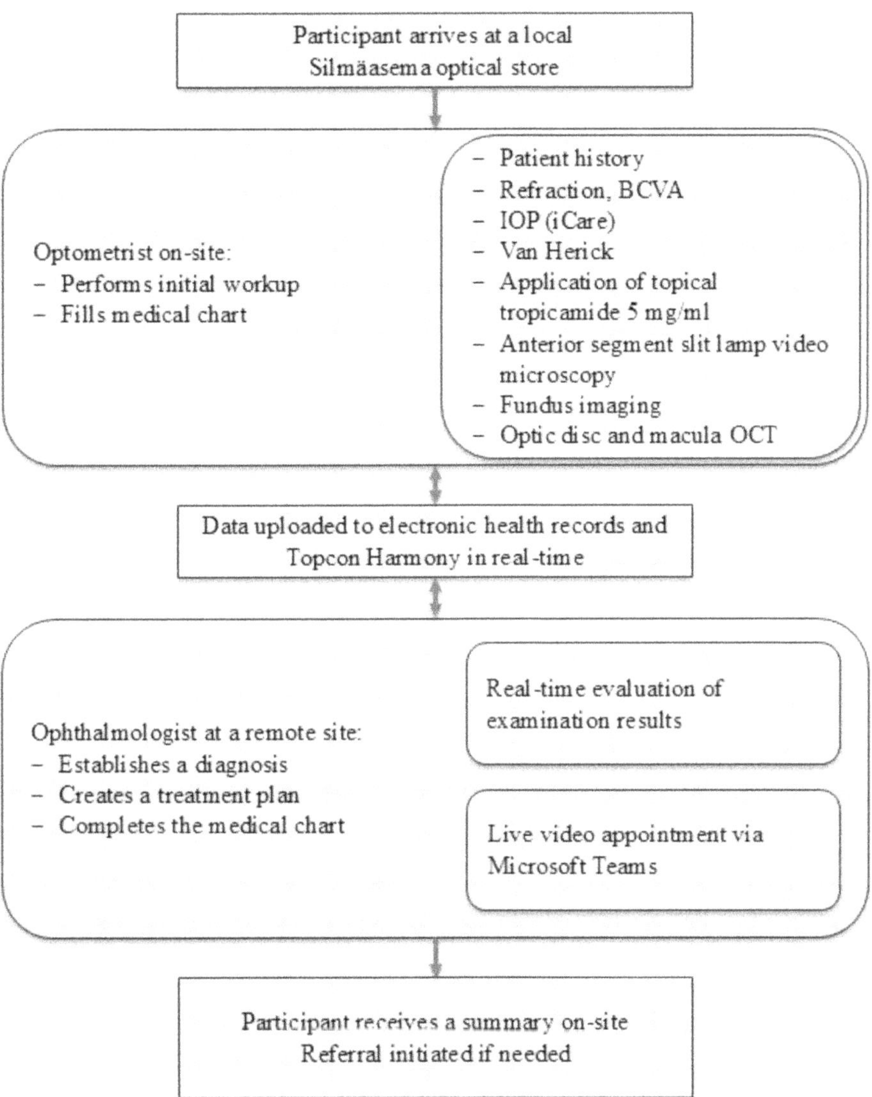

Fig. 1. Workflow of the hybrid teleophthalmology model.

3   Results

A total of 105 participants (210 eyes) were enrolled across two optical stores that participated in this study. The mean age of participants was 69.2 ± 9.8 years and 65% (n = 68) of all participants were females. A total of 67% (n = 70) had a history of cardiovascular disease, while 14% (n = 15) had previously been diagnosed with either type 1 or 2 diabetes. Almost half of the participants (43%, n = 45) had previously been diagnosed with an ophthalmological condition and 13% (n = 14) of participants had never visited an ophthalmologist. Study characteristics are presented in Table 1.

Table 1. Baseline characteristics of participants in the teleophthalmology pilot.

Characteristic	Description (n)
Number of participants	105
Mean age, years [min-max]	69.2 ± 9.8 [39–93]
Females	68 (65%)
Systemic conditions	
Diabetes mellitus	15 (14%)
Cardiovascular disease	70 (67%)
Dyslipidemia	39 (37%)
History of prior ocular disease	
Age-related macular degeneration	5 (5%)
Glaucoma or ocular hypertension	8 (8%)
Refractive laser surgery	7 (7%)
Intraocular lens (at least in one eye)	25 (24%)
Previous ophthalmologist visit	
Within 12 months	4 (4%)
Over 12 months	87 (83%)
Never	14 (13%)

In this teleophthalmology pilot, all participants were examined and no appointments had to be cancelled due to technical issues. However, one participant (1%) failed anterior segment slit lamp microscopy due to technical issues. Fundus photography had the lowest success rates. Complete imaging with five images per eye was obtained in 79% of participants (n = 83), of whom 69% (n = 72) were of full diagnostic quality. Furthermore, OCT scans from the optic disc and macula were successful in 94% (n = 99) of cases (Fig. 2). If the quality of one imaging modality was below full diagnostic standard, another modality compensated for the missing information, ensuring that no participant experienced complete failure of the hybrid teleophthalmology model.

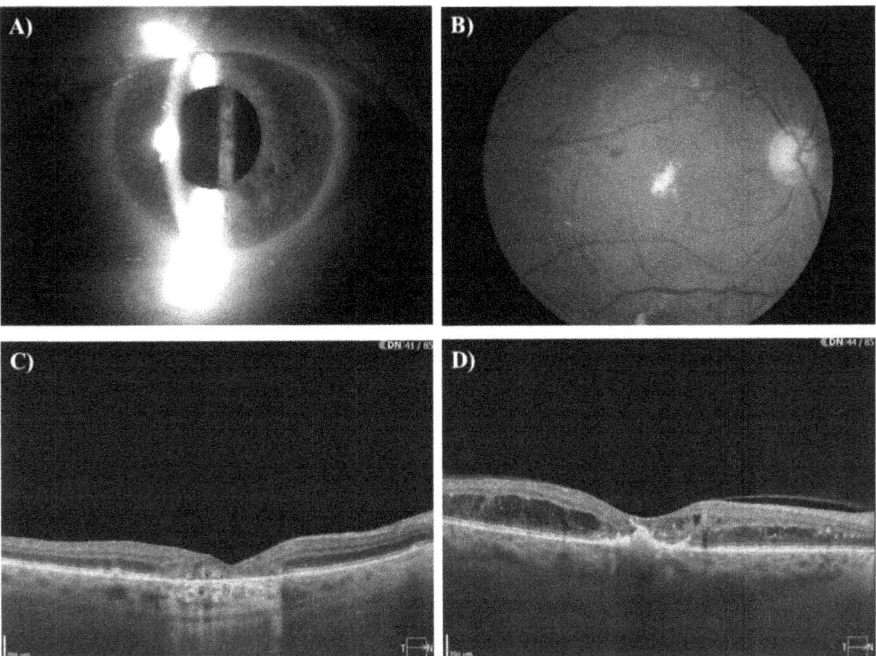

Fig. 2. Representative clinical findings obtained during teleophthalmology examinations. **a** Still frame from anterior segment slit-lamp video microscopy demonstrating secondary cataract in an eye with a previously implanted intraocular lens. **b** Fundus photograph showing moderate diabetic retinopathy with diabetic macular edema. **c** Macular optical coherence tomography (OCT) scan demonstrating retinal pigment epithelium atrophy in age-related macular degeneration. **d** Macular OCT scan showing cystoid macular edema.

Participants in this pilot had mean BCVA of 0.975 ± 0.31 in Snellen with normal mean IOP of 13.1 ± 3.7 mmHg, and only 3% (n = 3) of participants had IOP over 21 mmHg. 34% (n = 36) of participants had decreased Snellen BCVA under 0.8. Using OCT, exact measurements of central subfield thickness (CST), cup-to-disk ratio (C/D), retinal nerve fiber layer (RNFL) and ganglion cell layer (GCL) were obtained and detailed results are presented in Table 2.

Table 2. Ophthalmological outcomes.

Outcome	Mean (SD) [min-max]
Best-corrected visual acuity, Snellen	0.975 (0.310) [0.01–2.00]
Intraocular pressure, mmHg	13.1 (3.7) [3–26]
Van Herick	3.6 (0.7) [2–4]
Central Subfield Thickness, μm	266.3 (42.0) [149–455]
Cup-to-disc (C/D) ratio	0.44 (0.23) [0.00–0.97]

(continued)

Table 2. (*continued*)

Outcome	Mean (SD) [min-max]
Retinal nerve fiber layer (3.5mm), μm	95.97 (29.24) [62–431]
Ganglion cell layer, μm	83.6 (8.7) [60–113]

The most prevalent diagnosis established during the teleophthalmology appointments was dry eye syndrome (26%, n = 27). Other ophthalmological pathologies included senile incipient cataract (14.8%, n = 26), senile nuclear cataract (12.5%, n = 22) and dry AMD (10.2%, n = 18). In addition, of all participants, 6.8% (n = 12) had glaucoma suspicion and the proportion of previously diagnosed glaucoma was 1.7% (n = 3). The most common treatments initiated during the appointments were artificial tears (26%, n = 27) and topical corticosteroid for dry eye (3%, n = 3). Referral to a hospital eye clinic occurred in 19% (n = 20) of cases, with cataract surgery (9%, n = 9) being the most frequent indication. A further 4% (n = 4) of participants had to be referred to an on-site ophthalmologist due to the limitation of examination of the retinal periphery, while two participants had high myopia and a further two participants had possible symptoms of a retinal tear. Participants who were not referred due to limitations of the teleophthalmology model were referred based on the same clinical indications as in a standard on-site ophthalmologist appointment. All clinical outcomes are presented in Table 3.

Table 3. Ocular diagnoses, initiated treatments and referrals following hybrid teleophthalmology appointments.

Outcome	Value, n (%)
All diagnoses (N = 186)	
Dry eye syndrome	27 (26)
Senile incipient cataract	26 (14.8)
Presence of intraocular lens	25 (14.2)
Senile nuclear cataract	22 (12.5)
Dry age-related macular degeneration	18 (10.2)
Degeneration of macula, unspecified	13 (7.4)
Glaucoma suspect	12 (6.8)
Presbyopia	10 (5.7)
Secondary cataract	8 (4.5)
Benign neoplasm of choroid	5 (2.8)
Hyperopia	3 (1.7)
Vitreous degeneration	3 (1.7)
Myopia	3 (1.7)

(continued)

Table 3. (*continued*)

Outcome	Value, n (%)
Glaucoma	3 (1.7)
Amblyopia	2 (1.1)
Diabetic macular edema	2 (1.1)
Eyelid hemangioma	1 (0.6)
Blepharochalasis	1 (0.6)
Diabetic retinopathy	1 (0.6)
Blepharitis	1 (0.6)
Initiated medication	
Artificial tears for dry eye syndrome	27 (26)
Topical corticosteroid for dry eye	3 (3)
IOP-lowering medication	1 (1)
Topical cyclosporine	1 (1)
Referral to hospital	
Cataract surgery	9 (9)
YAG capsulotomy	4 (4)
Visual field testing	4 (4)
Blepharoplasty	1 (1)
Macular pucker vitrectomy	1 (1)
Acute cystoid macular edema	1 (1)

To compare participants who had never visited an ophthalmologist with those who had previous visits, a subgroup analysis was performed (Table 4). Baseline characteristics were similar between the groups and statistically significant differences were observed in the prevalence of senile nuclear cataract and dry age-related macular degeneration: 1 (7%) vs. 21 (23%) (p = 0.026) and 1 (7%) vs. 17 (19%) (p = 0.047) in the never visited and previously visited groups, respectively. Interestingly, there were no significant differences in glaucoma suspicion or dry eye syndrome (all p > 0.05).

Table 4. Comparison of baseline characteristics and clinical outcomes by prior ophthalmologist visit history.

	Never visited (n = 14) n (% or SD)	Visited previously (n = 91) n (% or SD)	p
Age, years	65.7 (9.6)	69.8 (9.8)	0.152
Sex, females	8 (57%)	60 (66%)	0.522
BCVA in worst eye	0.986 (0.384)	0.881 (0.326)	0.276

(*continued*)

Table 4. (continued)

	Never visited (n = 14) n (% or SD)	Visited previously (n = 91) n (% or SD)	p
Senile incipient cataract	6 (43%)	20 (22%)	0.397
Senile nuclear cataract	1 (7%)	21 (23%)	**0.026**
Dry age-related macular degeneration	1 (7%)	17 (19%)	**0.047**
Dry eye syndrome	4 (29%)	23 (25%)	0.793
Glaucoma suspicion	1 (7%)	11 (12%)	0.119
Complete fundus photography imaging acquired, n (%)	12 (86%)	71 (78%)	0.510
Referral required	4 (29%)	20 (22%)	0.584

4 Discussion

This pilot study demonstrates that a hybrid teleophthalmology model combining trained optometrists with a synchronous live video ophthalmologist appointment can deliver a comprehensive ophthalmological evaluation with high technical feasibility in underserved settings. Furthermore, this hybrid teleophthalmology model represents a valuable addition to ophthalmology services in areas where traditional on-site ophthalmologist appointments are scarce. The vast majority of participants (96%) were successfully examined using the workflow described, while the remaining participants required referral to an on-site ophthalmologist for further evaluation. Even when individual imaging was suboptimal, the combination of anterior segment video microscopy, OCT and real-time interaction with an ophthalmologist provided sufficient diagnostic information in all cases.

Previously, teleophthalmology models have largely focused on single-disease screening or virtual clinics, such as diabetic retinopathy, age-related macular degeneration and glaucoma [2, 6, 9, 10]. Although teleophthalmology has been shown to reduce healthcare resources and costs, it has also been shown to be as effective as on-site examinations [2, 6, 11]. For example, Heilenbach et al. demonstrated that rural areas and difficulties in accessing eye care services are risk factors for loss to follow-up [12], highlighting the importance of accessible ophthalmological care. Moreover, in Finland, ophthalmologist appointments in private optical stores are covered through a combination of patient out-of-pocket payments and partial reimbursement from the national health insurance system.

To ensure proper patient selection for hybrid teleophthalmology appointments, several exclusion criteria were applied to account for known limitations of teleophthalmology. Participant eligibility was assessed through interview; however, in larger-scale implementations with online booking available, ensuring appropriate patient selection may be more challenging. Furthermore, it is well recognized that individuals with disabilities may require additional support and tailored arrangements to ensure equitable access to teleophthalmology services [13]. Despite preliminary assessments prior to participation in the pilot, four participants required on-site evaluation of the peripheral retina due to symptoms suggestive of retinal tears and high myopia, underscoring the importance of strict exclusion criteria and training of local staff.

Most participants had previously visited an ophthalmologist, while 13% were first-time visitors. A history of refractive laser or cataract surgery was present in 31% of the participants. Following the hybrid teleophthalmology examination, the predominant diagnoses were dry eye syndrome (26%), senile incipient or nuclear cataract (27%), macular degeneration (18%) and glaucoma suspicion (7%). This heterogeneous participant population demonstrates that the hybrid teleophthalmology model is feasible across diverse patient groups, including those with systemic diseases, and is capable of detecting a wide range of ocular conditions.

Although Blais et al. reported that optometrist-led teleoptometry examinations were non-inferior to in-person examinations, for example in terms of subjective refraction, the prevalence of ocular pathology in that study was low [14]. Within the current model, the ophthalmologist participated in the live video appointment in real time, reviewed all examination findings, interacted directly with the participant and could direct the on-site optometrist to perform additional assessments as needed. This supports the role of optometrists as members of the telehealth team, rather than a technician [15]. Moreover, 19% of participants required referral to hospital eye care, most commonly for cataract surgery (9%). This emphasizes that the teleophthalmology model enables not only diagnosis but also appropriate treatment planning and referral to specialized care, including surgical interventions, when indicated. However, several factors have to be acknowledged before implementing a teleophthalmology model, including the time-consuming nature of the setup process, training of the front desk staff and optometrists, and procurement of new equipment. All these aspects also affect the cost-benefit of setting up a teleophthalmology site, resulting in higher patient-related costs compared to traditional on-site ophthalmologist appointments. Moreover, despite the higher cost of teleophthalmology appointments, patients have lower travelling costs when the service is provided locally.

In Finland, primary healthcare is based on general practitioners, while specialized ophthalmological services are centralized in regional or university hospitals. Individuals with eye care concerns often seek initial assessment at optical stores or private ophthalmologists rather than through primary healthcare providers. Consequently, teleophthalmology services integrated into optical stores may be particularly valuable in regions with limited availability of ophthalmologists, a challenge also reported internationally [16, 17]. By enabling direct ophthalmologist assessment, teleophthalmology may reduce the burden on primary healthcare and expedite appropriate referrals [18]. For example, in a Finnish study of 75 patients referred to a hospital eye clinic via primary healthcare physicians following optometrist's recommendation, only 1.3% had a clinically significant condition requiring further treatment, whereas 52% had completely normal findings on fundus photography at the ophthalmologist's evaluation [19]. The detection of clinically relevant pathology among participants without prior ophthalmological visits further highlights the potential of teleophthalmology to improve access to specialist eye care. Additionally, reducing the need for long-distance travel to centralized hospitals decreases patient-related costs, time away from work and logistical barriers to care [1, 6]. Moreover, decreased travel contributes to lower carbon emissions, supporting the ecological sustainability of teleophthalmology models [20, 21].

This study presents a comprehensive hybrid teleophthalmology eye examination model that, although not superior to conventional on-site slit-lamp biomicroscopy performed by an ophthalmologist, offers a valuable alternative. Limitations include the retrospective nature and the inability to fully assess the peripheral retina in a remote setting. Consequently, participants with symptoms or signs suggestive of peripheral retinal pathology were appropriately referred for in-person evaluation. Only two sites participated in this pilot and to further evaluate feasibility and scalability, future studies should include more sites, which would also give better geographical and population coverage for greater generalizability of the study results. Key strengths of this study include the use of pretrained optometrists performing standardized, high-quality examinations as members of the teleophthalmology team, combined with reliable nationwide broadband and 5G connectivity and a flexible electronic patient record system enabling seamless real-time data transfer and clinical collaboration. The diagnostic spectrum closely resembled that of conventional outpatient ophthalmology clinics, supporting the clinical relevance of this model. Importantly, this level of clinical judgment relies on synchronous ophthalmologist involvement, allowing real-time assessment of the overall clinical picture, an approach not achievable through optometrist-only evaluation without direct ophthalmologist participation. Moreover, despite the lack of a structured patient satisfaction survey, participants reported high satisfaction with the appointments.

In conclusion, this pilot study demonstrates that the described teleophthalmology model is feasible, clinically meaningful and scalable within a real-world eye care network. Future studies should address the current limitations of teleophthalmology examinations, particularly regarding peripheral retinal assessment, and evaluate outcomes in larger populations. With targeted training, the model could be extended to selected acute ophthalmic presentations. Further technological advances, including improved imaging modalities, automated diagnostic devices and artificial intelligence–assisted decision support, may enhance diagnostic accuracy and efficiency, ultimately helping to expand access to high-quality eye care.

Acknowledgments. The authors wish to thank all participating optometrists for their valuable contributions to participant examinations and cooperation at Silmäasema. We also extend our sincere appreciation to the members of the pilot project group for their collaboration, insights, and commitment throughout the development and implementation of this teleophthalmology model.

Disclosure of Interests The authors have no competing interests to declare that are relevant to the content of this article.

References

1. Dolar-Szczasny, J., Barańska, A., Rejdak, R.: Evaluating the efficacy of teleophthalmology in delivering ophthalmic care to underserved populations: a literature review. J. Clin. Med. **12**, 3161 (2023). https://doi.org/10.3390/jcm12093161

2. Mercer, R., Alaghband, P.: The value of virtual glaucoma clinics: a review. Eye (Lond.) **38**, 1840–1844 (2024). https://doi.org/10.1038/s41433-024-03056-7

3. Woś, R., Sys, D.: The role of tele-ophthalmology in modern eye care: a mixed-methods investigation of patient satisfaction and effectiveness. Eur. J. Ophthalmol. **35**, 1967–1978 (2025). https://doi.org/10.1177/11206721251366734

4. Walsh, L., Hong, C.Y., Chalakkal, R., Hong, S.C., O'Keeffe, B., Ogbuehi, K.: A systematic review of teleophthalmology services Post-COVID-19 pandemic in New Zealand, the United Kingdom, Australia, the United States of America, and Canada. Telemed. J. E Health **30**, 2795–2804 (2024). https://doi.org/10.1089/tmj.2024.0258

5. Hautala, N., et al.: Marked reductions in visual impairment due to diabetic retinopathy achieved by efficient screening and timely treatment. Acta Ophthalmol. **92**, 582–587 (2014). https://doi.org/10.1111/aos.12278

6. Weng, C.Y., et al.: Effectiveness of conventional digital fundus photography-based Teleretinal screening for diabetic retinopathy and diabetic macular edema: a report by the American academy of ophthalmology. Ophthalmology **131**, 927–942 (2024). https://doi.org/10.1016/j.ophtha.2024.02.017

7. Christopher, M., Hallaj, S., Jiravarnsirikul, A., Baxter, S.L., Zangwill, L.M.: Novel technologies in artificial intelligence and telemedicine for glaucoma screening. J. Glaucoma **33**, S26–S32 (2024). https://doi.org/10.1097/IJG.0000000000002367

8. Kapoor, R., et al.: Detecting common eye diseases using the first teleophthalmology GlobeChek Kiosk in the United States: a pilot study. Asia Pac. J. Ophthalmol. (Phila). **9**, 315–325 (2020). https://doi.org/10.1097/APO.0000000000000295

9. Sim, S.S., et al.: Digital technology for AMD management in the post-COVID-19 new normal. Asia Pac. J. Ophthalmol. (Phila). **10**, 39–48 (2021). https://doi.org/10.1097/APO.0000000000000363

10. Kato, A., et al.: Remote screening of diabetic retinopathy using ultra-widefield retinal imaging. Diabetes Res. Clin. Pract. **177**, 108902 (2021). https://doi.org/10.1016/j.diabres.2021.108902

11. Curran, D.M., Kim, B.Y., Withers, N., Shepard, D.S., Brady, C.J.: Telehealth screening for diabetic retinopathy: economic modeling reveals cost savings. Telemed. J. E Health **28**, 1300–1308 (2022). https://doi.org/10.1089/tmj.2021.0352

12. Heilenbach, N., et al.: Novel methods of identifying individual and neighborhood risk factors for loss to follow-up after ophthalmic screening. J. Glaucoma **33**, 288–296 (2024). https://doi.org/10.1097/IJG.0000000000002328

13. Shukla, K.: Running an inclusive and accessible teleophthalmology service for people with disabilities. Commun. Eye Health. **35**, 8–9 (2022)

14. Blais, N., Tousignant, B., Hanssens, J.-M.: Comprehensive primary eye care: a comparison between an in-person eye exam and a tele-eye care exam. Clin. Optom. (Auckl). **16**, 17–30 (2024). https://doi.org/10.2147/OPTO.S436659

15. Massie, J., Block, S.S., Morjaria, P.: The role of optometry in the delivery of eye care via telehealth: a systematic literature review. Telemed. J. E Health **28**, 1753–1763 (2022). https://doi.org/10.1089/tmj.2021.0537

16. Casazza, M., Bolz, M., Huemer, J.: Telemedicine in ophthalmology. Wien. Med. Wochenschr. **175**, 153–161 (2025). https://doi.org/10.1007/s10354-025-01081-z

17. Barrero-Castillero, A., Corwin, B.K., VanderVeen, D.K., Wang, J.C.: Workforce shortage for retinopathy of prematurity care and emerging role of telehealth and artificial intelligence. Pediatr. Clin. North Am. **67**, 725–733 (2020). https://doi.org/10.1016/j.pcl.2020.04.012

18. Jørgensen, E.P., et al.: Implementing teleophthalmology services to improve cost-effectiveness of the national eye care system. Eye (Lond.) **38**, 2788–2795 (2024). https://doi.org/10.1038/s41433-024-03156-4

19. Määttä, M., Talvensaari, K., Saari, J., Patja, K., Paterno, J.: Optometristien silmänpohjaku-vauksista ei juuri terveyshyötyä [Health benefits of optometrists' fundus scans are minimal]. Suom Lääkäril. **80** (2025)
20. Wong, Y.L., Aslam, T.M., Chang, D.F., Erny, B.: Sustaining ophthalmic practices for the future: a high-value care approach to environmental responsibility. Ophthalmol Ther. **14**, 1199–1218 (2025). https://doi.org/10.1007/s40123-025-01146-7
21. Rani, P.K., et al.: Teleophthalmology at a primary and tertiary eye care network from India: environmental and economic impact. Eye (Lond.) **38**, 2203–2208 (2024). https://doi.org/10.1038/s41433-024-02934-4

Development of Health Promotional Support Service Based on the Mobile Personal Health Record Application to Prevent Heart Failure

Hiromasa Ito[(✉)] [iD], Naoki Fujimoto [iD], and Kaoru Dohi [iD]

Mie University, Edobashi 2-174, Tsu, Mie, Japan
h-ito@med.mie-u.ac.jp

Abstract.

Background Heart failure (HF) is a chronic and progressive condition associated with frequent exacerbations and a high risk of hospital readmission. Sustained patient self-management is essential for long-term disease control; however, maintaining daily self-care and recognizing early signs of deterioration remain challenging in routine practice. Mobile health (mHealth) technologies may help support continuous self-management, but evidence focusing on patient-centered approaches remains limited, particularly in Japan.

Methods: We conducted a multicenter, prospective study at five hospitals in Mie Prefecture, Japan, between March 2022 and March 2023. Patients hospitalized for HF were enrolled and asked to use a smartphone-based personal health record application ("Heart Sign") for six months after discharge. Participants recorded daily blood pressure, pulse rate, body weight, and HF-related symptoms. The application provided patient-facing feedback using a simplified three-level HF status assessment algorithm. Adherence was evaluated using effective input rates, patient-reported outcomes were assessed with the Kansas City Cardiomyopathy Questionnaire (KCCQ), and user experience was evaluated using a structured questionnaire.

Results: A total of 56 patients were enrolled (mean age 61.8 years; 23.3% aged $\geq$ 70 years). Forty-nine patients (87.5%) continued application use for six months, reflecting sustained engagement. No deaths occurred, and HF-related rehospitalization was observed in three patients (5.4%). Multiple KCCQ domains, including symptoms, physical limitation, and quality of life, showed significant improvement (p < 0.001).

Conclusions: The Heart Sign application demonstrated good feasibility, sustained engagement, and improved patient-reported outcomes. Patient-centered mHealth solutions may support scalable HF self-management, particularly in aging societies with regional healthcare disparities.

Keywords: Mobile health · Personal health record · Chronic heart failure

M. Särestöniemi et al. (Eds.): NCDHWS 2026, CCIS 3009, pp. 103–110, 2026.
https://doi.org/10.1007/978-3-032-28812-7_9

1 Introduction

1.1 Heart Failure and the Role of Mobile Health

Heart failure (HF) is a chronic and progressive condition characterized by recurrent exacerbations and a high risk of hospital readmission [1–3]. Preventing avoidable readmissions remains a major challenge in HF care, and sustained patient self-management is widely recognized as an essential component of long-term disease control.

In routine clinical practice, however, maintaining effective self-management is difficult for many patients with HF. Common challenges include limited disease awareness, difficulty maintaining daily self-care behaviors, and reduced ability to recognize early signs of symptom worsening. Handwritten HF logbooks are commonly used to record daily parameters such as blood pressure, heart rate, body weight, and symptoms. However, these tools have several limitations. Incomplete recordings, forgotten entries, and difficulty interpreting long-term trends often prevent timely recognition of HF deterioration.

In recent years, mobile health (mHealth) technologies and personal health record (PHR) have attracted attention as tools to support continuous self-management in HF [4–8]. Although several digital interventions have been developed, evidence focusing on patient-centered self-management support—particularly within the Japanese healthcare setting—remains limited.

1.2 Regional Healthcare Challenges

The importance of digital self-management support is particularly evident in regions with limited access to specialized cardiovascular care. Mie Prefecture, located in central Japan, has a relatively high aging population and marked regional disparities in population density. In some areas, access to medical institutions is limited, making remote, technology-enabled approaches to the management of chronic diseases, including heart failure, increasingly important.

These regional characteristics highlight the potential value of mobile health (mHealth) solutions that enable patients to engage in daily self-management and share health information without relying on frequent in-person visits [5]. From a broader perspective, such challenges are not unique to Japan and are becoming increasingly relevant in aging societies worldwide.

1.3 "Heart Sign" Project and Study Objectives

To address these challenges, Mie University and Curecode Inc. (Toyama, Japan), have collaboratively developed a mobile PHR application to support self-management among patients with HF since 2020 (**Fig. 1**). Rather than functioning solely as a passive data-recording tool, the application was designed to empower patients to actively manage their condition and recognize early signs of HF exacerbation based on their own daily data.

In 2022, a clinical study was conducted to evaluate the feasibility and utility of this digital self-management approach. Since 2023, the project has been supported by the

Japan Agency for Medical Research and Development (AMED), enabling the implementation of multiple randomized controlled studies and accelerating real-world deployment efforts between 2024 and 2026.

This paper aims to introduce the HF management mobile application "Heart Sign," summarize findings from prior studies, and discuss future perspectives for scalable digital self-management and social implementation in HF care.

2   Methods

2.1   Study Design and Digital Intervention

This multicenter, prospective study was conducted at five hospitals in Mie Prefecture, Japan, between March 2022 and March 2023 to evaluate the feasibility and utility of a smartphone-based self-management application for patients with HF. Patients hospitalized for HF were enrolled and asked to install a dedicated mobile application ("Heart Sign") on their personal smartphones.

Participants were instructed to record daily blood pressure, pulse rate, body weight, and HF-related symptoms at home for six months after discharge. Based on the entered biometric data and symptoms, the application provided patient-facing feedback using a simplified three-level HF status assessment algorithm derived from prior clinical research [9]. The primary purpose of the application was to support daily self-management and increase patient awareness of potential HF deterioration.

2.2   Evaluation of Adherence, Outcomes, and User Experience

Adherence to application-based self-management was assessed using the effective input rate, defined as the proportion of days per month with complete data entry for all required parameters. Discontinuation was defined as cessation of application use within three months.

Patient-reported outcomes were evaluated using the Kansas City Cardiomyopathy Questionnaire (KCCQ) [10] at baseline and after six months of application use. User experience and perceived usefulness of the application were assessed using a structured, paper-based questionnaire administered at the end of the study. Changes in KCCQ scores were analyzed using nonparametric statistical methods.

User experience and perceived usefulness were assessed using a structured questionnaire developed specifically for this study. The questionnaire consisted of 10 items covering usability, perceived usefulness, satisfaction, and self-management awareness.

Each item was rated on a 5-point Likert scale (1 = strongly disagree to 5 = strongly agree). Example items included ease of daily data entry, clarity of feedback, and perceived improvement in disease understanding.

Although the questionnaire was not formally validated, its content was developed based on prior digital health usability studies and reviewed by clinical experts to ensure face validity.

2.3 Ethical Considerations

This study conformed to the principles of the Declaration of Helsinki and was approved by the Institutional Review Board of Mie University Graduate School of Medicine and each participating hospital ethics committee (Reference number H2021–144).

Written informed consent was obtained from all participants prior to enrollment. Participants were informed about the purpose of the study, data collection procedures, and their right to withdraw at any time without affecting their clinical care.

All collected data were anonymized and stored on secure servers in accordance with institutional data protection policies. Access to identifiable information was restricted to authorized study personnel only.

3 Results

3.1 Study Population and Application Use

A total of 56 patients were enrolled in the study, with a mean age of 61.8 years; 23.3% were aged 70 years or older. All participants were able to use the application independently on their personal smartphones without external assistance. During the six-month follow-up period, no deaths were observed, and three patients (5.4%) experienced HF-related rehospitalization.

3.2 Adherence and Continuation

Seven patients (12.5%) discontinued application use within three months, while 49 patients (87.5%) continued using for the full six-month period (Fig. 2). Among continuing users, high effective input rates were maintained throughout the study period, indicating sustained engagement in daily self-management.

3.3 Improvements in Health Status and User Experience

Significant improvements were observed in HF-related health status after six months of application use. KCCQ-overall summary (OS), KCCQ-clinical summary (CS), KCCQ-total symptom (TS), KCCQ-physical limitation (PL), and KCCQ-quality of life (QoL) scores were significantly improved at 6 months compared with baseline ($p < 0.001$) (Fig. 2). User experience questionnaires were completed by 46 participants (82.1%). Most respondents reported high satisfaction with the ease of daily data entry, and more than 90% indicated that the application improved their understanding of HF and its management.

4 Discussion

4.1 Feasibility and Implementation Potential of mHealth for HF Management

This multicenter prospective study demonstrated that a smartphone-based HF self-management application can be feasibly implemented in real-world clinical settings, with high continuation rates and favorable user engagement. Notably, all participants, including older adults, were able to use the application independently on their personal smartphones, suggesting a low barrier to adoption [11].

Our findings are consistent with prior studies demonstrating that mHealth interventions can improve patient-reported outcomes and support self-management in heart failure [8, 12, 13] In particular, the observed improvements in KCCQ scores align with previous trials reporting enhanced quality of life associated with digital health interventions.

However, unlike many previous studies that relied on structured telemonitoring systems led by healthcare providers, the present study emphasizes patient-centered self-management through a simple and intuitive interface. This approach may explain the high adherence observed in our cohort.

In addition, our findings extend previous work by demonstrating feasibility in a real-world, multicenter setting in Japan, where regional disparities in healthcare access remain a major challenge. This supports the potential scalability of PHR-based interventions in aging societies.

Sustained effective input rates over six months indicate that daily self-monitoring using a mobile application is achievable beyond short-term intervention periods. Improvements observed across multiple domains of the KCCQ further suggest that continuous digital self-management support may contribute to better patient-perceived health status. Together, these findings support the practical utility of patient-centered mHealth solutions as a complement to conventional outpatient HF care, particularly in settings where frequent in-person follow-up is challenging.

4.2 Clinical and Methodological Considerations

Several limitations should be considered when interpreting these findings. First, this study used a single-arm observational design, which limits causal conclusions regarding the effectiveness of the intervention. Although improvements in patient-reported outcomes were observed, they may partly reflect recovery after hospitalization or increased clinical attention.

Second, the study included only patients who owned and could use smartphones, which may introduce selection bias and limit generalizability to individuals with lower digital literacy. In addition, adherence and satisfaction were partly assessed using self-reported measures, which may be subject to response bias. Finally, the small sample size and regional focus require caution when applying the results to broader healthcare settings.

Despite these limitations, the study provides useful real-world evidence on usability, engagement, and patient acceptance—key factors for successful digital health implementation that are often underreported in early-phase studies.

4.3 Implications for Digital Health Implementation

The findings of this study are relevant beyond the Japanese healthcare context. Many European countries face similar challenges related to population aging, unequal access to healthcare, and growing demands for chronic disease management. Patient-centered mHealth applications that promote self-awareness and daily engagement may offer a scalable approach to HF management across different healthcare systems.

From an implementation perspective, the "Heart Sign" project demonstrates a stepwise development process, from application design and feasibility testing to randomized studies and real-world implementation, supported by collaboration between academia and industry. This approach aligns with current European priorities in digital health, including the generation of real-world evidence, user-centered design, and integration into routine care.

Future studies should examine comparative effectiveness, long-term clinical outcomes, and integration with existing digital health systems. Understanding how patient-driven self-management tools can be incorporated into multidisciplinary HF care pathways will be important to maximize their impact at both the patient and healthcare system levels.

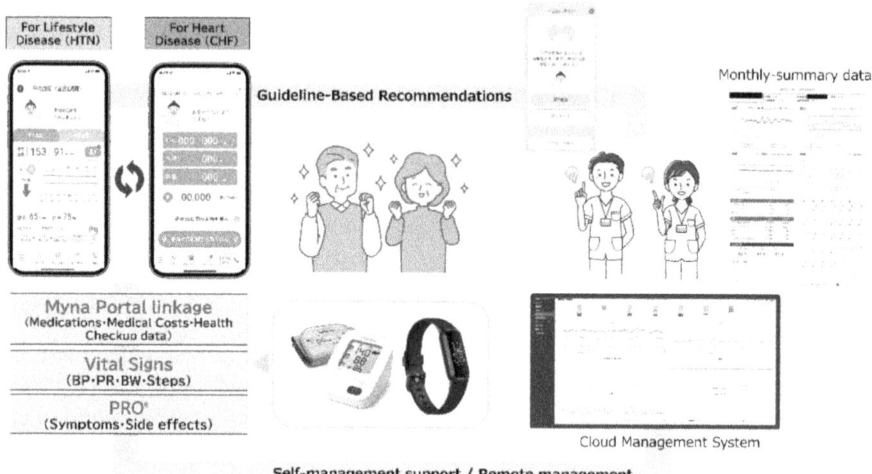

Fig. 1. Heart Sign mHealth system for heart failure management. The figure shows the "Heart Sign" mobile health system for heart failure self-management. The application collects daily vital signs and symptoms, provides guideline-based feedback, and shares data with a cloud platform for remote monitoring by healthcare professionals.

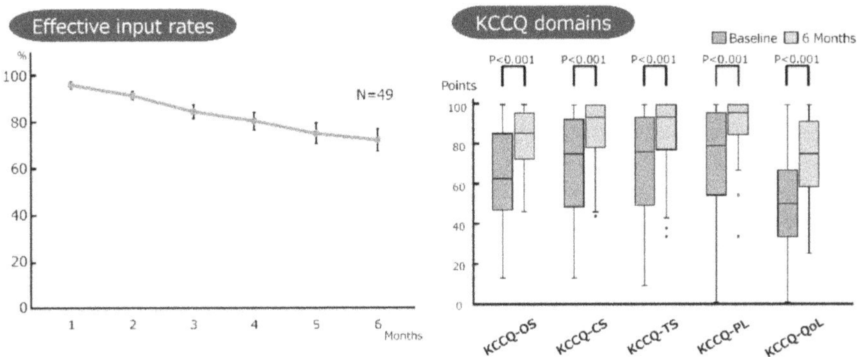

Fig. 2. Results of the preliminary study. Effective input rates remained high over six months, and Kansas City Cardiomyopathy Questionnaire (KCCQ) scores significantly improved from baseline to six months among app users.

5 Conclusion

The Heart Sign application demonstrated good feasibility, sustained engagement, and improved patient-reported outcomes. Patient-centered mHealth solutions may support scalable HF self-management, particularly in aging societies with regional healthcare disparities.

Acknowledgments. This study was funded by the AMED under Grant Number 25le0110026h0003.

Disclosure of Interests The authors have no competing interests to declare that are relevant to the content of this article.

References

1. Shiraishi, Y., et al.: 9-Year trend in the management of acute heart failure in japan: a report from the national consortium of acute heart failure registries. J. Am. Heart Assoc. **7**(18), e008687 (2018)
2. McDonagh, T.A., Metra, M., Adamo, M., Gardner, R.S., Baumbach, A., Böhm, M., et al.: 2021 ESC Guidelines for the diagnosis and treatment of acute and chronic heart failure. Eur. Heart J. **42**, 3599–3726 (2021)
3. Savarese, G., Becher, P.M., Lund, L.H., Seferovic, P., Rosano, G.M.C., Coats, A.J.S.: Global burden of heart failure: a comprehensive and updated review of epidemiology. Cardiovasc. Res. **118**, 3272–3287 (2023)
4. Saleh, Z.T., Elshatarat, R.A., Elhefnawy, K.A., Helmi Elneblawi, N., Abu Raddaha, A.H., Al-Za'areer, M.S., et al.: Effect of a home-based mobile health app intervention on physical activity levels in patients with heart failure: a randomized controlled trial. J. Cardiovasc. Nurs. **38**(2), 128–139 (2023)
5. Kitsiou, S., Vatani, H., Paré, G., Gerber, B.S., Buchholz, S.W., Kansal, M.M., et al.: Effectiveness of mobile health technology interventions for patients with heart failure: systematic review and meta-analysis. Can. J. Cardiol. **37**(8), 1248–1259 (2021)

6. Inglis, S.C., Clark, R.A., Dierckx, R., Prieto-Merino, D., Cleland, J.G.: Structured telephone support or non-invasive telemonitoring for patients with heart failure. Cochrane Database Syst. Rev. **2015**, Cd007228 (2015)
7. Widmer, R.J., Collins, N.M., Collins, C.S., West, C.P., Lerman, L.O., Lerman, A.: Digital health interventions for the prevention of cardiovascular disease: a systematic review and meta-analysis. Mayo Clin. Proc. **90**, 469–480 (2015)
8. Cajita, M.I., Hodgson, N.A., Lam, K.W., Yoo, S., Han, H.R.: Facilitators of and barriers to mHealth adoption in older adults with heart failure. Comput. Inform. Nurs. **36**, 376–382 (2018)
9. Nakane, E., Kato, T., Tanaka, N., Kuriyama, T., Kimura, K., Nishiwaki, S., et al.: Association of the induction of a self-care management system with 1-year outcomes in patients hospitalized for heart failure. J. Cardiol. **77**(1), 48–56 (2021)
10. Green, C.P., Porter, C.B., Bresnahan, D.R., et al.: J. Am. Coll. Cardiol. **35**(5), 1245–1255 (2000)
11. Ito, H., Fujimoto, N., Mori, H., Kirii, Y., Kimura, T., Takeuchi, M., et al.: Unveiling the new era of heart failure management using mobile health: a pilot study of "heart sign" focusing on user experience and quality of life. J. Cardiol. **84**(4), 276–278 (2024)
12. Koehler, F., Koehler, K., Deckwart, O., Prescher, S., Wegscheider, K., Winkler, S., et al.: Telemedical Interventional Management in Heart Failure II (TIM-HF2), a randomised, controlled trial investigating the impact of telemedicine on unplanned cardiovascular hospitalisations and mortality in heart failure patients: study design and description of the intervention. Eur. J. Heart Fail. **20**, 1485–1493 (2018)
13. Seto, E., Leonard, K.J., Cafazzo, J.A., Barnsley, J., Masino, C., Ross, H.J.: Mobile phone-based telemonitoring for heart failure management: a randomized controlled trial. J. Med. Internet Res. **14**, e31 (2012)

Health Technology Assessment and Impact Evaluation

Development of an Assessment and Reimbursement Model for Digital Therapies in the Finnish Healthcare System

Jari Haverinen$^{(\boxtimes)}$, Raija Järvinen, Teemu Mustola, and Petra Falkenbach

Finnish Coordinating Center for Health Technology Assessment (FinCCHTA), Oulu University Hospital, Oulu, Finland
`jari.haverinen@pohde.fi`

Abstract. Digital treatment modalities, particularly digital therapeutics (DTx) and remote patient monitoring (RPM), are increasingly recognized for their potential to improve clinical outcomes and healthcare system efficiency. Some European countries have established national health technology assessment (HTA) and reimbursement frameworks to support their integration into routine care, with Germany, France, and Belgium serving as frontrunners. Finland has been an early developer of HTA methodologies for digital health technologies (DHTs) through the Digi-HTA model, published in 2019 and implemented as part of the routine assessment activities of the Finnish Coordinating Center for Health Technology Assessment (FinCCHTA). Despite this methodological readiness, Finland has lacked a national reimbursement model for digital treatments, limiting their systematic adoption in healthcare. Recognizing the growing role of digital treatments and the need for evidence-informed reimbursement mechanisms, the Finnish Ministry of Social Affairs and Health launched a national Digital Therapy Trial for 2025–2026. Based on the outcomes of this trial, the goal is to develop a proposal for the next government program outlining an assessment and reimbursement model for digital treatments suitable for integration into the Finnish healthcare system. The trial is implemented by DigiFinland, with Kela, Sitra, and FinCCHTA serving as key expert partners. Within the project, FinCCHTA is responsible for conducting Digi-HTA assessments of the applications selected for the trial and for producing a summary of the assessed digital therapies, as well as a proposal for a future assessment model for digital therapies within the context of the Finnish healthcare system.

Keywords: Health technology assessment · Digital health · Digital therapeutics · Reimbursement

1 Introduction

Digital health technologies (DHTs), particularly digital therapeutics (DTx) and remote patient monitoring (RPM), are increasingly recognized for their potential to improve clinical outcomes and healthcare efficiency [1, 2]. These interventions include self-care

M. Särestöniemi et al. (Eds.): NCDHWS 2026, CCIS 3009, pp. 113–117, 2026.
https://doi.org/10.1007/978-3-032-28812-7_10

guidance, cognitive behavioral therapy, and RPM, and have demonstrated benefits in conditions such as chronic pain, diabetes, and insomnia, as well as in weight management [3–6]. However, evidence regarding their superiority over conventional treatments remains inconsistent and condition-specific [4, 5, 7]. Effectiveness may depend on how the intervention is implemented within care pathways [8]. Methodological limitations, variability in study quality, and contextual factors such as patient digital literacy and engagement further complicate the evaluation and implementation of digital interventions [5, 7, 9].

Wang et al. [10] emphasized that, in addition to research evidence, the adoption of digital interventions requires evidence-based health technology assessment (HTA) frameworks and clear approval and reimbursement procedures. Consequently, several European countries have already implemented, or are in the process of developing, HTA frameworks specifically for digital interventions [1, 2]. Finland has also been a pioneer in this field. Since 2019, the Finnish Coordinating Center for Health Technology Assessment (FinCCHTA) has conducted independent Digi-HTA assessments for DHTs, which some wellbeing service counties have already used as part of decision-making related to DHTs [1–3, 11–14].

Germany, France, and Belgium are European leaders in reimbursement models for digital therapies, all linking reimbursement to independent HTA assessment. Germany's 2019 Digital Healthcare Act introduced the Fast Track pathway for DTx classified as low-risk, CE-marked medical devices (class I and IIa), referred to as "Digitale Gesundheitsanwendungen" (DiGAs). France's Prise en charge anticipée numérique (PECAN) model, launched in 2023, enables reimbursement for DTx and RPM across all risk classes. Belgium launched an assessment and reimbursement model in 2018, named the Validation Pyramid, which applies to all CE-marked mHealth medical devices (all risk classes). [1, 2, 6].

Despite HTA methodological readiness for DHTs, Finland has lacked a national reimbursement model, limiting their adoption [3]. To address this, the Ministry of Social Affairs and Health launched a national Digital Therapy Trial (2025–2026) to inform a future assessment and reimbursement model. Twelve applications from different Finnish companies have now been selected for the trial. These include digital therapies classified as medical devices for treatment or secondary prevention, as well as wellness applications. The trial is implemented by DigiFinland, with Kela, Sitra, and FinCCHTA as key expert partners, each assigned a specific role in developing the future assessment and reimbursement model [15].

FinCCHTA's role is to conduct Digi-HTA assessments of the applications selected for the trial. In addition to conducting the assessments, FinCCHTA's role in the pilot is to produce a summary of the assessed digital therapies as well as a proposal for a future assessment model for digital therapies within the context of the Finnish healthcare system.

The research questions of this study are:

1. Are the applications selected for the Digital Therapy Trial effective based on research evidence, and do they meet the key requirements of the Digi-HTA assessment criteria?
2. What is the most suitable assessment model for digital therapies in the Finnish healthcare context?

2   Materials and Methods

The case study related to the trial project will be based on observational data collected from the Digi-HTA assessments of the applications selected for the trial. The findings emerging from the assessments will be analyzed using inductive content analysis. The trial is now underway, and 12 products from different companies have been selected to participate. Two of these selected applications have already been assessed using the Digi-HTA methodology prior to the start of the trial project. For these products, a new Digi-HTA assessment will not be required during the trial. However, the findings from the assessments of these two previously assessed products will be included in the overall analysis conducted within the project.

The study conducted during the trial will assess the extent to which the applications selected for the trial meet the core requirements of the Digi-HTA framework. A key aspect to be observed from an HTA perspective will be the strength of the research evidence supporting the assumed benefits of the applications selected for the trial, and whether this evidence could serve as a basis for granting preliminary or permanent reimbursement in the future. In addition, the findings will highlight observations related to other key domains assessed by the Digi-HTA methodology, namely safety, costs, usability and accessibility, and data security and protection. Some of the applications selected for the trial will utilize artificial intelligence (AI), so observations related to AI and its use will also be highlighted.

The proposal for a future Finnish assessment model will be based on a synthesis of the findings from the trial project, as well as the knowledge and best practices already established in the assessment models of pioneering countries such as Germany, France, and Belgium. From international assessment models, their key characteristics will be considered, as well as how they could be applied to the Finnish healthcare context. The proposal should also take into account the upcoming changes in HTA activities in Finland.

3   Discussion

In Finland, as in other EU countries, the potential of various digital treatment modalities has been recognized, along with the need to establish a systematic assessment and reimbursement model to support their adoption [1]. Germany, France, and Belgium have been pioneers in this area by developing national reimbursement models linked to HTA assessments for digital therapies [1, 2]. A common feature of these countries is that only applications classified as medical devices are accepted into the process. A key aspect of these models is that the starting point for assessments is the health benefits that digital therapies provide to patients, rather than the benefits to healthcare service organizations [1–3]. In addition, all models allow either permanent reimbursement or preliminary reimbursement, enabling companies to collect additional evidence in real-world settings [2].

Finland's Digital Therapy Trial is now underway, and a total of 12 products from different companies have been selected for the pilot [15]. One of the pilot's objectives is to determine whether the models already implemented in pioneering countries and the lessons learned from them can be applied directly to the Finnish healthcare system or whether national fine-tuning is required. Since only applications provided by Finnish companies were accepted into the trial, the results will provide insights into the capability of Finnish companies to deliver digital therapies that are effective within the context of the Finnish healthcare system.

Unlike the models in Germany, France, and Belgium, which accept only applications classified as medical devices, the Finnish trial also includes applications that are not classified as medical devices, such as a digital lifestyle intervention and an application intended for monitoring the nutrition of a patient with diabetes [1, 2, 15]. Based on the trial results, it will be possible to better assess whether applications not classified as medical devices could also fall within the scope of reimbursement in Finland.

In the Digital Therapy Trial project, different expert organizations have been assigned specific roles in developing a future assessment and reimbursement model for integration into the Finnish healthcare system. For example, Kela (the Social Insurance Institution of Finland) is examining in the trial what possibilities exist for establishing reimbursement for the applications in Finland. FinCCHTA's role is to conduct Digi-HTA assessments of the selected applications and to produce a proposal for a future assessment model for digital therapies in Finland, drawing on the trial results and international experience. Compared internationally, the Digi-HTA method is already very comprehensive; however, the trial may still bring forward new perspectives that should be implemented in future versions of the Digi-HTA framework [3, 14]. As the trial is still in its early phase and collaboration with the wellbeing services counties is just beginning, findings related to the Digi-HTA assessments performed during the trial will not be available until late 2026.

Acknowledgments. The digital therapy trial is part of the Ministry of Social Affairs and Health's national research, development and innovation program in the health and welfare sector.

Disclosure of Interests None

References

1. Mezei, F., Horváth, K., Pálfi, M., Lovas, K., Ádám, I., Túri, G.: International practices in health technology assessment and public financing of digital health technologies: recommendations for Hungary. Front. Public Health **11**, 1197949 (2023)
2. Tarricone, R., Petracca, F., Weller, H.M.: Towards harmonizing assessment and reimbursement of digital medical devices in the EU through mutual learning. NPJ Digital Medicine **7**(1), 268 (2024)
3. Haverinen J, The Digi-HTA, a new health technology assessment model for digital health technologies. Doctoral thesis (2024). https://urn.fi/URN:NBN:fi:oulu-202409125818
4. HLi, C., Luo, Q., Wu, H.: Digital therapeutics for insomnia: an umbrella review and meta-meta-analysis. NPJ Digit. Med. **8**, 554 (2025)
5. Seo, Y.G., Salonurmi, T., Jokelainen, T.: Lifestyle counselling by persuasive information and communications technology reduces prevalence of metabolic syndrome in a dose-response manner: a randomized clinical trial (PrevMetSyn). Ann. Med. **52**, 321–330 (2020)

6. SVDGV: DiGA-Report 2024: Market development of digital health applications. Berlin: Spitzenverband Digitale Gesundheitsversorgung (2024). https://www.digitalversorgt.de/en/news/diga-report-2024. Last accessed 31 Jan 2026

7. Tayshete, I., McCarthy, C., Ademoyegun, A., Gebrye, T., Fatoye, F., Mbada, C.: Effectiveness of smartphone-based applications in low-back pain rehabilitation: a systematic review and meta-analysis. Bull. Fac. Phys. Ther. **30**, 29 (2025)

8. Kendziorra, J., Seerig, K.H., Winkler, T.J., Gewald, H.: From awareness to integration: a qualitative interview study on the impact of digital therapeutics on physicians' practices in Germany. BMC Health Serv. Res. **25**, 568 (2025)

9. Koller, C., Blanchard, M., Hügle, T.: Assessment of digital therapeutics in decentralized clinical trials: a scoping review. PLOS Digit. Health **4**, e0000905 (2025)

10. Wang, C., Lee, C., Shin, H.: Digital therapeutics from bench to bedside. NPJ Digit. Med. **6**, 38 (2023)

11. Haverinen, J., Keränen, N., Falkenbach, P., Maijala, A., Kolehmainen, T., Reponen, J.: Digi-HTA: health technology assessment framework for digital healthcare services. Finnish J. EHealth EWelfare **11**(4), 326–341 (2019)

12. Jääskelä, J., et al.: Digi-HTA, assessment framework for digital healthcare services: information security and data protection in health technology—initial experiences. Finnish J. EHealth EWelfare **14**(1), 19–30 (2022)

13. Haverinen, J., Turpeinen, M., Falkenbach, P., Reponen, J.: Implementation of a new Digi-HTA process for digital health technologies in Finland. Int. J. Technol. Assess. Health Care **38**(1), e68 (2022)

14. Haverinen, J., et al.: Finnish Digi-HTA assessment model for digital health and an international comparison. In: Särestöniemi, M., et al. (eds.) Digital Health and Wireless Solutions, NCD-HWS 2024, Communications in Computer and Information Science, vol. 2084, pp. 309–321. Springer, Cham (2024)

15. DigiFinland. Digital therapy trial. https://digifinland.fi/digihoidot/. Last accessed 27 Jan 2026

Post-implementation Monitoring of CE-Marked AI-CDS in Radiology: A Longitudinal Mixed-Methods Evaluation of Spread, Scale-Up, and Sustainability

Line Silsand[1,2]([envelope]) [ORCID] and Gro-Hilde Severinsen[1] [ORCID]

[1] Norwegian Centre for E-Health Research, Sykehusvn. 23, 9019 Tromsø, Norway
`Line.Silsand@ehealthresearch.no`
[2] UiT The Arctic University of Norway, Hansine Hansens Veg 18, 9019 Tromsø, Norway

Abstract. This paper presents a longitudinal mixed-methods evaluation study of a CE-marked AI clinical decision support system (AI-CDS) for fracture detection implemented across four hospitals in a Norwegian hospital trust. Drawing on 85 interviews, observations, and operational monitoring data (2021–2025), the study examines how AI-CDS reshapes diagnostic workflows, redistributes responsibilities, and influences patient flow after deployment. Using the Non-adoption, Abandonment, Scale-up, Spread, and Sustainability (NASSS) Framework and Information Infrastructure (II) theory, we show that the static nature of CE-marked AI-CDS requires organisational adaption, involving infrastructuring work, new routines, and continuous governance. Findings reveal site-level variation in discharge practices and workflow design, shaped by geography, organisational maturity, and existing infrastructures. We argue that spread, scale-up, and sustainability unfold as non-linear, context-dependent processes that require ongoing post-implementation monitoring. The study highlights the need for lifecycle-oriented, socio-technical evaluation to ensure safe, meaningful, and sustainable integration of AI-CDS in healthcare.

Keywords: AI clinical decision support (AI-CDS) · Post implementation monitoring · Spread · Scale · Sustainability · Information infrastructure theory

1 Introduction

Today's healthcare systems are under increasing pressure to deliver high-quality care during rising demand, workforce shortages, and constrained budgets. In this context, artificial intelligence (AI) has emerged as a promising tool to address these challenges, of balancing the needs of patients, improving population health, enhancing cost-effectiveness, and improving efficiency in clinical workflows—also referred to as the quadruple aim of healthcare [1–3].

Radiology has been at the forefront of AI adoption in healthcare, with nearly 300 Conformité Europèenne (CE)-marked AI-based clinical decision support (AI-CDS)

© The Author(s) 2026
M. Särestöniemi et al. (Eds.): NCDHWS 2026, CCIS 3009, pp. 118–137, 2026.
https://doi.org/10.1007/978-3-032-28812-7_11

products now available for clinical use across Europe [4, 5]. These tools are designed to support radiologists in tasks such as image interpretation and anomaly detection. Despite significant technological advancements and substantial investments, the anticipated widespread integration of AI-CDS into clinical radiology workflows has not materialized as expected [6]. Even with intense commercialization, empirical evidence supporting claims of improved patient outcomes, healthcare effectiveness, and efficiency remains limited. One of the key barriers to adoption is the limited transparency and generalizability of performance data from commercial AI-CDS products. Regulatory standards, such as CE-marking, confirm compliance with safety and quality requirements, but they do not guarantee effectiveness or usability in diverse clinical environments [4]. Moreover, CE-marking does not provide insight into how AI-CDS impacts radiologists' workflows, decision-making processes or time efficiency [6–8]. Research indicates that CE-marking alone is insufficient to ensure successful implementation and adoption in real-world settings [3, 4].

Understanding these broader implications is essential because new technologies often reshape practice in ways that are difficult to predict. AI-CDS has the potential to fundamentally trigger changes to how clinical diagnostic and treatment processes are carried out. Current AI-CDS applications are not primarily designed to support the existing diagnostic pathway; rather, predictive AI-CDS tools typically aim to deliver a definitive output, often a diagnostic label, by addressing a binary question such as whether a patient has a specific condition or not. Instead of replacing traditional diagnostic processes, expert clinicians are increasingly adapting to AI-CDS by integrating and transforming these processes to leverage AI-CDS -driven outputs [9].

While there is significant uncertainty surrounding the effects of AI-CDS, one thing is becoming increasingly evident: fully realizing its potential will require fundamental changes in how we evaluate its deployment in clinical practice [9, 10]. Current evaluations of AI-CDS have primarily focused on system performance in controlled settings and short-term outcomes, neglecting longer-term impacts and unintended consequences. To inform evidence-based decision-making, there is a growing recognition that evaluations must consider real-world outcomes of AI-CDS systems as an assistive tool embedded in complex clinical workflows [3]. To address these gaps, this paper seeks to address the following research question:

How can longitudinal, mixed-methods process evaluations reveal the contextual, organizational, and infrastructural factors that shape the barriers, benefits, and evolving work practices following the implementation of CE-marked AI-CDS in radiology?

Drawing on a multi-year empirical collaboration between a Norwegian hospital trust and our research institution, we examine the post-implementation phase of an AI-CDS application for fracture detection in X-rays. The AI-CDS application is regulatory approved, and CE-marked as a CDS tool to support healthcare professionals' clinical decisions through image analysis.

This paper contributes to the existing AI research by highlighting the importance of longitudinal, mixed-methods process evaluations in understanding the spread, scale-up, and sustainability of AI solutions. By exploring how to address barriers and leverage benefits at multiple levels within healthcare organizations, we offer insights into aligning AI-CDS implementation with clinical and organizational goals.

2 Theory

As emphasized in the introduction, the added value of AI-CDS in radiology is today insufficiently understood [6, 10]. Existing studies indicate that many radiologists do not experience a substantial reduction in workload following the implementation of AI-CDS systems [6, 7, 11]. This suggests that evaluation approaches must extend beyond conventional performance metrics such as validating sensitivity and specificity. Evaluation approaches should address the actual clinical added value by considering dimensions such as patient impact, influence on clinical decision-making, workflow implications, and the overall benefit for patients [10]. Without a comprehensive understanding of these dimensions, the adoption and scaling of AI-CDS systems will probably continue to remain limited, even though more than 300 CE-marked products are available on the market [6, 8].

2.1 Evaluating and Implementing AI in Digital Health: From Metrics to Context and Complexity

Research on the implementation of digital health technologies, including AI-CDSs, shows that technological transformations are difficult to capture if evaluation is limited to immediate improvements, efficiency gains, or "*support*" effects [3, 12, 13]. Systems that appear promising in one environment often fail to reproduce in another, reflecting the influence of local workflows, infrastructures, and professional practices [2, 3]. Moreover, systematic performance measurement and publication of outcomes remain relatively uncommon in current implementation efforts [3].

Against this backdrop, evaluation should extend beyond traditional performance metrics to examine long-term effects, potential downsides, and unintended consequences, like loss of professional skills, increases in unnecessary referrals or tests, and biases that affect specific groups or conditions [3, 13, 14]. When technologies are implemented in an organization, they rarely fit seamlessly into existing work practice; rather, they contribute to changing work practices, shift organizational attention, and introduce new uncertainties. Implementation is therefore best understood as an evolving negotiated process rather than a straightforward linear transition [13].

Many of the observed challenges stem from issues like contextual differences in needs, existing work processes, health information infrastructures, care practices, interorganizational relationships, ethnic characteristics, and organizational cultures [3]. In addition, only a few studies of AI-CDS in healthcare sufficiently address how algorithms can be incorporated into clinicians' workflows, even though contextual organization of work (and the changes that follow the introduction of new tools) can materially affect algorithm performance [2, 3]. To improve implementations, organizational, technological, and user contexts should be treated as core components of evaluations; to enhance the generalizability of results and clarify requirements for adaptation when moving systems across settings [2, 3].

The implementation literature often uses the concepts of spread, scale-up, and sustainability to describe trajectories beyond initial pilots [15]. However, these terms are not always defined consistently and are sometimes used interchangeably to denote implementation beyond the original site. Following Papoutsi et al. [15], we use the terms as follows:

- **Spread** refers to the replication of practices across sites. It has often been conceptualized as the cumulative result of multiple implementations, and rather than as a separate phenomenon. There is limited discussion of adoption strategies for successful implementations transferred across settings.
- **Scale-up** denotes the organizational and infrastructural capacity required to underpin, support, and extend improvement interventions to widespread use across additional settings.
- **Sustainability** refers to maintaining and adapting improvements and their benefits over time in response to diverse and changing local contexts.

These are often defined and addressed as separate phases to be addressed in a linear process. Still, in real-life implementation processes, they are most often intertwined. These highlights spread, scale-up, and sustainability as elements of a complex adaptive system rather than as separate, sequential phases. The interdependence of these phases and the mutual reinforcement of results in them contribute to shaping and reshaping the context where they are implemented. Papoutsi et al. [15] outline a shift from attempting to perfect an intervention in isolation to growing it organically within its real-world context. Such an approach is better suited to the local context's social, cultural, and organizational complexities enabling adoption of local preconditions encompassing negotiations and discussions, rather than inflexible rule-based implementations [15]. In sum, robust evaluation and successful implementation of AI-CDS systems require shifting the focus from single-site linear performance metrics to assessments that include focusing on context, complexity, and change over time. The expectations for how spread, scale-up, and sustainability will unfold may significantly influence both the way these processes are studied and how they are operationalized in practice [15].

2.2 Addressing Context and Lifecycle in AI-CDS Implementation

To improve adoption of AI-CDS in real-world clinical practice, research must systematically address context-related barriers and facilitators at multiple levels of healthcare organizations [14]. This requires evaluating the full lifecycle of AI-CDS solutions, from procurement and pilot testing to post-implementation monitoring and long-term integration [14]. Lifecycle approaches emphasize socio-technical dynamics and stakeholder engagement throughout implementation, ensuring that evaluation captures both technical performance and organizational adaptation. A range of frameworks has emerged to guide the evaluation and implementation of such technologies, e.g. Consolidated Framework for Implementation Research (CFIR) [16], Technology, People, Organizations, and Macroenvironmental factors (TPOM) by Cresswell et al. [17]), Non-Adoption, Abandonment, Scale-Up, Spread, and Sustainability (NASSS) by Greenhalgh et al. [18], the Health Information Technology Evaluation Toolkit by Cusack and Poon [17], and the Technological–Organizational–Environmental (TOE) framework by Tornatzky [18]. These frameworks provide a structured lens for assessing not only the performance of AI-CDS tools but also the broader conditions that shape their adoption, use, and impact.

Accordingly, regardless of the selected framework, several evaluative dimensions remain critical [12, 16, 20]. Attention to context, including organizational, technological, and user factors:

- **Designing assistive tools** that help users understand system logic.
- **Optimizing systems** for ethics and equity.
- **Continuous evaluation and monitoring** of processes and outcomes.

These considerations remain relevant across health systems and infrastructures, as they shape both adoption and sustainability. Systematic use of detailed evaluation frameworks can support transferability of learning across settings, while revealing how unique aspects of different AI programs become co-shaped by their implementation environments [12, 16, 20].

In this paper, the NASSS framework by Greenhalgh et al. [12, 18] is applied to an empirical case (see the method chapter). NASSS was originally developed to study and guide real-time implementation of digitally enabled care, but it has since also become useful for evaluating AI-CDS implementations. NASSS provides a structured way to examine the micro-, meso-, and macro-level factors that influence implementation and its outcomes.

The framework's seven domains: condition, technology, value proposition, adopters, organization, wider context, and adaptation over time, help to identify where complexity and value arise. Because NASSS is both theoretically grounded and flexible, it supports formative evaluation throughout a project's lifespan by guiding the mapping of values, barriers, and evolving sources of complexity [12, 15, 18]. While NASSS enables a structured understanding of the complexity surrounding adoption and implementation, it does not fully account for the historically embedded, evolving nature of the technological environments into which AI-CDS systems are introduced. To address this, we also draw on Information Infrastructure (II) theory [21–24].

In this regard, II theory offers a valuable lens for understanding the interaction between technology and organizational context [21, 22]. Infrastructures are always built on existing practice, systems, and users—the installed base accumulating organically over time [22, 23]. This embeddedness means infrastructures are entirely intertwined with organizational routines and often remain invisible until interruptions occur, such as the implementation of a new system, e.g., AI-CDSs. II theory emphasizes relational and historical dimensions, highlighting how micro-level practices (e.g., clinical workflows) connect to macro-level structures (e.g., cross-organizational networks) [15]. It supports multiple, interdependent activities rather than isolated tasks, which is why a change in one component can ripple across the wider organisation [22, 23]. Consequently, understanding AI-CDSs as part of the II, the new technology will influence organizational hierarchies, redistribute responsibilities, and introduce new roles and routines [24].

"Growth" is an important part of *"infrastructuring,"* as it involves actively shaping and sustaining systems through customization and integration. Successful implementation requires balancing local variations with interoperability across sites, ensuring continuity while accommodating change. This perspective underscores the importance of socio-technical approaches to design and evaluation, recognizing infrastructures as dynamic, context-sensitive constellations that co-evolve with organizational

settings [21–23]. The impact of new technologies and calls for process-oriented, context-sensitive evaluations are essential to capture both intended and unintended consequences of AI-CDS deployment in healthcare [2, 3, 15].

Unlike adaptable systems such as Electronic Health Records (EHRs), CE-marked AI-CDS applications are static products that cannot be modified without undergoing a new CE-marking. This rigidity places greater demands on organizations to adjust work-flows and practices through organizational change processes alongside implementations to accommodate the technology and realize its intended benefits. Therefore, research designs must explore the relationship between intervention and context beyond diagnostic performance, investigating how AI-CDS contributes to patient value, influences clinical decision-making, and reshapes workflows in specific settings [3, 10].

3 Methods

3.1 Research Setting

This study was conducted in collaboration with a Norwegian hospital trust comprising Bærum, Drammen, Ringerike, and Kongsberg hospitals. The trust serves approximately 10% of the Norwegian population (500, 000 citizens). It includes one imaging diagnostics department across the four hospitals, where the radiology units vary in organizational structure and on-call radiologist availability. In 2023, the trust deployed a CE-marked AI-CDS application, BoneView from Gleamer, for detecting bone fractures in X-ray images. The procurement was motivated by increasing imaging volumes and radiologist workload. The initial expectations for the AI-CDS were to enhance the efficiency of the diagnostic process.

3.2 Data Collection

This study employed a mixed-methods approach, combining qualitative and quantitative data collected from 2021 to 2025 (see Table 1).

The qualitative data was collected at four different phases of the procurement and implementation process (see Fig. 1). The interview guide was adapted to each phase of the implementation process. The interview guides and data analysis were guided by the NASSS framework [12, 18].

The Quantitative Data was collected separately from each hospital's monitoring dashboard to enable a descriptive comparative analysis (See Table 1). The monthly data extracts are manually prepared by one person at the Hospital Trust. The dashboard distinguishes data for each hospital (see Table 1). The dashboard and figures have been used in follow-up meetings with individual hospitals to further enhance their impact.

3.3 Data Analysis

Qualitative Analysis

For this paper, only the interview data from the post-implementation phase (January 2025) were analyzed. The remaining interviews were used solely to describe the

Table 1. Qualitative and quantitative data collection

Qualitative data collection	Quantitative data collection
• Extensive data collection from 2021–2025 including 85 interviews at four different stages of the process • Observations of the AI solution in use at two hospitals • Observations - in the dialogue-based procurement, - in pre implementation workshops - meetings at all stages of the process • Ongoing status meetings with the project group and the Directorate of health every 3 weeks	• Operational data were collected by each hospital from October 2023 to May 2025 • Monthly data extracts from RIS are done manually by one person in Hospital Trust • Variables included: - Number of patients and examinations analysed by AI - Referral sources (e.g., general practitioners, ERs) - AI result categories (negative, uncertain, positive) - Patient outcomes (e.g., discharged home, referred to ED) • Data was collected separately for each hospital to enable comparative analysis

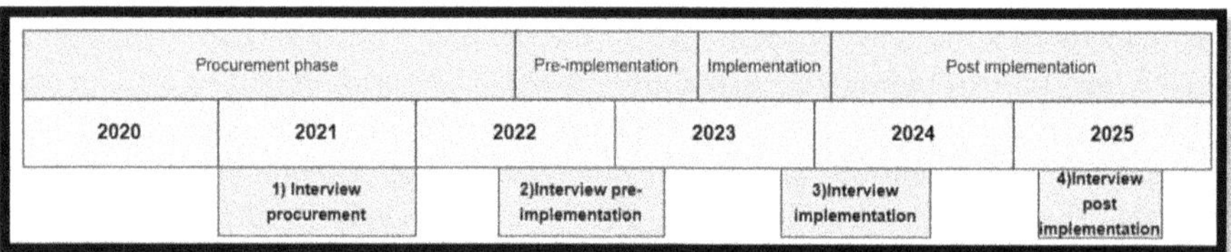

Fig. 1. The different phases of the qualitative data collection

workflows before and after AI implementation and to provide contextual background for understanding the AI-CDS implementation. The workflow description is presented in Chap. 4.1.

The post-implementation data includes 19 interviews with 12 radiographers: 4 radiologists and 3 clinical managers. The interviews explored how the AI-CDS reshaped work practices, redirected organizational attention, and introduced new risk factors influencing the spread, scale-up, and sustainability of the AI system. A two-step analysis was conducted, using the NASSS framework [12, 20] as the first step to sort the data into the seven NASSS categories. In the second step, we used a reflexive thematic data analysis [25], guided by the theoretical lenses described in Sect. 2.0 and with a particular focus on the II theory as the guiding analytical framework. II theory emphasizes relational and historical dimensions, linking micro-level practices (e.g., clinical workflows and handovers) to macro-level structures (e.g., cross-organizational networks, certification regimes, and governance). This perspective allowed us to examine the AI-CDS not as an isolated tool but as a component within a broader socio-technical infrastructure. We operationalized II in our coding by combining deductive codes (micro–macro linkages, installed base constraints, infrastructuring work, growth, interoperability) with inductive codes derived from interviews and observations. Theme development followed an abductive approach, resulting in three key themes: Diagnostic Uncertainty in AI-Assisted Radiology; Workflow and Logistical Adaptations; and Redistribution of Responsibilities, in which each of the themes reflects how infrastructural relations shape and are shaped by AI-CDS implementation. The three key themes are presented in 4.0 Result.

Quantitative Descriptive Analysis.

For the quantitative descriptive analyses, we compared the numbers from the hospitals' monitoring dashboards. These numbers are continuously updated and provide an overview of the distribution of total examinations, negative findings, and discharge decisions across the four hospitals, including percentages for negative exams and patients discharged after negative results. In this paper, we included the numbers from the hospital's monitoring dashboard from October 2023 to April 2025 (see Table 1). In 4.0 Result, the numerical data are systematically presented using tables, bar charts, and graphs to facilitate clear visualization and interpretation. Each table and figure is accompanied by a descriptive narrative that explains the key findings and contextualizes the data.

4   Results

In this section, we first present the workflow description before and after implementing the AI-CDS (Chap. 4.1). Then we present a descriptive analysis comparing the numbers from each hospital's monitoring dashboard, along with the main findings from the three key themes that emerged from the qualitative analysis. By combining quantitative presentation with qualitative explanation, the approach enhances transparency and complements the other, providing a more comprehensive understanding of the post-implementation phase. Qualitative approaches offer depth and context, while quantitative approaches contribute breadth and generalizability.

4.1   Workflow Description Based on Qualitative Data

To understand the potential barriers and benefits arising from the introduction of AI-CDS, it is necessary to conduct a qualitative baseline description of the existing technologies, work practices, and users (the installed base) [22, 23]. New technologies such as AI-CDS influence hierarchies, redistribute responsibilities, and introduce new roles and routines, addressing the need to provide follow-up descriptions of work practices when the technology is deployed in clinical settings (a life-cycle approach) [3, 14, 15]. The following is a brief description of work practices before and after the implementation of the AI-CDS.

Before AI Implementation

Prior to AI deployment, patients with suspected fractures were referred to radiology by general practitioners, from the municipalities' Emergency Rooms (ER), or emergency departments (ED). Radiographers performed X-rays, while radiologists checked images quality and interpreted the images during daytime hours. When the day shift ends, the number of radiologists available for acute X-ray cases drops to just a few at the two large hospitals and no radiologists are present at the two small ones (see Fig. 2).

Before AI was introduced, the established workflow at Bærum Hospital allowed radiographers to send patients without suspected fractures back to the municipality's ER since they shared the location. Similar practices for the radiographer's workflow existed at Kongsberg Clinic and Ringerike Clinic, where radiologists were not present during evenings and nights. Here, radiographers could refer patients to the ED or, in cases where images clearly indicate no fracture, send them home, with radiologists interpreting images the following day. Drammen Hospital, however, had a different workflow, and the hospital and the municipality's ER are not located at the same site. Patients referred to imaging with suspected fractures were always directed to the hospital's ED after X-rays were taken. Here, radiographers lacked delegated authority to send patients home, even when images clearly showed no fracture. Outside of dayshifts, the physicians working in the ED, often with limited radiological expertise, were responsible for image interpretation, leading to delays, increased patient waiting times, and potential diagnostic uncertainty.

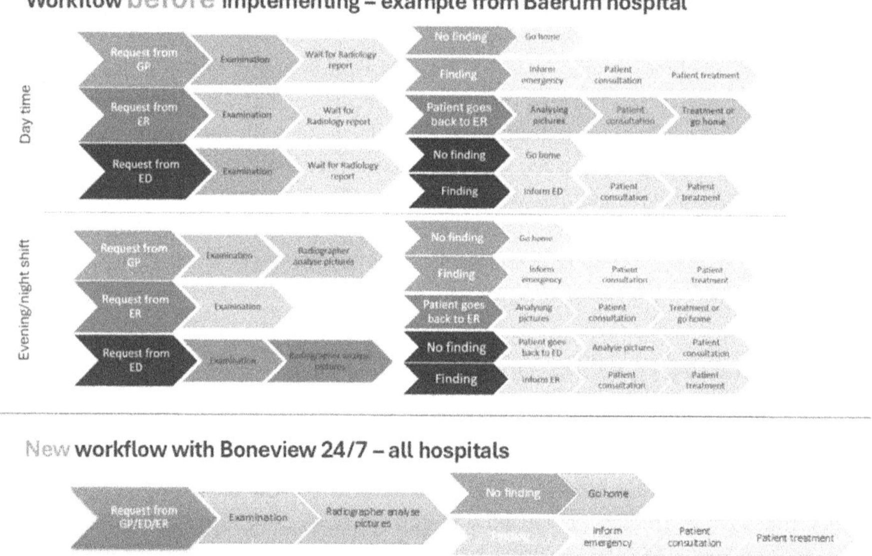

Fig. 2. The workflow before and after the AI system was implemented (Fig. 1 is by Vestre Viken HF)

After AI Implementation

Using BoneView as AI-CDS in the workflow, radiographers now perform an X-ray, then upload anonymized images to the cloud-based BoneView solution, which provides a preliminary result within minutes. The results were flagged in the Radiology Information System (RIS) as follows:

- **Green (no fracture)**
- **Red (fracture)**
- **Yellow (uncertain)**.

Based on the referral, the AI-CDS output, and clinical interpretations, the radiographers decided whether to discharge the patients, refer them to the orthopaedics or refer them to the ED. The radiologists continue to interpret all images retrospectively to ensure diagnostic quality and patient safety.

4.2 Presentation of Data from the Monitoring Dashboards

Table 2 gives an overview of each hospital's total examinations where the AI-CDS is used and the total number of patients having their examination assessed by the AI-CDS system. The total number of examinations exceeded the total number of patients. The main reason is that multiple images are taken for each patient to capture different angles of the suspected fracture. These differences were also reflected in the ratio of negative examinations to patients with negative results. The differences between the two comparable categories were distributed roughly equally across the hospitals. Moreover, the percentage of negative examinations was almost equally distributed across hospitals, with approximately 50% of the total examinations at each hospital being negative. The proportion of patients with negative examinations who were sent home varied across hospitals, with Bærum Hospital sending home the highest rate at 71.5% (see Table 2).

Table 2. Overview of numbers related to the use of AI technology

Hospital	Total images	Total patients	Negative images	Patients negative	Patients sent home	% negative image	% negative patients sent home
Bærum	26 403	21 922	13 401	10 277	7 347	50.8	71.5
Drammen	19 946	16 726	10 981	8 464	2 982	55.1	35.2
Kongsberg	7 849	6 294	4 257	3 032	1 494	54.2	49.3
Ringerike	8 801	7 332	4 444	3 360	1 727	50.5	51.4

The numbers presented in Fig. 3 demonstrate notable variation in patient management following negative AI-CDS results across the four hospitals. For patients with an AI-CDS negative result, Bærum Hospital had the highest direct-discharge rate at 72%, with the remaining 28% referred for additional follow-up. The patients who require further follow-up are distributed as follows: 10% were referred to the municipality emergency room (ER), 5% to the hospital's acute unit or outpatient clinic, and 13% received other kinds of follow-up. This reflected a streamlined workflow enabled by proximity to emergency services, both in the hospital and the municipality. In contrast, for patients with an AI-CDS negative result, Drammen discharged 35%, while 37% were referred to the hospital's outpatient clinic or ED, and 27% received other forms of follow-up. None were referred to the municipality's Emergency Room.

These numbers indicate a more cautious approach, differences in workflow integration, and a greater physical distance to the ER. Kongsberg and Ringerike showed intermediate patterns: 49% and 51% of patients without fractures were discharged home, respectively, while 31% and 15% were referred to hospital services. Ringerike additionally referred 2% of patients to the municipality's ER. These differences suggest that organizational priorities and geographical factors influence how negative AI-CDS findings are managed, even when no fractures were detected.

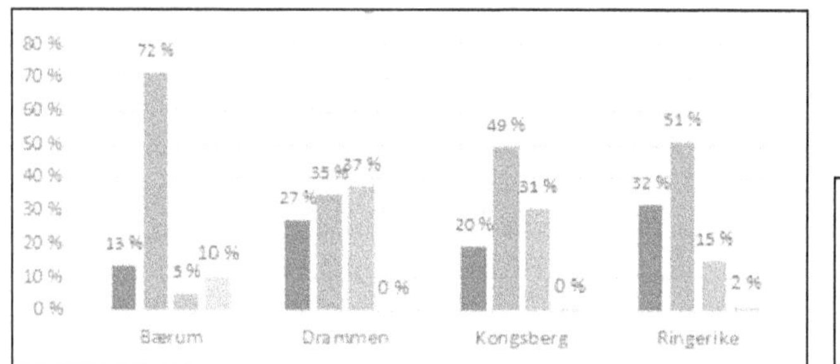
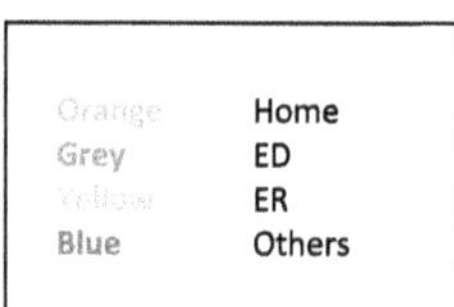

Fig. 3. Distribution of Patients with no fracture detected by the AI-CDS

Over time, the proportion of patients with no fracture detected by the AI-CDS discharged home remained relatively stable across most hospitals. However, a slight increase was observed in Bærum, Drammen, and Ringerike, whereas Kongsberg shows an increase between November 2024 and February 2025, after which the proportion of patients sent home dropped again to around 40% (See Fig. 4). These trends indicated that while overall patterns stabilized, local workflow adjustments and organizational strategies continued to shape discharge practices.

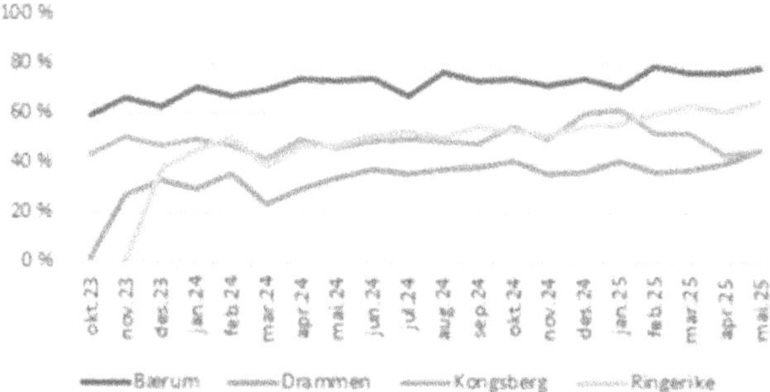

Fig. 4. Trend in the number of patients discharged home after AI-CDS detects no fracture (October 2023–May 2025)

4.3 Diagnostic Uncertainty in AI-CDS Assisted Radiology

Following the implementation of the AI-CDS for fracture detection, diagnostic uncertainty remained a concern. While the algorithm demonstrated high performance on simple fractures, its limitations became evident in complex cases and examinations affected by e.g., the quality of the images or injuries where it was important to compare to historical injuries and images. Interview data illustrated these challenges: *«Just today, there was a severe talus fracture that the AI-CDS didn't flag as red"* (Radiologist 7).

False negatives and positives persist, underscoring the need for human oversight even when AI-CDS outputs were classified as *"green (negative)."* Radiographers and radiologists reported that discrepancies between AI-CDS results and clinical presentation often triggered manual review and escalation, especially when the AI-CDS result was negative, but the patient remained in significant pain. Technical factors, such as skin folds and old fractures, further compromised algorithmic accuracy, leading to misread or flagged results labeled *"yellow"* (uncertain).

However, before using AI-CDS, at most locations, patients who were referred to fracture X-rays from the municipalities' ERs after regular hours had to proceed to an examination in the hospital's ED, most often waiting hours in line. Even if the radiographers had clearly observed that the X-ray showed no fracture. Today, using AI-CDS has changed this workflow: patients are sent home directly if the referral does not specify any other action, and radiographers don't suspect a fracture. Accordingly, the responsibilities for follow-up after negative AI-CDS results shifted, necessitating clearer referral instructions and standardized procedures, as much more responsibility has fallen on the referring physician, specifically the radiographers, to decide what should happen after the X-ray examination.

These limitations raised patient safety concerns, as negative AI-CDS results risked premature discharge without adequate clinical assessment. However, this limitation has been addressed by implementing additional review procedures (a radiologist always interprets the images the next day) and ensuring medical approval for decisions when AI-CDS results are negative or uncertain. *"The AI-CDS only currently focuses on interpreting bone fractures, which means many musculoskeletal injuries that previously received clinical assessment, such as joint fluid accumulation or ligament damage in arms and legs, may now go undetected"* (Radiologist 7). Professional judgment remained essential when AI outputs deviated from clinical impressions: *"If AI-CDS says there's nothing, but I think it is something there, I add the image to the radiologist's acute response list"* (Radiographer 4).

This vignette illustrates that, despite efficiency gains, AI-CDS integration introduces new risks that necessitate sustained human oversight and adaptive workflows to safeguard diagnostic quality.

4.4 Workflow and Logistical Adaptations Following AI-CDS Integration

The integration of AI-CDS into radiology workflows has introduced significant changes to patient distribution and interdepartmental coordination. The system provided rapid image analysis, typically within minutes, enabling direct discharge of patients from the radiology department when no fracture was detected. These adjustments significantly reduced pressure on ED consultations and patients' waiting time. Radiographers reported that AI-CDS improved the overall fracture workflow by streamlining routines and enhancing mutual understanding among departments.

While AI-CDS adoption has improved the overall workflow, new logistical challenges have emerged. Taking the images for each patient took more time for the radiographers because they had to wait several minutes for the AI-CDS result, then inform patients of the result, and direct them further based on the AI-CDS result and the clinical status of the patient. Responsibility for delivering results has shifted from radiologists to AI-CDS-assisted radiographers, and patient logistics from office staff to radiographers. In the latter changes were particularly noticeable during evenings and weekends when staffing was limited, prompting practical adjustments such as relocating patients to wait outside the imaging lab rather than in the main waiting area.

In cases of uncertainty, radiographers frequently consult orthopedic specialists or radiologists, which can introduce delays in the patient flow: *"In the evening or at night, I can call and ask if the orthopedic specialist can take a look at an image"* (Radiographer 4).

This vignette demonstrates that while AI-CDS enhances efficiency, it simultaneously redistributes responsibilities and creates new logistical dependencies.

4.5   Redistribution of Responsibilities in AI-Assisted Radiology

The implementation of AI-CDS for fracture detection has led to a notable redistribution of responsibilities within the clinical team. Radiographers received a more active role in patient management, including communicating imaging results directly to patients and, in certain cases, determining whether discharge was appropriate based on AI outputs. This represented a significant departure from previous practice, where such decisions were primarily made by radiologists or emergency physicians. As one radiographer observed: *"The workflow for radiographers has changed because we now provide results directly to the patient"* (Radiographer 18).

Following the implementation of the AI-CDS system, radiographers became the last point of contact for patients before discharge, increasing expectations that they provide home-care advice. One radiographer noted the challenge of answering questions such as: *"Do I need to see a GP? Is it safe to use my leg? How often can I take painkillers?"* These are issues that typically require medical expertise beyond their scope. Despite these changes, radiologists remained ultimately responsible for image interpretation, patient follow-up, and X-ray quality assurance.

Radiologists reported minimal direct workload reduction from the AI-CDS implementation; still, they acknowledged that AI-CDS offered opportunities to plan their workdays more effectively. Now they can prioritize and focus on interpreting complex emergency examinations without interruptions from simple X-ray evaluations. The redistribution of tasks has blurred traditional role boundaries and introduced new expectations for collaboration and decision-making. The introduction of AI-CDS shifted responsibility for post-imaging decision-making to referring physicians, as previously mentioned. The responsibility for patient distribution and home sending advice was now increasingly on radiographers.

This vignette illustrates that AI-CDS integration not only alters diagnostic workflows but also reconfigures professional roles, requiring clear protocols and interprofessional communication to ensure patient safety and continuity of care.

5 Discussion

5.1 Evaluating AI Beyond Performance Metrics

Evaluating the implementation and impact of AI-CDS in clinical practice requires moving beyond conventional diagnostic performance metrics (e.g., validation of sensitivity and specificity) to capture organizational, workflow, and clinical value. The findings from this study illustrate that while AI-CDSs, such as BoneView, increase efficiency, they also create new uncertainties and complexities that challenge traditional workflows and decision-making. This aligns with the argument for assessing actual clinical added value, including the impact on patient clinical pathways, the influence on clinical decision-making, workflow implications, and unintended consequences, rather than focusing solely on algorithmic accuracy [3, 10]. One important example from this case was how most radiographers appreciated their new role in patient distribution following the AI-CDS implementation.

Still, their workload increased in complexity, as they had to assess where to send the patients and when to discharge them. The criteria and challenges varied from hospital to hospital, depending on whether radiographers had discharged patients before the AI-CDS implementation, the location of the municipality's ER, and the number of radiologists on call. Without such qualitative contextual knowledge, evaluation results from quantitative data, e.g., dashboards, risk being misinterpreted or failing to generalize properly across settings, particularly given the heterogeneity of healthcare environments and infrastructures [3]. To anchor these points in our quantitative data, approximately half of all examinations were negative across sites, yet the proportion of negative-result patients discharged varied significantly (Bærum 71.5%, Drammen 35.2%, Kongsberg 49.3%, Ringerike 51.4%; see Table 2), demonstrating how organizational context and geographic factors substantially shape realized benefits.

Moreover, because CE-marking assures regulatory compliance but not context-specific effectiveness or usability, local post-implementation monitoring was necessary to verify vendor claims, quality, and outline unintended consequences. The site-level dashboards and mixed-methods evaluation complemented pre-market evidence by revealing how workflow integration and role redistribution influence patient flow and clinical quality. Finally, the observed effects reflected all dimensions of the Quadruple Aim. Patients experienced shorter waiting times and fewer ED visits. Process efficiency improved through smoother clinical pathways and a redistribution of workload. Cost and value gains were realized downstream, extending beyond the radiology department. Staff experiences also improved, as radiographers assumed expanded responsibilities and radiologists were better able to prioritize complex cases.

5.2 Lifecycle Evaluation and Socio-Technical Dynamics

In healthcare services, there is a focus on immediate value and cost savings; however, it is important to recognize that AI-CDS are unlikely to deliver these immediately after implementation. A reason is that AI-CDSs, as part of a larger socio-technical information infrastructure II, require "growth" in actively shaping and sustaining systems through customization and integration to enable AI-CDSs to deliver value and cost-benefit savings [24]. In this case, the AI-CDS generates savings primarily in later stages of the implementation process, and the observed benefits are not immediate or uniformly distributed; instead, they accumulate at different points along the patient pathway and across professional roles.

While the AI-CDS system provides benefits for clinicians, these benefits do not necessarily benefit those who were the original target group. For instance, time savings and throughput benefits are more pronounced in emergencies and orthopedic contexts than in radiology. Still, the cost of investing in the AI-CDS system is borne by the image diagnostics department. Such patterns underscore the importance of lifecycle evaluation, which spans pilot testing, implementation, post-implementation monitoring, and long-term integration, focusing on socio-technical barriers and facilitators, in addition to stakeholder engagement [3, 14]. The socio-technical evaluation outlined extensive values generated by the implementation process, even if the main goal was not achieved shortly after the implementation ended. Benefit realization from such processes takes time and depends on the organization's maturity, as well as on systematic post-implementation monitoring. This is a new way of governing digital solutions in healthcare organizations, as it demands continuous monitoring, as such solutions constantly impact the evolving II [3, 22–24].

In practice, lifecycle monitoring should operate at multiple levels (e.g., counts of AI-assisted examinations, discharge rates after negative results, downstream utilization, and time saved), enabling periodic recalibration as routines, roles, and inter-departmental dependencies evolve. How organizations manage to adapt to new workflows unsurprisingly correlates with the nature of the original workflow. Greater deviations between old and new workflows require more effort to change and optimize. These changes influence the implementation outcome and affect the effects that can be monitored in the post-implementation phase.

It is important to note that interpreting benefits from the post-implementation quantitative data depends on the availability of high-quality pre-implementation baselines. For example, the dashboard data show that Bærum discharges more than 70% of patients, whereas Drammen discharges approximately 35%. Without comparable pre-implementation data, however, it is impossible to determine which hospital achieved the greatest improvement. Some relevant insights can nevertheless be derived from the qualitative interviews. In Drammen, radiographers and leaders reported that, prior to implementation, all patients were sent to the hospital's ED, even when radiographers identified clear fractures. In contrast, radiographers in Bærum had already been discharging patients either directly home or to the municipality's ER, located in the same building, before implementing the AI-CDS. Consequently, the change in work practice was more substantial for Drammen, as they had to establish an entirely new workflow, including delegating discharge responsibilities to radiographers. Their discharge rate, therefore, increased from 0% to approximately 35%. Bærum had no pre-implementation data on discharged patients before implementing AI-CDS. Accordingly, it is not possible to determine how much their discharge rate exactly increased. It is, however, reasonable to conclude that the implementation caused less disruption to existing workflows at Bærum than at Drammen.

Rather than treating spread, scale-up, and sustainability as linear, fixed stages, they are better understood through a complex systems lens, where implementation evolves in nonlinear ways shaped by local adjustments, situational factors, and ongoing negotiation [3, 15]. Post-implementation monitoring depends on the process in place prior to deployment. In practice, this means monitoring at multiple levels (e.g., number of AI-CDS-assisted examinations, discharge rates, and downstream time saved) and recalibrating benefits as organizational routines evolve.

5.3 CE-Marked Rigidity Challenges Organizational and Contextual Heterogeneity: Implications for Spread, Scale-Up, and Sustainability

CE-marked AI-CDS applications are static products that cannot be adapted without costly recertification, meaning clinical workflows must adjust to the technology [7, 11]. From an Information Infrastructure (II) perspective, this rigidity underscores the need for local workflow redesign, task redistribution, and coordination across departments [22, 24]. This geographical reality seems to affect decision-making when deciding whether to send the patient with no fracture home or not. These patterns reflect contextual heterogeneity, differences in local needs, work processes, infrastructures, and organizational cultures that materially influence adoption and outcomes [3].

Extending the AI-CDS across the trust required supporting infrastructure, such as monitoring dashboards, as well as new role configurations, including radiographers communicating results and directing patient flow. The effort and staffing implications varied by site, showing that scale-up depends on each hospital's installed base and capacity to integrate new routines (digital and organizational maturity).

Finally, sustainability is shaped by ongoing adjustments. Trends over time (e.g., Kongsberg's decline from ~60% to ~40% home discharges) indicate that benefits are not static; they evolve with local adjustments, governance routines, and infrastructuring work. Sustained value thus requires ongoing monitoring and recalibration of workflows, responsibilities, and interfaces. This demonstrates that sustained value relies on continuous monitoring, governance, and infrastructuring work rather than a one-time implementation.

Within II theory, information infrastructures grow from an installed base of existing technologies and routines, and new components must be fitted into that base with minimal disruption while maintaining interoperability [22, 24]. In our case, the AI-CDS's rigidity places greater demands on workflow redesign, role redistribution, and boundary-spanning coordination to realize intended benefits. Static CE-marked AI-CDS applications make organizational adaptation and change management the primary focus for value realization. This contrasts with the evolving nature of II, e.g., in traditional technology implementation, configurable Electronic Health Record (EHR) systems that can be adapted to specific users' needs [8]. The process mirrors other digital innovations: open-ended, adaptive, and shaped by local negotiations and constraints [7, 11, 21–23]. Consequently, clinical practice must adapt to the technology rather than the other way around. This case illustrates that the implementation of CE-marked AI-CSDs faces many of the same challenges as other digital innovation processes and can be characterized as an open-ended, experimental, and conflict-ridden negotiation process in which work practices are reshaped, organizational attention is redirected, and new risks emerge [13].

5.4 AI-CDS Value Realization Through Workflow Reconfiguration and Infrastructuring

Justifying the use of AI-CDS requires looking beyond diagnostic accuracy to understand its impact on the broader patient pathway and the organization's capacity to manage shifting workloads, decision points, and downstream activity. AI-CDS outputs shape patient distribution, resource use, and workflow coordination; thus, evaluating value requires assessing not only whether the system detects findings correctly, but also how it alters the flow of patients and work across departments. Implementing AI-CDS often necessitates redesigning or discontinuing existing practices to avoid an additive workload and ensure that the technology contributes meaningfully to service performance rather than shifting tasks unevenly between professional groups.

Although the radiology department bears the cost of AI-CDS procurement and operation, many downstream benefits, such as reduced ED load and faster patient throughput, accrue. In our data, differences in discharge rates and follow-up destinations across hospitals illustrate how benefits are redistributed along the patient pathway rather than being retained within radiology alone. To meaningfully articulate return on investment (ROI), it is therefore necessary to consider system-level value, including reductions in waiting times, relief of ED pressure, and changes in staff workload. This requires acknowledging that value realization is growing, context-dependent, and distributed unevenly across organizational units over time.

Evaluation frameworks that link AI deployment to clinically meaningful outcomes, workflow impacts, and organizational adaptation are essential for revealing this broader value [3, 10, 21]. Monitoring must therefore extend beyond radiology throughput to capture effects on waiting times, discharge decisions, and downstream service utilization [3, 6].

Clinical decision-making itself is multifactorial, involving professional judgment, contextual interpretation, and coordinated work across roles. A CE-marked AI-CDS is trained for a narrow task and cannot be adapted to local clinical nuances without recertification, which limits its direct diagnostic contributions. However, indirect effects, such as improved patient flow, reduced bottlenecks, redistributed workload, and altered pathways, can be substantial.

Consistent with socio-technical perspectives, these effects depend on how tasks are redistributed across roles and how workflows are reconfigured in practice. Continuous evaluation is required to document these consequences, refine responsibilities, and ensure that evolving routines support safe and effective care [3, 13, 14]. Tracking AI-CDS use over time and mapping its ripple effects allows organizations to identify where new burdens or risks emerge and how roles should be adjusted across different stages of implementation. Realizing the full value of AI-CDS, therefore, demands organizational awareness and recognition that implementation is not a fixed end-state, but an ongoing process shaped through continuous infrastructuring and alignment of technology, workflows, and professional practices [3, 22].

6 Conclusion

Our findings show that the success of CE-marked AI-CDS implementations cannot be evaluated at the point of deployment but must be understood as a continuous, context-sensitive process of infrastructuring. Because CE-marked systems are static and cannot be locally adapted without recertification, organizations must adjust workflows, redistribute tasks, and recalibrate benefits over time. This requires evaluation approaches that extend beyond diagnostic performance to capture workflow effects, pathway changes, redistributed responsibilities, unintended consequences, and downstream value.

Although radiology carries the investment, benefits such as reduced ED pressure and faster throughput materialize elsewhere in the patient pathway. Differences in discharge rates and follow-up destinations across hospitals demonstrate that value is redistributed across service lines rather than confined to radiology. This underlines the need for a system-level view of ROI, recognizing that value realization is increasing, unevenly distributed, and shaped by local context.

Three interconnected trajectories shape long-term impact: First, practice changes did not replicate uniformly across sites. Differences in discharge rates and co-location with ERs show that spread is highly context-dependent, shaped by geography, installed base, and local workflows. Second, scaling the AI-CDS required site-specific infrastructure and new role configurations, which demonstrated that scale-up depends on organizational and digital maturity. Finally, benefits changed over time rather than stabilizing. Shifts in discharge patterns underscore that sustainability requires continuous monitoring and recalibration, supported by ongoing governance and infrastructuring work.

All together, these findings highlight the need for lifecycle-oriented, theory-informed evaluation that integrates, e.g., NASSS, II theory, and complex systems thinking. Implementing AI-CDS sustainably requires tracking a small set of pathway-level indicators, pairing them with qualitative insight into evolving work practices, and maintaining feedback loops to support spread, scale-up, and long-term value across heterogeneous healthcare settings.

Acknowledgments. This study was a collaboration between our research group and the project in Vestre Viken Hospital trust. We would like to thank the project management for their important feedback on our findings, input to empirical knowledge, as well as being gate-openers with the first informants.

References

1. Petersson, L., et al.: Challenges to implementing artificial intelligence in healthcare: a qualitative interview study with healthcare leaders in Sweden. BMC Health Serv. Res. **22**(1), 850 (2022)
2. Alami, H., Lehoux, P., Papoutsi, C., Shaw, S., Fleet, R., Fortin: Understanding the integration of artificial intelligence in healthcare organisations and systems through the NASSS framework: a qualitative study in a leading Canadian academic centre. BMC Health Serv. Res. **24**(1), 701 (2024)

3. Cresswell, K., et al.: The need to strengthen the evaluation of the impact of artificial intelligence-based decision support systems on healthcare provision. Health Policy **136**, 104889 (2023)
4. EU. CE marking. https://europa.eu/youreurope/business/product-requirements/labels-mar kings/ce-marking/index_en.htm. Last accessed 14 Dec 2025
5. HealthAIregister. Products, health AI register radiology. https://healthairegister.com/radiol ogy/products. Last accessed 16 Dec 2025
6. Paalvast, O., Sevenster, M., Hertgers, O., de Bliek, H., Wijn, V., Buil, V., Knoester, J., Vosbergen, S., Lamb, H.: Radiology AI lab: evaluation of radiology applications with clinical end-users. J. Imaging Inform. Med. 1–9 (2025)
7. Silsand, L., Kannelønning, M., Severinsen, G.-H., Ellingsen, G.: Enabling AI in radiology: evaluation of an AI deployment process. Stud. Health Technol. Inform. **316**, 580–584 (2024)
8. van Leeuwen, K., et al.: Comparison of commercial AI software performance for radiograph lung nodule detection and bone age prediction. Radiology **310**(1), 230981 (2024)
9. D'Adderio, L., Bates, D.: Transforming diagnosis through artificial intelligence. npj Digit. Med. **8**(1), 54 (2025)
10. Boverhof, B., et al.: Radiology AI Deployment and Assessment Rubric (RADAR) to bring value-based AI into radiological practice. Insights Imaging **15**(1), 34 (2024)
11. Severinsen, G.-H., Silsand, L.: Implementing commercial AI for radiology in a Norwegian health trust—Experiences from using the NASSS framework for Formative Process evaluation. 43 anonym (2026)
12. Greenhalgh, T., et al.: Beyond adoption: a new framework for theorizing and evaluating nonadoption, abandonment, and challenges to the scale-up, spread, and sustainability of health and care technologies. J. Med. Internet Res. **19**(11), e8775 (2017)
13. Vikkelsø, S.: Subtle redistribution of work, attention and risks: electronic patient records and organisational consequences. Scand. J. Inf. Syst. **17**(1), 10 (2005)
14. Hogg, H., Brittain, K., Talks, J., Keane, P.A.: Intervention design for artificial intelligence-enabled macular service implementation: a primary qualitative study. Implement. Sci. Commun. **5**(1), 131 (2024)
15. Papoutsi, C., Greenhalgh, T., Marjanovic, S.: Approaches to spread, scale-up, and sustainability. Cambridge University Press (2024)
16. Gray, C., Shen, N., Pham, Q., Wiljer, D.: Evaluating digitally enabled health services. In: Handbook of Health Services Evaluation: Theories, Methods and Innovative Practices. Springer, pp. 309–330 (2025)
17. Cresswell, K., Williams, R., Sheikh, A.: Developing and applying a formative evaluation framework for health information technology implementations: qualitative investigation. J. Med. Internet Res. **22**(6), e15068 (2020)
18. Greenhalgh, T., et al.: The NASSS-CAT tools for understanding, guiding, monitoring, and researching technology implementation projects in health and social care: protocol for an evaluation study in real-world settings. JMIR Res. Protoc. **9**(5), e16861 (2020)
19. Tornatzky, L.: The processes of technological innovation. Lexington/DC Heath & Company (1990)
20. Cresswell, K., et al.: Theoretical and methodological considerations in evaluating large-scale health information technology change programmes. BMC Health Serv. Res. **20**, 1–6 (2020)
21. Hanseth, O., Lyytinen, K.: Design theory for dynamic complexity in information infrastructures: the case of building internet. In: Enacting Research Methods in Information Systems. Springer, pp. 104–142 (2016)
22. Hanseth, O., Monteiro, E., Hatling, M.: Developing information infrastructure: the tension between standardization and flexibility. Sci. Technol. Human Values **21**(4), 407–426 (1996)
23. Aanestad, M., Grisot, M., Hanseth, O., Vassilakopoulou, P.: Information Infrastructures within European Health Care: Working with the Installed Base. Springer International (2017)

24. Hanseth, O., Lyytinen, K.: Design theory for dynamic complexity in information infrastructures: the case of building internet. J. Inf. Technol. **25**(1), 1–19 (2010)
25. Braun, V., Clarke, V.: Using thematic analysis in psychology. Qual. Res. Psychol. **3**(2), 77–101 (2006)

Waiting Times from the Real-World Earliest Contacts to Realized Visits to Public Primary Healthcare in 2019–2025 in Finland: A National Register Study

Vesa Jormanainen[(✉)] [iD]

Medical Faculty, Department of Public Health, Doctoral School of Health Sciences, Doctoral Programme in Population Health, University of Helsinki, Tukholmankatu 8 B, 00014 Helsinki, Finland

`vesa.jormanainen@fimnet.fi, vesa.jormanainen@gov.fi`

Abstract. In primary healthcare, waiting times are less often considered a policy concern than for elective care, and waiting times have scarcely been measured in primary healthcare. Our data were obtained from the Finnish Institute for Health and Welfare (THL) open web pages on national level non-urgent public primary healthcare monthly waiting times to physician and nurse visits in 2019–2025. THL classified distributions of non-urgent public primary healthcare waiting times in five classes. We compared annual waiting times of 0–7 days (within one week) and 0–14 days (within two weeks) in overall, physician and nurse visit datasets. In 2021–2025, data from real-world earliest contacts to realized visits were based on 88 million visits, out of which 59 million (68%) were evaluated for need of care and treatment. Overall waiting time was realized within one week in 71 per cent (81% in two weeks), whereas within one week in 56 per cent (69% in two weeks) in physician, and within one week in 82 per cent (89% in two weeks) in nurse visit datasets. Monthly data on realized physician visits in 2019–2025 suggest a decreasing trend for shorter waiting times, and thus, longer overall waiting times. Waiting times for physician and nurse visits were shorter in summer holiday months.

Keywords: Primary healthcare · Waiting times · Finland

1 Introduction

In many national healthcare systems, waiting times and lists generally arise as the result of an imbalance between the demand for and the supply of healthcare services [1–4]. In some countries maximum waiting times have been used as a target for providers and/or a guarantee for patients [1]. In primary healthcare, waiting times are less often considered a policy concern than for elective care, and only a few countries have implemented maximum waiting times to get an appointment with a general practitioner (GP) or other primary healthcare providers.

M. Särestöniemi et al. (Eds.): NCDHWS 2026, CCIS 3009, pp. 138–150, 2026.
https://doi.org/10.1007/978-3-032-28812-7_12

Waiting times have scarcely been measured and reported in primary healthcare [1, 5–7]. Most common information made available to the public is on waiting times for hospital treatment [8]. The first systematic review on interventions designed to reduce waiting times for primary healthcare appointments suggested that open access scheduling and other patient-centered interventions may reduce waiting times [5]. Prior to the COVID-19 pandemic, many countries saw improvements in waiting times in general [3]. However, international and national comparisons of the reasons for long waiting times are complicated [9, 10].

1.1 Legislation and Waiting Time to Treatment in Finland Since 2002

In 2002 in Finland, a Decision in Principle by the Council of State on securing future of healthcare stated that the principle of access to treatment within a reasonable period would be embodied in legislation by 2005 [11, 12]. Legislation was set in five Acts (a national Healthcare Guarantee) in Finland in March 2005. According to the legislation, persons should assume of immediate contact with their public primary healthcare centre during official opening hours, and their non-urgent needs for health must be assessed by a healthcare professional within three weekdays after the contact. The person must get access to appropriate medical or dental treatment within three months in primary healthcare. In specialized hospitals, need for care assessment must be started within three months after the referral has been received. Medical or dental specialist hospital care must be started within six months after the need for care has been assessed. For children and youth, medical care must be started within three months after the need for care has been assessed.

Before 2007, Healthcare Guarantee data were gathered and monitored by the Ministry of Social Affairs and Health by using questionnaire data on numbers of patients who had waited for specialist hospital care over six months in nine specialties [13]. The Finnish Institute for Health and Welfare (THL) continued questionnaire-based data gathering three times annually in 2007–2011. THL Avohilmo Register includes much electronic data from real-world primary healthcare in Finland as part of the Care Registers for Social Welfare and Health Care. THL Avohilmo Register has been utilized partly in 2011–2013 and in its full extent since 2014.

During the first years of Healthcare Guarantee access to services was improved and it was associated with a EUR 380 million increase in costs of the municipalities in 2002–2007 [14, 15]. Specialized hospitals were granted 70 per cent of the additional costs, whereas primary healthcare received 30 per cent of the additional cost. However, the Healthcare Guarantee did not bring along a new service form, but it gave population right to have access to medically qualified care in certain time and to receive only evidence-based care [15].

In a series of nine questionnaire surveys (1998–2011) among patients attending within one week in September in 65 primary healthcare centres in the Tampere University Hospital catchment area in Finland, a total of 147 394 responses were evaluated [16]. This first longitudinal, systematic inquiry showed that overall satisfaction diminished, and fewer patients reported good access to and continuity of care in Finland.

In 2011, the previous legislation on the Healthcare Guarantee was refined and transferred to the new Finnish Health Care Act (1326/2010) [17]. This legislation introduced patients' freedom-of-choice concept in healthcare services: persons may choose their healthcare centres' unit in which they would receive their healthcare within their home municipality. This freedom-of-choice was also extended to the choice of specialist hospital care. All choices of treatment places were to be done in consensus with medical or dentist doctors who make the referral to the specialized hospitals.

Essentially, urgent healthcare must be provided immediately irrespective of the person's place of residence [17]. These emergency healthcare situations were set on responsibilities and to be organized by the municipalities and hospital districts. In cases of emergent situations, it was the responsibility of the municipality that the patient could make an immediate contact in official open hours during weekdays. The municipalities had the duty to organize off-hours emergency services. The healthcare professional must assess the patient's need for care within the third weekday after the patient made the contact to the primary healthcare if it was not possible to assess during the initial contact. Based on the need of care assessment, medically or dentally justified care must be provided within three months after the need for care was assessed. In specialized hospitals, need for care assessment must be started within three months after the referral has been received. Medical or dental specialized hospital care must be started within three weeks after the referral was received. In case the need for care assessment requires specialist physician evaluation, or special radiological or laboratory tests, assessment and tests must be done within three months after receiving the referral. For children and youth, mental health services in specialist hospitals must be started within three weeks after the need for care has been evaluated. In case the need for care assessment requires specialist physician evaluation or special tests, assessment and tests must be done within six weeks after receiving the referral. Appropriate care must be organized and started within six months after the need of care was assessed.

In 2012, approximately half of the respondent patients had obtained a GP appointment within a week according to a questionnaire study [18]. Younger age and more urgent reason for contact were the most significant factors associated with faster access to GP appointments. Patients with non-urgent matters waited longer than those with illness.

Currently access to first aid and emergency treatment must be provided immediately, regardless of the patient's place of residence. Non-urgent medical care is provided at primary healthcare centres. Primary healthcare should be reachable without delay by telephone or digital means during working week office hours. Reachability by telephone means that, in addition to making an appointment, persons are provided with advice and a preliminary plan for procedures, and information about how to deal with an ailment, a symptom or a problem. Persons can also visit the primary healthcare in person.

The need for care must be assessed the same day a person contacts healthcare. The need for care can also be assessed by a healthcare professional other than a physician. The government relaxed rules of waiting time limits in 2024, re-establishing a maximum three months (90-day) waiting for non-urgent primary healthcare after assessment, instead of the tighter two week or one-week limits previously implemented or planned. Actual waiting times vary significantly by wellbeing services counties (WBSs) and City of Helsinki and patient demographic.

1.2   The Year 2023 Reform of Healthcare, Social Welfare and Rescue Services

Finland is known to be one of the few countries with the fundamental structure of public primary healthcare since the early 1970s. The healthcare system in Finland was one of the most decentralized in the OECD [13, 20, 21]. The primary healthcare has been universal and taxation-based, mainly provided earlier before 2023 by municipality-arranged, multidisciplinary healthcare centres. The Finnish healthcare services offer universal coverage over a comprehensive range of health needs implemented primarily by public owned and operated organizations since year 1972.

Finland undertook an extensive healthcare, social welfare and rescue services Reform in 2023 with the most drastic changes in the nation's post-World War II history [20]. The 2023 Reform is still underway, with significant revision of legislation. As part of the changes, the 300 municipalities no longer organize healthcare, social welfare and rescue services' activities. This responsibility was shifted to regional level of 21 WSCs, City of Helsinki and HUS Group that organize social welfare, healthcare and rescue services for the entire country. Along with current reforms, budget and human resource cuts have been introduced by the WSCs and city of Helsinki.

1.3   Study Objectives

In the Finnish legislation, waiting times as Healthcare Guarantee have been set to public primary healthcare as well as to specialized hospital healthcare. According to the Healthcare Act, non-urgent primary healthcare services' waiting time is calculated from an evaluated admission visit to a registered realized visit in public primary healthcare. We have observed that these legally defined waiting times may well be based on rather small amounts of data, and thus, may not reflect good quality waiting time estimates of public primary healthcare in Finland.

Our study objective was to utilize real-time primary healthcare data in a national data repository for waiting time from the earliest time stamp to realized visits in monthly and annual time series in 2019–2025 in Finland.

2   Materials and Methods

Waiting time for non-urgent primary healthcare services is calculated from an evaluated admission visit to a registered visit in public primary healthcare in Finland. However, not all primary healthcare service providers in Finland can provide comprehensive and good quality time stamps, e.g. service data are missing in place to place in substantial amounts. This is why we chose to maximize available data by utilizing waiting times calculated from recorded earliest contact in the primary healthcare (electronic health record system) to recorded visits. In our material, earliest time stamp can be a contact, an evaluated admission visit, or an appointment booking, which ever became first.

Material. We utilized national level non-urgent public primary healthcare monthly real-world waiting times in 2019–2025 published at the open THL internet websites (data accessed 18 January 2026). THL Avohilmo Register is part of the Care Registers for Social Welfare and Health Care [22, 23]. Distributions of non-urgent public primary healthcare waiting times were classified by the THL in five classes: 0–7 days, 8–14 days, 15–30 days, 31–90 days, and over 90 days.

Methods. Monthly numbers of persons waiting in each class were aggregated (100%). The class proportion (number in a class [n] divided by the month sum [N]) was expressed as a per cents (%):

We compared national level annual waiting times of 0–7 days (within a week) and 0–14 days (within two weeks) from the earliest time stamp to registered visits in annual and monthly data in 2019–2025 by public primary healthcare overall material, physician and nurse (nurse, registered nurse or midwife) visits.

The results are presented in absolute numbers, per cents (%), means, figures and tables.

3   Results

There were totally 88.0 million (13.5 million in 2019 and 12.6 million in 2025) registered non-urgent visits from the earliest contact to the non-urgent realized visits to public primary healthcare in 2019–2025 in Finland. Among evaluated admission visits (59.4 million; 68%), the overall waiting time realized within one week in 71 per cent and two weeks in 81 per cent, respectively (Fig. 1, Table 1).

Monthly data on 2019–2025 suggest a longer waiting time trend for public primary healthcare since the start of COVID-19 epidemic in March 2020 in Finland. However, the overall waiting time in 2025 seem to be at the same level than before the COVID-19. The waiting times have been shorter in summer holiday months (e.g. July and August).

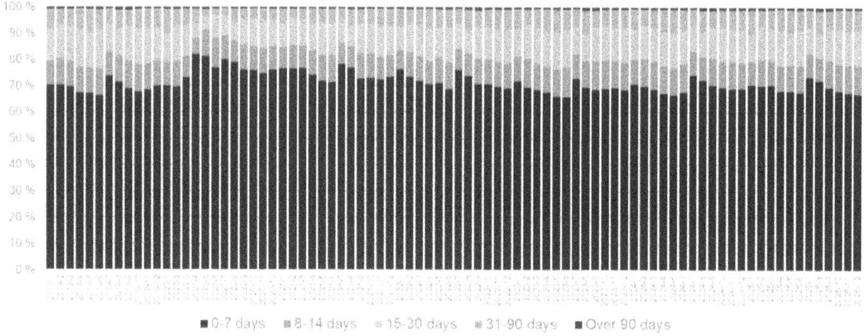

Fig. 1. Distributions of national level non-urgent public primary healthcare waiting times from earliest contact to a realized visit by waiting time classification (0–7 days, 8–14 days, 15–30 days, 31–90 days, and over 90 days) in 2019–2025 in Finland. The monthly class proportions are presented as percentages (%). *Source* THL Avohilmo Register

Annual national level non-urgent public primary healthcare waiting time data suggest that overall waiting times during 2023–2025 were longer than in 2019–2022 (Table 1).

Table 1. Annual distributions of national level non-urgent public primary healthcare waiting times from earliest contact to a realized visit in 2019–2025 in Finland. The annual class proportions are presented as percentages (%). *Source* THL Avohilmo Register

Year	All (number)	Waiting time from earliest contact to a realized primary healthcare visit (%)				
		0–7 days	8–14 days	15–30 days	31–90 days	Over 90 days
2019	8 894 311	69.2	9.8	13.0	7.2	0.8
2020	8 987 547	76.0	8.9	9.7	4.7	0.6
2021	8 668 920	74.5	8.8	10.6	5.4	0.6
2022	7 895 655	71.8	9.1	11.4	6.9	0.8
2023	7 810 192	68.9	10.3	12.6	7.4	0.8
2024	8 603 518	69.5	10.0	12.1	7.5	0.9
2025	8 551 657	69.3	9.8	12.1	7.9	0.9
All	59 411 800	71.4	9.5	11.7	6.7	0.8

3.1   Visits and Waiting Time to Primary Healthcare Physician and Nurses

Visits to Primary Healthcare Physicians. In 2019–2025 in Finland, there were totally 28.9 million (5.4 million in 2019 and 3.2 million in 2025) registered non-urgent visits to public primary healthcare physicians. Among evaluated admission visits (24.3 million; 83%), the overall waiting time realized within one week in 56 per cent and two weeks in 69 per cent, respectively (Fig. 2, Table 2).

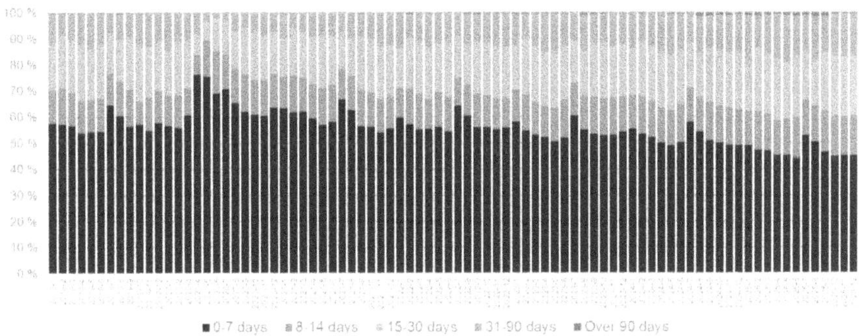

Fig. 2. Distributions of national level non-urgent public primary healthcare waiting times from earliest contact to a realized physician visit by waiting time classification (0–7 days, 8–14 days, 15–30 days, 31–90 days, and over 90 days) in 2019–2025 in Finland. The monthly class proportions are presented as percentages (%). *Source* THL Avohilmo Registry

Monthly data on realized public primary healthcare physician visits in 2019–2025 suggest a decreasing waiting time trend in shorter waiting times and an increasing trend

Table 2. Annual distributions of national level non-urgent public primary healthcare waiting times from earliest contact to a realized physician visit in 2019–2025 in Finland. The annual class proportions are presented as percentages (%). *Source* THL Avohilmo Registry

		Waiting times from earliest contact to a realized physician visit (%)				
Year	All (number)	0–7 days	8–14 days	15–30 days	31–90 days	Over 90 days
2019	4 346 142	56.9	12,5	19.4	10.7	0.6
2020	4 017 535	64.3	12.9	15.3	7.1	0.4
2021	3 610 920	59.3	13.2	18.1	8.9	0.4
2022	3 262 935	56.9	12.4	18.7	11.2	0.7
2023	3 141 135	53.9	13.4	19.9	12.0	0.7
2024	3 089 320	51.7	13.8	20.3	13.2	0.9
2025	2 772 657	46.8	14.4	22.2	15.4	1.3
All	24 240 644	56.3	13.2	18.9	10.9	0.7

in longer waiting times since the start of COVID-19 epidemic in March 2020 in Finland. Waiting time in 2025 seem to be longer than before the COVID-19. Waiting times to physician visits have been shorter in summer holiday months (e.g. July and August).

Annual national level non-urgent public primary healthcare waiting time from earliest contact to a realized physician visit data show an overall decreasing trend of number of visits since 2019. These data also indicate that waiting times were longer during 2023–2025 than during 2019–2022.

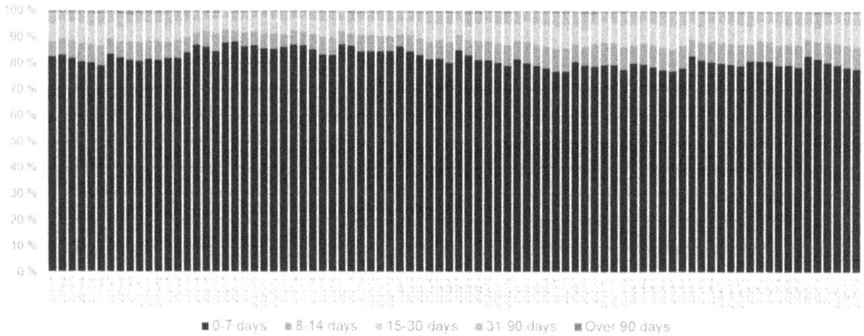

Fig. 3. Distributions of national level non-urgent public primary healthcare waiting times from earliest contact to a realized nurse, registered nurse or midwife visit by waiting time classification (0–7 days, 8–14 days, 15–30 days, 31–90 days, and over 90 days) in 2019–2025 in Finland. The monthly class proportions are presented as percentages (%). *Source* THL Avohilmo Registry

Visits to Primary Healthcare Nurses, Registered Nurses and Midwives. In 2019–2025 in Finland, there were totally 59.9 million (8.1 million in 2019 and 9.4 million in 2025) registered non-urgent visits to public primary healthcare nurses (nurse, registered nurse or midwife). Among evaluated admission visits (35.2 million; 59%), the realized overall waiting time was one week in 82 per cent and two weeks in 89 per cent, respectively (Fig. 3, Table 3).

Monthly data 2019–2025 suggests a smoothly decreasing trend among shorter waiting times for public primary healthcare nurse visits. In 2025, the waiting times seem to be approximately on the same level than before COVID-19. The observed waiting times were shorter for nurse visits in summer holiday months (e.g. July and August).

Table 3. Annual distributions of national level non-urgent public primary healthcare waiting times from earliest contact to a realized nurse, registered nurse or midwife visit in 2019–2025 in Finland. The annual class proportions are presented as percentages (%). *Source* THL Avohilmo Registry

Year	All (n)	Waiting times from earliest contact to a realized nurse, registered nurse or midwife visit (%)				
		0–7 days	8–14 days	15–30 days	31–90 days	Over 90 days
2019	4 526 338	85.2	7.1	7.2	4.0	1.1
2020	4 969 556	85.5	5.7	5.3	2.8	0.7
2021	5 058 615	85.4	5.7	5.3	3.0	0.7
2022	4 630 386	82.3	6.7	6.3	3.8	0.8
2023	4 669 255	79.0	8.2	7.7	4.3	0.9
2024	5 514 115	79.5	7.8	7.6	4.2	0.8
2025	5 782 086	80.1	7.6	7.3	4.3	0.7
All	35 150 351	81.8	6.9	6.6	3.8	0.8

Annual national level non-urgent public primary healthcare waiting time from earliest contact to a realized nurse, registered nurse and midwife visit data show an overall increasing trend of number of visits since 2019. These data also show the lowest numbers of annual nurse visits took place during 2022–2023, whereas the highest during 2024–2025. Number of annual nurse visit data also indicate that waiting times were longer during 2023–2025 than during 2019–2022.

Comparison of non-urgent primary healthcare physician and nurse visit waiting times. In 2019–2025 in Finland, there were 2.1 times more non-urgent visits to primary healthcare nurses than to physicians. Numbers of evaluated admissions showed 1.4 times more visits to nurses than to physicians. However, proportions of evaluated admissions were higher in physician (83%) than in nurse (59%) visit datasets.

3.2 COVID-19 Epidemic and the Year 2023 Reform

From the earliest contact to the realized visits to a public primary healthcare physician and nurse before, during and after the COVID-19 epidemic in 2019–2022 in Finland, there were totally 34.4 million non-urgent visits (mean 8.6 million per year), whereas 25.0 million (mean 8.3 million per year) in 2023–2025.

Before the year 2023 Reform in 2019–2022, there were totally 18.6 million (mean 4.7 million per year) registered non-urgent visits to public primary healthcare physicians and 33.6 million (mean 8.4 million) to nurses. In the physician admission visits, waiting time in 2019–2022 was less than a week in 59 per cent (84% in nurses) and less than two weeks in 72 per cent (90% in nurses), whereas 50 per cent (77% in nurses) and 65 per cent (88% in nurses) in 2023–2025 after the 2023 Reform, respectively.

In waiting time data from earliest time stamp to realized visits in 2019–2025, physician visits decreased from 4.4 million in 2019 to 2.8 million in 2025 suggesting a decreasing trend. However, nurse visits increased from 4.5 million in 2019 to 5.8 million in 2025 suggesting an increased trend.

4 Discussion

To the best of our knowledge, our national register study is the first to report non-urgent primary healthcare real-world monthly and annual waiting times from the earliest time stamp to realized physician and nurse visit in Finland in a 7-year long time series (2019–2025). Our register data analyses were based on 88.0 million realized visits.

Among 59 million assessed admissions, the overall primary healthcare waiting time to physicians and nurses in 2019–2025 was realized within one week in 71 per cent and two weeks in 81 per cent. Monthly data on realized public primary healthcare waiting time proportions suggest a decreasing long-term trend in physician visits, whereas a slightly decreasing trend in nurse visits. Based on our data, decreasing trends suggest longer waiting times. Waiting times to physician and nurse visits were constantly shorter in summer holiday months, when there is usually less demand for visits and possibly less supply of services, too. Waiting time observations may be due to increase in service demand after the COVID-19 epidemic, enhanced registration of visits after the year 2023 Reform and increased nurse online service provision working patterns, or their combinations.

On a national primary healthcare service providers' questionnaire study in spring 2025, 76 per cent of the nurse first contacts and 41 per cent of the physician contacts were online [22, 23]. However, not all access data to public primary healthcare were comprehensive, thus causing uncertainty to register data analyses.

A questionnaire-based survey in 11 high-income countries revealed that data made available to the public are on waiting times for hospital treatment (though not primary healthcare), being reported for major hospitals in seven countries [8]. Information on patient experience at hospital level is also made available in many countries, but it is not generally available in respect of primary care services. Public reporting of waiting times aggregate measures of quality and safety, as well as of outcomes of individual physicians, remain relatively uncommon. This is likely to be due to both unresolved methodological and ethical problems and concerns that public reporting may lead to unintended consequences.

Reducing waiting time from referral to first visit for community outpatient services may contribute to better health outcomes [24]. However, the modest benefits in health outcomes observed in reducing wait time for community outpatient services suggest that other possible benefits such as increasing patient flow should be explored.

Few countries (Finland, Norway and Spain) have implemented maximum waiting times to get an appointment with a primary healthcare provider [1, 3]. Policies focused on increasing supply of general practitioners, nurses and appointment slots. These are justified as primary healthcare is the first access point for the patient to the health system where inequalities may arise. Some countries (Australia, Luxembourg and Estonia) used new technologies such as teleconsultations to increase supply and to better manage demand (applications to find available doctors). Finland has also developed, launched and uses new technologies (e.g. MyKanta) to increase supply and better demand management for inhabitants [25].

In a comprehensive systematic review on interventions designed to reduce waiting times for primary healthcare appointments, dedicated telephone calls for follow-up consultation, presence of nurse practitioners on staff, nurse and general practitioner triage, and email consultations were effective at reducing wait times [5]. All above mentioned interventions are in use in Finland except email consultations that are not allowed due to current legislation. Instead in Finnish primary healthcare, online services utilize chat services for first timely access [26].

A patient's need for non-emergency care in primary healthcare in Finland is usually made by nurses [18, 27]. Access to primary healthcare centres have deteriorated in past years despite several government acts aiming to develop Finnish healthcare system. In 2007, 72 per cent of the Finnish study population estimated that an appointment could be obtained within three days [28]. In 2015, the percentage of patients reporting easy access to primary healthcare decreased from 38 to 18 per cent over a 15-year study period [16].

Since the start of COVID-19 pandemic in March 2020 in Finland, vaccination strategies were organized to protect population against the virus infection and its likely health consequences [29]. Vaccinations were organized by municipalities and offered free of charge. These massive vaccinations were carried out mainly by nurses, registered nurses and various other healthcare professionals. Due to these organizational changes within primary healthcare organizations, it may have had effects on nurse contact registrations during 2020–2022.

Data coverage of the waiting time registry is considered good except Southern Finland's Vantaa and Kerava WSC and City of Helsinki, who changed their electronic records data systems recently: Vantaa in 2019 and Kerava and City of Helsinki in 2021. Due to these changes, total number of care contacts has decreased significantly [30]. In City of Helsinki situation seem to be back to normal state. However, in Vantaa and Kerava WSC there still exist problems and in 2024 there were a deficit of approximately 350 000 care contacts which would contribute one percentage of the whole country's care contacts. Different types of electronic health record data systems and their version that are used in primary healthcare in Finland may contribute to waiting time recording and their connection to respective care contacts. Legislation changes in September 2023 brought up structured recording responsibility for the healthcare professionals, and that may have had effects also on year 2024 data.

Proportion of face-to-face contacts of primary healthcare physicians of all care contacts has increased from 20 per cent in 2021 to over 30 per cent in 2024 [30]. At the same timeframe online physician contacts have increased from five per cent to almost 40 per cent. During 2021–2024 number of waiting time registered online contacts have increased from less than 100 000 to 450 000. Among primary healthcare nurses, registered nurses and midwifes, proportion of care contacts during 2021–2024 have increased more than those of physicians. Proportion of face-to-face contacts of nurses of all care contacts has increased from approximately 10 per cent to over 30 per cent. Online contacts have increased from approximately five per cent to 50 percent during 2021–2024. During the same timeframe number of nurse online contacts has increased 10-fold from 300 000 contacts to 2.5 million contacts. These changes at least partly reflect the effects of COVID-19 pandemic has had in Finland.

Since the start of the year 2023 Reform, primary healthcare is provided through three overlapping channels: WSC-owned health centres, the occupational health care scheme (which uses many private contracted providers) and private providers which supply services directly to private patients [20]. In addition, the Finnish Student Health Services provides primary healthcare services, including mental and dental health care services, for students in higher education. Public primary healthcare centres usually employ GPs, nurses and other professionals, depending on the size and needs of the population.

In spring 2020, the national health insurance reimbursements were extended to cover digital services, which at least partly may explain their rapid expansion across primary healthcare since the COVID-19 pandemic and more recently WSCs have been investing in various digital services [31]. For instance, WBCs introduced digital clinics which work as a first point of contact for clients, and through which needs assessment as well as certain services can be provided. Both digital platforms (software) and digital services are often supplied by private providers. The rapid expansion of digital services is a response to the budgetary and recruitment challenges faced by WSCs. Digital services such as chats, remote consultations and digital clinics are also widely used in the private sector, with accelerated provision during and after the COVID-19 pandemic.

5   Conclusions

In our seven-year (2019–2025) time series register study in Finland, our descriptive analyses show that it is possible to develop and maintain national level primary healthcare waiting time compilations and report them via internet webpages. In Finland, waiting times are calculated centrally in a standardized way by the THL utilizing recorded time stamps. Our study results suggest different waiting time trends for realized primary healthcare physician and nurse visits and contacts.

Creating situational pictures on service system will remain essential to continue monitoring the progress of digitalization in healthcare and social welfare services at both WSCs, City of Helsinki and national level. Information on the current situation can and will be utilized, among other things, in developing the operations of WSCs and City of Helsinki and selecting development targets for guidance.

Disclosure of Interests. The author has no competing interests to declare that are relevant to the content of this article. The author is currently Medical Counsellor at the Ministry of Social Affairs and Health of Finland, Department of Clients and Services in Healthcare and Social Welfare, Service System Unit.

References

1. OECD: Waiting times for health services: next in line. OECD Health Policy Studies. Paris: OECD Publishing (2020)
2. Moir, M., Barua, B.: Waiting your turn. Wait times for health care in Canada, 2024 report. Fraser Institute (2024)
3. OECD: Health at a glance 2025: OECD indicators. Paris: OECD Publishing 2025:110–111
4. Siciliani, L.: Waiting times for health services, health, and labour. Eur. J. Public Health (2025)
5. Ansell, D.E., Crispo, J.A.G., Simard, B., Bjerre, L.M.: Interventions to reduce wait times for primary care appointments: a systematic review. BMC Health Serv. Res. **17**, 295 (2017)
6. Pfell, J.N., et al.: A telemedicine strategy to reduce waiting lists and time to specialist care: a retrospective cohort study. J. Telemed. Telecare **29**, 10–17 (2020)
7. Nwagbara, U.I., Hlongwana, K.W., Chima, S.C.: Mapping evidence on factors contributing to long waiting times and interventions to reduce waiting times within primary health care facilities in South Africa: a scoping review. PLoS ONE **19**, e0299253 (2024)
8. Rechel, B., et al.: Public reporting on quality, waiting times and patient experience in 11 high-income countries. Health Policy **120**, 377–383 (2016)
9. Viberg, N., Forsberg, B.C., Borowitz, M., Molin, R.: International comparisons of waiting times in health care-limitations and prospects. Health Policy **112**, 53–61 (2013)
10. Siciliani, L., Moran, V., Borowitz, M.: Measuring and comparing health care waiting times in OECD countries. Health Policy **118**, 292–303 (2014)
11. Pelttari, H., Kaila, M.: Kiireettömän hoitoon pääsyn selvitys: nykytila ja toimenpide-ehdotuksia. STM raportteja ja muistioita 2014:27. Helsinki: Sosiaali- ja terveysministeriö (2014) [In Finnish]
12. Government proposal to the Parliament on changing several Acts (HE 77/2004 vp). [In Finnish]. https://www.finlex.fi/fi/hallituksen-esitykset/2004/77
13. Jonsson, P.M., Häkkinen, P., Järvelin, J., Kärkkäinen, J.: Finland. In: Siciliani, L., Borowitz, M., Moran, V. (eds.): Waiting time policies in the health sector. OECD Health Policy Studies. Paris: OECD Publishing, pp. 133–146 (2013)
14. Pekurinen, M., Mikkola, H., Tuominen, U. (eds.): The economics of the health care quarantee: impact on healthcare costs, activities, and reimbursement from the national health insurance. Report 5/2008. Helsinki: Stakes (2008) [In Finnish]
15. VTV.: Hoitotakuu. VTV toiminnantarkastuskertomus 167/2008. Helsinki: Valtiontalouden tarkastusvirasto (2008) [In Finnish]
16. Raivio, R., Jääskeläinen, J., Holmberg-Marttila, D., Mattila, K.J.: Decreasing trends in patient satisfaction, accessibility and continuity of care in Finnish primary health care: a 14-year follow-up questionnaire study. BMC Fam. Pract. **15**, 98 (2014)
17. Goverment proposal for Health care act (HE 1326/2010 vp). [In Finnish]. https://www.finlex.fi/fi/lainsaadanto/saadoskokoelma/2010/1326#OT5_OT5
18. Tolvanen, E., Koskela, T.H., Mattila, K.J., Kosunen, E.: Analysis of factors associated with waiting times for GP appointments in Finnish health centres: a QUALICOPC study. BMC. Res. Notes **11**, 220 (2018)
19. Kokko, S.: Towards fragmentation of general practice and primary health care in Finland? Scand. J. Prim. Health Care **25**, 131–132 (2007)
20. Keskimäki, I.: Development of primary health care in Finland. The Lancet Global Health Commission on Financing Primary Health Care. Working Paper 9. London (U.K.): London School of Hygiene & Tropical Medicine; April (2022)

21. Karanikolos, M., Tynkkynen, L.K., Keskimäki, I.: Finland: Health system summary, 2024. Copenhagen: European Observatory on Health Systems and Policies, WHO Regional Office for Europe (2024)
22. Marttila, T., Mahkonen, R.: Access to primary healthcare in 2024. Statistical report 24/2025. Helsinki: Finnish Institute for Health and Welfare (THL) (2025) [In Finnish]
23. THL Primary Healthcare Homepage. Last accessed 2 Jan 2026
24. Lewis, A.K., Harding, K.E., Snowdon, D.A., Taylor, N.F.: Reducing wait time from referral to first visit for community outpatient services may contribute to better health outcomes: a systematic review. BMC Health Serv. Res. **18**, 869 (2018)
25. Jormanainen, V.: Regional use of open notes via nationwide web-based MyKanta patient portal in 2017–2024 in Finland. Stud. Health Technol. Inform. **327**, 909–913 (2025)
26. Ruotanen, R., Kangas, M., Tuovinen, T., Keränen, N., Haverinen, J., Reponen, J.: Finnish e-health services intended for citizens: national and regional development. Finnish J eHealth eWelfare **13**(3), 283–301 (2021)
27. Jokelin, E., Piirainen, L., Mustonen, E., Torkki, P.: Improving access, mixed continuity: effects of multidisciplinary teams on primary healthcare in Finland: a quasi-experimental study. Scand. J. Prim. Health Care **43**, 745–758 (2025)
28. Mäntyselkä, P., Halonen, P., Vehviläinen, A., Takala, J., Kumpusalo, E.: Access to and continuity of primary medical care of different providers as perceived by the Finnish population. Scand. J. Prim. Health Care **25**, 27–32 (2007)
29. Tiirinki, H., Viita-aho, M., Tynkkynen, L.-K., Sovala, M., Jormanainen, V., Keskimäki, I.: COVID-19 in Finland: vaccination strategy as part of the wider governing of the pandemic. Health Policy Technol **11**, 100631 (2022)
30. THL Access to Primary Healthcare Homepage. [In Finnish]. Last accessed 23 Mar 2026
31. Kärkkäinen, E., Virtanen, L., Kainiemi, E., Heponiemi, T., Vehko, T.: Digitalization and its strategic management in the organization of social and health services. A picture of the situation more than a year after the welfare areas started operating. Discussion Paper 45/2024. Helsinki: Finnish Institute for Health and Welfare (2024) [In Finnish, abstract in English]

Clinical Investigation of Health Technologies: A Scoping Review of Evaluation Methods

Axa Saukkonen[1], Henna Härkönen[1], Jenna Syrjälä[1], Minna Vanhanen[2], Elina Laukka[3,4], Paulus Torkki[3], Kirsi Talman[5,6], Monira Yesmean[1], and Miia Jansson[1,7,8(✉)]

[1] Research Unit of Health Sciences and Technology, University of Oulu, Oulu, Finland
`miia.jansson@oulu.com`
[2] Research and Innovation, Oulu University of Applied Sciences, Oulu, Finland
[3] Department of Public Health, Faculty of Medicine, University of Helsinki, Helsinki, Finland
[4] School of Wellbeing and Culture, Oulu University of Applied Sciences, Oulu, Finland
[5] Sailab—MedTech Finland, Helsinki, Finland
[6] Department of Nursing Science, University of Turku, Turku, Finland
[7] RMIT University, Melbourne, VIC, Australia
[8] Medical Research Center Oulu, Oulu, Finland

Abstract. The aim of this scoping review was to synthesize and map recommended evaluation methods for the clinical investigation of health technologies. A database search was conducted in January 2025 in the Scopus, Ovid MEDLINE, and CINAHL databases, and grey literature was searched in the Mednar database. Publications from 2015–2024 were included if they described the clinical investigation of health technologies at various maturity levels, as assessed using the Technology Readiness Level (TRL) framework. Nine studies were included in the review. Recommended evaluation methods varied across different TRLs, with considerable overlap observed between evaluation domains. In addition, these methods exhibited an evolutionary progression, becoming increasingly rigorous and incorporating broader contextual and social considerations as technological maturity advanced. At TRLs 5–6, clinical investigations focused on efficacy; at TRLs 7–8, on effectiveness and clinical validity; and at the highest maturity level, on implementation and clinical utility. Notably, evaluation methods were not recommended by device risk class. The clinical investigations of health technologies remains fragmented, and no consistent approach has been established. The application of the TRL framework provided a novel and structured approach to map evaluation methods according to the stage of maturity. There is a need for harmonized evaluation frameworks that support clinical investigations in line with EU regulations.

Keywords: Clinical Evaluation · Clinical Validation · Health Technology · In Vitro Diagnostic Medical Devices · Medical Device · Technology Readiness Level

M. Särestöniemi et al. (Eds.): NCDHWS 2026, CCIS 3009, pp. 151–165, 2026.
https://doi.org/10.1007/978-3-032-28812-7_13

1 Introduction

According to WHO [1], *"Health technologies include medicines, medical devices, assistive technologies, techniques and procedures developed to solve health problems and improve the quality of life"*. In this study, the term "health technology" refers to both medical devices (MD) used for medical purposes [2] and in vitro diagnostic medical devices (IVD) used for analyses of specimens outside the human body [2].

Health technologies are a key part of modern healthcare, providing devices for disease prevention, diagnosis, and treatment [3, 4]. Advances in digitalization and artificial intelligence (AI) have accelerated innovation and created new opportunities to address global healthcare challenges, which has increased interest in assessing the effectiveness of health technologies [5–7].

Market access is regulated, for example in the European Union (EU), with the sectoral EU regulations and national legislation, which aim to sneer the safety and performance of the device throughout product lifecycle. Before entering the market, manufacturer must demonstrate the device's safety and performance for its intended purpose; the higher the risk class, the more robust the clinical evidence required [2, 8, 9].

Clinical investigation is required for medical devices, covering both the clinical evaluation of MDs and the predictive performance of IVDs. Regardless of the device type, the overarching objective is the same: to demonstrate that the device fulfills the essential requirements for safety and performance. The literature underscores the importance of structured and transparent evaluation frameworks that enable reliable and comparable assessment across technologies [10–13].

The application of Technology Readiness Levels (TRLs) in clinical investigations provides a systematic framework for assessing the maturity of health technologies throughout their lifecycle. Originally developed by NASA in the 1970s to evaluate technology's readiness for deployment in space missions [14], the TRL framework has since been widely adopted across various industries, including healthcare and MDs [15–17]. Its use in clinical investigations is particularly important, as it allows evaluation efforts to be aligned with the technology's stage of maturity, ensuring that assessments are both relevant and targeted.

Earlier reviews have proposed several evaluation domains (e.g., clinical assessment, economics, ethics, safety, and usability) for clinical investigation and emphasized the importance of aligning evaluation methods with technology maturity [18–20]. However, these reviews have not mapped evaluation methods according to specific TRLs and evaluation stages (e.g., efficacy, effectiveness, implementation), which limits their practical applicability. This review addresses that gap by synthesizing and mapping recommended evaluation methods to support the generation of clinical evidence on safety, performance, and clinical benefit, thereby providing clearer guidance for future assessments and facilitating implementation.

2 Material and Methods

2.1 Aims and Objectives

The aim of this scoping review was to synthesize and map recommended evaluation methods for the clinical investigation of health technologies. Research question was as follows: *What evaluation methods are recommended by the literature for the clinical investigation of health technologies across TRLs 5–9 and various risk classes?*

2.2 Design

This study was conducted in accordance with the JBI manual for scoping reviews [21]. The study protocol was pre-registered in the Open Science Framework registry on 18th of Jan 2025 (DOI: 10.17605/OSF.IO/U9FZC).

2.3 Eligibility Criteria

Given the rapid development of health technologies, the review included only peer-reviewed studies written in English or Finnish and published within the last decade (2015–2024). The studies were selected according to predefined inclusion criteria:

- Population: health technology.
- Concept: methods applied to clinical evaluation of MDs and to performance evaluation of IVDs.
- Context: TRLs 5–9 and risk class.

   When available, expert perspectives, consensus statements, reports, guidelines, and evaluation frameworks were considered appropriate to support the synthesis and mapping of recommended evaluation methods for the clinical investigation of health technologies. Empirical studies, post-market studies, and economic evaluations and technologies at TRLs 1–4 were excluded, due to their focus on pre-clinical or post-market settings. Publications focusing on Health Technology Assessment (HTA) were also excluded, as their system-level scope extends beyond primary clinical evidence needed to assess safety, performance, and clinical benefit during device development and pre-market regulation.

2.4 Search Strategy

The search strategy was planned in collaboration with an information specialist. A preliminary search was conducted in November 2024 in the Scopus and Ovid MEDLINE databases. The screening of titles, abstracts, and keywords served as the basis for identifying key search terms and formulating the final search queries. The final search was conducted in January 2025 using the Scopus, Ovid MEDLINE, and CINAHL databases. The MeSH terms, free-text terms, and proximity operators were used to build a sensitive search strategy. Grey literature was searched via Mednar. The search strategy and search results are presented in Table 1.

Table 1. Studies characteristics.

Database (date of search)	Search string	Number of results
Scopus (22.1.2025)	(TITLE-ABS-KEY("medical device*" OR "medical technology" OR "biomedical technology" OR "health technology" OR "Equipment and Supplies") AND TITLE-ABS-KEY((((evaluat* OR assess*) W/3 (method* OR instrumen* OR indicator* OR tool OR framework* OR model*))) AND TITLE-ABS-KEY((((effect* OR performance OR efficacy OR impact OR affect* OR cost OR benefit*)))) AND PUBYEAR >2014 AND PUBYEAR <2025	3914
Ovid MEDLINE (24.1.2025)	exp Biomedical Technology/ or exp. "Equipment and Supplies"/ or ("medical device*" or "medical technology" or "health technology").ab,kf,ti. AND ((evaluat* or assess*) adj4 (method* or instrumen* or indicator* or tool or framework* or model*)).ab,kf,ti. AND ((evaluat* or assess*) adj4 (effect* or performance or efficacy or impact or affect* or cost or benefit*)).ab,kf,ti. AND limit 4 to yr. = "2015–2024"	4211

(continued)

Table 1. (continued)

Database (date of search)	Search string	Number of results
CINAHL (22.1.2025)	(((MH "Equipment and Supplies+") OR (MH "Technology, Medical") OR (MH "Digital Technology+") OR (MH "Surgical Technology")) OR ("medical device*" or "medical technology" or "health technology")) AND ((evaluat* or assess*) N3 (effect* or performance or efficacy or impact OR affect* OR cost OR benefit*)) AND ((evaluat* or assess*) N3 (method* or instrumen* or indicator* or tool OR framework* OR model*))	2583
Mednar (24.1.2025)	("medical device*" OR "medical technology" OR "biomedical technology" OR "health technology" OR "Equipment and Supplies") AND (evaluat* OR assess*) AND (effect* OR performance OR efficacy OR impact OR affect* OR cost OR benefit*) AND (method* OR instrumen* OR indicator* OR tool OR framework* OR model*)	581

2.5 Study Selection

The screening at all stages was conducted independently by two researchers (AS, MJ, HH, JS, MV, EL, MY). Disagreements were resolved by a third researcher [21]. The screening process was conducted using the Covidence software tool (https://www.cov idence.org/).

The database search yielded 11 289 results. After screening titles and abstracts, 200 records were assessed in full text. Of these, 191 records were excluded for the following reasons: did not evaluate device performance, lacked an evaluation method, were preclinical, published in non-eligible languages, focused on post-market evaluation, lacked full text, or were unrelated to health technologies. The study selection process is summarized in the PRISMA flow diagram (see Fig. 1).

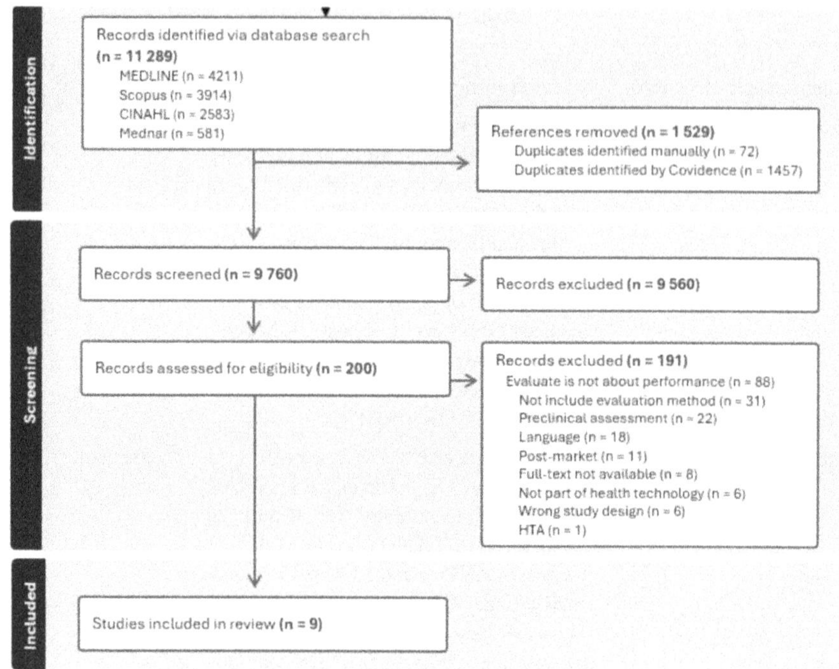

Fig. 1. PRISMA flowchart of the database search process.

2.6 Data Extraction

Two researchers (AS, MJ) independently extracted data using tables developed during the protocol stage to capture key information (e.g., authors, year) and main findings, including evaluation domains (broad frameworks), topics of assessment (specific considerations), and evaluation measures (detailed criteria). Throughout the review, AS and MJ collaboratively and iteratively refined the extraction tables to ensure a comprehensive and coherent synthesis of the evidence. The review was reported in accordance with the Preferred Reporting Items for Systematic Reviews and Meta-Analyses extension for Scoping Reviews (PRISMA-ScR) guidelines [22].

2.7 Analysis

Evaluation methods were categorized using TRL framework [14], which is a widely accepted approach for maturity assessment of health technologies [16, 17]. The TRL framework comprises nine levels, ranging from early conceptual development to full deployment [15]. In this study, however, we focused specifically on the clinical validation stages: TRL 5 (model validation), TRL 6 (real-time model testing), TRL 7 (workflow implementation), TRL 8 (clinical outcome evaluation), and TRL 9 (model integration).

Overlaps between the evaluation domains were addressed by categorizing the recommended evaluation methods according to evaluation stages (including efficacy, effectiveness, and implementation). The extracted data were then synthesized descriptively in accordance with scoping review guidelines and are presented in the Results section.

3 Results

3.1 Study Characteristics

We included seven evaluation frameworks [23–29], one expert perspective [30], and one methodological guide [31] in the final review to synthesize and map recommended evaluation methods for the clinical investigation of health technologies (Table 2).

Table 2. Studies characteristics.

Author(s), Year	Type of study	Regulation
Ding et al. [23]	Evaluation framework for conversational agents	Not reported
Chapel et al. [24]	Assessment framework for telerehabilitation	Not reported
Kukhareva et al. [25]	Evaluation framework for electronic health record integrated innovations	Not reported
Tanguay et al. [26]	Validation and evaluation framework of radiology AI-software	Not reported
Larson et al. [27]	Regulatory framework for AI-based diagnostic imaging algorithms	EU—MDR USA—FDA
Graziadio et al. [28]	Evaluation framework for a diagnostic point of care test	EU—MDR/IVDR USA—FDA
Chouvarda et al. [29]	Evaluation framework for impact assessment	Not reported
Nagle [30]	Expert perspective	Not reported
Park and Han [31]	Methodological guide	USA—FDA

The evaluation frameworks were derived from the World Health Organization's [32] recommendations for digital health interventions, which outline existing study designs, outcome measures, and sample size considerations [23]; the National Institute for Health and Care Excellence framework [33], which defines evidence standards for digital health technologies [27]; and the Health Technology Assessment Core Model [34], which specifies domains related to safety, accuracy, clinical effectiveness, costs, and economic evaluation [24].

Forty-four percent of the included evaluation frameworks originated in the United States of America [25–27, 30]. Additionally, 66.7% focused exclusively on Medical Device Software (MDSW) [23, 25–27, 30, 31].

Recommended user characteristics included age, gender, nationality, ethnicity, religion, education and socioeconomic status, health conditions, and devices used. Measures of usage, adherence, and uptake encompassed indicators such as conversation duration, dropout rates, follow-up rates, completion of questionnaires, and average daily reach time [23].

Primary data sources included laboratory tests, as well as observational (e.g., cross-sectional, and case-control studies) and experimental (e.g., quasi-experimental studies, randomized controlled trials) designs [23, 28]. User experience and clinical/health outcomes were recommended to be assessed by using validated tools [23]. Diagnostic accuracy studies included both interventional (e.g., randomized controlled trials, cluster-randomized trials, stepper wedge designs, adaptive designs, umbrella designs) and observational designs (e.g., feasibility studies, case-control designs), in which the performance of a novel test is compared with a reference standard in a defined population [28].

For MDs, *feasibility* referred to the ability of a device to function as intended; *efficacy* denoted its capacity to achieve the intended results under controlled research conditions or clinical trials; and *effectiveness* described the attainment of those outcomes in real-world settings. *Implementation* encompassed the adoption, integration, and sustainability of MDs within specific contexts, including existing policies and practices [23]. For IVDs, *clinical validity* referred to performance in real-world clinical practice, whereas *clinical utility* denoted the extent to which use of the IVD improved clinical decision-making and patient outcomes [28].

3.2 Clinical Investigation of Health Technologies at Different TRLs

Recommended evaluation methods varied across different TRLs, with considerable overlap observed between evaluation domains. In addition, these methods exhibited an evolutionary progression, becoming increasingly rigorous and incorporating broader contextual and social considerations as technological maturity advanced (See Fig. 2).

An evolutionary pattern of evaluation methods

Potential Value Propositions	Efficacy and Clinical Validity (TRL 5–6)	Effectiveness and Clinical utility (TRL 7–8)	Implementation and Connected Health Outcomes (TRL 9)	Actual Value Propositions
Human interaction	User experience	Barriers to adoption	Facilitators of adoption	
Economic assessment	Cost analysis	Value assessment	Budget impact analysis	

Fig. 2 An evolutionary pattern of evaluation methods at different TRLs.

At TRLs 5–6, clinical investigations primarily focused on efficacy. For MDs, efficacy encompassed [23–27, 30, 31]:

- **Capability**, such as accuracy (e.g, sensitivity, specificity, predictive value, transparent logic, transparent degree of confidence), reliability (e.g., deterministic), and safety (e.g., risk of harm);
- **Clinical performance**, including discrimination (e.g., sensitivity, specificity) and calibration (e.g., Calibration plot, Hosmer–Lemeshow goodness-of-fit);

- **Functionality**, such as response accuracy, voice, and device control;
- **Utilization**, including applicability and acceptability across settings;
- **Social acceptability**, such as task (e.g., time to complete task, keystrokes, mouse clicks, screen changes) and process (e.g., task completion) efficiency and organizational fit (e.g., billing, or regulatory requirements);
- **System quality**, such as security, functionality, and performance;
- **Technical acceptability**, such as data readiness (e.g., availability, accuracy completeness, quality and granularity of data), functional requirements (e.g., test coverage), software performance (e.g., system load and response time acceptability), information quality (e.g., accuracy, relevance), interoperability (e.g., portability, standards compliance), and regulatory compliance (e.g., legal compliance, data encryption and backup, vulnerability testing);
- **Use and user satisfaction**, including use, self-reported use, intention to use, competency, ease of use, and satisfaction;
- **User acceptability**, such as cognitive load (e.g., cognitive effort), usability (e.g., ease of use, ease of learning), content quality, and integration with electronic health records;
- **User experience**, such as usability, feasibility, ease of use, satisfaction, engagement, working alliance, acceptance/preference, usefulness/helpfulness, perceived quality and trust, intention to use, and suggestions for improvement.

For IVD, efficacy encompassed clinical validity [28]:

- **Diagnostic accuracy,** including number of false negative and positive rates, true positive and negative counts, positive and negative predictive values, as well as sensitivity and specificity;
- **Human and workflow factors**, such as usability.

At TRLs 7–8, clinical investigations focused on the effectiveness of MD and the clinical utility of IVD. For MDs, clinical effectiveness encompassed [23–27, 29–31]:

- **Health care process**, such as diagnosis, treatment, prevention, and stratification;
- **Health economic evaluations**, such as unit costs (e.g., technology acquisition or action-specific costs), reduction of costs of care (e.g., reduction in hospital days and number of hospitalizations), and health economic evaluations (e.g., cost-utility, cost-effectiveness, cost-minimization, and cost-benefit analyses).
- **Personal intermediate outcomes**, such as health literacy, behaviour change, self-efficacy, knowledge, and skills;
- **Personal health outcomes**, such as disease onset, disease deterioration, hospitalization rate;
- **Performance metrics**, such as detection, triage, radiomics, segmentation, augmentation, classification, prediction;
- **Productivity measures**, including efficiency, resource reduction/reallocation, care coordination, cost-savings;
- **Service access**, including improved and cost-efficient access to services;
- **Service quality**, such as performance, responsiveness, and usability;
- **Safety and information quality**, such as risk of unintended harms;

- **User experience**, such as initial usability, user acceptance and satisfaction, perceived effectiveness, working alliance;
- **Quality of care**, including appropriateness of care, clinical outcomes, incidence of adverse events, care transitions.

For IVD, clinical utility included [28]:

- **Efficiency measures**, including work process and information flow;
- **Health economic evaluation**s, including resource use, costs, and quality adjusted life years (QALYs);
- **Performance measures**, including diagnostic accuracy;
- **Patient outcomes**, such as recovery, survival, and quality of life (QoL);
- **Quality of care**, such as clinical decision-making.

At TRL 9, clinical investigations focused on the implementation and clinical utility. For MDs, implementation encompassed [24, 25, 27, 29, 30]:

- **Access**, such as access to services/clinicians and patient/care-giver participation;
- **Clinical effectiveness**, including health outcomes in short, medium, and/or long term (e.g., clinical results, mortality, quality of life), patient satisfaction (e.g., willingness to reuse technology and recommend technology), and comparative accuracy of replacement technology;
- **Communication**, including quality of patient-caregiver interaction and stimulation of user-engagement, motivation, and involvement over time;
- **Business growth,** such as industrial activity and business growth related to new services and products;
- **Durability**, such as periodic quality control checks, ongoing monitoring of individual, and aggregated cases;
- **Economic outcomes**, including costs, cost-effectiveness, cost saving, and return on investment;
- **Environmental context**, such as organizational culture, risk tolerance, leadership, system design, and implementation processes;
- **Ethical analysis**, including principal question about the ethical aspects of technology (e.g., privacy and data security);
- **Human interaction and relations**, including patient-to-provider communication, shared decision-making, and patient-carer dependency;
- **Investments and tools required to use the technology,** such as type of operating system and its availability;
- **Regulation compliance**, including legal regulation of novel techniques;
- **Regulation of market**, such as reimbursement of intervention;
- **Safety**, such as technology- (e.g., number of adverse effects of intervention), use-, and user-dependent (e.g., misinterpretation of information sent) safety risks;
- **Social implementation**, such as readiness for wide clinical use (e.g., performance, accuracy, usability, workflow integration), implementation and maintenance costs, implementation strategies (e.g., facilitators and barriers in both individual and system levels), short-and long-term adoption, reach and fidelity, and innovation normalization;

- **Social outcomes**, such as process outcomes (e.g., completion of desired tasks under real-world conditions), health outcomes (e.g., patient health, equity, safety), health equity (e.g., impact across gender/minority groups), and dissemination value (e.g., value for another organization);
- **Technical implementation**, such as integration, installation, maintenance (e.g., software integration and configurability), technical support, and real-world technical performance (e.g., software stability and downtime);
- **Technical portability**, such as integration requirements;
- **Training and information needs,** including protocols, educational materials, and recommendations;
- **User satisfaction**, such as long-term usability, user acceptance, and satisfaction;
- **Value proposition**, including desirability, feasibility, and viability.

For IVD, implementation included:

- **Cost analysis**, such as cost-minimization and cost-consequences analyses;
- **Budget impact analysis**, assessing the effects on a defined budget, including both costs and revenues;
- **Value assessment**, including cost-effectiveness analysis (e.g., incremental cost-effectiveness ratio) and value of information analysis.

3.3 Clinical Investigation of Health Technologies at Different Risk Classes

Recommended evaluation methods were not reported by device risk class. Although information on the intended use of the health technologies was extracted from the studies, determining the risk category based solely on this information—without detailed manufacturer documentation—would have been unreliable.

4 Discussion

According to our findings, recommended evaluation methods varied across different TRLs, with considerable overlap observed between evaluation domains. In addition, these methods demonstrated a clear evolutionary progression, becoming progressively more rigorous and incorporating broader contextual and social considerations as technological maturity advanced (See Fig. 2).

Early evaluations focused on efficacy under controlled or ideal conditions. As technologies matured, the focus expanded to effectiveness in real-world settings, and ultimately to implementation, encompassing the adoption, integration, and sustainability of health technologies within specific contexts. At this stage, evaluations also addressed broader impacts, including influence on public health policies, organizational practices, and business outcomes, reflecting the widening societal and contextual relevance of the technology.

Consistent with previous studies [10, 11], clinical investigations of health technologies remain fragmented, and a standardized evaluation framework has yet to be established. Furthermore, the specific research instruments or operationalized outcome measures were infrequently reported, and notable inconsistencies in terminology were observed. In line with previous studies [35, 36], economic assessments and health economic evaluations were limited in the existing frameworks.

Classifying digital health technologies by function, as recommended by NICE and the Department of Health and Social Care, enables stratification into evidence tiers based on potential risk to users [28]. However, none of the included studies reported the risk classification of the health technologies, which precluded any analysis of evaluation methods according to risk level. A probable reason for this may be that the definition of health technology was inconsistent across studies, as some included MDs defined under EU regulations, while others examined broader technological solutions.

The intended use of health technologies was classified according to the EU Medical Device Regulation [8] and the In Vitro Diagnostic Regulation [2]. In some studies, the intended use was clearly described within the study, while in others it had to be inferred from the content of the publication and the description of the technology. Determining the risk class based solely on researchers' interpretations without official manufacturer documentation was considered too unreliable and could have led to incorrect conclusions.

Although the evaluation domains varied, the application of the TRL framework provided a novel and structured approach to map evaluation methods according to the stage of maturity. This review extends previous literature, which has primarily examined evaluation from methodological or technology-specific perspectives [18, 19, 37], by highlighting the phased progression of evaluation and the systematic shift in evaluation targets in accordance with technological maturity, demonstrating a clear evolutionary trajectory.

Only limited elements of generalizability, robustness, and reproducibility were reflected in the evaluation methods identified in this review. Future evaluations would benefit from more detailed recommendations that more explicitly articulate how the FAT paradigm—as well as robustness, reproducibility, and generalizability—should be systematically incorporated into the evaluation procedures [37].

4.1 Limitations and Future Recommendations

This scoping review has several limitations. First, only nine studies were included, most of which focused on MDSW, potentially overemphasizing evaluation methods for AI-based systems. Evaluation methods also varied across TRLs, with notable overlap between domains. Thus, these findings should be viewed as preliminary and require further investigation. Second, the search strategy focused on health technologies, which may explain the considerable number of database hits; future studies could benefit from focusing specifically on MDs and/or IVD. Third, time and language restrictions may have led to the exclusion of relevant studies. Fourth, the boundaries between TRLs were often blurred, reflecting the iterative nature of health technology development. However, the TRL approach appears to be a promising tool for structuring and harmonizing the clinical investigation of health technologies. However, its connection to existing regulatory requirements requires further exploration.

Entering into the market, manufactures need to meet considerable technical, financial, managerial, and regulatory challenges. Most studies were conducted in the United States, which may explain the regulatory focus, as only a few explicitly referenced EU

Regulations [2, 8], suggesting limited alignment between clinical evaluation and regulatory assessment in practice. The gap between regulation and research practice appears unclear, which may slow down the safe and effective implementation of new health technologies.

Although the health economic evaluations evolved, future studies should focus on different risk classes and comprehensive health economic evaluations. In addition, systematic literature reviews are needed to evaluate the state of the art of the clinical investigation performed at TRLs 1–4. The role of HTA should also be examined, as it provides a structured framework to assess the clinical, economic, organizational, and social impacts of health technologies, thereby informing evidence-based decision-making and supporting the adoption, integration, and sustainability of innovations in healthcare.

5   Conclusions

Based on this scoping review, the clinical investigation of health technologies remains fragmented. Notably, evaluation methods were not recommended by device risk class. The application of the TRL framework provided a novel and structured approach to map evaluation methods according to the stage of maturity. There is a need for harmonized evaluation frameworks that support clinical investigations in line with EU regulations.

Acknowledgments. We would like to acknowledge Informational Specialists Sirpa Grekula for her assistance with the search strategy.

Disclosure of Interests The authors have no competing interests to declare that are relevant to the content of this article.

References

1. World Health Organization. (2023) Health technologies. World Health Organization (2023). https://www.who.int/europe/news-room/fact-sheets/item/health-technologies
2. EU, European Union; Regulation (EU) 2017/746 of the European parliment and of the council. L_2017117EN.01017601.xml (2017)
3. Bitkina, O.V., Park, J., Kim, H.K.: Application of artificial intelligence in medical technologies: a systematic review of main trends. Digit. Health. **9**, 20552076231189331 (2023)
4. Endalamaw, A., Zewdie, A., Wolka, E., Assefa, Y.: A scoping review of digital health technologies in multimorbidity management: mechanisms, outcomes, challenges, and strategies. BMC Health Serv. Res. **25**, 382 (2025)
5. Abbasian, M. et al.: Foundation metrics for evaluating effectiveness of healthcare conversations powered by generative AI. NPJ Digit. Med. **7**, 82 (2024)
6. Alhussain, G., Kelly, A., O'Flaherty, E.I., Quinn, D.P., Flaherty, G.T.: Emerging role of artificial intelligence in global health care. Health Policy Technol. **11**(3), 100661 (2022)
7. Koebe, P.: How digital technologies and AI contribute to achieving the health-related SDGs. Int. J. Inf. Manag. Data Insights. **5**(1), 100298 (2025)
8. EU, European Union; Regulation (EU) 2017/745 of the European parliment and of the council. L_2017117EN.01000101.xml (2017)

9. Talman, K., Keinänen, A., Heikkinen, E., Rahkola, M., Weinitschke, T., Hollanti L. Terveyste-knologian sääntelyn käsikirja. (2024). https://www.sailab.fi/wp-content/uploads/2024/06/sai lab_terveysteknologiankasikirja-web-40.pdf

10. Beams, R. et al.: Evaluation challenges for the application of extended reality devices in medicine. J. Digit. Imaging. **35**(5), 1409–1418 (2022)

11. Hendrix, N., Veenstra, D.L., Cheng, M., Anderson, N.C., Verguet, S.: Assessing the economic value of clinical artificial intelligence: challenges and opportunities. Value Health: J. Int. Soc. Pharmacoeconomics Outcomes Res. **25**(3), 331–339 (2022)

12. Schachner, T., Keller, R., Wangenheim, V.: F.: artificial intelligence-based conversational agents for chronic conditions: systematic literature review. J. Med. Internet Res. **22**(9), e20701 (2020)

13. Maaß, L. et al.: Challenges and alternatives to evaluation methods and regulation approaches for medical apps as Mobile medical devices: international and multidisciplinary focus group discussion. J. Med. Internet Res. **26**, e54814 (2024)

14. Mankins, J.: Technology readiness levels. http://www.artemisinnovation.com/images/TRL_White_Paper_2004-Edited.pdf

15. Fleuren, L.M., Thoral, P., Shillan, D., Ercole, A., Elbers, P.W.G.: Machine learning in intensive care medicine: ready for take-off? Intensive Care Med. **46**(7), 1486–1488 (2020)

16. Jansen-Kosterink, S., Broekhuis, M., Van Velsen, L.: Time to act mature: gearing eHealth evaluations towards technology readiness levels. Digit. Health. **8**, 20552076221113396 (2022)

17. Ruiz Seva, R., Tan, A.L.S., Tejero, L.M.S., Salvacion, M.L.D.S.: Multi-dimensional readiness assessment of medical devices. Theor. Issues Ergon. Sci. **24**(2), 189–205 (2023)

18. Bonten, T.N. et al.: eHealth evaluation research group.: online guide for electronic health evaluation approaches: systematic scoping review and concept mapping study. J. Med. Internet Res. **22**(8), e17774 (2020)

19. Fajkis-Zajączkowska, N., Zawada, A., Bojko, M., Kolasa, K.: Comprehensive analysis of frameworks for evaluating artificial intelligence solutions in healthcare: a descriptive review. Comput. Biol. Med. **196**(Pt B), 110750 (2025)

20. Rauwerdink, A. et al.: Approaches to evaluating digital health technologies: scoping review. J. Med. Internet Res. **26**, e50251 (2024)

21. Peters, M., Godfrey, C., McInerney, P., Munn, Z., Tricco, A., Khalil, H.: Scoping Reviews. In: Aromataris, E., Lockwood, C., Porritt, K., Pilla, B., Jordan, Z. (eds.) JBI Manual for Evidence Synthesis. (2020)

22. Tricco, A.C. et al.: PRISMA extension for scoping reviews (PRISMA-ScR): checklist and explanation. Ann. Intern. Med. **169**(7), 467–473 (2018)

23. Ding, H., Simmich, J., Vaezipour, A., Andrews, N., Russell, T.: Evaluation framework for conversational agents with artificial intelligence in health interventions: a systematic scoping review. J. Am. Med. Inform. Assoc. **31**(3), 746–761 (2024)

24. Chapel, B. et al.: Standardization of the assessment process within telerehabilitation in chronic diseases: a scoping meta-review. BMC Health Serv. Res. **22**, 984 (2022)

25. Kukhareva, P.V. et al.: Evaluation in life cycle of information technology (ELICIT) framework: supporting the innovation life cycle from business case assessment to summative evaluation. J. Biomed. Inform. **127**, 104014 (2022)

26. Tanguay, W. et al.: Assessment of radiology artificial intelligence software: a validation and evaluation framework. Can. Assoc. Radiol. J. = J. l'Association Can. Radiol. **74**(2), 326–333 (2023)

27. Larson, D.B., Harvey, H., Rubin, D.L., Irani, N., Tse, J.R., Langlotz, C.P.: Regulatory frameworks for development and evaluation of artificial intelligence-based diagnostic imaging algorithms: summary and recommendations. J. Am. Coll.E Radiol.: JACR. **18**(3 Pt A), 413–424 (2021)

28. Graziadio, S. et al.: How to ease the pain of taking a diagnostic point of care test to the market: a framework for evidence development. Micromachines. **11**(3), 291 (2020)
29. Chouvarda, I. et al.: ENJECT working group 1 network: connected health services: framework for an impact assessment. J. Med. Internet Res. **21**(9), e14005 (2019)
30. Nagle, L.M.: The evaluation imperative. Stud. Health Technol. Inform. **225**, 88–92 (2016)
31. Park, S.H., Han, K.: Methodologic guide for evaluating clinical performance and effect of artificial intelligence technology for medical diagnosis and prediction. Radiology. **286**(3), 800–809 (2018)
32. World Health Organization: Monitoring and Evaluating Digital Health Interventions: A Practical Guide to Conducting Research and Assessment (2016). https://apps.who.int/iris/handle/10665/252183
33. National Institute for Health and Care Excellence (NICE): Evidence standards framework for digital health technologies. (2022). https://www.nice.org.uk/what-nice-does/digital-health/evidence-standards-framework-esf-for-digital-health-technologies
34. Lampe, K., Pasternack, I. (eds.): HTA Core Model for Diagnostic Technologies v 1.0. Work Package 4: The HTA Core Model. https://urn.fi/URN:NBN:fi-fe2020092475757 (2008)
35. Härkönen, H., Lakoma, S., Torkki, P., Laukka, E., Pennanen, P., Leskinen, R-L., Jansson, M.: Impact of digital services in healthcare and social welfare—an umbrella review. Int. J. Nurs. Stud. **152**, 104692 (2024)
36. Laukka, E. et al.: Effectiveness of interactive digital health services in non-communicable diseases: an umbrella review and evidence synthesis from 26 meta-analyses. Int. J. Nurs. Stud. **174**, 105277 (2025)
37. Recht, M.P. et al.: Integrating artificial intelligence into the clinical practice of radiology: challenges and recommendations. Eur. Radiol. **30**, 3576–3584 (2020)

HTA and Ethical Impact Assessment—Preliminary Perspectives

Jaakko Hakula$^{(\boxtimes)}$

90450 Kempele, Finland
jaakko.hakula@dnainternet.net

Abstract. Health technology assessment (HTA) is defined as a multidisciplinary process the explicit methods of which determine the value of products and systems throughout the entire lifecycle. Equity, efficiency, and high-quality reflect ethical, legal, and socio-economic values and norms. Subcategories of assessments steer the discussion towards general and AI ethics. AI-driven technologies present a whole new context where facts and values challenge communities of stakeholders. Ethical impact assessment as a study scenario leads the reader to a impact framework. A case of the sleep apnea digital care pathway by Pohde is backed up by the principles of digi-HTA. The positivist way of describing a process of ethical impact assessment is of a suggestive nature. Policies, practices, processes, and products and services are in the center of ethical HTA impact assessment. Hopefully the essay will nourish future discussions on the subject-matter.

Keywords: Health technology assessment · (AI) ethics · (AI) ethical impact assessment

1 Introduction

The aim of the study is to evaluate interdependencies between health technology assessment (HTA), HTA impact evaluation, and ethical argumentation, with preliminary views on a real-world example. Readers are reminded that the article is totally based on publicly available materials, except for some pieces of information about the author's own sleep apnea treatment. No insider (business) information has been at hand or made use of. Too specific comments or conclusions on complex process models are avoided for fear of possible mistakes and misunderstandings. The toolbox of the European Patients' Academy on Therapeutic Innovation (EUPATI) [1], and the impact framework of the Commonwealth Scientific and Industrial Re-search Organization (CSIRO), guide understanding of the subject matter. Overall outlines for moral assessment can be found in Crockett [2] —later complemented by several references on applied ethics in healthcare, medicine, and AI.

The idea of connecting HTA and (AI) ethical impact evaluation (or assessment) derives from the main topics of the Nordic Conference on Digital Health and Wire-less Solutions 2026 (NCDHWS2026) [3]. Results of several literature searches showed that

© The Author(s) 2026
M. Särestöniemi et al. (Eds.): NCDHWS 2026, CCIS 3009, pp. 166–178, 2026.
https://doi.org/10.1007/978-3-032-28812-7_14

focusing solely on a theoretical essay no novel aspects would be given to potential readers. Especially recent literature on AI ethics is abundant while that on impact assessment not as prominent. Combinations of the two are quite rare. Various ethical assessments have been made by ethics committees of research and healthcare organizations supporting studies. The rules of national boards and EU legislation have also been followed (e.g. cf. [4]). However, there is scarce knowledge whether processes of digital HTA and HTA impact evaluation − software and hard-ware planning, implementation and production included − have had ethical walkthroughs as a coordinated whole. For example, contractual restrictions of multi-stakeholder projects may hinder open access to relevant information to all participants or governmental authorities.

The inspiration to choose the real-world example from contexts of Digi-HTA [6–8] and sleep apnea [9–10] stems from the author's personal, multidisciplinary and professional interests, elaborated by own patient experiences. Both theoretical and practical choices made by the author presumably effect and affect the results and conclusions of the study. In the end, this essay ought to be seen as a suggestive opening for further discussions.

2 Literature Review

2.1 HTA in General

Health technology assessment (HTA) as a systematic discipline was launched in the mid-1970's by the U.S. Office of Technology Assessment. Thereafter, alternative definitions have been discussed. According to the latest (new) definition "HTA is a multidisciplinary process that uses explicit methods to determine the value of a health technology at different points in its lifecycle. The purpose is to inform decision-making in order to promote an equitable, efficient, and high-quality health system." The guiding principles of the new definition are to make it more understandable worldwide, accepted in multi-stakeholder cooperation [11–13]. The core definitional text is clarified with the aid of four notes. Notes 1 and 2 refer to interventional properties of health technologies, utilized in processes with the best available evidence. Note 3 encompasses dimensions of multiple values of health technologies (e.g. clinical effectiveness, ethical, legal, socio-economic, cultural, and organizational issues, with multiple stakeholders' interests). Note 4 emphasizes the lifecycle view of health technologies in relation to HTA processes [5].

The old definition of HTA referred by O'Rourke et al. [5] was more diffuse compared with the new version with its explanatory notes. The old version was more general and concentrated mainly around items around technology itself. Although the new definition is also built around technological issues it is further specified by its notes. The content of the notes explicates at least twofold changes that have taken place in recent decades. Multidisciplinary scientific progress has produced an immense growth of knowledge and know-how, which has improved people's health and welfare around the world, though mostly in western societies. In healthcare more evidence is gathered from scientific studies to be applied in practice. In democratic societies welfare standards have supported patient participation (e.g. cf. [1]). Con-currently, many negative impacts have occurred.

Complexities of international development on people's lives have given rise to socio-economic malaise. Malware in digitalized contexts is a fact. The aforementioned lines illuminate the applicability of the new definition of HTA to respond to present-day requirements. HTA is a multifaceted, evolutionary process focusing on multi-stakeholder cooperation in the limits of ethical, cultural, societal, legal, and economic principles. Constant discussion on values and norms in relation to HTA and its impacts are needed. The lifecycle view attains realistic goals to be set. HTA development processes in every phase of a lifecycle seek for a balanced solution (cf. [5, 6]).

Key prerequisites for successful diffusion of HTA thinking locally, nationwide and globally are based on joint visions of policy-driven and political debates on healthcare. In global contexts the focus of ethical thinking in HTA has given birth to several insights. HTA implementation has moral effects, which justify ethical evaluation in addition to preferring economic parameters. Values carried by technology may disrupt traditional moral principles and rules of society, also applying to HTA. The central idea of HTA is to strive for better healthcare, and as healthcare with its values attempts to improve health and welfare, the same is also valid for HTA. Likewise, healthcare and health policy are expected to share evidence-based principles and transparency in decision-making [7]. Both facts and values matter in the HTA contexts [8].

Recent studies on HTA of complex health technologies reveal somewhat contradictory results. Problems often arise because of insufficient research data — not necessarily in connection with technical complexities of the products themselves [9]. Health technology companies around the world confront inadequate resources and economic turbulence in the competitive markets. The goals of adaptive health technology assessment (aHTA) may compromise those of full-fledged deployment of HTA. Policy makers' priority-settings demand agile services from HTA agencies and health technology companies. aHTA methods are widely used in various contexts, but more precise definitions are expected from both researchers and practitioners [10].

2.2 On Healthcare and AI Ethics

Without exaggeration, artificial intelligence-based technologies (AIHT) pose a major challenge to multidisciplinary HTA projects [11]. AIHT's differ from traditional health technologies in many respects. They have translational impact widely on health and healthcare systems, and they may provoke increased expectations in everyday field-work. New ethical, legal and social controversies emerge. The opaque complexity of AIHT's puts pressure on regulators, policy-makers, and HTA agencies when evaluating and approving AI products [19–21]. Despite AI in healthcare having huge potential to access high-quality medical services, product teams in health technology companies are faced with multiple conundrums in clinical validation, regulatory affairs, data strategy and model development [12]. Standardization-related and ethical dilemmas in AI have perplexed legislatures to enact in complex environments [23–26]. The ecosystem view of healthcare decision-making might support stakeholders to comprehend the interconnected complexities across disciplines and practices [13].

The importance of digital technology as a modern norm setter in relation to traditional actors in politics and legislature is underlined by researchers in sociology of law [14]. Algorithms in a technical sense differ significantly from those of a social-science view. Hydén [14] defines algo norms as second-order entities, and as a sub-category of technical norms. Algo norms emerge when algorithms are faced with the surrounding society. They have indirect societal consequences. Legal norms share the same pattern of two-level properties with technical and algo norms. Strictly speaking legal norms instruct actors to correct interpretation and application of legal rules. They have also a second-order influence on societal issues. Algo norms often create uncertainties in legal regulation. AI-driven technologies are used in decision-making, learning, and executing tasks where data may be complex and laborious to interpret. Ignorance about the potential of new technology transforms a practical problem into a value one. Ambivalence in deep tech regulation may lead to a trial-and-error mode of norm setting. Policymakers prefer to debate on primary legal issues in the spirit of ethical arguments. Legislative procedures may be postponed until future governmental programmes are negotiated [14] (e.g. cf. [15]).

The fundamentals of healthcare / medical ethics and general AI ethics date back to the three main schools of normative ethics: virtue ethics, deontological ethics, and consequentialism (e.g. utilitarianism) [16, 17]. The main principles of medical ethics – beneficence, nonmaleficence, autonomy, and justice and equity – are intermingled with engineering and business ethics to produce versions of applied ethics of technology and AI [7, 16, 18]. Globally the digital world ethics of applied AI in healthcare resides in the centers of both theoretical and practical debates [32–34]. There are several reasons for the present situation. Firstly, epistemic concerns refer to evidence-based inconsistencies of AI in medicine and healthcare. Secondly, normative concerns reflect the justifiable fears that AI shall transform basic conceptions of health, healthcare and medical practice. Thirdly, traceability concerns raise questions about 'the black-box' properties of AI systems development that may deteriorate rules of accountability [19]. Multiple biases related to AI and machine learning (ML) systems prevail. Ethical dilemmas of injustice, bad output/outcome, restricted autonomy, transformation of basic concepts and values, and defects of accountability emerge [20]. Generative AI, and more specifically, large language models (LLM) applied in versatile autonomous systems with agentic properties enhance the potential availability of high-tech product spectrum, increasing ethical challenges also in healthcare [21, 34–36].

The crux of AI ethics is a systematic framework of interconnected concepts beginning from transparency, fairness, and privacy. The goal of ethical activity is to reach responsible AI use, supported by user trust, accountability, and non-discriminatory data practices [22]. In healthcare AI developers are provided with operationalizable guidelines to be utilized in design and applications. Human-centered and holistic views are respected in AI development. The basics of the ethical AI framework in healthcare rely on professional best practices, where the AI lifecycle stands for data management, model development, deployment and monitoring. Governance as organizational and regulation as legal policies are built on the aforementioned basics. The whole framework can be called ethical AI [23, 37–38]. In practice, mere summaries of theoretical principles and general guidelines do not solve individual or organizational ethical problems in HTA. More sophisticated, context-specific tools are needed [7, 24, 25].

Yet one more complex concept regarding AI ethical question remains. AI (value) alignment is a process, where values or principles are formally encoded in AI systems with the purpose of reflecting instructions, intents or preferences of the primary or wider stakeholders. AI alignment consists of technical and normative aspects, and its goals can differ significantly according to the interest groups. Instead of trying to find genuinely moral principles of alignment, fair principles might suffice. Both sociotechnical, interpersonal (macro) and socioaffective, intrapersonal (micro) perspectives broaden the technical emphasis of the alignment concept [41–43].

2.3   (Ethical) Technology and Impact Assessment

There is no single, omnivalid definition of impact assessment. The context and stakeholders' worldviews and goals of the projects determine the alternatives to be chosen [26]. In a philosophical stance, five ideal types can be discerned. Different assumptions can be considered about the nature of knowledge (i.e. ontology) and the possibility of finding out and understanding that very knowledge (i.e. epistemology). In impact assessment of health research paradigms are diverse. Evidence-based medicine (EBM) and (health) economical models represent mainly positivist methodologies while the remaining four types of constructivist, realist, critical, and performative origins broaden the scope of impact evaluation towards social sciences [27]. One practical definition of impact refers to"an effect on, change or benefit to the economy, society and/or environment, beyond those contributions to academic knowledge." [28].

Researchers [29] present four interconnected approaches of impact assessment. Technology assessment (TA), with subcategories of health TA, industrial TA or participatory TA, has introduced most comprehensive and multidisciplinary evaluations of safe and suitable technologies. Impact assessment (IA) strives analytically to predict or at least forecast future realizations of key effects. Its subsets are environmental impact assessment (EnIA) and societal impact assessment (SIA). The difference between the occurrence and non-occurrence of action can be defined as an impact or effect. Possible decisions should be based on the best available information, bearing in mind IA's adaptivity to react to changes during the whole project [29].

The counterparts of TA and IA are ethical technology assessment (eTA) and ethical impact assessment (eIA), respectively. The relevance of eTA involves systematic argumentation by ethicists during the whole lifecycle of a technology project, and that of eIA is to encourage developers and decision-makers to participate in the ethical assessment of their projects. In general, all of the aforementioned approaches have several mutual aims, but they also differ in some respects. All of them facilitate participation and produce social shaping of research and innovation (IA with certain constraints). TA, IA and eIA can be utilized to predict consequences of societal developments, also with the aim of avoiding harms from technology and infrastructural programmes. TA and eIA address societal challenges. Many overlapping and partly contradictory definitions of evaluation methods can be found even in the one and the same publication [29]. Impact assessment projects can be compromised in many ways. There may be remarkable time lag between active phases of (research) projects and impacts to be evaluated. Impacts are often complex and dynamic – not easily attributable to some specified item or stakeholder. Confounding factors may arise when new data, information or evidence achieved in earlier phases of a project intermingle with accepted outcomes, thus making it difficult to reach reliable conclusions on impacts [26].

3 Ethical Impact Assessment as a Study Scenario

3.1 Ethical Impact Assessment

Ethical impact assessment (EIA) can be defined as a structured, anticipatory process which identifies and evaluates the ethical contributions of emerging technologies, planned research or innovation projects, and legislation, with priorities to inform primary stakeholders in design, governance and policy-makers. EIA focuses on ethical analysis as an essential part of assessment. EIA is applied amongst wide range of technologies, preferring the idea of life-cycle involvement [47,48; cf. [5], Note 4].

EIA shares the systematic analysis of ethically relevant subject matter with traditional ethical evaluation methods, but differs from the traditional ones in several respects. One core property of EIA is lifecycle orientation, reminding stakeholders of the importance to apply ethical reflecting through the entire developmental project. Much emphasis is put on anticipatory approach. EIA underlines ethics-guided governance. Ethical evaluation is integrated into responsible practices. The deployment of systematic, anticipatory, and context-sensitive methodology guarantees a qualified ethical reflection across the entire technological development. Responsiveness to new knowledge from operational environment and alignment with societal values [30–32].

EIA utilizes methodologies according to its primary objective: identification and evaluation of the ethical criteria for novel technologies and projects. Various step-by-step methods are applied depending on the context [31, 32]. Ethical impacts (i.e. ethical implications of emerging technologies) originate in development, introduction, or appliance of technologies that can be evaluated as morally positive or negative following ethical principles, values, or societal norms [31]. To succeed in an EIA, sufficient capacity is needed to identify possible future consequences of technologies, concurrently with the ability to arrange ethically significant consequences to be evaluated in a proper manner. The capacity-ability pair sets the methodological foundation of EIA: foresight analysis and ethical analysis as methods of choice. An understanding of the technologies with their social, legal, and institutional context is imperative [31].

3.2 AI Ethical Impact Assessment

Multidisciplinarity and multimodality represent a modern way of defining the concepts of AI and algorithmic impact assessment (AIA). Focusing on merely technical matters escapes the potential of both multifarious benefits and harms. As multidisciplinarity broadens the scope of investigation within AIAs, multimodality leads communities of stakeholders to learn of knowing the capabilities, restrictions, ethical issues, and societal effects of AI systems. Societal risks, impacts, and harms can be identified cooperatively across disciplines, thus ending up with promising results [33]. Both positive and negative aspects of impacts of AI systems help the HTA industry to survive [34].

Kazim and Koshiyama [35] emphasize the intimate connection between data and AI ethics. They present the evolution of AI ethics in three consecutive phases — principle-based, ethical-by-design, and standardization-operationalization ones. Trust-worthy AI ethics as applied ethics stands for 'the psychological, social and political impact of AI,' and is further expanded towards human-centric AI ethics defined as 'the development and deployment of AI systems that respect human dignity and autonomy'. AI impact assessment should be prioritized over data protection. More-over, it should remain independent of data protection due to special properties of AI technology irreducible to principles of data security [35].

4 A Case Description

4.1 The Digi-HTA Context

Finnish Coordinating Center for Health Technology Assessment (FinCCHTA) is the national HTA coordination unit that steers health technology assessment work in Finland. Digi-HTA is a method developed for digital products and services for social and health care and well-being by FinCCHTA. The suitability of a product or service is evaluated for the use of customers and employees in IT. The items of assessment consist of effectiveness, costs, safety, data protection and security, along with usability and accessibility. Especially conditions of commissioning of a digital product (e.g. the care process and changes in IT), are examined. High technology companies are offered opportunities to demonstrate the suitability of their digital products or services for the use in social and health care or in promoting well-being [36, 37].

Digi-HTA has advanced, for example, generation of various digital health applications, artificial intelligence (AI), and robotics. The emphasis of developmental activities in HTA is on harmonization and coordination of pan-European and global perspectives [37]. Interestingly, all but one of the four HTA models evaluated and compared to each other had ethics issues systematically covered: the global CEN ISO/TS 82304–2 framework. In the other three − the Finnish Digi-HTA, the German DiGAV, and the NordDEC of the Nordic countries – systematic ethical aspects were not available [38].

4.2 The Case of Sleep Apnea Digital Care Pathway (SA-DCP)

The prevalence of obstructive sleep apnea (OSA) has been increasing globally in recent years. Sleep apnea is linked to multiple morbidity, especially metabolic, car-diovascular, and musculosceletal diseases in various combinations [39]. Continuous positive airway pressure (CPAP) therapy is the treatment of choice for moderate or severe sleep apnea. CPAP therapy reduced the apnea-hypopnea index (AHI) and daytime sleepiness. Physical activity improved the quality of life of the OSA pa-tients [40]. The economic benefits of CPAP were connected to potential decline in healthcare use, and also to parameters of quality of life [41]. CPAP was cost-effective compared to the non-treatment group with OSA [42]. More studies are needed in relation long-term outcomes and combination therapies [37].

In 2019 a sleep apnea digital care pathway (SA-DCP) was launched at Oulu University Hospital (OUH). It is an example of an application produced according to digi-HTA principles [4, 43–45]. The CPAP therapy starts with initial guiding on the use of the device. SA-DCP consists of information and instructions about CPAP therapy. The idea is to encourage patients to explore digital material in advance. The aim of the procedure is to enhance the initial guiding session, and presumably re-duce the amount of later contacts by phone or face-to-face. Electronic messaging via the SA-DCP technology is also available between patients and healthcare per-sonnel. Study results on SA-DCP use were promising but further follow-up is needed [4].

5 Results and Discussion

Figure 1 illustrates a modified impact framework on a general level [28]. It represents the positivist (consequentalist or utilitarian) school of impact evaluation [27]. Alternatively, teleological (virtue ethical), and deontological moral assessment can be placed in the same context. The idea to use the framework is try to clarify some very preliminary suggestions of ethical impact assessment, leaving systematic HTA themes in the background. However, HTA is backing up the presentation.

The impact framework depicted in Fig. 1 can resemble a lifecycle according to the new definition of HTA [5]. On the other hand, ethical impact assessment process in the five phases with the feed-back loop and additional project specifications can be imagined in the form of a lifecycle. The ethical impact assessment process starts from the input phase, where ethics personnel have the capabilities and abilities needed to delve into ethical argumentation (cf. [33]). The activities phase is presented as a AI-driven process in this case, and in the output phase contains ethical material about the activities. Changes – both positive and negative – are summarized in the outcomes phase. The whole lifecycle proceeds in time and space [1, 26, 28].

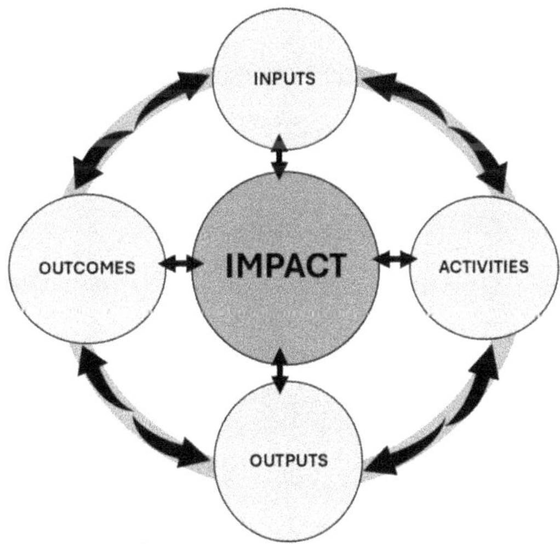

Fig. 1. Impact framework (modified by ideas from [1, 28])

The impact phase is a complex, multidisciplinary and multidimensional bunch of ethical reflections. Longe-range temporal involvement can be described as repetitive rounds of feedback between the entities of the impact framework in Fig. 1 [28, 44–45]. The phases of input-activities-output produce the scheduled and controllable action, and those of output-outcomes-impact represent results, with direct and indirect possibilities of influence. The whole of five phases with the feedback stand for planning and evaluation, while the first three ones are called monitoring [28].

With reference to Sect. 4 contents of the digi-HTA and SA-DCP are to fit in the (AI ethical) impact framework presented in Fig. 1. A new determinant of ethical impact assessment could be added to the key assessment domains. The requirements for the procedure should be multidisciplinary and multimodal (cf. [33]). In an ideal world the whole process and lifecycle of the SA-DCP could be morally assessed according to three main schools of normative ethics. Virtuous persons as decision-makers and representatives of institutions aim to common good, with no intentions of immorality or self-interest. Deontic ethics emphasizes free will and rational capacity to judge between right and wrong decisions. Economic issues must be viewed as systems of equal rights and defined duties. The dominant practice, consequentalism, pinpoints the importance of outcomes. Individual interests and desires are acceptable [2, 16].

From a patient perspective perhaps the most contradictory issue is associated with trust and (AI) transparency of the SA-DCP. The various black boxes in the process might trigger mistrust and suspicions towards professionals and health organizations. Can one rely on digital facilities? On what premises should one trust?

6 Conclusions

The aim of the study is to provoke discussion on the necessity of connecting ethical impact assessment to HTA projects both locally and nationally −even globally. Especially there is a true need to expand AI ethical (impact) assessment transdisciplinarily. Policies, practices, processes, and products and services are in the center of ethical HTA impact assessment [46].

Disclosure of Interests. None declared.

References

1. European Patients' Academy on Therapeutic Innovation (EUPATI): Health Technology Assessment process: Fundamentals. https://toolbox.eupati.eu/resources/health-technology-assessment-process-fundamentals. (2026) Last accessed March 29 2026
2. Crockett, C.: The cultural paradigm of virtue. J. Bus. Ethics. **62**(4), 191–208 (2005). https://doi.org/10.1007/s10551-005-0190-8
3. Nordic Conference on Digital Health and Wireless Solutions 2026 (NCDHWS) homepage. https://nordic-digihealth.com. Last accessed 30 March 2026
4. Haverinen, J., Harju, T., Mikkonen, H., Liljamo, P., Turpeinen, M., Reponen, J.: Digital care pathway for patients with sleep apnea in specialized care: mixed methods study. JMIR Hum. Factors. **11e47809** (2024). https://doi.org/10.2196/47809
5. O'Rourke, B., Oortwijn, W., Schuller, T.: The new definition of health technology assessment: a milestone in international collaboration. Int. J. Technol. Assess. Health Care. **36**(3), 187–190 (2020). https://doi.org/10.1017/S0266462320000215

6. Urbina, I., Adams, R., Fernandez, J., Willemsen, A., Hedberg, N., Rüther, A.: Advancing cooperation in health technology assessment in Europe: insights from the EUnetHTA 21 project amidst the evolving legal landscape of European HTA. Int. J. Technol. Assess. Health Care. **40**(1), e75 (2024). https://doi.org/10.1017/S0266462324004689

7. Saarni, SI., Hofmann, B., Lampe, K., Lühmann, D., Mäkelä, M., Velasco-Garrido, M., et al.: Ethical analysis to improve decision-making on health technologies. Bull. World Health Organ. 86(8), 617–623 (2008). doi:https://doi.org/10.2471/BLT.08.051078

8. Hofmann, B., Bond, K., Sandman, L.: Evaluating facts and facting evaluations: on the fact-value relationship in HTA. J. Eval. Clin. Pract. **24**, 957–965 (2018). https://doi.org/10.1111/jep.12920

9. Hogervorst, M.A., et al.: Reported challenges in health technology assessment of complex health technologies. Value Health. **25**(6), 992–1001 (2022). https://doi.org/10.1016/j.jval.2021.11.1356

10. Nemzoff, C., et al.: Adaptive health technology assessment: a scoping review of methods. Value Health. **26**(10), 1549–1557 (2023). https://doi.org/10.1016/j.jval.2023.05.017

11. Alami, H. et al.: Artificial intelligence and health technology assessment: anticipating a new level of complexity. J Med Internet Res. **22**(7), e17707 (2020). https://doi.org/10.2196/17707

12. Higgins, D., Madai, V.I.: From bit to bedside: a practical framework for artificial intelligence product development in healthcare. Adv. Intell. Syst. **2**, 2000052 (2020). https://doi.org/10.1002/aisy.202000052

13. Schünemann, H.J., et al.: The ecosystem of health decision making: from fragmentation to synergy. Lancet Public Health. **7**(4), e378–e390 (2022). https://doi.org/10.1016/S2468-2667(22)00057-3

14. Hydén, H.: AI, norms, big data, and the law. Asian J. Law Society. **7**(3), 409–436 (2020). https://doi.org/10.1017/als.2020.36

15. Värri, A.O.: Harmonised standards to the AI act—for medical devices, too. FinJeHeW 17(2), 235–240 .https://doi.org/10.23996/fjhw.159722. https://eur-lex.europa.eu/eli/reg/2024/1689/oj/eng. (2025) Last accessed 26 Jan 2026

16. Kazim, E., Koshiyama, A.: A high-level overview of AI ethics. Patterns. **2**(9), 100314 (2021). https://doi.org/10.1016/j.patter.2021.100314

17. Ortega-Bolaños, R., Bernal-Salcedo, J., Germán Ortiz, M., et al.: Applying the ethics of AI: a systematic review of tools for developing and assessing AI-around systems. Artif. Intell. Rev. **57**, 110 (2024). https://doi.org/10.1007/s10462-024-10740-3

18. Varkey, B.: Principles of clinical ethics and their application to practice. Medical principles and practice: international journal of the Kuwait University, Health Science Centre. **30**(1), 17–28 (2021). https://doi.org/10.1159/000509119

19. Morley, J., Floridi, L.: The ethics of AI in health care: an updated mapping review. **1−31** (2024). https://doi.org/10.2139/ssrn.4987317

20. Hofmann, B.: Biases in AI: acknowledging and addressing the inevitable ethical issues. Front Digit Health, 20(7), 1614105. doi:10.3389/fdgth.2025.1614105

21. Stahl, B.C., Eke, D.: The ethics of ChatGPT–exploring the ethical issues of an emerging technology. Int. J. Inf. Manag. **74**, 102700 (2024). https://doi.org/10.1016/j.ijinfomgt.2023.102700

22. Solanki, P., Grundy, J., Hussain, W.: Operationalising ethics in artificial intelligence for healthcare: a framework for AI developers. AI Ethics. **3**(1), 223–240 (2023). https://doi.org/10.1007/s43681-022-00195-z

23. Radanliev, P.: AI ethics: integrating transparency, fairness, and privacy in AI development. Appl. Artif. Intell. **39**(1), 1–42 (2025). https://doi.org/10.1080/08839514.2025.2463722

24. Iniesta, R.: The human role to guarantee an ethical AI in healthcare: a five-facts approach. AI Ethics. **5**, 385–397 (2025). https://doi.org/10.1007/s43681-023-00353-x
25. Kemell, K.K., Floréen, P., Raatikainen, M., et al.: Implementing AI ethics in practice and the question of 'who?' A framework and a multiple case study. AI Ethics. **6**, 45 (2026). https://doi.org/10.1007/s43681-025-00870-x
26. Penfield, T., Baker, M.J., Scoble, R., Wykes, M.C.: Assessment, evaluations, and definitions of research impact: a review. Res. Eval. **23**(1), 21–32 (2014). https://doi.org/10.1093/reseval/rvt021
27. Raftery, J., Hanney, S., Greenhalgh, T., Glover, M., Blatch-Jones, A.: Models and applications for measuring the impact of health research: update of a systematic review for the health technology assessment programme. Health Technol. Assess. **20**(76) (2016). https://doi.org/10.3310/hta20760
28. Commonwealth Scientific and Industrial Research Organization (CSIRO). How CSIRO ensures it delivers impact. https://www.csiro.au/en/about/Corporate-governance/Ensuring-our-impact/A-CSIRO-wide-approach-to-impact. Last accessed 30 Jan 2026
29. Nielsen, R.Ø.; Gurzawska, A., Brey, P.: Principles and Approaches in Ethics Assessment. Ethical Impact Assessment and Conventional Impact Assessment. SATORI, European Commission's Seventh Framework Programme (FP7/2007–2013) (2015). https://satoriproject.eu/media/1.a-Ethical-impact-assessmt-CIA.pdf
30. Gabriel, I.: Artificial intelligence, values, and alignment. Minds Mach. **30**, 411–437 (2020). https://doi.org/10.1007/s11023-020-09539-2
31. Brey, P.A.E.: Ethical impact assessment: theoretical foundations, methodology, and applications. Sci. Eng. Ethics. **32**, 6 (2026). https://doi.org/10.1007/s11948-025-00574-9
32. Reijers, W., Brey, P., Rodrigues, R., Koivisto, R., Tuominen, A.: A Common Framework for Ethical Impact Assessment. SATORI, European Commission's Seventh Framework Programme (FP7/2007–2013) (2016). https://satoriproject.eu/media/D4.1_Annex_1_EIA_Proposal.pdf
33. Becerra Sandoval, J.C., Jing, F., Alvarado Garcia, A., Berger, S.E., Candello, H., Lustig, C.: Opportunities and challenges of multidisciplinary algorithmic impact assessments. J. Responsible Innov. **12**(1), 2499302 (2025). https://doi.org/10.1080/23299460.2025.2499302
34. Rahman, M.A., Victoros, E., Ernest, J., Davis, R., Shanjana, Y., Islam Md, R.: Impact of artificial intelligence (AI) Technology in Healthcare Sector: a critical evaluation of both sides of the coin. Clin. Pathol. **17** (2024). https://doi.org/10.1177/2632010X241226887
35. Kazim, E., Koshiyama, A.: The interrelation between data and AI ethics in the context of impact assessments. AI Ethics. **1**, 219–225 (2021). https://doi.org/10.1007/s43681-020-00029-w
36. FinCCHTA (the Finnish Coordinating Center for Health Technology Assessment): Digi-HTA. https://fincchta.fi/en/digi-hta-eng/about-digi-hta. Last accessed 30 March 2026
37. Haverinen, J., Keränen, N., Falkenbach, P., Maijala, A., Kolehmainen, T., Reponen, J.: Digi-HTA: health technology assessment framework for digital healthcare services. Finn. J. Ehealth Ewelfare. **11**(4), 326–341 (2019). https://doi.org/10.23996/fjhw.82538
38. Haverinen, J., et al.: Finnish Digi-HTA Assessment Model for Digital Health and an International Comparison. In: Särestöniemi, M. et al. (eds.) Digital Health and Wireless Solutions: NCDHWS 2024. Springer Cham; 2024:309–332. Last accessed 30 Sep 2025. https://doi.org/10.1007/978-3-031-59091-7_20
39. Palomäki, M., Saaresranta, T., Anttalainen, U., Partinen, M., Keto, J., Linna, M.: Multimorbidity and overall comorbidity of sleep apnea: a Finnish nationwide study. ERJ Open Res. **8**(2), 1–12 (2022). https://doi.org/10.1183/23120541.00646-2021

40. Figard, C., et. al.: Effect of sleep apnea interventions on multiple health outcomes: an umbrella review of meta-analyses of randomised controlled trial. **eClinicalMedicine 89**, 103529 (2025). https://doi.org/10.1016/j.eclinm.2025.103529
41. McMillan, A., Bratton, D.J., Faria, R., Laskawiec-Szkonter, M., Griffin, S., Davies, R.J., et al.: A multicentre randomised controlled trial and economic evaluation of continuous positive airway pressure for the treatment of obstructive sleep apnea syndrome in older people: PREDICT. Health Technol. Assess. **19**(40) (2015). https://doi.org/10.3310/hta19400
42. Robles, A., et al.: Cost-utility and budget impact analysis of CPAP therapy compared to no treatment in the management of moderate to severe obstructive sleep apnea in Colombia from a third-party payer perspective. Expert Rev. Pharmacoecon. Outcomes Res. **23**(4), 399–407 (2023). https://doi.org/10.1080/14737167.2023.2181792
43. Haverinen, J.: The Digi-HTA, a new health technology assessment model for digital health technologies. Doctoral dissertation, University of Oulu. Acta Universitatis Ouluensis. D, Medica 1803 (2024). https://urn.fi/URN:NBN:fi:oulu-202409125818
44. The Wellbeing County of Northern Ostrobothnia (Pohde). Evaluation of methods. https://pohde.fi/tietoa-meista/kehittaminen-ja-innovaatiot/menetelmien-arviointi/ (SIC!Translate from Finnish into English), Last accessed 30 March 2026
45. The Wellbeing County of Northern Ostrobothnia (Pohde).: Pohde uniapnean digi-hoitopolku. https://www.terveyskyla.fi/omapolku/digihoitopolut/pohde-uniapnea-digihoito polku. Last accessed 30 March 2026
46. Graham, K.E.R., Langlois-Klassen, D., Adam, S.A.M., Chan, L., Chorzempa, H.L.: Assessing Health Research and innovation impact: evolution of a framework and tools in Alberta Canada. Front. Res. Metr. Anal. **3**, 25 (2018). https://doi.org/10.3389/frma.2018.00025
47. FinCCHTA (the Finnish Coordinating Center for Health Technology Assessment) homepage. https://fincchta.fi/en/fincchta. Last accessed 30 March 2026
48. WHO: Health Technology Assessment of Medical Devices. WHO Medical Device Technical Series, 2nd edn. World Health Organization, Geneva (2025)
49. Di Bidino, R., Daugbjerg, S., Papavero, S.C., Haraldsen, I.H., Cicchetti, A., Sacchini, D.: Health technology assessment framework for artificial intelligence-based technologies. Int. J. Technol. Assess. Health Care. **40**(1), e61 (2024). https://doi.org/10.1017/S0266462324000308
50. Bélisle-Pipon, J.-C., Couture, V., Roy, M.-C., Ganache, I., Goetghebeur, M., Cohen, I.G.: What makes artificial intelligence exceptional in health technology assessment. Front. Artif. Intell. **4**, 736697. https://doi.org/10.3389/frai.2021.736697
51. Laux, J., Wachter, S., Mittelstadt, B.: Three pathways for standardisation and ethical disclosure by default under the European union artificial intelligence act. Comput. Law Secur. Rev. **53**, 105957 (2024). https://doi.org/10.1016/j.clsr.2024.105957
52. Pham, T.: Ethical and legal considerations in healthcare AI: innovation and policy for safe and fair use. R. Soc. Open Sci. **12**(5), 241873 (2025). https://doi.org/10.1098/rsos.241873
53. Corfmat, M., Martineau, J.T., Régis, C.: High-reward, high-risk technologies? An ethical and legal account of AI development in healthcare. BMC Med. Ethics. **26**, 4 (2025). https://doi.org/10.1186/s12910-024-01158-1
54. Acharya, D.B., Kuppan, K., Divya, B.: Agentic AI: autonomous intelligence for complex goals—a comprehensive survey. IEEE Access 13, 18912–18936 (2025). doi:https://doi.org/10.1109/ACCESS.2025.3532853
55. Sapkota, R., Roumeliotis, K.I., Karkee, M.: AI agents vs. Agentic AI: a conceptual taxonomy, applications and challenges. Inf. Fusion. **126B, 103599** (2026). https://doi.org/10.1016/j.inffus.2025.103599

56. Elia, M., Ziethmann, P., Krumme, J., et al.: Responsible AI, ethics, and the AI lifecycle: how to consider the human influence? AI Ethics. **5**, 4011–4028 (2025). https://doi.org/10.1007/s43681-025-00666-z
57. Dahlgren Lindström, A., Methnani, L., Krause, L., et al.: Helpful, harmless, honest? Sociotechnical limits of AI alignment and safety through reinforcement learning from human feedback. Ethics Inf. Technol. **27**, 28 (2025). https://doi.org/10.1007/s10676-025-09837-2
58. Kirk, H.R., Gabriel, I., Summerfield, C., et al.: Why human-AI relationships need socioaffective alignment. Hum. It Soc Sci Commun. **12**, 728 (2025). https://doi.org/10.1057/s41599-025-04532-5

User Experience, Acceptance and Adoption of Health Information Systems

Determinants of Citizen Adoption of the EUDI Wallet for Health Services in Finland: A Scoping Review and Conceptual Framework

Khaled Md Saifullah[1]([✉])(iD), Mohammad Rahman[2](iD),
Miguel Bordallo López[2](iD), Timo Koivumäki[1](iD), Kristina Mikkonen[3](iD),
Minna Isomursu[4](iD), Olli Silvén[2,5](iD), and Constantino Álvarez Casado[2,5]([✉])(iD)

[1] Martti Ahtisaari Institute, Oulu Business School, University of Oulu,
Oulu, Finland
[2] Center for Machine Vision and Signal Analysis (CMVS), University of Oulu,
Oulu, Finland
constantino.alvarezcasado@oulu.fi
[3] Research Unit of Health Sciences and Technology, University of Oulu,
Oulu, Finland
[4] Empirical Software Engineering in Software, Systems and Services (M3S),
University of Oulu, Oulu, Finland
[5] Candour Oy, Oulu, Finland

Abstract. By late 2026, the mandate for European Digital Identity Wallets (EUDI Wallets) under the revised eIDAS framework will fundamentally affect the interaction model of the Finnish national *Kanta* ecosystem. This study presents a scoping review of 74 studies, following the PRISMA-ScR reporting guideline, to map the determinants of citizen adoption when health-related authentication and attribute presentation are mediated through the wallet paradigm. We propose a descriptive conceptual framework that integrates the Unified Theory of Acceptance and Use of Technology (UTAUT2) with Privacy Calculus Theory to explain user behavior across three interacting layers: citizen-level psychology, the functional wallet paradigm, and the institutional governance ecosystem. Our findings reveal that adoption in Finland is not a struggle for basic digitization, but a complex migration of established habits into a decentralized model. The framework distinguishes between the wallet as an identity and consent broker for cloud-based services (Role A) and as a secure local container for verifiable credentials like e-prescriptions, vaccinations and the European Health Insurance Card (Role B). We analyze the "Root of Trust" established by national authorities, including the Digital and Population Data Services Agency (DVV), the Finnish Transport and Communications Agency (Traficom), and the National Police Board, and contrast this with the psychological impact of systemic data breaches, such as the Vastaamo incident. Beyond technical utility, the synthesis highlights the role of "Warm Experts" in bridging the digital divide for citizens over age 75. To our knowledge, this is the

M. Särestöniemi et al. (Eds.): NCDHWS 2026, CCIS 3009, pp. 181–213, 2026.
https://doi.org/10.1007/978-3-032-28812-7_15

first review focused specifically on determinants of Finnish citizen adoption of the EUDI Wallet for health services and on translating those determinants into a wallet-specific conceptual framework. The resulting synthesis provides a roadmap for service designers to use selective disclosure and purpose-limited requests to strengthen perceived safety and digital equity in the high-sensitivity domain of healthcare.

Keywords: EUDI Wallet · Digital Health Adoption · Finland · eIDAS 2.0 · Privacy Calculus · UTAUT2 · Verifiable Credentials

1 Introduction

Digital health services require strong electronic identification and controlled sharing of sensitive information. The revised eIDAS framework (Regulation (EU) 2024/1183), often referred to as "eIDAS 2.0" [1], establishes the European Digital Identity Wallet (EUDI Wallet) as an EU interaction model for the identification and presentation of verifiable attributes. In parallel, the European Health Data Space (EHDS) increases the policy relevance of interoperable and accountable digital access to health information across Member States. Healthcare is treated as a priority sector, and designated public and private providers are required to accept the wallet for authentication [1]. Beyond technical interoperability, the framework introduces a reliance model with relying party registration and transparency expectations, including justification and proportionality of requested attributes, which is relevant for health data under GDPR [1,9]. This enables a wallet-based presentation of health-related attestations that are currently physical or distributed across portals, including the European Health Insurance Card (EHIC), e-prescriptions, and medical certificates [1,58]. While this implies a transition toward interoperable digital identification in many Member States, the Finnish case is shaped by an already mature digital health ecosystem and established authentication routines.

The EUDI Wallet is intended to complement national infrastructures. In Finland, nationwide services are provided through *Kanta* Services and the *MyKanta* portal (*OmaKanta* in Finnish), which cover prescriptions and health records across public and private providers and pharmacies [24,50]. Strong identification in routine access is commonly mediated through bank-based credentials [24,50]. Under eIDAS 2.0, the wallet introduces a state-governed channel for identification and attribute presentation under the common EU model [1]. The national preparation is coordinated by the Ministry of Finance and the Digital and Population Data Services Agency (DVV) is responsible for the technical implementation of the wallet application [6,42]. Under a coexistence approach, *MyKanta* remains a primary interface for domestic workflows, while the wallet can add an authentication channel and, where implemented, a holder for

---

K. M Saifullah and C. Á Casado—These authors contributed equally to this work.

selected health credentials issued by authoritative sources. In this setting, adoption can be interpreted as a migration in which wallet-based access is compared to learned *Kanta* and bank-based routines, and outcomes are sensitive to perceived effort, predictability, and role clarity [25]. Inclusion remains relevant in this coexistence setting. Adoption gaps have been reported among older adults and groups with lower digital competence [24], and older users report barriers to mobile health applications that are related to usability, device access, perceived effort, and perceived financial risk [48]. Sensitivity to health-data misuse can also affect willingness to adopt new access models. Previous incidents, including the *Vastaamo* data breach, in which a private psychotherapy provider suffered unauthorized access to patient records affecting tens of thousands of citizens [18], can increase perceived risk and reduce tolerance for ambiguity in disclosure and accountability [45]. At the same time, effective use often depends on practical assistance from family members or frontline personnel, which can be in tension with wallet interaction models that bind credentials and consent to an individual device [28,39,54]. Finnish work on warm experts suggests that informal support can enable first successful completion, but can also shift decisions away from the citizen when support becomes over-delegation [19,32]. These factors motivate assessing wallet-based access not only in terms of security, but also in terms of perceived effort, perceived control, and trust, including how citizens interpret the responsibilities of the issuer, the wallet provider, and the relying party [1].

Cross-border scenarios provide an additional motivation. The revised eIDAS regulation addresses cross-border authentication and recognizes offline authentication in sectors such as health, for example through e-prescription verification with QR codes or related mechanisms [1]. The EUDI Wallet Architecture and Reference Framework (ARF) specifies interfaces between wallets, issuers, and relying parties to support interoperability and selective disclosure, including in proximity and offline settings [15]. For example, a Finnish citizen could obtain medicines based on an e-prescription in another Member State or confirm insurance coverage through wallet-based verification without relying on country-specific portals [1,15]. Evidence from Finland and Estonia indicates that cross-border e-prescription journeys still depend on operational interoperability and clear responsibilities across actors [47]. Professional identity credentials are also relevant because access to records and prescription issuance depend on verifiable professional status and authorization [1,15].

The Finnish rollout requires decisions on institutional roles, accountability, and operational responsibilities across authorities, healthcare providers, and market actors. These decisions include relying party onboarding, how attribute requests and consent are communicated, and how wallet-based authentication is integrated into existing service entry points. Workforce readiness is relevant because healthcare and pharmacy professionals often mediate digital support, and competence gaps can affect the completion of wallet-mediated steps [40]. This paper examines adoption determinants in Finnish digital health by integrating citizen-level determinants with enabling conditions defined by public authorities and service delivery actors, while accounting for wallet interaction roles that mediate authentication and attribute presentation. The study follows a scoping review and synthesizes determinants that are addressable through service design and governance prior to large-scale deployment. The study is also timely in light of the EHDS, which entered into force in 2025 and strengthens the strategic relevance of interoperable identification, authentication, and consent mechanisms in cross-border digital health services [43]. To our knowledge, this is the first study to apply a wallet-specific adoption framework that integrates the Unified Theory of Acceptance and Use of Technology (UTAUT2) and Privacy Calculus with the functional roles defined by the EUDI Wallet architecture in the Finnish digital health context. The main contributions are:

- A scoping review that maps adoption determinants from the literature relevant to wallet-mediated access to digital health services in Finland
- A three-layer conceptual framework that links citizen-level determinants, wallet interaction mechanisms, and institutional governance conditions to adoption outcomes
- An illustrative application of the framework to a high-sensitivity e-prescription dispensing workflow

The remainder of the paper is organized as follows. Section 2 presents the background on the EUDI Wallet, the Finnish digital health context, and the theoretical foundations. Section 3 describes the review methodology. Section 4 introduces the conceptual framework. Section 5 presents the findings of the literature synthesis, and Sect. 6 discusses their implications for Finnish digital health services. Finally, Sect. 7 concludes the paper and outlines directions for future research.

2   Background

2.1   EUDI Wallet and Healthcare Context

The EUDI Wallet is an electronic identification means that supports storage and presentation of person identification data (PID) and electronic attestations of attributes (EAA) under the revised eIDAS framework [1,57]. In healthcare, strong identification and controlled disclosure are necessary for access to sensitive records and for regulated transactions such as prescribing and dispensing [4,57]. The framework also covers proximity and offline scenarios through short-range communication mechanisms, including Near Field Communication (NFC) and Bluetooth Low Energy (BLE), which are relevant for face-to-face interactions in pharmacies, hospitals, and public offices [1,3,14].

A central healthcare use case is the digitization of the European Health Insurance Card (EHIC). The EHIC currently exists mainly as a physical card and is used to access medically necessary state-provided care during temporary stays within the Union [14]. The wallet-based EHIC introduces a digital issuance and verification process intended to support verification of insurance status and reimbursement coordination, aligned with the European Social Security Pass (ESS-PASS) initiative [14]. The wallet paradigm also supports e-prescription related scenarios, where a health identity attestation can support identification at the pharmacy and enable retrieval of prescription data through cross-border infrastructures such as MyHealth@EU [13,16]. Work on digital identity wallets and self-sovereign identity (SSI) in health and social services suggests that attribute-based presentation can increase user control, while also introducing dependencies that depend on governance, integration, and operational practices [20]. These observations motivate domain-specific analysis of adoption conditions in healthcare settings.

2.2   Finnish Digital Health Context and Identity Infrastructure

Finland has a mature nationwide digital health infrastructure through *Kanta* Services and the *MyKanta* portal, supporting electronic prescriptions, health records, and citizen access across public and private providers and pharmacies [11]. *MyKanta* is used by more than 2.5 million citizens annually, and the infrastructure processes tens of millions of e-prescriptions per year [24]. This scale creates a baseline where new access mechanisms are evaluated against established routines and where perceived benefits must outweigh transition effort. The wallet also changes the interaction logic, since portal-based access is centered on viewing and managing records through centralized services, while wallet-based access can be organized around holding and presenting verifiable credentials on the user device. Table 1 summarizes differences that are relevant for perceived effort and perceived control.

Access to *MyKanta* and related public services is mediated through *Suomi.fi* e-Identification, which functions as a shared identification broker for public administration services. Users select an identification method, and the identification service operates through a brokerage model where the broker can be provided by an operator such as Telia Finland Oyj [55]. After authentication, the service transmits the personal identity code and name to the service provider [55]. In practice, the Finnish Trust Network and bank-based credentials remain the dominant authentication method in routine use [24]. This creates a stable mental model in which strong digital identification is closely associated with a banking relationship and familiar sign-in patterns across sectors. Post-adoption research indicates that satisfaction with an established system can increase resistance to alternatives, consistent with status quo bias and habit formation in continued use [29,59]. For wallet adoption, this implies that citizens can weigh installation, initial identity setup, and learning a new access model against the marginal benefit over existing portal and bank-based routines.

The relationship between effort and trust is also shaped by workforce capability. Recent cross-national evidence shows differences in digital health competence among healthcare professionals, and links higher competence to organizational and managerial support and to integration of digital solutions in routine practice [40]. In a wallet-mediated setting, these competence differences are relevant because professionals and pharmacy staff often provide digital counseling and practical support that can affect whether citizens complete authentication and

Table 1. Structural comparison between the current Kanta ecosystem and the EUDI Wallet interaction paradigm in healthcare.

Feature	Current Kanta ecosystem	EUDI Wallet paradigm
Data location	Centralized national repositories accessed through *MyKanta* and connected services	Credentials and attestations can be held on the user device, while clinical repositories remain in national systems and are accessed through service-specific backends [1,15]
Access model	Portal-based access to prescriptions and records	Attribute presentation for a stated purpose, with selective disclosure when applicable [1,15]
Authentication	Strong electronic identification commonly mediated through bank-based credentials in routine use	Wallet-based PID and attestations under the eIDAS 2.0 framework [1]
Verification	Backend queries to national repositories after authentication	Cryptographic verification of credential validity, offline or online depending on the use case, combined with backend access when retrieval from registries is required [1,15]
Delegation	*Suomi.fi* e-Authorizations support acting on behalf under defined mandates	Representation depends on national implementation choices, including how mandates are expressed and verified in wallet-mediated transactions [1,15]

consent steps successfully and whether the interaction is perceived as trustworthy.

Despite the maturity of the system, studies report adoption gaps and uneven user experience. Older adults, especially those aged 75 years and older, report barriers related to digital competence, usability, technical problems, and motivation, and multi-step authentication can be experienced as a burden [35]. Broader user studies report that digital services are valued for convenience and accessibility, while shortcomings remain in usability, engagement, affordability, and communication with healthcare providers [31]. These findings imply that changes in authentication and consent handling should be assessed in terms of perceived control and support, not only in terms of security properties. In parallel, Finnish policy suggests the expansion of technology assisted service pathways in primary healthcare, including a legislative proposal for technology assisted assessment of the need for care under defined conditions while preserving access to evaluation by a healthcare professional [52]. In this policy context, strong identification and clear consent remain necessary because both automated pathways and professional services require a reliable link between the person and entitlements and records.

Within this baseline, the EUDI Wallet can be analyzed as an additional identification and credential presentation layer that interfaces with existing infrastructures rather than replacing them. Since strong identification is commonly mediated through bank-based credentials, the wallet introduces a state-governed alternative and supports presentation of selected health credentials in domestic and cross-border scenarios [13,14,24]. Under a coexistence model, *MyKanta* remains a primary domestic interface, while the wallet can act as an entry method and a user controlled channel for verifiable credentials issued from authoritative sources [13,14].

2.3   Adoption, Trust, and Privacy Determinants in Digital Health and Implications for Wallet-Based Access

Finnish studies indicate that perceived usefulness supports the adoption of digital health services, while barriers include usability problems, multi-step authentication, and limited digital skills, particularly among older adults [24,31,35]. Consumer-focused research also links preventive eHealth adoption intent to effort expectancy, self-efficacy, and threat evaluations, while perceived barriers remain a central challenge [30]. These observations align with acceptance models that connect performance expectancy, effort expectancy, habit, and facilitating conditions to continued use and show that complex terminology and unclear guidance can increase perceived effort [31,35,38].

The EUDI Wallet further changes the interaction model by structuring access around explicit attribute requests and user controlled presentation decisions under relying party registration and transparency expectations [1,15]. In healthcare, this can shift perceived effort and perceived control because sharing is framed as presenting specific attributes for a stated purpose rather than granting broad account-level access [1]. Adoption therefore depends on usability and consistent communication of roles, responsibilities, and request practices between issuers, relying parties, and public authorities [1,15].

From a privacy calculus perspective, users balance convenience against misuse risks [4]. In Finland, the *Vastaamo* case has been analyzed as a failure in sociotechnical governance and accountability, suggesting that breach experiences can recalibrate perceived risk and trust beyond immediate incident response [18,37]. Clinical analyses further describe cybersecurity incidents as patient-safety relevant events that can discourage care seeking and increase sensitivity to confidentiality failures [37]. Privacy concerns can limit use even when services are available [35]. The wallet addresses this by supporting selective disclosure and cryptographic minimization, enabling verification of validity without exposing full records [15]. For example, a pharmacy can verify a prescription without accessing broader medical history [13].

2.4   Research Objective and Questions

Existing research characterizes user behavior within centralized platforms such as *Kanta*, while evidence remains limited on how established habits transfer to a wallet-mediated interaction model. In parallel, healthcare wallet and SSI studies discuss attribute disclosure and user control, but their implications depend on governance arrangements and on how services integrate wallet flows into existing workflows [20,57].

This study synthesizes determinants that may shape Finnish citizen adoption of wallet-based healthcare access. It constructs a conceptual framework that integrates UTAUT2 acceptance constructs with privacy calculus trade-offs [4,38]. UTAUT2 was selected because it captures consumer-oriented acceptance constructs, including performance expectancy, effort expectancy, habit, social influence, and facilitating conditions, that are relevant for citizen-facing digital health services. Privacy Calculus Theory was selected because wallet-mediated health interactions involve explicit attribute disclosure decisions where users weigh expected benefits against perceived risks under uncertainty. The integration of these two frameworks is motivated by the observation that adoption in this domain cannot be explained by usability and functional utility alone (UTAUT2), nor by privacy risk-benefit trade-offs alone (Privacy Calculus), but requires both lenses to account for the interaction between acceptance determinants and disclosure decisions in a high-sensitivity setting. The study addresses three research questions: how acceptance determinants and privacy-related trade-offs may shape adoption of wallet-mediated health access in Finland, how institutional and ecosystem factors may condition these determinants through governance and integration choices, and how the determinants can be organized into a unified model and interpreted through a high-sensitivity work-flow using e-prescription dispensing as the reference case [13].

3   Methodology

This study follows a scoping review design as defined by the Arksey and O'Malley framework [2], with methodological refinements recommended by Levac et al. [36]. A scoping review was selected because the objective is to map the extent, characteristics, and conceptual structure of the evidence on EUDI Wallet adoption determinants in Finnish healthcare, rather than to estimate a pooled effect for a narrowly defined intervention outcome. The evidence base is heterogeneous in study designs, populations, and outcome types, and the topic remains institutionally and technically emergent. The scoping approach supports a structured mapping of adoption determinants, governance conditions, and privacy-related trade-offs, while identifying research gaps that can motivate later systematic reviews once implementation contexts and empirical constructs are more stable. The review synthesizes empirical and review-based evidence on adoption determinants, while complementary normative and policy-relevant sources were used to contextualize the Finnish healthcare setting and to derive the wallet-mediated healthcare access framework. Reporting follows the PRISMA-ScR (Preferred

Reporting Items for Systematic Reviews and Meta-Analyses extension for Scoping Reviews) guideline [46,56]. The review targets determinants of adoption and non-adoption of wallet-mediated access to digital health services, with Finland as the primary context. Normative and technical sources were consulted only to define concepts, roles, and workflows for the wallet interaction model, including the revised eIDAS regulation and EUDI Wallet health-related specifications [1,13–15]. These framework documents were not included in the scoping review study count and were not treated as empirical evidence of adoption determinants.

3.1   Search Strategy and Information Sources

Evidence identification followed a two-track approach. The search was conducted in January 2026 and covered publications from 2015 to 2025. *Google Scholar* was the primary search engine to cover health informatics, information systems, and digital identity research. Records were restricted to English and filtered by publication year. The English-language restriction supported transparent and consistent screening but may exclude relevant Finnish or Swedish evidence. Because *Google Scholar* does not provide a consistent peer-review filter, peer-review status was assessed during selection based on venue and document type. In parallel, the *Elicit* platform was used as an AI-assisted discovery tool to propose candidate studies from prompts derived from the research questions. Elicit retrieves records from large multidisciplinary scholarly indexes, including Semantic Scholar (over 200 million publications across all fields), OpenAlex (243 million publications from over 260,000 sources), and PubMed (over 33 million biomedical citations). This combined corpus covers major publishers (Springer Nature, Elsevier, Wiley, Taylor & Francis, SAGE), university presses, professional societies (IEEE, ACM), and open-access publishers (PLOS, Frontiers, MDPI) [10]. Recent coverage analyses indicate that OpenAlex achieves 98.6% coverage of guideline-cited articles and provides approximately 28–29% more records than Web of Science or Scopus, which supports using Elicit as a broad-coverage retrieval tool for scoping reviews [49]. Elicit supported discovery only; it did not automate inclusion decisions, critical appraisal, or synthesis. Because AI-assisted retrieval is less transparent and less reproducible than a fully specified database search, all Elicit-suggested records were manually verified before inclusion [34]. Records from *Elicit* were exported, merged with the *Google Scholar* set, deduplicated, and screened using the same eligibility criteria.

To support transparency and consistency, the following structured search query was used in Google Scholar: ("EUDI Wallet" OR "European Digital Identity Wallet" OR "eIDAS 2.0" OR "digital identity") AND ("healthcare" OR "e-prescription" OR "eHealth" OR "MyKanta" OR "Kanta") AND ("adoption" OR "trust" OR "privacy" OR "usability") AND ("Finland" OR "Europe"). Search queries were iteratively refined to capture citizen-level determinants of digital health use, institutional and regulatory determinants, and identity-mediated healthcare scenarios. Example query phrases included "user determinants of MyKanta and digital health adoption in Finland", "barriers to e-health adoption", "institutional and government determinants of EUDI Wallet adoption in Europe", and "policy-level barriers to digital health adoption in Finland".

Forward snowballing was carried out through the *Cited by* feature in *Google Scholar* to identify newer studies and interdisciplinary work connected to the included evidence base [60].

3.2   Eligibility Criteria

Studies were eligible if they were empirical sources focused on adoption or governance determinants for digital health services or digital identity frameworks in a European healthcare context, and if they analyzed citizens or public, institutional, or market actors as relevant determinants of adoption. Studies were excluded if they were non-empirical, outside Europe, outside the healthcare domain, or limited to technical protocol properties without linkage to adoption, trust, privacy, usability, accountability, or governance. The criteria were applied holistically and refined iteratively during familiarization with the retrieved literature, consistent with scoping review practice [2,36].

3.3   Selection Process and PRISMA-ScR Flow

The records were identified through *Google Scholar* and *Elicit* (n=167). After initial de-duplication and eligibility filtering, 71 records were removed and 96 records proceeded to title and abstract screening.The duplication rate between the two platforms was notably low (n=3). This is attributed to the complementary nature of the search mechanisms, where Google Scholar captured a broad range of academic indexing, while Elicit semantic search identified distinct interdisciplinary papers. Because the intersection of digital health adoption and the emerging EUDI wallet infrastructure is highly nuanced, titles and abstracts frequently lacked sufficient detail to definitively determine if a study met the eligibility criteria. For instance, it was often challenging to differentiate at the abstract level whether a paper focused solely outside the given scope or if it offered relevant insights into socio-technical adoption, governance, or usability. To avoid accidentally excluding relevant evidence, a highly conservative screening approach was taken. Consequently, no records were excluded during the initial title and abstract screening phase, and all 96 records were sought and successfully retrieved for full-text assessment.

During the full-text evaluation, 22 reports were excluded (9 did not focus on Finland, 3 were duplicates, and 10 were not relevant to the EUDI Wallet context). The final qualitative synthesis included 74 studies. This high final inclusion ratio (74 out of 96) reflects the broad exploratory scope of the scoping review, where diverse methodologies, ranging from policy analyses to qualitative citizen studies were considered relevant if they addressed the intersection of digital health adoption and identity infrastructure. Screening decisions were made by the first author and reviewed by the co-authors, with disagreements resolved through discussion. Figure 1 reports the selection flow and exclusion reasons.

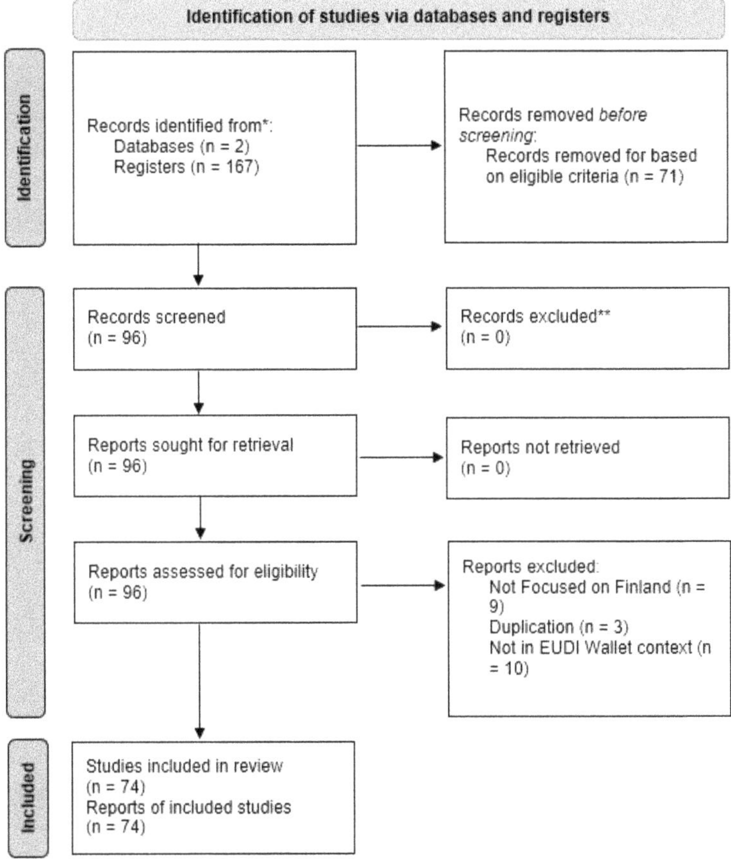

Fig. 1. PRISMA-ScR Flow Diagram for the scoping review.

3.4 Data Extraction and Quality Considerations

In the context of this scoping review, the synthesized data comprises extracted textual findings, qualitative themes regarding socio-technical behaviors, reported quantitative metrics (e.g., adoption barriers), and policy directives from the included literature. This diverse conceptual and empirical data was systematically extracted to map the determinants of wallet adoption. A structured extraction template captured author, year, country, study design, population, the health service or identity system under analysis, and findings related to adoption or non-adoption. Definitions and operationalization of trust and privacy were also extracted to support conceptual consistency. Data extraction was performed by the first author and checked by co-authors. Bibliometric extraction results are not presented because the primary objective of this review is to qualitatively synthesize socio-technical adoption determinants to build a conceptual framework, rather than to conduct a quantitative analysis of publication metadata.

Consistent with scoping review methodology, and given the heterogeneity of the study designs, the quality assessment focused on internal validity and relevance [2,56]. Each empirical study was assessed for clarity of design, sampling description, and analysis transparency [22]. These assessments were used to weigh evidence during synthesis rather than to apply a strict exclusion threshold.

3.5 Synthesis and Framework Development

A hybrid theory mapping combining deductive and inductive approaches was applied, following established methodological guidance for theory-driven qualitative synthesis [17]. This theory mapping approach integrates inductively derived macro-level institutional conditions with deductively mapped micro-level psychological constructs. This approach is appropriate when a review is guided by established theoretical constructs. In the deductive phase, findings extracted from the included studies were mapped to pre-defined constructs from UTAUT2 and privacy calculus theory [5,59]. The UTAUT2 constructs included performance expectancy, effort expectancy, social influence, facilitating conditions, hedonic motivation, price value, and habit. The Privacy Calculus included perceived benefits, perceived risks, trust, and perceived control. Each extracted finding was assigned to one or more constructs based on definition-based alignment with the original theory.

Inductive thematic analysis captured wallet-specific patterns, including transparency of attribute requests, clarity of issuer and relying party responsibilities, and the implications of selective disclosure and offline presentation in healthcare interactions under the revised framework [1,15]. Themes were organized into three streams aligned with the research questions: citizen-level determinants, institutional and regulatory determinants, and identity-mediated high-sensitivity healthcare workflows. Thematic synthesis integrated findings across streams into a conceptual framework linking wallet roles and ecosystem conditions to user perceptions and adoption outcomes. The interpretation of the framework was illustrated through the cross-border e-prescription dispensing workflow described in the EUDI Wallet documentation [13].

4   Conceptual Framework

This section proposes a descriptive framework that organizes the determinants identified in the scoping review synthesis into a wallet-specific adoption model for the Finnish digital health context [46,56]. The framework is integrative rather than causal and is not intended for statistical estimation or protocol-level evaluation of the EUDI Wallet technical stack [1,15]. The proposed framework is conceptual and descriptive in nature and is not empirically validated within this study. The core intention is to organize and interpret available evidence. Its purpose is to structure how determinants reported in Finnish digital health research and healthcare-oriented wallet studies may interact when identification, authentication, and attribute presentation are mediated through a wallet in healthcare [24,51]. The framework clarifies the socio-technical conditions under which established access habits may transfer into a decentralized interaction model [25,52]. It should therefore be read as a testable conceptual scaffold for later empirical work, not as an already validated explanatory model.

The framework separates the determinants into three interacting layers. The citizen layer covers acceptance, capability, and trust determinants that shape engagement with digital health services, including digital competence and support needs, usability frictions, and concerns related to access to sensitive health information [21,28,54]. The wallet-paradigm layer captures interaction mechanisms that condition user experience and user control and distinguishes two functional roles in healthcare: wallet-based authentication and consent for access to services, and local presentation of verifiable health-related credentials in proximity or offline settings [13,14]. The institutional and governance layer captures the enabling conditions defined by national implementation choices and the EU trust and reliance framework, including responsibilities of the competent authority, supervision, relying party on-boarding, and cross-border interoperability constraints. In Finland, this includes DVV as the wallet implementation actor and Traficom as a supervisor within the national arrangement [1,15].

The framework links these layers to outcomes along care and pharmacy journeys, including first successful completion, continued use, and perceived safety. Perceived safety refers to confidence in accountable handling and confidence that attribute sharing is understandable and proportionate to the stated purpose, so that the interaction can be completed without unintended disclosure [5,8].

4.1   Scope and Modeling Assumptions

The framework targets healthcare settings where identification, authentication, and attribute presentation follow the interaction model defined by the revised eIDAS trust framework and its interoperability specifications [1,15]. The scope is limited to determinants that can be shaped through service design, governance choices, and stakeholder communication in the Finnish digital health ecosystem. Technical properties are considered only when they condition perceived effort, perceived control, trust, or perceived safety, or when they affect accountability obligations for relying parties under the trust and supervision model [1].

A core assumption is coexistence with established Finnish infrastructures. The framework does not assume replacement of *Kanta* or *MyKanta*, but treats the wallet as an additional interaction layer integrated into existing access points and pharmacy workflows [11,24]. This matters because learned routines influence whether wallet steps are experienced as simplification or added friction, and because adoption gaps related to digital competence and support needs persist even in a mature national system [21,28,54].

Two wallet roles are used throughout to separate interaction patterns. Role A is identity and consent brokering for access to online services, where a relying party requests attributes and the user decides whether to present them under a stated purpose [1]. Role B is local presentation of verifiable credentials in proximity or offline settings, including e-prescription dispensing and EHIC verification [13,14]. These roles can co-occur within a single journey, but the determinants are interpreted through the role that is active at each step [23]. The unit of analysis is completion of concrete journeys in which the wallet mediates a health-related transaction with a relying party. Therefore, the framework focuses on the first successful completion, continued use, and perceived safety as outcomes at the interaction-level [5,8,27]. Clinical outcomes and protocol-level security performance are outside scope and are discussed only when they constrain the interaction model through governance requirements or user-relevant assurances [1,15]. Figure 2 summarizes the boundary conditions by separating the citizen layer, the wallet-paradigm layer with two roles, and the Finnish ecosystem layer where responsibilities and supervision are defined.

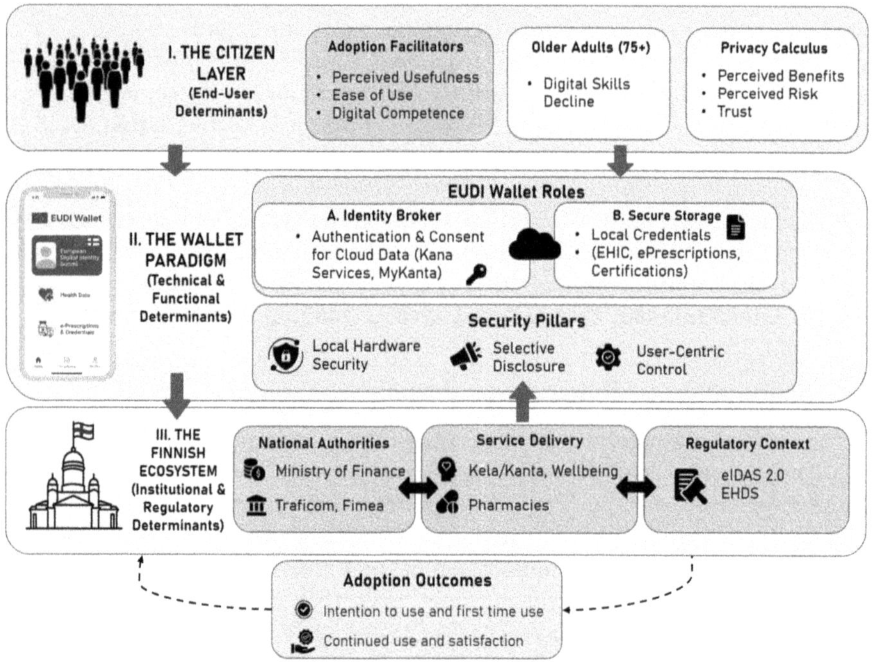

Fig. 2. Layered conceptual view of EUDI Wallet adoption in Finnish healthcare. The figure separates determinants into three interacting layers: (I) citizen determinants (acceptance, digital competence, and privacy-calculus trade-offs), (II) the wallet paradigm with two functional roles that can co-occur within a single journey (identity and consent brokering for access to services, and local presentation of verifiable health-related credentials), and (III) the Finnish ecosystem layer (authorities and supervision, service delivery actors, and the regulatory context under eIDAS 2.0 and the EHDS).

4.2   Citizen-Level Adoption Determinants

The citizen layer comprises constructs that reflect psychological, experiential, and capability factors expected to influence engagement with wallet-mediated healthcare interactions. Determinants are grouped into acceptance factors and privacy-related trade-offs [5,59]. The synthesis is used to populate these constructs with determinants observed in Finnish digital health services and in healthcare-oriented wallet settings.

UTAUT2 provides acceptance constructs related to perceived benefit, perceived effort, enabling resources, social context, and learned routines, but does not account for privacy-related disclosure decisions that are central to health data interactions [59]. In wallet-mediated journeys, performance expectancy refers to the expected benefit of using the wallet for identification and attribute presentation, for example, when access steps are perceived as simpler, more portable across contexts, or more consistent across relying parties. Effort expectancy refers to the perceived ease of completing the wallet steps, including prompt clarity, number of actions, and predictability. Facilitating conditions cover resources and support for completion, including digital competence, access to suitable devices, and assistance when problems occur [28]. Social influence reflects the encouragement and practical help of important others, which can enable first successful completion for users with support needs [39]. Habit captures established digital health routines and their transfer to wallet interaction patterns, which is central in Finland because routine use of national services can increase sensitivity to added steps [25]. Hedonic motivation and price value are not treated as primary constructs because access to public health services is mainly utilitarian and not typically priced at the point of use [59]. Indirect burdens, including time cost and cognitive load, are reflected through effort expectancy, facilitating conditions, and habit.

Privacy calculus describes disclosure decisions as a trade-off between expected benefits and perceived risks under uncertainty [5]. In healthcare, the trade-off is salient because interactions can involve special categories of personal data and attributes that reveal health status, entitlements, or treatment-related information. Perceived benefits include reduced authentication friction, faster completion, continuity of care, and cross-border recognition when credentials are accepted across Member States. Perceived risks include unintended disclosure, secondary use beyond the stated purpose, and security incidents that reduce confidence in the surrounding ecosystem [8,27]. Trust is treated as a condition that reduces perceived risk and supports disclosure and continued use. In wallet-mediated healthcare, trust concerns the issuer, the relying party, and the governance arrangements responsible for supervision and accountability. Perceived control captures agency at the point of use, including whether the user can understand and influence attribute sharing, with clear information on what is requested, by whom, and for what purpose. It also reflects whether selective disclosure supports meaningful choice rather than broad account-level consent [1,15]. In the framework, perceived benefits, perceived risks, trust, and perceived control interact with acceptance determinants to shape first successful completion, continued use, and perceived safety [5,8,27].

4.3 Wallet-Paradigm Mechanisms as Interaction Mediators

Citizen-level determinants translate into outcomes through interaction mechanisms defined by the trust and interoperability framework [1,15]. These mechanisms mediate how acceptance and privacy-related determinants shape journeys. Two roles capture the main patterns, separating identity and consent brokering from local credential presentation.

4.3.1 Role A: Identity and Consent Brokering for Access to Online Health Services

Role A covers wallet-based identification and authentication for access to online services, structured around a relying party request for defined attributes and a user-controlled presentation decision under a stated purpose [1]. In Finland, Role A is relevant for access points to services such as *MyKanta*, where the wallet can act as an additional channel alongside existing identification methods [24]. Effort and facilitating conditions depend on reliability and predictability, including number of actions, failure recovery, and prompt clarity. A central mediator in Role A is transparency of the attribute request. The interaction is framed as a request for specific attributes under an explicit purpose statement, aligned with transparency and proportionality expectations in the revised framework [1,15]. In healthcare, this framing can strengthen perceived control and trust through the intelligibility of the purpose statement, proportionality of requested attributes, and the ability to distinguish the roles of issuer, wallet provider, and relying party [1,5]. The framework therefore treats request transparency and purpose clarity as mediators that can reduce perceived effort and support perceived safety by reducing uncertainty about what is shared and why [27]. To make the mediator role operational in later reporting, the framework treats request transparency as consisting of three observable elements: attribute list clarity, purpose clarity, and relying party identity clarity at the time of consent.

4.3.2 Role B: Local Presentation of Verifiable Health-Related Credentials

Role B refers to local presentation and verification of health-related credentials in proximity or offline settings, including e-prescription dispensing and EHIC verification [13,14]. In this role, perceived safety and risk are shaped by whether users understand which attributes are held locally and which are disclosed during the interaction. Standardized mechanisms, such as QR codes or proximity communication through NFC and BLE, support face-to-face presentation and verification [15]. Effort determinants are influenced by usability in time-constrained settings, where a fast scan can reduce authentication friction at service counters. The wallet paradigm also supports selective disclosure, allowing users to present proof of a specific requirement, such as a valid prescription or insurance eligibility, without exposing broader records [1,15]. Perceived benefits depend on whether local presentation supports continuity in cross-border and offline contexts without requiring access to national backends during the encounter. For Role B, the framework distinguishes between user-facing disclosure transparency and operational reliability, because failure recovery and fallback procedures can affect perceived effort and perceived safety in face-to-face service encounters. Role B links decentralized storage and selective disclosure to user-relevant outcomes, including confidence in the interaction and perceived safety when sensitive health data are involved.

4.4 Institutional and Governance Determinants as Enabling Conditions

Wallet-mediated interactions depend on enabling conditions defined by institutional roles, governance choices, and operational practices. In the framework, these determinants act mainly through trustworthiness, transparency, reliability, and access to support rather than as direct psychological predictors. This layer follows the reliance and accountability model of the revised eIDAS framework, where responsibilities are distributed across wallet providers, issuers, and relying parties under supervision and defined liability [1,15].

Public governance determinants describe how competent authorities define roles and supervision practices and enforce expectations for relying party onboarding and registration [1]. In Finland, DVV is a central actor in technical implementation and in the state-governed delivery model that can support perceived legitimacy [6,42]. Supervision can involve authorities such as Traficom, contributing to the assurance environment in which wallet and relying party behavior is monitored [1]. These determinants condition adoption by clarifying accountability and constraining attribute request practices. The revised framework emphasizes registration and transparency expectations, including purpose limitation and proportionality of requested attributes, which is salient in healthcare [1]. Clear supervision and liability can reduce perceived risk by supporting responsibility attribution when failures occur and by increasing confidence that requests follow predictable rules, which is relevant in contexts shaped by previous incidents, including the Vastaamo breach [45].

Service delivery determinants describe how healthcare providers, pharmacies, and digital service operators integrate wallet interaction patterns into entry points and workflows, and how they organize support when authentication or verification fails. In Finland, this includes actors in the *Kanta* ecosystem and related public service structures, such as wellbeing services counties and Kela, where integration quality shapes whether the wallet is experienced as simplification or added friction [24]. Integration also depends on the digital health competence of frontline staff, since professionals support users, resolve common failures, and embed wallet steps into routine workflows [40]. This layer also captures inclusion safeguards for persistent support needs. Evidence indicates that many users, including older adults and vulnerable groups, rely on human assistance in practice [28,39]. The availability of support and accessible alternatives conditions whether wallet-mediated access improves equity or reinforces exclusion [28,54]. Support needs are role-dependent: Role A places weight on onboarding and device continuity, while Role B places weight on assisted completion at the point of service and on recovery paths under time pressure.

4.5 Outcome Model and Feedback over Time

Outcomes are defined at the journey level: first successful completion, continued use, and perceived safety. Perceived safety captures confidence in accountable handling and confidence that disclosure is understandable and proportionate to the stated purpose [5,8]. Feedback captures how post-use experiences update expectations. Successful completion can reduce perceived effort and strengthen habit. Repeated failures, unclear requests, or weak transparency can increase perceived risk and reduce willingness to rely on the wallet in high-sensitivity healthcare interactions.

4.6 Synthesis and Mapping to Healthcare Journeys

The framework summarizes an adoption model in which institutional and governance conditions shape operational constraints and interaction mechanisms, which in turn shape citizen evaluations of benefit, effort, risk, perceived control, and trust. The framework is interpreted through journeys that make the wallet roles explicit. Role A covers wallet-based access to online services structured around attribute requests and user-controlled consent. Role B covers face-to-face presentation and verification in settings such as e-prescription dispensing and EHIC verification [13,14]. The scoping review results are reported by layer and mapped to the constructs and mediators, to clarify which determinants are likely to dominate across journeys and at which step of the interaction the role changes.

5 Results and Synthesis

5.1 Citizen-Level Determinants: Acceptance and Risk-Benefit Trade-Offs

The scoping review synthesis identifies that the acceptance of the Finnish citizen is a negotiation between functional utility, friction between the interface, and systemic trust. In the included evidence base, these determinants are not only interface-level perceptions but also reactions to authentication routines, consent practices, and expectations of institutional accountability in high-sensitivity health transactions. Empirical evidence provides a baseline for how these constructs will likely respond to the introduction of a wallet-based interaction model. Since large-scale EUDI Wallet deployment in Finnish healthcare is not yet established, the synthesis interprets evidence from Finnish digital health and pharmacy as the domestic baseline and uses wallet and SSI studies to anticipate which determinants can be transferred to wallet-based interaction patterns and which may change.

5.1.1   Performance Expectancy and Effort Expectancy Evidence suggests that performance expectancy is consistently associated with the value of location-independent health management. In pharmacies, 93% to 95.8% of customers report high satisfaction when digital services support remote prescription management and renewals [25,33]. This utility is counterbalanced by expected effort. Although 94.6% of users report that current login procedures are easy, reflecting familiarity with bank-based identification, studies still report usability frictions, including many interaction steps during authentication and added cognitive load related to complex medical terminology [35,50,61]. Across the evidence base, these findings imply that wallet-based access will be judged against a well-learned routine, and that perceived effort will depend on interaction predictability, clear error recovery, and integration into existing service entry points rather than a parallel step.

The role distinction clarifies the reference points for both constructs. For online access (Role A), the wallet is compared against bank-based routines, so the perceived benefit depends on whether the flow reduces steps, reduces repeated confirmations, or improves recovery after failures. For proximity and offline presentation (Role B), the reference point is physical presentation or counter-based verification. In this case, performance expectancy depends on the transaction time, the reliability of offline availability, and the clarity of what is disclosed during presentation [14].

5.1.2   Facilitating Conditions and Social Influence Digital competence is a key condition for independent use. Older adults, particularly those aged 75 years and older, and users with physical limitations such as poor eyesight, are less likely to perceive benefits of digital tools or to complete tasks without support [21,54]. In this context, social influence is expressed mainly as practical assistance from warm experts, including family members and healthcare professionals, which supports first successful completion [28,39]. Evidence on "Warm Experts" in Finland also shows a risk that support shifts privacy decisions from the citizen to the helper, which can reduce perceived control if wallet interactions do not support assisted use with clear boundaries and safe recovery [19,32]. In Role A, assisted use is most visible during installation, initial identity setup, and account recovery. In Role B, assisted use is most visible at service counters, where time pressure makes error recovery and clear handover between citizen and helper relevant.

Facilitating conditions also extend to the professional environment. In pharmacies and other face-to-face touchpoints, completion depends partly on the competence of the staff to verify credentials and to resolve validation failures without long delays [40]. These findings link adoption with the availability of support pathways and with clear responsibility boundaries when support is provided, since wallet-based interaction introduces explicit attribute requests and presentation decisions for a stated purpose [1].

5.1.3   Habit and the Mature Ecosystem Unlike emerging digital markets, the Finnish context is characterized by high habituation. E-prescriptions reached 100% saturation by 2017, and the *MyKanta* portal recorded 179 million sign-ins by 2022 [23,26]. This suggests that for the EUDI Wallet to be adopted, it must successfully migrate these established routines into the new paradigm rather than attempting to create entirely new behaviors. The synthesis therefore treats habit as a structural determinant that can amplify both positive effects of simplification and negative effects of added steps, since even small deviations from established authentication and dispensing routines can be experienced as net friction.

5.1.4   Privacy Calculus: Transparency Versus Trauma The synthesis indicates that perceived risk and trust are tightly coupled in Finnish digital health. Breach experiences, including the Vastaamo case, are associated with a higher perceived risk and a lower tolerance of ambiguity in disclosure and accountability [18,45]. Misunderstandings about consent and information sharing also remain common, as reflected by more than 93,000 users who have set prohibitions to block data sharing between providers [25]. In wallet-based access, these patterns translate into a focus on perceived control at the point of use, meaning the ability to understand what attributes are requested, why they are requested, and which party requests them, and to make a proportionate presentation decision under relying party transparency expectations [1]. The evidence base also suggests that consistent request practices, clear attribution of responsibility, and understandable disclosures can strengthen perceived safety in routine care and pharmacy transactions [5,27]. Role A is most sensitive to request transparency and purpose clarity across relying parties, because these features condition whether users can distinguish legitimate requests and form stable expectations. Role B is most sensitive to disclosure transparency during presentation and to clarity on what is held locally versus disclosed, together with operational reliability at the point of care, because failures and unclear fallback can increase perceived effort and reduce confidence in face-to-face encounters.

5.2   Institutional and Governance Enablers

The synthesis indicates that institutional and governance factors act primarily as enabling conditions that shape trust, perceived control, and completion reliability, rather than as direct psychological predictors. In Finland, these conditions reflect national implementation choices, supervision arrangements, and service integration decisions that affect how wallet-based interactions are experienced in high-sensitivity journeys [1,6,15,42]. The governance layer is characterized by a "multi-authority" model where the Ministry of Finance guides the national implementation project (2024–2026), ensuring alignment with the European Health Data Space and the broader digitalization of public services [41,43]. Table 2 summarizes the main governance enablers identified in the synthesis and their expected links to citizen-level determinants.

Table 2. Governance enablers and their expected links to citizen-level determinants in wallet-based health interactions

Enabler category	Institutional action	Citizen determinant influenced
Legal certainty and liability	Definition of roles, obligations, and reliance conditions for wallets, issuers, and relying parties under the revised eIDAS framework	Perceived risk, institutional trust, perceived safety
Supervision and registration	Relying party registration and supervision arrangements, including the competence authority responsibilities in the national setup	Trust, perceived control, expectation of proportionate attribute requests
Interoperability baseline	Adoption of the common architecture and interfaces specified in the ARF for cross-border and multi-actor transactions	Performance expectancy, perceived reliability of completion
Inclusion safeguards and alternatives	Requirements and practices for assisted use, offline or proximity modes, and support services in high-sensitivity journeys	Facilitating conditions, effort expectancy, first successful completion
National health infrastructure integration and certification	Operational responsibilities and certification processes that condition reliable integration with *Kanta* and related services, including national requirements for information systems and certification or registration practices around health sector systems	Perceived reliability of completion, effort expectancy, perceived safety
Data protection and cyber security oversight	GDPR supervision and the supervision of strong electronic identification and trust services, including expectations on compliance, auditing, and incident handling	Institutional trust, perceived risk, perceived safety

5.2.1 Trust Infrastructure, Supervision, and Legal Validity

The synthesis indicates that perceived safety in wallet-based health access is closely linked to structural assurance. The revised eIDAS framework frames the wallet as part of a regulated trust and reliance model, defining responsibilities for wallet providers and expectations for relying parties [1]. In the Finnish implementation, DVV plays a central role in the technical delivery of the wallet application, while the National Police Board provides the official electronic identity (eID) as a digital equivalent to a passport, reinforcing the "Root of Trust" for citizens [7]. Sector-specific supervision is divided between the Finnish Supervisory Agency for Welfare and Health (Valvira), which monitors healthcare professionals and units, and the Finnish Medicines Agency (Fimea), which regulates the pharmaceutical workflows essential for e-Prescription dispensing [44]. This regulatory density supports a high "perceived safety" environment, but also requires seamless coordination to avoid "accountability gaps" during cross-border attribute sharing [61]. These governance arrangements condition adoption by clarifying liability when failures occur and supporting predictable relying party behavior in attribute request practices, which directly influences perceived control and trust.

5.2.2   Interoperability, Legacy Integration, and Inclusion Safeguards

Interoperability requirements defined in the ARF aim to ensure consistent wallet-to-issuer interaction patterns, which affects perceived reliability in cross-border health journeys [15]. In the healthcare domain, this is further enabled by Kela and THL, who act as the primary data holders for the national Kanta registries. By integrating the wallet with the existing Kanta-based authentication, the transition leverages the high habituation of the population to domestic digital health services [24,53].

Implementation strategies that layer wallet-based access onto existing entry points, rather than introducing parallel or inconsistent paths, are positioned as enablers that protect habit while reducing perceived effort. Finally, inclusion safeguards remain critical. The Finnish implementation includes mandates for "digital-first but not digital-only" access, ensuring that pharmacies and wellbeing services counties provide human-mediated support for the "warm expert" network [28,41]. This ensures that presentation of wallet-based identities does not increase exclusion in vulnerable groups [14,54].

Figure 3 consolidates these findings by mapping the governance enablers and citizen-level determinants identified in the scoping synthesis to the expected direction of influence on behavioral intention in wallet-based health access. In the figure, the labels "+ve" and "-ve" indicate the hypothesized direction of influence between constructs. A "+ve" label denotes an expected positive relationship, meaning that a stronger presence of the source condition is expected to strengthen the target determinant or increase behavioral intention. A "-ve" label denotes an expected negative relationship, meaning that a stronger presence of the source condition is expected to reduce the target determinant or decrease behavioral intention. For example, stronger supervision and legal clarity are expected to reduce perceived risk, whereas higher perceived risk is expected to reduce behavioral intention. By contrast, stronger facilitating conditions, trust, perceived control, and perceived benefits are expected to increase behavioral intention. These directions are interpretive and theory-informed rather than empirically estimated, and they are included to make the logic of the proposed framework explicit for later testing. This theory-mapping step links the inductively synthesized governance and adoption themes to deductively organized acceptance constructs, providing a structured visual explanation of the expected relationships without claiming statistical causation.

6   Discussion

This study examined determinants that can influence citizen adoption of the
EUDI Wallet for healthcare access in Finland before large-scale deployment.
The contribution is twofold. First, the work consolidates evidence from Finnish
digital health and healthcare-oriented wallet literature through a scoping review
synthesis and maps it to acceptance and privacy constructs. Second, it extends a
generic UTAUT2 plus Privacy Calculus framing with wallet-specific interaction
mechanisms and an enabling-conditions layer that reflects the eIDAS 2.0 reliance
and accountability model [1,15]. The resulting framework distinguishes citizen
determinants, wallet-paradigm roles, and Finnish ecosystem determinants, and
links them to observable outcomes along high-sensitivity journeys, as depicted
in Fig. 2. The framework was derived directly from the scoping review evidence
through the hybrid coding process described in the methodology: deductive coding mapped findings to UTAUT2 and Privacy Calculus constructs, inductive thematic analysis identified wallet-specific interaction patterns, and the three-layer
structure emerged from grouping the coded determinants by their level of origin

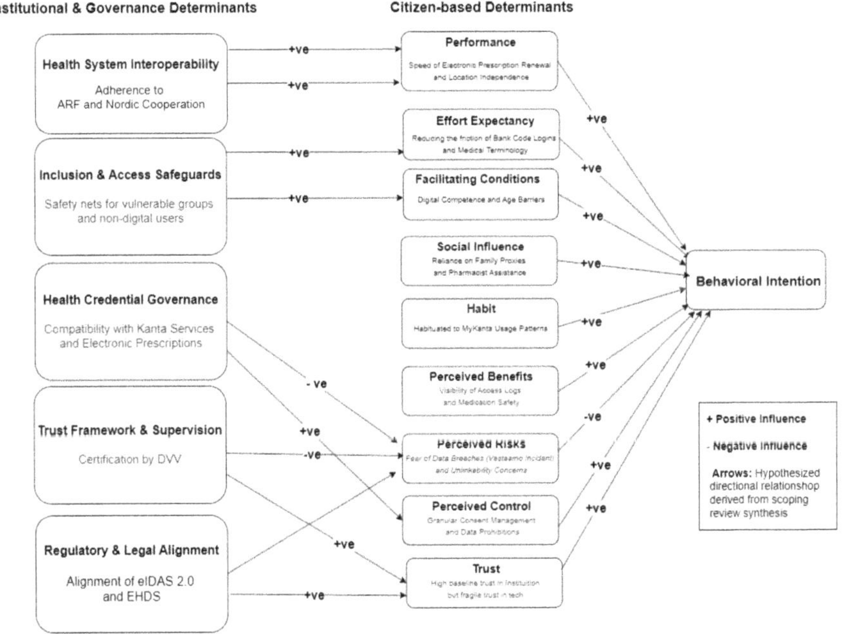

Fig. 3. Synthesis map linking institutional and governance enablers to citizen-level
determinants and behavioral intention in wallet-based health access. Box contents summarize determinants identified in the PRISMA-ScR synthesis. Arrow labels indicate the
hypothesized direction of influence derived from the qualitative synthesis and theory
mapping: "+ve" denotes an expected positive influence and "-ve" denotes an expected
negative influence. These links are interpretive and conceptual, not statistically estimated causal effects.

(citizen, wallet paradigm, governance). The arrows in Fig. 3 represent hypothesized directions of influence derived from this theory-guided coding, where an enabler is linked to a citizen-level determinant when the reviewed evidence indicates a conditioning or strengthening relationship. This positions the framework as an evidence-informed synthesis rather than a standalone theoretical contribution. In policy terms, the EUDI Wallet introduces a shift from account-centric access to an interaction model centered on attribute requests and user-controlled presentations, which can change how citizens interpret access to health services even when back-end registries remain unchanged.

A central implication is that citizen adoption in Finland is likely to be evaluated against an already mature baseline rather than against an absence of digital services. The evidence indicates high perceived utility for remote prescription management and routine use of *MyKanta*, but it also shows that perceived effort remains sensitive to small frictions, particularly when authentication and navigation require repeated steps or when health information is difficult to interpret [24,33,50,61]. This matters for the EUDI Wallet because Role A (identity and consent brokering for access to online health services) is not replacing a weak system, but competing with familiar bank-based routines. The most immediate adoption motivation is therefore a perceived reduction in authentication friction in high-frequency tasks, such as *MyKanta* access and e-Prescription renewals, combined with the expectation that a state-governed wallet provides a stable public anchor of assurance under eIDAS 2.0. Adoption therefore depends less on introducing a new capability and more on whether wallet-based access can integrate into existing entry points with predictable completion, clear recovery after failure, and a stable user experience across relying parties. In this setting, habit acts as an amplifier: when wallet steps are experienced as a simplification, continued use can consolidate quickly, but when wallet steps add uncertainty, even small additional burdens can be perceived as net friction [23,25].

Privacy-related findings further indicate that adoption cannot be explained only through functional utility. The synthesis suggests that perceived risk and trust are tightly coupled in Finnish healthcare, with persistent concerns about data misuse and secondary access, shaped by prior incidents and by analyses that frame the Vastaamo case as a governance and accountability failure that can recalibrate trust beyond the immediate incident response [5,18,45]. This implies a trauma-informed adoption context in which improvements in usability alone are unlikely to offset uncertainty about disclosure and accountability. This strengthens the motivation for wallet mechanisms that increase perceived control through clearer attribute requests, explicit purpose statements, and disclosure that is understandable and proportionate to the service need. The framework treats these elements as interaction-level mediators rather than abstract principles, because users experience them at the point of decision, during authentication and consent (Role A) or during in-person presentation of credentials (Role B). Therefore, the discussion supports a design priority on user-facing transparency that is consistent across services, since inconsistent request phrasing or unclear party roles can increase perceived risk even when the underlying trust framework is strong [1,15]. An additional uncertainty is how citizens will interpret the difference between a government-controlled wallet and the current bank-based model, including whether misperception about surveillance or centralized control could reduce uptake and increase preference for physical alternatives even when formal assurance is higher.

The enabling-conditions layer highlights that citizen determinants will be shaped by governance and service delivery practices that citizens may not observe directly but experience through reliability, support, and accountability. In the Finnish context, the distribution of responsibilities across authorities and service delivery actors is a potential point of fragility if it results in unclear support paths or inconsistent relying party behavior. The revised eIDAS framework introduces relying party registration and expectations on proportionality and transparency, which can support predictable attribute request practices and thereby reduce perceived risk and increase perceived control [1]. However, these expectations must be translated into operational guidance, monitoring, and incident handling that is visible to service operators and intelligible to citizens. This is especially relevant in a multi-authority environment where strategic coordination and implementation responsibilities are distributed, for example across the Ministry of Finance as the national coordination actor, DVV as the technical delivery actor, sector regulators and supervisors, and health-sector actors responsible for operational workflows. In parallel, service delivery actors determine whether wallet-based access works in practice at critical touchpoints, such as pharmacies and regional service portals, where time pressure, error recovery, and assisted use shape perceived effort and perceived safety. Evidence on digital competence barriers and reliance on warm experts indicates that inclusion safeguards are not an auxiliary concern but a condition for first successful use in vulnerable groups [28,39,54]. Since warm expert support can both enable adoption and create over-delegation, assisted pathways should be treated as part of the service design and governance problem, including clear support boundaries, safe fallback options, and interaction steps that preserve citizen understanding of what is being presented and why [19,32]. Given evidence of a sharp competence threshold in older age groups, a digital-first rollout that is perceived as digital-only would risk reinforcing exclusion unless assisted pathways are resourced and operationally safe. This implies that wallet adoption should be evaluated not only by uptake metrics, but also by whether assisted pathways remain safe, comprehensible, and realistic in routine settings.

The framework also points to opportunities and open questions for market actors. Although the current analysis focuses mainly on public-sector entry points and regulated healthcare workflows, the operational readiness of private market actors remains a critical uncertainty. The current evidence base provides limited insight into how individual pharmacies, private clinics, or occupational healthcare providers will handle wallet interactions at the service edge. These actors are relevant because they can become issuers of certain domain credentials and not only relying parties, for example when producing attestations for private laboratory results, medical certificates, or wellness-related documents, subject to the evolving credential governance model. These actors can also extend wallet-based use beyond *MyKanta* login. Plausible near-term use cases include pharmacy pickup and proxy scenarios, cross-border e-Prescription dispensing, EHIC presentation, appointment check-in, and presentation of professional credentials for staff access to systems. Each use case shifts which wallet role dominates and which determinants are most salient. For instance, counter-service flows make usability under time pressure and fallback procedures central, while remote care flows make request transparency and party-role clarity central. Future extensions of the framework should therefore include market and service operator determinants more explicitly, including onboarding pathways for relying parties, the consistency of purpose statements, and the handling of failures and disputes at the service edge.

Several uncertainties and limitations follow from the study design. First, this study follows a scoping review design, which maps the evidence landscape but does not assess the weight or quality of evidence for specific interventions. The framework is descriptive and integrative rather than predictive, and the absence of formal quality appraisal of individual sources is a known limitation of the scoping review approach. Empirical validation of the framework through expert interviews, stakeholder consultation, or survey-based testing remains a necessary next step. The review synthesizes heterogeneous evidence, and the EUDI Wallet is not yet deployed at scale in Finnish healthcare. As a result, the results indicate likely drivers and barriers, but do not estimate effect sizes or causal relations. Some determinants may also shift after deployment due to learning effects, media attention, early incidents, or changes in relying party practices. In addition, the search strategy relied on Google Scholar and the Elicit AI-assisted discovery platform rather than discipline-specific bibliographic databases such as Scopus or Web of Science. Elicit draws from Semantic Scholar, OpenAlex, and PubMed, which provides broad coverage, but the AI-driven retrieval process is not as transparent or reproducible as a fully specified Boolean search strategy executed on traditional subscription databases. This is a recognized limitation of scoping reviews that use AI-assisted workflows. Furthermore, the review excluded Finnish and Swedish publications, which may have reduced coverage of national reports and practice-oriented studies. The bibliometric data extracted during the charting process are not presented in this paper due to space constraints but are available from the corresponding author on request. The synthesis is also design-centered on Finland, and cross-border behavior will depend on how other Member States implement issuer processes, relying party onboarding, and proximity or offline verification patterns [15]. Transferability is likely highest to Member States with mature digital health portals and routine strong electronic identification, while determinants may differ where identification is less embedded in everyday care workflows. These limitations are the reason the framework is positioned as descriptive and integrative rather than predictive.

Future work should therefore prioritize empirical validation in realistic settings and should examine both citizen experience and operational readiness.

A first direction is the formative evaluation of the user journeys of Role A and Role B with special attention to older adults and users with support needs, measuring perceived effort, perceived control and perceived safety before and after repeated use. A second direction is service-level evaluation with pharmacies and portal operators, focusing on failure recovery, customer support load, and the consistency of attribute request practices across relying parties. A third direction concerns market-player onboarding and governance: studies should examine how relying party registration, purpose descriptions, and auditing practices influence request proportionality and user trust over time. Further work can also examine professional identity and authorization scenarios, for example, whether staff credentials anchored in professional registries can support cryptographically verifiable role assertions for remote care workflows, and how such mechanisms affect both staff burden and citizen trust. These evaluations should be longitudinal, since the framework assumes feedback effects where successful journeys strengthen habit and trust, while repeated failures increase perceived effort and perceived risk.

Technical and operational research questions also remain important because they shape user experience and institutional accountability. Priorities include secure and usable account recovery and device change, handling of lost devices, the clarity of consent and prohibition management, and the reliability of proximity and offline verification in real service counters. For proximity-based use, empirical testing should quantify transaction time, failure rates, and recovery paths for QR, NFC, and BLE flows in pharmacy and clinic environments where time pressure is high. Further work should also address how wallet-based attribute presentation integrates with existing health system components, including identity binding, logging and transparency views that users can understand, and incident response procedures that avoid accountability gaps across actors. These technical topics are not separate from adoption, because they condition whether wallet-based journeys are perceived as safe, predictable, and supportable in routine care.

In general, the study supports a cautious interpretation. Finland has high baseline adoption of digital health services, but this does not guarantee adoption of a new access paradigm. The likely success conditions are consistent wallet-based journeys that respect existing habits, interaction-level transparency that increases perceived control, and operational governance that ensures predictable relying party practices and accessible support. Under these conditions, the EUDI Wallet can become a meaningful additional channel for health access and credential presentation, including cross-border scenarios where interoperability under the ARF and EHDS-related pathways can function as a practical bridge for care continuity, while reducing reliance on a single credential ecosystem and improving clarity of attribute sharing in high-sensitivity transactions.

7 Conclusion

The transition to the EUDI Wallet represents a socio-technical change in how health data is accessed and shared. In the Finnish context, adoption will not be driven by the introduction of new capabilities but by the refinement of existing ones. For a population already habituated to a mature national infrastructure, the wallet must prove its value not as a replacement but as a state-governed alternative that reduces authentication friction and strengthens perceived agency over sensitive information. The scoping review and the resulting framework suggest that the success of the deployment rests on three interdependent conditions.

First, the wallet paradigm, through selective disclosure and local storage, provides a mechanism to address the heightened privacy sensitivity that follows from previous data breaches. By shifting from account-centric access to attribute-based presentation, the framework supports a reconstruction of institutional trust. This is consistent with analyses of the Vastaamo case as a governance and accountability failure and with clinical framing of confidentiality incidents as patient-safety relevant events [18,37]. Second, digital health equity depends on treating adoption as a human process. The role of warm experts shows that digital competence functions as a threshold condition, and that success will be shaped by how well institutional governance supports the most vulnerable citizens through assisted use and accessible onboarding. Evidence indicates that informal support enables first successful completion but can also shift privacy decisions to helpers if assisted pathways are not designed with clear boundaries [19,32]. Third, the multi-authority model of the Finnish ecosystem requires coordinated responsibilities across policy-makers, technical agencies (DVV, Traficom), and health-sector operators (Kela, wellbeing counties). This coordination is necessary to ensure that attribute requests remain proportionate, transparent, and accountable across both domestic and cross-border journeys, consistent with EU-level emphasis on cybersecurity and operational assurance in healthcare [12,47].

The EUDI Wallet functions as a consent-brokering layer for a high-sensitivity domain. If implemented with consistent attention to transparency, interaction-level clarity, and inclusion safeguards, it can serve as a practical bridge for care continuity and cross-border access in the Finnish healthcare system.

Acknowledgments. The research was supported by the University of Oulu, the 6G Flagship (369116), Profi5 HiDyn programme (326291), SViSenS Academy Project Funding 2025 (370277) and Profi7 Hybrid intelligence program (352788), funded by the Research Council of Finland. The authors wish to acknowledge the use of AI-assisted tools for language editing, with a focus on grammar checking and improving readability. In addition, the Elicit platform was used during the literature search as an AI-assisted discovery aid for candidate records. All inclusion decisions, exclusions, data extraction, synthesis, interpretation, and final writing decisions were performed by the authors.

References

1. Regulation (eu) 2024/1183 of the european parliament and of the council of 11 april 2024 amending regulation (eu) no 910/2014 as regards establishing the european digital identity framework (2024). http://data.europa.eu/eli/reg/2024/1183/oj, official Journal of the European Union
2. Arksey, H., O'malley, L.: Scoping studies: towards a methodological framework. Int. J. Soc. Res. Methodol. **8**(1), 19–32 (2005)
3. Commission, E., Directorate-General for Employment, S.A., Inclusion, Leuven, H.K.: The European Health Insurance Card – Reference year 2015. Publications Office (2016). https://doi.org/10.2767/630740
4. Dang, Y., Guo, S., Guo, X., Wang, M., Xie, K., et al.: Privacy concerns about health information disclosure in mobile health: questionnaire study investigating the moderation effect of social support. JMIR Mhealth Uhealth **9**(2), e19594 (2021)
5. Dienlin, T.: Privacy calculus: Theory, studies, and new perspectives. In: The Routledge Handbook of Privacy and Social Media, pp. 70–79. Routledge (2023)
6. Digital and Population Data Services Agency: European digital identity wallet (2024). https://dvv.fi/en/european-digital-identity-wallet, Accessed 24 Jan 2026
7. Digital and Population Data Services Agency: Digital identity wallet will add efficiency and security to finnish daily life - new app to be introduced at the end of 2026 (October 2025). https://dvv.fi/en/-/digital-identity-wallet-will-add-efficiency-and-security-to-finnish-daily-life-new-app-to-be-introduced-at-the-end-of-2026
8. Dinev, T., Hart, P.: An extended privacy calculus model for e-commerce transactions. Inf. Syst. Res. **17**(1), 61–80 (2006)
9. Eichacker, M., Hajric, A., Moll, T., Möllers, F., Vogelgesang, S.: Report on the architecture of the eudi-wallet. Technical Report 2024-0393, Defendo IT GmbH, Saarbrücken, Germany (Nov 2024), prepared on behalf of the Bundesverband der Verbraucherzentralen und Verbraucherverbände – Verbraucherzentrale Bundesverband e.V
10. Elicit: Elicit's source for papers (2025). https://support.elicit.com/en/articles/553025, updated October 29, 2025. Elicit searches over 138 million academic papers from Semantic Scholar, PubMed, and OpenAlex
11. Eriksson-Backa, K., Hirvonen, N., Enwald, H., Huvila, I.: Enablers for and barriers to using my kanta-a focus group study of older adults' perceptions of the national electronic health record in finland. Inform. Health Soc. Care **46**(4), 399–411 (2021)
12. European Commission: Communication from the commission to the european parliament, the council, the european economic and social committee and the committee of the regions: European action plan on the cybersecurity of hospitals and healthcare providers. Tech. Rep. COM/2025/10 final, European Commission, Brussels (January 2025). https://eur-lex.europa.eu/legal-content/EN/TXT/?uri=celex:52025DC0010, accessed: 2026-02-01
13. European Commission: The ePrescription Manual. EU Digital Identity Wallet - Digital Building Blocks (2025), https://ec.europa.eu/digital-building-blocks/sites/spaces/EUDIGITALIDENTITYWALLET/pages/930452930/ePrescription, Accessed 24 Jan 2026. Last updated 22 Dec 2025
14. European Commission: The European Health Insurance Card (EHIC) use case manual. EU Digital Identity Wallet - Digital Building Blocks (2025), https://ec.europa.eu/digital-building-blocks/sites/spaces/EUDIGITALIDENTITYWALLET/pages/930453001/EHIC, Accessed 24 Jan 2026. Last updated 22 Dec 2025

15. European Commission, eIDAS Expert Group: European digital identity wallet: Architecture and reference framework (arf) (2025), https://github.com/eu-digital-identity-wallet/eudi-doc-architecture-and-reference-framework/releases/tag/v2.7.3, Accessed 24 Jan 2026

16. European Parliament and Council: Regulation (EU) 2025/327 of the european parliament and of the council of 11 february 2025 on the european health data space and amending directive 2011/24/eu and regulation (EU) 2024/2847. Official Journal of the European Union **L Series**, OJ L 2025/327 (2025), http://data.europa.eu, published on 5 March 2025

17. Fereday, J., Muir-Cochrane, E.: Demonstrating rigor using thematic analysis: a hybrid approach of inductive and deductive coding and theme development. Int J Qual Methods **5**(1), 80–92 (2006)

18. Ghanbari, H., Koskinen, K.: When data breach hits a psychotherapy clinic: the vastaamo case. J. Inform. Technol. Teaching Cases (2024). https://doi.org/10.1177/20438869241258235

19. Hänninen, R., Taipale, S.: Warm experts among us: conceptualising the challenges of informal digital support for older adults. New Media Soc., 14614448251385087 (2025)

20. Harrell, D.T., et al.: Technical design and development of a self-sovereign identity management platform for patient-centric health care using blockchain technology. Blockchain Healthcare Today **5**, 10–30953 (2022)

21. Heponiemi, T., Virtanen, L., Kainiemi, E., Saukkonen, P., Reponen, J., Lääveri, T.: Health information systems' support for management and changing work: survey study among physicians. JMIR Med. Inform. **13**, e65913 (2025)

22. Hong, Q.N., et al.: The mixed methods appraisal tool (mmat) version 2018 for information professionals and researchers. Educ. Inf. **34**(4), 285–291 (2018)

23. Jormanainen, V.: Large-scale implementation and adoption of the finish national kanta services in 2010–2017: a prospective, longitudinal, indicator-based study. Finnish J. eHealth eWelfare **10**(4), 381–395 (2018)

24. Jormanainen, V., Lindgren, M., Keskimäki, I., Kaila, M.: Use of my kanta in finland 2010–2022. In: Healthcare Transformation with Informatics and Artificial Intelligence, pp. 448–451. IOS Press (2023)

25. Jormanainen, V., Parhiala, K., Niemi, A., Erhola, M., Keskimäki, I., Kaila, M.: Half of the finish population accessed their own data: comprehensive access to personal health information online is a corner-stone of digital revolution in finnish health and social care: Englanti. Finnish J. eHealth eWelfare **11**(4), 298–310 (2019)

26. Jormanainen, V., Vehko, T., Lindgren, M., Keskimäki, I., Kaila, M.: Implementation, adoption and use of the kanta services in finland 2010–2022. In: Caring is Sharing–Exploiting the Value in Data for Health and Innovation, pp. 227–231. IOS Press (2023)

27. Juga, J., Juntunen, J., Koivumäki, T.: Willingness to share personal health information: impact of attitudes, trust and control. Rec. Manag. J. **31**(1), 48–59 (2021)

28. Kaihlanen, A.M., et al.: Towards digital health equity-a qualitative study of the challenges experienced by vulnerable groups in using digital health services in the covid-19 era. BMC Health Serv. Res. **22**(1), 188 (2022)

29. Kim, H.W., Kankanhalli, A.: Investigating user resistance to information systems implementation: a status quo bias perspective. MIS Q. , 567–582 (2009)

30. Koivumäki, T., Pekkarinen, S., Lappi, M., Väisänen, J., Juntunen, J., Pikkarainen, M.: Consumer adoption of future mydata-based preventive ehealth services: an acceptance model and survey study. J. Med. Internet Res. **19**(12), e429 (2017)

31. Komarova, A.: User experience of digital healthcare services in Finland from the customer perspective (2024)
32. Korpela, V., Pajula, L., Hänninen, R.: Investigating the multifaceted role of warm experts in enhancing and hindering older adults' digital skills in Finland. Int. J. Lifelong Educ. **43**(5), 509–522 (2024)
33. Lämsä, E., Timonen, J., Ahonen, R.: Pharmacy customers' experiences with electronic prescriptions: cross-sectional survey on nationwide implementation in Finland. J. Med. Internet Res. **20**(2), e68 (2018). https://doi.org/10.2196/jmir.9367
34. Lau, O., Golder, S.: Comparison of elicit ai and traditional literature searching in evidence syntheses using four case studies. Cochrane Evid. Synth. Methods **3**(6), e70050 (2025)
35. Laukka, E., Lakoma, S., Harjumaa, M., et al.: Older adults' preferences in the utilization of digital health and social services: a qualitative analysis of responses to open-ended questions. BMC Health Serv. Res. **24**, 1184 (2024). https://doi.org/10.1186/s12913-024-11564-1
36. Levac, D., Colquhoun, H., O'brien, K.K.: Scoping studies: advancing the methodology. Implement. Sci. **5**(1), 69 (2010)
37. Looi, J.C., et al.: Cybersecurity lessons from the vastaamo psychotherapy data breach for psychiatrists and other mental healthcare providers. Australas. Psychiatry **33**(1), 106–110 (2025)
38. Mezei, J., Sell, A., Walden, P.: Technology readiness, UTAUT2 and continued use of digital wellness services-A configurational approach (2022). https://doi.org/10.24251/HICSS.2022.181
39. Mielonen, J., Kuusisto, H., Kinnunen, U.M., Kemppi, A., Saranto, K.: Older adults' experiences of ehealth in health and social care. Finnish J. eHealth and eWelfare **15**(3), 276–286 (2023)
40. Mikkonen, K., et al.: Digital health competence among healthcare professionals: a cross-sectional cluster analysis across 19 countries and regions. Inter. J. Nursing Stud., 105348 (2026)
41. Ministry of Finance: Project to implement the reformed eidas regulation nationally (2024). https://vm.fi/en/eidasregulation, Accessed 26 Jan 2026
42. Ministry of Finance, Finland: European digital identity wallet (2024). https://vm.fi/en/european-digital-identity-wallet, Accessed 24 Jan 2026
43. Ministry of Social Affairs and Health: Ehds regulation implementation in finland (2026). https://stm.fi/en/ehds-regulation
44. Ministry of Social Affairs and Health: Supervision of healthcare in Finland (2026). https://www.eu-healthcare.fi/healthcare-in-finland/healthcare-system-in-finland/supervision-of-healthcare-in-finland/, reflecting Valvira and Fimea roles in 2026 context
45. Ntangee, J.: Cybersecurity threat in cloud computing in the finnish healthcare sector: a case study in the finnish healthcare (2025)
46. Page, M.J., et al.: The prisma 2020 statement: an updated guideline for reporting systematic reviews. bmj **372** (2021)
47. Palma, F.N.S.: Interoperability challenges and critical success factors in the deployment of cross-border digital medical prescriptions in Finland and Estonia. In: 2022 IEEE International Conference on Digital Health (ICDH), pp. 60–65. IEEE (2022)
48. Pan, J., Dong, H., Bryan-Kinns, N.: Perception and initial adoption of mobile health services of older adults in london: mixed methods investigation. JMIR Aging **4**(4), e30420 (2021)

49. Rajit, D., McDonald, S., Tay, C.T., Du, L., Enticott, J., Teede, H.: Assessing the coverage of pubmed, embase, openalex and semantic scholar for automated single database searches in living guideline evidence surveillance: a case study of the international pcos guidelines 2023. J. Clin. Epidemiol., 111789 (2025)
50. Sääskilahti, M., Ahonen, R., Timonen, J.: Pharmacy customers' experiences of use, usability, and satisfaction of a nationwide patient portal: survey study. J. Med. Internet Res. **23**(7), e25368 (2021)
51. Schwalm, S., Alamillo-Domingo, I.: Self-sovereign-identity & eidas: a contradiction? challenges and chances of eidas 2.0. Wirtschaftsinformatik **58**, 247–270 (2021)
52. Sosiaali- ja terveysministeriö: Hallitus esittää mahdollisuutta teknologia-avusteiseen hoidon tarpeen arviointiin perusterveydenhuollossa. Tiedote (Jan 2026). https://stm.fi/-/hallitus-esittaa-mahdollisuutta-teknologia-avusteiseen-hoidon-tarpeen-arviointiin-perusterveydenhuollossa, Accessed 24 Jan 2026. Julkaistu 22.1.2026
53. TEHDAS Joint Action: Finland country visit factsheet - european health data space development. Tech. rep., Finnish Institute for Health and Welfare (THL) and Kela (2023). https://tehdas.eu/app/uploads/2023/04/finland-country-visit-factsheet-04-2023.pdf
54. Torkki, P., et al.: The use and perceived benefits of digital health services among Finnish older adults: survey study. Health Inform. J. **32**(1), 14604582261416860 (2026). https://doi.org/10.1177/14604582261416861
55. Tossavainen, A.: Means of digital personal identification and authentication to digital services in Finland (2025)
56. Tricco, A.C., et al.: Prisma extension for scoping reviews (prisma-scr): checklist and explanation. Ann. Intern. Med. **169**(7), 467–473 (2018)
57. Van Roijen, D.: The European digital identity wallet: a healthcare perspective. Blockchain Healthcare Today **7** (2024). https://doi.org/10.30953/bhty.v7.344, PMID: 39649413; PMCID: PMC11624493
58. Vanella, A.: Evolution of Digital Identity in Europe: Experimenting with the eIDAS 2.0 Framework and the EU Digital Identity Wallet, Master's thesis, Politecnico di Torino (2025). https://webthesis.biblio.polito.it/35272/
59. Venkatesh, V., Thong, J.Y., Xu, X.: Consumer acceptance and use of information technology: extending the unified theory of acceptance and use of technology. MIS Q., 157–178 (2012)
60. Wohlin, C.: Guidelines for snowballing in systematic literature studies and a replication in software engineering. In: Proceedings of the 18th International Conference on Evaluation and Assessment in Software Engineering, pp. 1–10 (2014)
61. Zuuring, E.: Digital healthcare solutions: evaluating the usability of ehrs on public health services in Finland (2024)

Paramedicine Speech Recognition Adoption: A Socio-Technical Ranking Study

Desmond Hedderson[1]([envelope]) [iD], Helen Monkman[1] [iD], Ian E. Blanchard[2,3] [iD],
and Karen L. Courtney[1] [iD]

[1] School of Health Information Science, University of Victoria, Victoria, BC V8P 5C2, Canada
dhedderson@uvic.ca
[2] Cumming School of Medicine, University of Calgary, Calgary, Canada
[3] Alberta Health Services, Emergency Medical Services, Calgary, Canada

Abstract. Speech recognition-aided documentation could improve paramedicine documentation and continuity of patient care. However, little research has been done to facilitate the development and implementation of technology, including speech recognition, in paramedicine. We asked Canadian paramedics to rank the dimensions most important to them overall when considering the adoption of speech-recognition technologies (n = 275) and to identify the value of different features of speech-recognition-aided documentation within each dimension of the Sittig and Singh socio-technical model (n = 323). Paramedics rated the product design and usability dimensions as more important than the broader system dimensions. However, all dimensions were represented by the top 10 most positively rated features, except Workflow & Communication, which had no features ranked higher than 12th. Individual features were scored on a scale of 1 (not valuable) to 5 (extremely valuable). Five of the top ten desired features were in the People or Human-Computer Interaction dimensions. In highest rank order, the top ten desired features included: Patient Interaction, Training, Compliance, Support, Durability, Accuracy, Continuous Improvement, Editing, Dictation, and Training Support. For the top ten listed features, 86–95% of the scores were 4 or 5. These results highlight Canadian paramedics' need for a purpose-built system. Understanding these priorities can help vendors and paramedic systems design and implement effective speech-recognition-aided documentation systems in paramedicine.

Keywords: Paramedicine · Socio-technical Model · Implementation · Technology Adoption · Speech Recognition

1 Introduction

Paramedics operate in time- and resource-constrained environments, where they provide life-saving interventions and patient assessments [1]. This leaves little time for documentation, and as data demands from stakeholders increase, it results in delays in completing and submitting electronic documentation to emergency departments and in inaccurate post-care charting [2]. The time and data volume pressures can contribute

© The Author(s) 2026
M. Särestöniemi et al. (Eds.): NCDHWS 2026, CCIS 3009, pp. 214–221, 2026.
https://doi.org/10.1007/978-3-032-28812-7_16

to documentation burden for paramedics. This documentation burden can lead to gaps in patient information during transfer of care to the emergency department and may negatively affect patient care and outcomes [3, 4].

Advancing technologies, such as speech recognition (SR)-aided documentation, can help address the documentation burden in paramedicine. SR-aided documentation has been shown to produce more complete notes, take less time, and be less error-prone than typed clinical documentation in other health care settings [5–8]. With advancements in natural language processing, algorithmic noise reduction, and artificial intelligence (AI), implementing SR-aided documentation in paramedicine is now feasible [1, 2, 6, 9, 10].

While well studied and understood in other healthcare contexts, the implementation of technologies, including SR-aided documentation, has not been adequately explored in paramedicine [11]. This lack of research means we lack understanding of the dimensions that influence paramedics' adoption, use, and acceptance of new technology. This lack of understanding could lead to suboptimal development, implementation, or use of technology in paramedicine [12]. The development and uptake of new technologies has been identified as an enabling factor for the future of paramedicine in Canada, but it remains critical to understand the paramedic perspective to take full advantage of these technologies [13].

One paradigm for studying and understanding health information technology, such as SR-aided documentation, is the Sittig and Singh socio-technical model [12]. The model includes eight dimensions: 1) Hardware and Software, 2) Clinical Content, 3) Human-Computer Interface, 4) People, 5) Workflow and Communication, 6) Internal Organizational Policies, Procedures, Environment and Culture, 7) External Rules, Regulations and Pressures, and 8) System Measurement and Monitoring [12]. The socio-technical model includes the characteristics of the technology and the interactions between a technology and the systems in which it operates. The socio-technical model has been used to classify perceptions and adoption needs in previous studies of smart glass technology in paramedicine [14]. Understanding which of these dimensions of the sociotechnical model paramedics found more relevant could help guide the implementation and development of new technology for paramedicine.

This study sought to identify which dimensions of Sittig and Singh's socio-technical model influence the adoption and implementation of SR-aided documentation in Canadian paramedicine.

2   Methods

The University of Victoria Human Research Ethics Board approved this explanatory mixed-methods study [15]. As part of a larger thesis, a voluntary web-based survey was distributed to Canadian paramedics across all 10 provinces through regulatory bodies, professional associations, and alumni groups. The survey included questions on attitudes, perceptions, and prior experience with SR technologies. This paper outlines one question which asked respondents, "Which sections' features would you trade off?" using a scale from one to eight, with one being the most important and eight the least. The rankings were then analyzed using Friedman's test, calculating the effect size using Kendall's W, and then a Pairwise Wilcox test for post hoc pairwise comparisons using the Bonferroni correction to determine any significance between rankings.

The questionnaire also included ranking questions on the value of 45 potential features of SR-aided documentation based on previous studies and technology available in other healthcare settings [11]. The features were classified by their relevance to each dimension, according to the definitions provided by Sittig and Singh [12]. The ranking scale ranged from one (not valuable) to five (extremely valuable). The features were categorized into the eight dimensions of the Sittig and Singh socio-technical model [12].

3   Results

The respondents included paramedics from every Canadian province, with an average age of 38 years. Respondents were asked to self-select their gender: 59% men, 37% women, and 5% non-binary or self-identified. Most respondents work as frontline staff (66%), however, educators (13%), supervisors (7%), executives (7%), students (4%), and researchers (3%) were also represented. Of all the responses (323) available for analysis, 275 answered the optional question ranking the dimensions of the socio-technical model. The results are presented in Fig. 1.

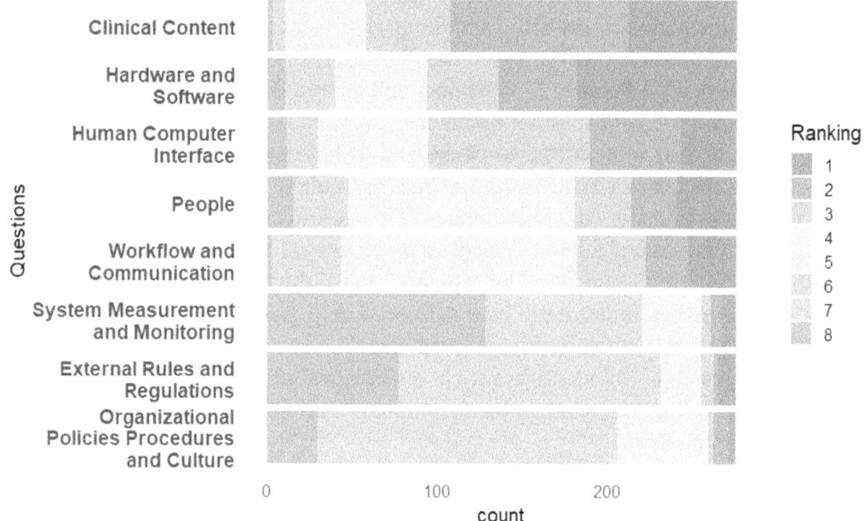

Fig. 1. Priority rankings of the Sittig and Singh socio-technical model dimensions, n = 275, with 1 being most important to keep and 8 being least important.

The Friedman test comparing the rankings of the dimensions was significant, $\chi 2 = 869.99$, df = 7, $P < 0.001$, with moderate-to-strong agreement (Kendall's W = 0.45), indicating that the ratings differed significantly between at least two dimensions. The Clinical Context dimension had more high rankings (1–3) and fewer low rankings (6–8), while the Hardware and Software dimension had the most top rankings; however, the difference between the two was not significant. The Human-Computer Interface dimension ranked third most important, with fewer top rankings but more high rankings and fewer low rankings. The People dimension had more higher rankings and the Workflow and Communication dimension had fewer lower rankings. While System Measurement and Monitoring received the highest number of the lowest rankings, External Rules, Regulations, and Pressures received the most overall low rankings. Internal Organizational Policies, Procedures, Environment and Culture ranked lowest overall with the fewest high rankings. The results of a pairwise Wilcox test (Table 1) show that most dimensions differed significantly. Hardware and Software compared to Clinical Content, Human-Computer Interface compared to Hardware and Software, People compared to Workflow and Communication, and System Measurement and Monitoring compared to External Rules, Regulations and Pressures were the exceptions and did not differ significantly.

Table 1. Pairwise Wilcox test p-values An (*) indicates a significant difference. Abbreviations (CC – Clinical Content, HS – Hardware and Software, HCI – Human-Computer Interface, Pe – People, WC – Workflow and Communication, SSM – System Measurement and Monitoring, ERRP – External Rules, Regulations, and Pressures, IOPPC – Internal Organizational Polices, Procedures, Environment, and Culture).

	CC	HS	HCI	Pe	WC	SSM	ERRP	IOPPC
CC	-							
HS	0.082	-						
HCI	< 0.001*	0.362	-					
Pe	< 0.001*	< 0.001*	0.003*	-				
WC	< 0.001*	< 0.001*	< 0.001*	1.000	-			
SSM	< 0.001*	< 0.001*	< 0.001*	< 0.001*	< 0.001*	-		
ERRP	< 0.001*	< 0.001*	< 0.001*	< 0.001*	< 0.001*	1.000	-	
IOPPC	< 0.001*	< 0.001*	< 0.001*	< 0.001*	< 0.001*	< 0.001*	< 0.001*	-

The ten features with the highest percent of total responses as positive ratings (4 or 5 on the scale) are shown in Fig. 2 and include features from all dimensions of the socio-technical model, except the Workflow and Communication dimension. Specifically, Three features were from the People dimension (Patient Interaction 95%, Training 92%, Support 91%), two from the Human-Computer Interface dimension (Accuracy 89%, Editing 86%), and one each from the remaining dimensions Hardware and Software (Durability 91%), Clinical Content (Dictation 86%), System Measurement and Monitoring (Continuous Improvement 88%), External Rules, Regulations and Pressures (Compliance 92%), and Internal Organizational Policies, Procedures, Environment and Culture (Training Support 86%). Workflow and Communications highest rated feature was 12th on the list and thus was not included.

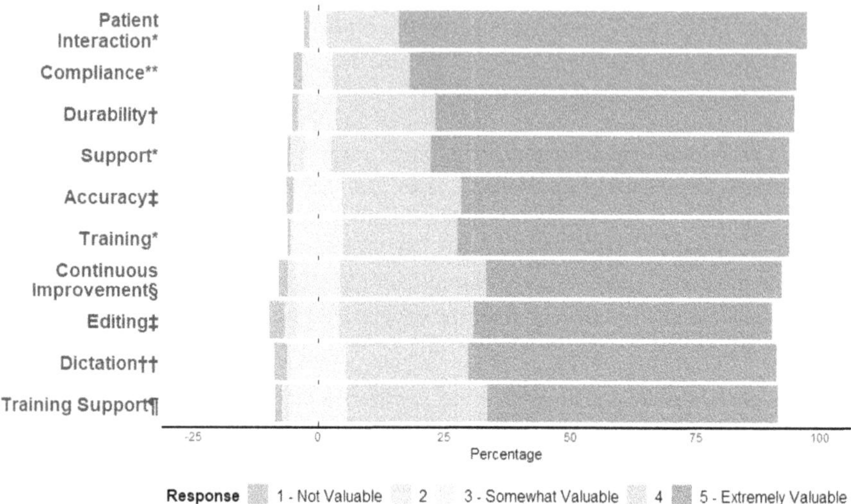

Fig. 2. The top ten highly valued features, n = 323, based on a 4 or 5 ranking. (†) Hardware and Software, (‡) Clinical Content, (††) Human-Computer Interface, (*) People, (¶) Internal Organizational Policies, Procedures, Environment, and Culture, (**) External Rules, Regulations, and Pressures, (§) System Measurement and Monitoring.

4   Discussion

The results from the questionnaire suggest that Canadian paramedics place a high value on the form and function of technology. Paramedics perceive the features of broader system aspects (System Measurement and Monitoring; Internal Organizational Policies, procedures, Environment; and External Rules, Regulations and Pressures) as less important, and the features included in the dimensions that affect the physical product and the technology's usability (Hardware and Software; Clinical Content; and Human-Computer Interface) as more important. This information highlights that paramedics require a product with high functionality. Developers can use this knowledge to focus development and prototype efforts on ensuring the product has high usability and functionality.

However, the system aspects of implementation were also heavily represented among the highest-valued features in the questionnaire. Specifically, paramedics place a high value on the system's medicolegal compliance and available technical support, as well as the organization's commitment to ensuring appropriate training support and investment, and a continuous improvement cycle that recognizes and acts on feedback. These results highlight Canadian paramedics' need for a purpose-built system when using technology and the importance of training and support. SR-aided documentation will need to be well-designed to integrate into the paramedicine environment and workflow and well supported by both the organization and the vendor.

Understanding which dimensions of the socio-technical model paramedics favour could provide benefits for future work. A better understanding of paramedics' priorities can help vendors tailor products to meet their needs. Similarly, organizations can use this information to ensure that their technology implementation plans focus on the factors paramedics value most. This knowledge can help prevent costly implementation failures and service corrections.

Currently, there is a paucity of research on paramedics' perceptions and requirements regarding technology adoption [11, 18]. This lack of empirical research has led to ill-fitting and underperforming technologies in paramedicine. The technologies employed in the paramedic profession, such as documentation and decision-support systems, are often adapted from other professions and practice environments [2, 14]. Understanding how to adopt technologies in paramedicine has been identified as a priority for the future of paramedicine in Canada [13].

Further research could clarify the importance of each dimension and help develop targeted implementation plans. For example, a full needs assessment of a Canadian paramedic service could help identify which dimensions of the socio-technical model could be most important for a new SR-aided documentation system. Using the socio-technical model, we could also explore the priorities of other stakeholders, such as IT or billing departments, or regulatory bodies [12]. Developing this knowledge framework for paramedicine could help improve how paramedicine functions.

A limitation of this study was that respondents were asked to rank the dimensions of the socio-technical model based on the selection of features listed in each dimension, rather than on the dimensions' definitions. To better understand why paramedics prioritize the dimensions, it would be best to conduct a follow-up, targeted interview to clarify the rankings provided.

5   Conclusion

This study sought to identify which dimensions of Sittig and Singh's socio-technical model could influence the adoption and implementation of SR-aided documentation in Canadian paramedicine. This work identifies that while paramedics favour form and function over broader system implications, they believe certain organizational and external pressures are critical for implementation. More research is required to fully clarify the rankings and determine whether they change based on role within the system or the type or purpose of the technology. The Sittig and Singh socio-technical model provides a tool for exploring paramedics' priorities regarding SR-aided documentation technology. There has been a dearth of research on what helps with the development, implementation, and use of technology in paramedicine.

References

1. Hedderson, D.R., Lai, C.: Integrated Hands-Free Electronic Patient Care Report (ePCR) Charting (IHeC): designing the architecture. AMIA Annu. Symp. Proc. **22**(2024), 533–540 (2025)
2. Meier L, Bauer JG, Denecke K. Speech-based documentation in emergency medical services with the electronic language interface for ambulance services. In: 2020 IEEE International Conference on Healthcare Informatics (ICHI) [Internet], Oldenburg, Germany, pp. 1–6. IEEE (2020). https://ieeexplore.ieee.org/document/9374336/, cited May 7 2023

3. Stiell, A., Forster, A.J., Stiell, I.G., van Walraven, C.: Prevalence of information gaps in the emergency department and the effect on patient outcomes. CMAJ Can Med Assoc J. **169**(10), 1023–1028 (2003)

4. Carter, A.J.E., Davis, K.A., Evans, L.V., Cone, D.C.: Information loss in emergency medical services handover of trauma patients. Prehosp. Emerg. Care **13**(3), 280–285 (2009)

5. Johnson, M., Lapkin, S., Long, V., Sanchez, P., Suominen, H., Basilakis, J., et al.: A systematic review of speech recognition technology in health care. BMC Med. Inform. Decis. Mak. **14**(1), 94 (2014)

6. Shagoury J.: "Multi-task": using speech to build up electronic medical records while caring for patients. In: Neustein, A (ed). Advances in Speech Recognition [Internet], pp. p. 247–73. Springer US; Boston, MA (2010). https://doi.org/10.1007/978-1-4419-5951-5_11, cited 6 June 2023

7. Blackley, S.V., Schubert, V.D., Goss, F.R., Al Assad, W., Garabedian, P.M., Zhou, L.: Physician use of speech recognition versus typing in clinical documentation: a controlled observational study. Int J Med Inf. **141**, 104178 (2020)

8. Blackley, S.V., Huynh, J., Wang, L., Korach, Z., Zhou, L.: Speech recognition for clinical documentation from 1990 to 2018: a systematic review. J Am Med Inform Assoc JAMIA. **26**(4), 324–338 (2019)

9. Kemppainen, A.: VISAC - Towards a Voice Interface for Swedish Ambulance Care [Master of Biomedical Engineering]. [Gothenburg, Sweden]: Charlmers University (2022)

10. Tanberk, S., Dağlı, V., Gürkan, M.K.: Deep learning for videoconferencing: a brief examination of speech to text and speech synthesis. In: 2021 6th International Conference on Computer Science and Engineering (UBMK), pp. 506–511 (2021)

11. Hedderson, D., Courtney, K.L., Monkman, H., Blanchard, I.E.: Speech recognition technology in prehospital documentation: a scoping review. Int J Med Inf. **193**, 105662 (2025)

12. Sittig, D.F., Singh, H.: A new socio-technical model for studying health information technology in complex adaptive healthcare systems. In: Patel, V.L., Kannampallil, T.G., Kaufman, D.R. (eds.) Cognitive Informatics for Biomedicine. Health Informatics. Springer, Cham (2015). https://doi.org/10.1007/978-3-319-17272-9_4

13. Tavares, W., Allana, A., Beaune, L., Weiss, D., Blanchard, I.: Principles to guide the future of paramedicine in canada. Prehosp Emerg Care. **26**(5), 728–738 (2022)

14. Zhang, Z., Ramiya Ramesh Babu, N.A., Adelgais, K., Ozkaynak, M.: Designing and implementing smart glass technology for emergency medical services: a sociotechnical perspective. JAMIA Open. **5**(4), ooac113 (2022)

15. Creswell, J.W., Plano Clark, V.L.: Designing and conducting mixed methods research, p. 275. SAGE Publications, Thousand Oaks, Calif (2007)

16. Oliver, D.G., Serovich, J.M., Mason, T.L.: Constraints and opportunities with interview transcription: towards reflection in qualitative research. Soc Forces Sci Medium Soc Study Interpret. **84**(2), 1273–1289 (2005)

17. Smith, C.P.: Motivation and Personality: Handbook of Thematic Content Analysis, p. 738. Cambridge University Press (1992)

18. Bijani, M., Abedi, S., Karimi, S., Tehranineshat, B.: Major challenges and barriers in clinical decision-making as perceived by emergency medical services personnel: a qualitative content analysis. BMC Emerg. Med. **21**(1), 11 (2021)

Towards Healthy Ageing: Design and Implementation of a Person-Centered Digital Health System

Michele Atzeni[1] , Margherita La Gamba[1], Laura Giani[1] ,
Gokce B. Laleci Erturkmen[2] , Erika Jarva[3] , Iiro Nerg[4] , Sylvain Sebert[4] ,
Teija Juola[4], and Maria Bulgheroni[1(✉)]

[1] Ab.Acus Srl, Via Francesco Caracciolo 77, 20155 Milan, Italy
mariabulgheroni@ab-acus.eu
[2] SRDC Software Research Development and Consultancy Corporation, Ankara, Turkey
[3] Research Unit of Health Sciences and Technology, Faculty of Medicine, University of Oulu, Oulu, Finland
[4] Research Unit of Population Health, Faculty of Medicine, University of Oulu, Oulu, Finland

Abstract. Digital health technologies offer promising opportunities for longitudinal health monitoring, yet their adoption in research settings faces significant barriers including usability concerns, participant burden, and data privacy issues. This paper presents the design, implementation, and usability evaluation of a person-centered digital health system for scalable, privacy-preserving longitudinal health monitoring in ageing populations. The system was developed within the STAGE project to support a two-year study (2026–2028) with approximately 10,000 participants from the Northern Finland Birth Cohort (NFBC1966). The system employs a modular, privacy-centered architecture comprising a cross-platform mobile application and a cloud backend infrastructure, all designed to be GDPR-compliant with comprehensive security measures. Development was guided by structured co-creation activities and patient and public involvement (PPI) through interviews, questionnaires, and workshops with diverse stakeholders including ageing citizens, caregivers, clinicians, and researchers. The mobile application enables periodic self-reported assessments of wellbeing, cognitive and physical functioning, mental health, nutrition, anthropometric measurements, falls, and mobility patterns, complemented by GPS-based mobility tracking during four-week monitoring periods. The system employs a foreground-first data collection approach requiring explicit user interaction to maintain transparency and trust. Two pilot studies demonstrated strong usability outcomes. Pilot #1 (N = 11) yielded high Single Ease Question scores (all means > 5.6/7). Pilot #2 (N = 17) achieved a System Usability Scale score of 87.95 (SD = 8.18), classified as "Excellent," with no critical issues reported. The platform includes FHIR-compliant data export capabilities (17 profiles, 12 valuesets) to facilitate healthcare system integration. While challenges remain regarding long-term engagement and digital literacy variability, the system provides a robust foundation for sustainable, participant-centered longitudinal health research in ageing populations.

Keywords: Digital health · System architecture · User-centered design

© The Author(s) 2026
M. Särestöniemi et al. (Eds.): NCDHWS 2026, CCIS 3009, pp. 222–233, 2026.
https://doi.org/10.1007/978-3-032-28812-7_17

1   Introduction

The pervasiveness of digital technologies in everyday human life has been substantially increasing over recent years. In 2024, more than 70% of the global population owned a smartphone, confirming a widespread diffusion across various demographic and socioeconomic groups [1]. This continuously expanding availability is reshaping the way services are designed and delivered, including health research and care. In particular, smartphones have enabled the large-scale adoption of self-tracking practices related to health outcomes, behaviors, and lifestyle habits. Through the combined use of digital survey delivery and embedded smartphone sensors, such as accelerometers, GPS, and usage logs, citizens can contribute valuable and high-frequency data in a quite unobtrusive manner. These technologies are expected to be key enablers of longitudinal health monitoring, capturing intra-individual variability, as well as long-term trends. Despite this potential, their widespread adoption and sustained acceptance within research settings remain limited [2]. Several challenges are still delaying their effective implementation, including issues related to usability, participant burden, trust, and data privacy. Among these factors, digital health literacy plays a key role, as it strongly influences both participants' ability to engage with digital health technologies and their long-term retention especially when addressing not digitally native populations, including the older ones.

Therefore, despite growing interest in mobile health platforms for longitudinal research, few systems have been specifically designed to meet the combined demands of large-scale cohort studies, older adult populations involvement, and GDPR-compliant data governance. Within the STAGE project, we have addressed these issues in a comprehensive multidisciplinary manner to set up a reliable digital health system, comprising a mobile application, a cloud infrastructure, and data interoperability layers, for longitudinal data collection in health research. The platform, GDPR compliant by design, includes both the digital delivery of periodic surveys and the continuous acquisition of smartphone sensors (GPS data) and its primary usage is to support structured and repeated data collection over a two-year period (2026–2028), complementing existing Northern Finland Birth Cohort (NFBC1966) [3] data, with an expected recruitment of approximately 10,000 participants, without duplicating or interfering with established clinical protocols.

2   Methods

2.1   Requirements and Design Principles

The design of the digital health system was informed by a structured, iterative requirements-gathering process based on co-creation and patient and public involvement (PPI), reflecting a person-centered approach that prioritizes active participant involvement and transparency throughout development. Such approaches have been widely adopted in comparable digital health initiatives, where participatory design has demonstrated improved alignment between system functionalities and user needs, as well as higher long-term adherence in longitudinal studies [4, 5]. Requirements were collected via a multidisciplinary co-creation working group using surveys and semi-structured interviews with ageing citizens, clinicians, and researchers [5]. The process identified functional, clinical, ethical, and legal requirements for developing tools to predict and prevent ageing with multi-morbidity, with particular focus on aligning data collection with clinically meaningful outcomes. In parallel, PPI activities, including interviews (n = 8), questionnaires (n = 9) and in-person workshops with representatives of different stakeholder groups (i.e., ageing citizens, informal caregivers, educators, policy makers and business-oriented actors), involving between six and twelve participants per session, were conducted to gather perspectives on the use of a health monitoring system within a long-term follow-up study.

Co-creation activities and PPI activities generated initial system requirements that guided development. Three primary requirements emerged from these consultations.

First, stakeholders emphasized robust data governance and management, including secure data collection, storage, and processing compliance with ethical and legal regulations to support controlled data sharing across research organizations and accommodate large-scale, longitudinal studies with sensitive health data.

Second, the approach required support for multimodal continuous data collection through mobile devices complementing periodic clinical examinations and questionnaires by capturing long-term lifestyle, behavioral, and environmental data to better reflect real-life conditions and fluctuating symptoms beyond single clinical visits.

Third, digital tools were needed to facilitate remote data collection and streamline study workflows. Specific capabilities included in-app questionnaire and tasks administration, and real-time access to results, all of them being essential for reducing time burden and improving data completeness.

As a final step in the definition of design principles, a cross-disciplinary working group was formed to agree on the clinical study protocol, data scope, core functionalities, and identify potential ethical and regulatory challenges.

Identifying which data to collect, we searched for a balance between participant burden and scientific value. The mobile app was designed to collect repeated self-reported and test-based measures, including general wellbeing, cognitive and physical functioning, mental health, nutrition, anthropometric measurements, falls, mobility, and life or health events. Continuous sensing via the smartphone was limited to GPS data to capture mobility patterns.

2.2 Architecture

We developed a modular, privacy-centered digital health architecture to support secure health data collection while maintaining user trust and regulatory compliance. The system follows a three-tier design comprising: a mobile application for user interaction, an API middleware for business logic, and a cloud backend for distributed storage and processing capabilities (see Fig. 1).

The design emerged from the requirements gathered from the co-creation and PPIs: first, the need for transparent data practices that keep users informed and in control; and second, compliance with healthcare data protection regulations, including (GDPR). These requirements shaped fundamental design decisions across all system components, which are described in more detail below.

Security measures include: (i) encryption, all data is encrypted both in transit using Transport Layer Security (TLS) 1.3 and at rest using 256 bit Advanced Encryption Standard (AES-256) encryption; (ii) authentication and authorization, the system implements secure Jason Web Token (JWT) authorization for user identity verification; (iii) Role-Based Access Control (RBAC), access permissions are managed through a comprehensive RBAC system that defines distinct roles (e.g., patient, clinician, administrator) with granular permissions.

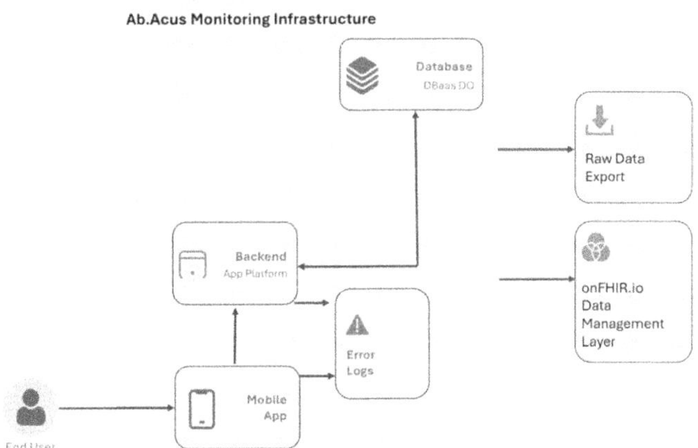

Fig. 1. System Architecture. The monitoring infrastructure integrates a mobile application, Flask backend API (App Platform), MySQL database, and error logging system. Data export is supported through both raw format and FHIR-compliant output.

The mobile application (App) has been developed in Flutter (version 3.24.5) [6], which is a cross-platform environment, hence targeting devices embedded with iOS or Android operating systems, and is available both in English and Finnish locales. The App is a tool that allows ageing citizens to monitor ageing lifestyle, cognitive functioning, and overall mental health in longitudinal settings (see Fig. 2). It includes four main sections.

Home Page with Scheduled Tasks. The homepage displays all the weekly assessments the user is asked to complete, following a specific timeline. These tasks are based on standardized literature assessments, either presented as questionnaires or interactive tasks of memory, cognitive response, and reasoning.

Progress Overview. The progress overview page provides users with a dashboard of their data. Key metrics displayed include overall data collection phase progress, recently logged mood entries, latest body metrics (e.g., weight, and waist circumference), the count of recorded life moments, and any fall reports. The page also features a map visualization showing the user's location data, and a "see more" option to access the complete list of all logged data entries (Fig. 3).

Diary Page for Spontaneous Logging. Users can record unplanned events such as fall, and relevant life events that may affect their health status.

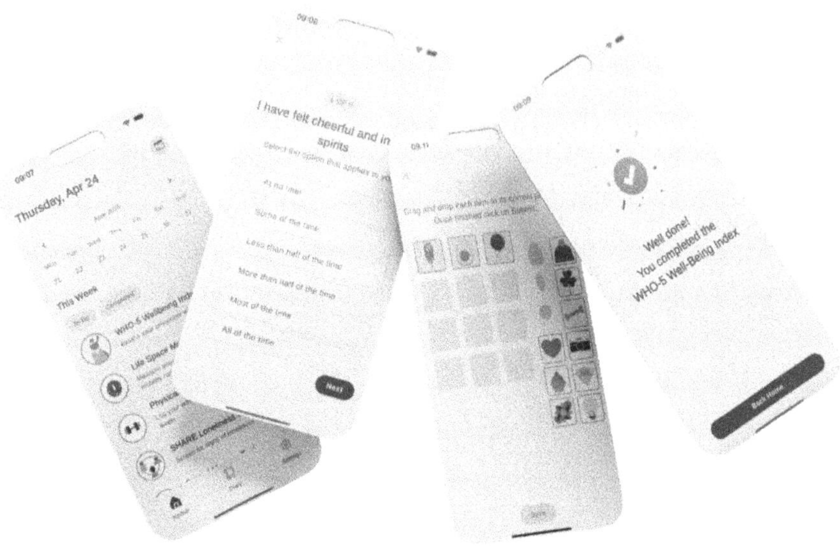

Fig. 2. TheApp Interface. Screenshots showing the main application features: daily task in Homepage (left), questionnaire and tasks interfaces (center), and feedback screen (right).

Settings and User Preferences. This section allows access to customizable settings such as reminders, accessibility options (e.g. dark mode, text size, language), the privacy policy, and send feedback messages.

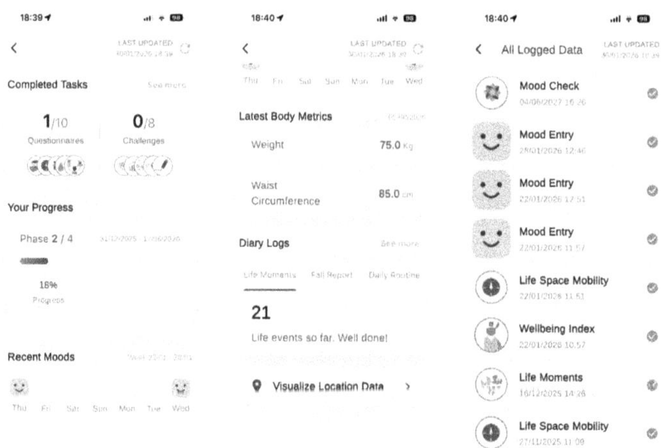

Fig. 3. Screenshots showing key application features: progress overview with completed tasks and study phase tracking (left), dashboard displaying latest body metrics, diary logs, and location data visualization option (center), and comprehensive logged data history including mood entries, wellbeing assessments, and life events (right).

Data collection employs a foreground-first approach for user awareness and build trust. Almost all data collection activities require explicit user interaction and are initiated only when the App is actively in use. Users receive clear notifications before any data collection event, with the ability to review, modify, or decline data submission.

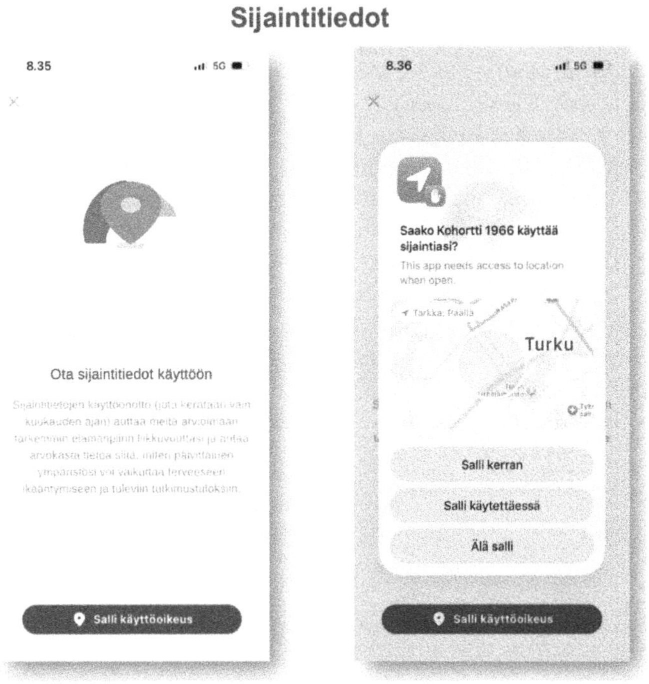

Fig. 4. The App Interface. Screenshots showing the request of location (iOS) clearly explaining (here in Finnish) the purpose and for how long the location monitoring will happen.

The only background information gathered is related to geospatial data. Users are explicitly asked to enable geospatial monitoring for four-week periods to collect data on their movement patterns. Location permission is requested explicitly with transparent disclosure of the data collection purpose (Fig. 4).

Cloud Backend leverages Digital Ocean [7] services for RESTful API, data storage, backup, and recovery. The RESTful API, developed using Python 3.13 [8] and Flask [9], serves as the middleware between the App and backend services. It handles request validation, business logic execution, data transformation, and access control. The API is documented using OpenAPI specifications, while data is stored in EU geographic regions for security and durability. The storage layer implements automated backup schedules.

For all errors or potential malicious data access, audit logs are stored and analyzed leveraging Better Stack [10].

Finally, to facilitate integration with existing healthcare systems, the platform includes a data export module that converts collected health data into Health Level

7 (HL7) Fast Healthcare Interoperability Resources (FHIR) format. The implementation follows the FHIR profiling approach, mapping application-specific data structures to standardized FHIR resources.

A total of 17 FHIR profiles were defined, comprising 11 Observation profiles and 6 Questionnaire profiles, to support a consistent and standardised representation of self-reported data, lifestyle measures, and contextual environmental parameters.

As a part of these profiles, we have created 12 valueset, by selecting matching codes from Logical Observation Identifiers Names and Codes (LOINC) [11], SNOMED CT [12] and ad-hoc STAGE codes to encode the semantics as a part of the common data model. The exported FHIR resources will be saved to the onFHIR.io [13] FHIR Repository via FHIR Restful API, which will be used as the common data repository enabling data exchange between different components of the STAGE Digital Platform.

The proposed architecture builds upon design paradigms validated through prior pilots (LongITools [14, 15]) and large-scale digital phenotyping studies (Youth-GEMs [16], HappyMums [17, 18]), managing comparable operational demands: participant populations above 1,000, longitudinal observation periods exceeding one year, and continuous high-frequency data acquisition. These precedent implementations demonstrated adequate system scalability, operational stability, and regulatory compliance throughout their deployment cycles, with no reported security compromises or significant service disruptions.

2.3 Assessment

A first demo version of the system (hereafter named Pilot #1) was tested earlier in the development by a group of voluntary users from STAGE project partners and researchers not directly related to the development of the system.

11participants provided feedback. A quantitative and standardized usability assessment was conducted using the Single Ease Question (SEQ) [19], applied to four key tasks regarding the completion of activities available in the Homepage and in the Diary. The SEQ is a 7-point rating scale to assess how difficult it is for users to find a task.

Following the development phase, the final App version was evaluated in a four-week pilot study with 17 participants (hereafter named Pilot #2). The participant cohort included volunteers from the University of Oulu STAGE researchers, cohort age group representatives involved in the App design and researchers and citizens not involved in the development of the App in Finland. Basic usage metrics and post-pilot feedback were collected and analyzed through both qualitative methods (open-ended questions) and quantitative assessment using the System Usability Scale (SUS).

The SUS is a 10-item attitude Likert scale questionnaire that allows to collect a global view of subjective assessments of usability [20]. Eleven participants responded to the SUS and open-ended questions relating to preferences and experiences of using the App. In addition, two remote feedback sessions were organized to provide the pilot users with a possibility to express and discuss the App feedback in more detail. The pilot users attended remote feedback sessions.

3   Results

The results, as shown in Table 1 and Fig. 5, present both the mean and the standard deviations of the SEQ scores for each task from Pilot #1, as well as a graphic plot of the SUS scores from Pilot #2.

Results from Pilot #1 were encouraging, with high average SEQ scores for most tasks. All average values were above 5.9 in a scale ranging from 1 (very difficult) to 7 (very easy) with lowest and highest Confidence Interval (C.I.) of 5.0 and 7.0 respectively. In addition to these results, open-ended questions provided useful feedback. Some users left general comments such as "It is a friendly application", while others offered constructive suggestions, including "It would be better to name the surveys with more layman terms" and "I felt that more feedback after a task was needed."

The App was further refined based on the initial feedback and re-evaluated in Pilot #2, which assessed the overall end-user experience. The participant group was nearly evenly distributed across operating systems, with 52.9% using Android and 47.1% using iOS.

Table 1. single ease question (SEQ) scores by task. Mean scores and 95% confidence intervals for each evaluated task. Scores range from 1 (very difficult) to 7 (very easy).

Task	Average	95% C.I
T1	6.89	[6.63,7.00]
T2	5.67	[4.8, 6.53]
T3	6.89	[6.63, 7.00]
T4	6.00	[5.23, 6.77]

Task completion rates showed that 12 users successfully completed the interactive tasks, while questionnaire completion was lower: 8 users completed all questionnaires, and 4 additional users completed at least 50%.

Notably, no participants reported critical issues or experiences that prevented continued use of the App.

Quantitative usability evaluation yielded a mean SUS score of 87.95 (SD = 8.18). This corresponds to a grade 'Excellent' and places the system in the highest percentile of evaluated digital products [21].

The score substantially exceeds both the neutral threshold (68) and the 'good' usability cutoff (71.4), demonstrating high user satisfaction with the interface design and functionality. This result indicates that the system can be adopted for broader deployment, expecting minimal usability barriers for the target user population.

Results from the open-ended questions and feedback sessions indicated that users appreciated the App's visual clarity, ease of use, pleasant color palette, and customizable functionalities (e.g., notification settings). Users perceived the App as highly intuitive and straightforward, while still incorporating gamified tests designed without flashy or visually overwhelming elements.

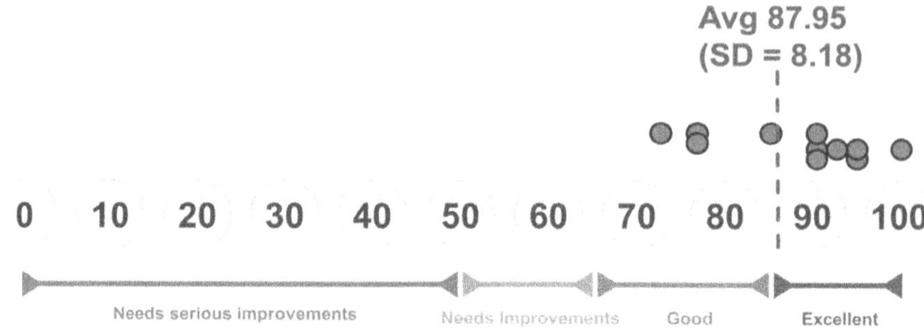

Fig. 5. System Usability Scale (SUS) Score Distribution. Individual participants with SUS scores plotted against the standardized SUS interpretation scale. The mean score was 87.95 (SD = 8.18), falling within the "Excellent" range (80–100).

The user interface allows the user to move easily between the tasks and sections. These elements were perceived to distinguish the App from other similar health monitoring apps.

The feedback also highlighted the contrasting aspect of the simplistic overview of the App, inducing discussion and reflection on how to ensure user engagement and interest throughout the two-year period.

Moreover, the pilot users recognized several minor linguistic errors (a mix of Finnish and English) and detailed issues to improve questionnaire or test functionalities and instructions. Some participants also raised concerns over the usage of the diary section, which does not include scheduled tasks for the monitoring period.

One of the main changes made according to the Pilot #2 feedback considered moving some of the activities (weight and waist circumference measurement, mood assessment and daily routines) from the diary section as scheduled tasks to be repeated every 6-month interval. This change contributes to a more systematic data collection of those specific parameters.

4   Discussion

The design and development of the platform required to face several methodological, technical, and human-centred challenges that represent well known key barriers to digital longitudinal health research.

From a technical perspective, appropriate robustness and interoperability across diverse smartphone devices and operating systems required thorough architectural choices and extensive testing. At the same time, balancing the demand for effective data collection with constraints related to battery consumption and data storage proved to be an additional challenge. Addressing these technical demands was essential to meet the requirements of a large-scale cohort study, where system instability or data loss would directly undermine the scientific integrity of the longitudinal dataset.

Significant effort was also devoted to addressing usability and accessibility issues, to cope with expected various digital health literacy among participants, directly influencing engagement, adherence, and long-term retention. This was particularly critical given the older adult target population, whose diverse digital health literacy represents a well-documented barrier to engagement and long-term retention in longitudinal digital health research. Therefore, the co-creation and PPI approach strongly improved the requirements-gathering process.

Furthermore, full GDPR compliance in terms of data privacy and security was another key element to improve acceptance by end users. In this context, GDPR-compliant data governance was not only a legal requirement but a fundamental design principle to ensure participant trust across a sensitive, large-scale health data collection effort.

Comparable digital health initiatives have demonstrated the feasibility of deploying smartphone-based platforms for longitudinal health data collection within large existing epidemiological cohorts [22, 23], supporting the viability of the approach adopted in the STAGE project. Relative to these initiatives, the proposed digital health system advances the state of the art through its foreground-first data collection philosophy, full FHIR-based interoperability, and the depth of its co-creation process, which engaged diverse stakeholder groups from the earliest design stages. Furthermore, the achieved SUS score of 87.95 compares favourably with the mean SUS benchmark of 76.64 reported across digital health applications [24], suggesting that the design choices adopted were effective in meeting the specific needs of the target population.

Despite these efforts, some limitations remain. First, the system's dependence on participant-owned smartphones introduces variability in hardware capabilities, operating system versions, and usage patterns, which may affect data consistency and completeness.

Second, although the system was designed to be inclusive, individuals with lower digital literacy or limited access to digital resources may still be underrepresented. Third, the long-term participant engagement cannot be yet fully assessed, and adherence may decline over time despite careful design choices.

Additionally, perceptions of data privacy and surveillance may continue to influence participant trust and willingness to engage with continuous digital monitoring without adequate educational efforts.

Future work will focus on addressing these limitations and further strengthening the system. Further integration of real-time monitoring and feedback mechanisms may support participant engagement and early detection of data quality issues.

Continued co-design with participants and stakeholders will remain central to future iterations of the system, ensuring that technological advancements stay aligned with ethical principles, user needs, and adapt to the evolving requirements of longitudinal health research.

Acknowledgments. This study was funded by the European Union's Horizon Europe Research and Innovation Programme (grant number 101137146). T.J., S.S., M.B. conceptualized the study and developed the research methodology. L.G., M.L.G. and E.J. led the co-creation activities and patient and public involvement process. M.A., L.G., and M.B. designed and developed the App and system architecture. M.A. managed the cloud infrastructure and backend implementation. M.A., G.B.L.E. developed the FHIR data export module and interoperability components. M.A., I.N., and E.J. coordinated and conducted the pilot studies. M.A. performed the data analysis and usability assessment. M.A., M.L.G, L.G., and M.B. drafted the manuscript. All authors contributed to manuscript revision, read, and approved the submitted version.

Disclosure of Interests. The authors have no competing interests to declare that are relevant to the content of this article. All authors contributed to the research in their professional capacities without any conflicts of interest, financial or otherwise, that could inappropriately influence or bias the content of this work.

References

1. Digital 2026 Global Overview Report. https://wearesocial.com/uk/blog/2025/10/digital-2026-global-overview-report/
2. Oliveri, S., et al.: Opportunities and challenges of web-based and remotely administered surveys for patient preference studies in a vulnerable population. Patient Prefer. Adherence **15**, 2509–2517 (2021). https://doi.org/10.2147/PPA.S327006
3. Taanila, H., et al.: Associations between cohort study participation and self-reported health and well-being: the Northern Finland Birth Cohort 1966 Study. J. Epidemiol. Community Health **76**, 1019–1026 (2022). https://doi.org/10.1136/jech-2022-219229
4. Goodday, S.M., Karlin, E., Brooks, A., Chapman, C., Harry, C., Lugo, N., Peabody, S., Rangwala, S., Swanson, E., Tempero, J., Yang, R., Karlin, D.R., Rabinowicz, R., Malkin, D., Travis, S., Walsh, A., Hirten, R.P., Sands, B.E., Bettegowda, C., Holdhoff, M., Wollett, J., Szajna, K., Dirmeyer, K., Dodd, A., Hutchinson, S., Ramotar, S., Grant, R.C., Boch, A., Wildman, M., Friend, S.H.: Value of engagement in digital health technology research: evidence across 6 unique cohort studies. J. Med. Internet Res. **26**, e57827 (2024). https://doi.org/10.2196/57827
5. Jarva, E., Yrttiaho, T., Isomursu, M.: Requirements elicitation for a health monitoring mobile application: a participatory design approach with clinicians and researchers. Finnish Journal of EHealth and EWelfare. **17**, 44–56 (2025). https://doi.org/10.23996/fjhw.154924
6. Google Flutter. https://flutter.dev/
7. Digital Ocean. https://www.digitalocean.com/
8. Van Rossum, G., Drake, F.L.: Python 3 Reference Manual. CreateSpace, Scotts Valley (2009)
9. Ronacher, A.: Flask. https://flask.palletsprojects.com/en/stable/
10. Better Stack. https://betterstack.com/
11. Logical Observation Identifiers Names and Codes (LOINC). https://loinc.org/
12. SNOMED CT terminology. https://www.snomed.org/
13. OnFHIR, HL7 FHIR Based Secure Health Data Repository. https://onfhir.io/
14. LongITools.: https://cordis.europa.eu/project/id/874739/results
15. Ronkainen, J., Nedelec, R., Atehortua, A., Balkhiyarova, Z., Cascarano, A., Ngoc Dang, V., Elhakeem, A., van Enckevort, E., Goncalves Soares, A., Haakma, S., Halonen, M., Heil, K.F., Heiskala, A., Hyde, E., Jacquemin, B., Keikkala, E., Kerckhoffs, J., Klåvus, A., Kopinska, J.A., Lepeule, J., Marazzi, F., Motoc, I., Näätänen, M., Ribbenstedt, A., Rundblad, A., Savolainen, O., Simonetti, V., de Toro Eadie, N., Tzala, E., Ulrich, A., Wright, T., Zarei, I., d'Amico, E., Belotti, F., Brunius, C., Castleton, C., Charles, M.A., Gaillard, R., Hanhineva, K., Hoek, G., Holven, K.B., Jaddoe, V.W.V., Kaakinen, M.A., Kajantie, E., Kavousi, M., Lakka, T., Matthews, J., Piano Mortari, A., Vääräsmäki, M., Voortman, T., Webster, C., Zins, M., Atella, V., Bulgheroni, M., Chadeau-Hyam, M., Conti, G., Evans, J., Felix, J.F., Heude, B., Järvelin, M.R., Kolehmainen, M., Landberg, R., Lekadir, K., Parusso, S., Prokopenko, I., de Rooij, S.R., Roseboom, T., Swertz, M., Timpson, N., Ulven, S.M., Vermeulen, R., Juola, T., Sebert, S.: LongITools: Dynamic longitudinal exposome trajectories in cardiovascular and metabolic noncommunicable diseases. Environ. Epidemiol. **6**, e184 (2022). https://doi.org/10.1097/EE9.0000000000000184
16. Youth-GEMs.: https://cordis.europa.eu/project/id/101057182/results

17. HappyMums.: https://cordis.europa.eu/project/id/101057390/results
18. Biaggi, A., Zonca, V., Anacker, C., Begni, V., Benedetti, F., Bramante, A., Braniecka, A., Brenna, V., Bulgheroni, M., Buss, C., Cavaliere, L., Cecil, C.A.M., Couch, A.C., de Barra, D., El Marroun, H., Entringer, S., Grassi-Oliveira, R., Jackowska, M., Korosi, A., Kwant, P.J.C., Lahti, J., Lekadir, K., Mansuy, I., Manuella, F., Marizzoni, M., Meyer, U., Monk, C., Nakić Radoš, S., Pariante, C.M., Pollux, B.J.A., Priestley, K., Räikkönen, K., Richetto, J., Riva, M.A., Rothmann, L.M., Simonetti, V., Vai, B., Vernon, A.C., Žutić, M., Cattaneo, A.: Understanding, predicting, and treating depression in pregnancy to improve mothers' and offspring's mental health outcomes: The HappyMums study. Brain Behav. Immun. Health **44**, 100961 (2025). https://doi.org/10.1016/j.bbih.2025.100961Capcan. P.: Single ease question. https://uxhints.com/user-testing/ux-metric-single-ease-question-seq/
19. Brooke, J.: SUS: a quick and dirty usability scale. In: Jordan, P.W., Thomas, B., McClelland, I.L., Weerdmeester, B. (eds.) Usability Evaluation in Industry. CRC Press, London (1996). https://doi.org/10.1201/9781498710411
20. Capcan, P.: Single ease question. https://uxhints.com/user-testing/ux-metric-single-ease-question-seq/
21. Bangor, A., Kortum, P., Miller, J.: Determining what individual SUS scores mean: Adding an adjective rating scale. J. Usability Studies. **4**, 114–123 (2009)
22. Yi, L., et al.: Measuring environmental and behavioral drivers of chronic diseases using smartphone-based digital phenotyping: intensive longitudinal observational mHealth substudy embedded in 2 prospective cohorts of adults. JMIR Public Health Surveill. **10**, e55170 (2024). https://doi.org/10.2196/55170
23. Giusti, M., Samuelsson, K.: Evaluation of a smartphone-based methodology that integrates long-term tracking of mobility, place experiences, heart rate variability, and subjective well-being. Heliyon. **9**, e15751 (2023). https://doi.org/10.1016/j.heliyon.2023.e15751
24. Hyzy, M., et al.: System usability scale benchmarking for digital health apps: meta-analysis. JMIR mHealth uHealth. **10**, e37290 (2022). https://doi.org/10.2196/37290

Assessing Community Health Workers' Experiences with Digital Rehabilitation: Usability, Barriers, and Implementation Needs in Primary Care Settings

Michael Oduor[1]([✉]) [iD], Gerard Urimubenshi[2] [iD], Juliette Gasana[2] [iD], Eeva Aartolahti[1] [iD], Nassib Tawa[3] [iD], David Tumusiime[2] [iD], and Katarina Korniloff[1] [iD]

[1] Institute of Rehabilitation, Jamk University of Applied Sciences, Jyväskylä, Finland
`michael.oduor@jamk.fi`
[2] College of Medicine and Health Sciences, University of Rwanda, Kigali, Rwanda
[3] College of Health Sciences, Jomo Kenyatta University of Agriculture and Technology, Juja, Kenya

Abstract. There is limited access to rehabilitation in many low-and middle-income countries where shortages of trained professionals, geographic barriers amongst other socio-economic factors hinder service delivery. Digital rehabilitation solutions may offer a scalable means of expanding access, yet little is known about their use by community health workers (CHWs) who play a central role in primary care delivery. This study examined CHWs' usability perceptions and experiences with a digital rehabilitation application piloted in Rwanda and Kenya. A qualitative study design was applied, combining semi-structured interviews with a quantitative usability evaluation. Thirty-five CHWs (Rwanda n = 21; Kenya n = 14) used the application for at least one month before participating in interviews (n = 21) and completing questionnaires on demographics, computer proficiency, attitudes toward digital technology (ITASH), and usability (System Usability Scale; SUS). Interviews were transcribed, coded, and analyzed, while descriptive statistics were used for quantitative measures. The CHWs reported positive experiences with the application, noting its ease of use, usefulness in supporting clients with common musculoskeletal conditions and strengthening their professional identity. The combined mean SUS score of 75.9 indicated good usability, with Kenyan CHWs reporting slightly higher scores. ITASH scores reflected generally positive attitudes toward digital technologies, though confidence and workload-related items scored lower. Key challenges included limited access to smartphones, connectivity, language constraints, and context-specific logistical barriers. The CHWs recommended additional exercise programs, enhancing local language support, and providing continuous training. Digital interventions can strengthen rehabilitation in resource-constrained settings, improving CHWs' skills, confidence, and ability to support clients. Addressing training needs and technology access barriers is essential for successful implementation and scale-up.

Keywords: Digital Rehabilitation · Usability · Attitudes Towards Technology · Community Health Workers · Primary Care

© The Author(s) 2026
M. Särestöniemi et al. (Eds.): NCDHWS 2026, CCIS 3009, pp. 234–249, 2026.
https://doi.org/10.1007/978-3-032-28812-7_18

1   Introduction

Globally, roughly one in three individuals will require rehabilitation during their lifetime because of illness or injury [1]. Demand for these services is greater than what is available, leaving large unmet needs, especially in low-and middle-income countries (LMICs) [2]. These regions also bear the greatest global burden of disease [3]. In Rwanda and Kenya, for example, the burden of disability is compounded by limited infrastructure, workforce shortages, and geographic barriers that hinder access to timely and quality rehabilitation care [4–7]. To improve rehabilitation services in resource-constrained settings, health systems need strengthening through technology, interprofessional teamwork, task shifting and task sharing [4, 8]. The latter point was also emphasized by Kenyan rehabilitation professionals [6].

As healthcare systems shift towards integrated, person-centred care, integrating high-quality rehabilitation into service delivery is crucial [9]. Digital technologies are key to health service delivery and in addressing access challenges [10–13]. Digital interventions have the potential to increase the accessibility, availability, and affordability of rehabilitation self-management support and services [14, 15]. For example, during the COVID-19 pandemic in South Africa, telerehabilitation initiatives examined whether remote physiotherapy could be feasibly delivered in resource-constrained public health settings to improve continuity of care and reduce patients' travel demands [16].

The delegation of tasks from specialized professionals to less specialized health workers through task shifting and task sharing is a strategic response to workforce shortages [8, 17, 18]. Community health workers (CHWs) promote health outcomes and are seen as a solution to addressing the shortage of health workers, the lack of a pervasive national health system, and a critical workforce to address health system strengthening [17, 19, 20]. Studies from Uganda and Kenya, for example, have shown that digital tools can support CHWs in delivering health services, provided that usability and contextual relevance are prioritized [21, 22].

Despite the potential benefits of digital services to augment conventional face-to-face rehabilitation programs, integrating digital rehabilitation into primary care remains underexplored. CHWs, who are often tasked with delivering essential health services at the primary care level, would benefit from initiatives that incorporate digital tools into rehabilitation, enhance their digital skills, improve client follow-up, support effective decision-making, and foster overall competence development [19–23]. However, their perceptions, experiences, and challenges with such technologies are not well documented. Furthermore, digital rehabilitation solutions must be culturally relevant, and accessible to users with varying levels of digital literacy. It is important to consider digital tools that are feasible, cost-effective, and tailored to the needs of end-users [15].

This study is part of a project that focused on improving access to rehabilitation services in primary care settings in LMICs [24] where challenges include provider shortages, limited knowledge, resource constraints and other social, environmental and technological challenges [4–7, 15, 22]. The lack of resources and shortage of trained personnel poses a threat to health and health equity worldwide [25], prompting the need for innovative approaches in delivering rehabilitation services. The study acknowledges the emergence of new healthcare roles particularly that of CHWs, highlighting the need to further explore avenues for task shifting and task sharing in rehabilitation. This study therefore investigates how Rwandan and Kenyan CHWs perceive a digital rehabilitation application, examining its usability, the challenges, and its perceived benefits, alongside the accessibility and availability of rehabilitation services. By combining usability data with qualitative findings on improvements to rehabilitation access, the research seeks to guide the implementation of digital rehabilitation solutions that are contextually relevant and scalable.

2   Materials and Methods

2.1   Study Design

A qualitative study using semi-structured interviews complemented by a quantitative usability assessment was applied. CHWs were interviewed about their clients' experiences accessing and using rehabilitation services and their usability perceptions and experiences of a digital rehabilitation application, the Inclusion App (Fig. 1).

The application was piloted among CHWs in Rwanda and Kenya. The application includes basic exercise programs for the most common rehabilitation needs identified in the respective countries. These exercises are based on a "do no harm" principle and include conditions such as knee pain, low back pain and other musculoskeletal conditions. The exercise programs included in the application are evidence based and from Physitrack's [26] content library.

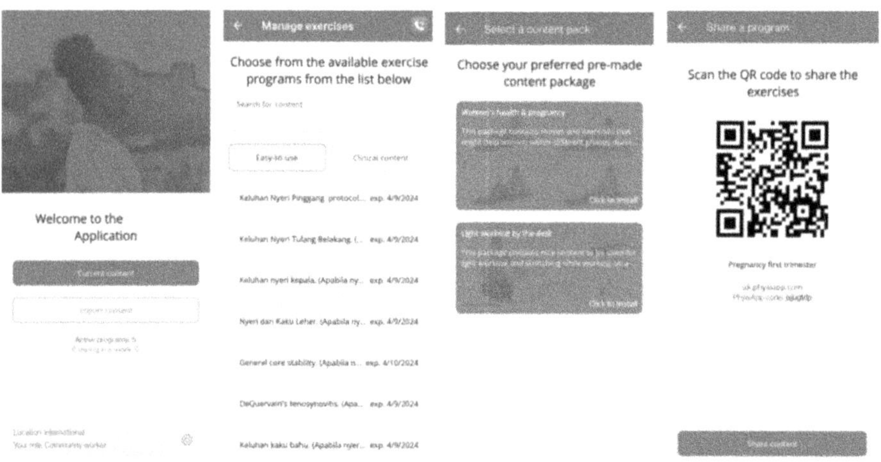

Fig. 1. Screenshot of the application

2.2   Study Setting and Participants

The study was primarily conducted in Rwanda and partly replicated in Kenya. The local research team consulted rehabilitation professionals who identified the most common conditions among rehabilitation service users, and ten different exercise programs for these conditions were pre-installed in the application. The CHWs were recruited across three districts in Rwanda, two in rural areas and one in an urban area, to ensure a comprehensive representation of the country's rehabilitation situation and the contextual challenges in access to rehabilitation services. In Kenya, CHWs were recruited across an urban and a rural county.

A real-world pilot started with deployment of the application in May 2023 in Rwanda and in December 2023 in Kenya. The CHWs received basic training on installing and using the application and sharing the pre-installed exercise programs with clients. They were also educated about the content of the exercise programs, how to guide clients in performing the exercises, and when to advise them to seek help from a rehabilitation or other health professional. In Rwanda, CHWs participated in an introductory workshop where they were introduced to the project and its objectives. They also received assistance in installing the application and were briefed on the exercise programs. Subsequently, monthly meetings were held for guidance and to share their experiences. In Kenya, two in-person training sessions were organized per location, with the remainder of the support provided remotely.

The study included CHWs ($n = 35$) who had used the digital rehabilitation application for at least 1 month prior to data collection. The CHWs were purposively recruited through contact from the local health administrations and their coordinators. They actively engaged in the delivery of basic preventive health services at the time and included individuals best positioned to provide insights into their clients. None of the respondents had previous knowledge of digital rehabilitation technologies and many had limited experience with digital services.

2.3 Data Collection

Data collection took place over a two-week period in November 2023 in Rwanda and April–May 2024 in Kenya. Data were collected through semi-structured interviews (n = 21) focusing on CHWs overall experiences of the digital rehabilitation application, the challenges they faced while using the application and those they identified in the community. A questionnaire (n = 35) was also included to collect demographic information on participants' age, gender, education, computer proficiency [27], professional background, usability of the application and their attitudes towards technology.

To assess the computer proficiency of the CHWs, we used the short form of the validated computer proficiency questionnaire (CPQ-12) [27]. The CPQ-12 asks respondents to rate their ability to perform a number of computer-related tasks (e.g., Using a computer/tablet to enter events into a calendar, finding information about community resources on the Internet) on a 5-point scale (1 = Never tried, 2 = Not at all, 3 = Not very easily, 4 = Somewhat easily, 5 = Very easily). The questionnaire consist of six subscales with two items each: (1) Computer basics, 2 Printer, (3) Communication, (4) Internet, (5) Calendar, and (6) Entertainment [27].

The CHWs attitudes towards information technology and the digital rehabilitation application were assessed using the short version of the Information Technology Attitude Scales for Health (ITASH) [28–31]. The ITASH is a validated instrument which was designed to measure healthcare workers' attitudes toward information technology. It consists of four scales comprising 19 items: (1) Care Value of digital technology (1–4), (2) Training of digital technology skills (5–10), (3) Digital technology confidence (11–14), and (15–19) Workload value of digital technology (five items) (see Table 3). The items are scored on a four-point Likert scale, where 1 = strongly disagree, and 4 = strongly agree with total scores ranging from 19 to 76 [28]. Participants responded to the question: *"What are your thoughts about using Information Communication Technology (ICT) solutions such as Inclusion App in rehabilitation?"*.

To assess perceived usability, participants completed the System Usability Scale (SUS). The SUS is a 10-item questionnaire that provides a global view of users' subjective ratings of a product's usability [32, 33]. It has been applied across a wide range of health-related domains [13, 14, 34]. Responses are scored on a five-point Likert scale, and the total SUS score ranges from 0 to 100, with higher scores reflecting greater perceived usability. Items included statements such as *"I think that I would like to use the Inclusion App frequently"* and *"I found the Inclusion App unnecessarily complex,"* rated on a 5-point Likert scale.

The interview guide and questionnaires were translated into Kinyarwanda by the local research team in Rwanda. In Kenya, the interviews were held in English and questions were clarified and/or translated to Kiswahili (Kenya's national language) during the interview process when needed.

2.4 Data Analysis

The interviews of Rwandan CHWs were audio-recorded, translated from Kinyarwanda to English and transcribed verbatim. All sensitive personal information was omitted, and each participant was assigned a code (starting from 200). Qualitative analysis was conducted by the second author. The first author interpreted the results and the other authors reviewed and approved them.

Qualitative data from open-ended responses were analyzed using directed qualitative content analysis. An initial coding framework was developed deductively based on the major themes of the interview guide. These predefined themes included perceived benefits of using the application, usability and confidence in use, benefits for clients and CHWs, challenges and barriers, and recommendations for improvement. All responses were reviewed and coded into these themes. Manual coding was conducted, and illustrative quotations for each theme were included. Regarding the trustworthiness of the qualitative data, credibility, dependability and confirmability were enhanced through a code-recode procedure.

Descriptive statistics were used to describe the participants' characteristics, their computer proficiency and attitudes towards technology. Negatively worded items (11, 14–19) in the ITASH scale were reversed scored to keep the values positively oriented so that higher scores reflect more positive attitudes toward ICT solutions (Table 3) [28, 30, 31]. The negatively worded items appear primarily in the Digital technology confidence and Workload value of digital technology subscales. Scores were summarized as mean ± SD and a total score was computed across all 19 items of the scale.

SUS evaluation was used to determine the overall usability score of the application. The descriptive statistics and SUS scores were analyzed using Microsoft Excel for

Microsoft 365 MSO (Version 2511). Mean scores were interpreted using Bangor et al.'s [34] usability benchmarks, where scores above 68 are considered above average.

2.5 Ethical Considerations

Research activities in Rwanda were in collaboration with the University of Rwanda and in Kenya with Jomo Kenyatta University of Agriculture and Technology (JKUAT). Ethical approval in Rwanda was obtained from the Rwanda National Ethics Committee (RNEC185/2023) and in Kenya from the JKUAT Institutional Scientific and Ethics Review Committee (JKU/ISERC/02316/0809) and a research license from the National Commission for Science, Technology and Innovation. In addition to seeking approval from the local district and county officials where we held the interviews. All participants were informed about the study's purpose, procedures, and their rights as research subjects. Written informed consent was obtained prior to participation, and confidentiality was maintained throughout.

3   Results

3.1   Respondent Characteristics

Majority of the participants were female (68.6%). Besides their roles as CHWs, some respondents engaged in entrepreneurial activities such as sales, adult teaching, farming, hairdressing, and tailoring. Kenyan CHWs reported using other digital tools in their work. These included the main application used by all CHWs in Kenya for household registrations, visit tracking, and assessments, as well as specialized apps for mental health, gender-based violence support, identifying issues among school-aged children, and recording elderly individuals' health information. Besides text messaging, Rwandan participants reported prior use of Babylon Health's digital platform (operating in Rwanda as Babyl at the time) before its discontinuation. An overview of respondent's characteristics is presented in Table 1.

Kenyan CHWs self-assessment of their computer proficiency was higher than that of Rwandans (Table 2). However, both groups highlighted the need for additional digital competence training and support.

3.2   Information Technology Attitude Scales for Health

The combined average sum of the ITASH scores was 66.3 ($\pm$3.5). The average sum for Rwandan CHWs was 67.4 ($\pm$2.6) and for Kenya CHWs it was 64.5 ($\pm$3.9). Rwandan CHWs had generally higher ITASH scores particularly in Care Value of ICT (items 1–4) and ICT confidence (items 11–14) subscales. Rwandan CHWs mostly agreed with the items 4, 10 and 15 (reverse scored) (Mean = 3.95 each) about ICT solutions helping to improve and personalize care, the need to learn and belief in the utility of ICT solutions. The items with the highest average ratings amongst Kenyan CHWs besides item 4 were 7 and 9 describing the necessity to improve professionals' digital skills and how using ICT solutions enhances professionals' knowledge (Mean = 3.86 each). They least agreed on items 11, 14 and 17 (Table 3).

Table 1. Demographic characteristics and self-reported technology experience and use

Variable	Rwanda	Kenya
Age	25–29, 1 (5.3%) 35–39, 3 (15.8%) 40–44, 5 (26.3%) 45–49, 7 (36.8%) 50–54, 2 (10.5%) $\geq$ 55, 1 (5,3%) (19 of 21 participants)	30–34, 3 (21.4%) 40–44, 2 (14.3%) 45–49, 2 (14.3%) 50–54, 5 (35.7%) $\geq$ 55, 2 (14.3%)
Gender	Male, 7 (33.3%) Female, 14 (66,7%)	Male, 4 (28.6%) Female, 10 (71.4%)
Education	At most secondary school, 16 (74.2%) At most technical diploma, (15.8%) (19 of 21 participants)	At most secondary school, 12 (85.7%) At most technical diploma, 2 (14.3%)
IT experience	Very Little, 3 (14.3%) Average, 14 (66.7%) Quite extensive, 4 (19%)	Average (7) (50%) Quite extensive (5) (35.7%) Very extensive (2) (14.3%)

Table 2. Mean subscales CPQ-12 scores for the CHWs

	Rwanda (N = 21) Mean(SD)	Kenya (N = 14) Mean(SD)
Computer basics	2.6 (1.2)	3.1 (1.7)
Printer	1.4 (0.9)	2.0 (1.4)
Communication	2.1 (1.3)	4.2 (1.2)
Internet	2.9 (1.3)	4.3 (1.2)
Calendar	2.1 (1.4)	4.1 (1.4)
Entertainment	3.6 (0.8)	4.4 (1.0)

3.3 System Usability Scale Scores

Overall, CHWs had a positive experience using the application. It was user-friendly and suitable for common conditions their clients experienced. Furthermore, the process of sharing exercise programs and learning about their clients' rehabilitation needs enhanced and enriched their interactions. The combined average SUS score was 75.9 ($\pm$9.1) indicating above average usability and the application's user-friendliness. The average usability rating for Kenyan CHWs (79.3, $\pm$7.4) was higher than that of their Rwandan counterparts (73.6, $\pm$9.6). The SUS scores correspond with a rating of "good" in the adjective rating scale [35].

Table 3. Responses to the information technology attitude scales for health (n = 35)

# ITASH	Rwanda (n = 21) Mean(SD)	Kenya (n = 14) Mean(SD)	Total (n = 35) Mean(SD)
1. Using ICT solutions is helping to improve client rehabilitation	3.9 (0.3)	3.6 (0.9)	3.8 (0.6)
2. The sort of information I can get from the ICT solutions helps me give better rehabilitation to clients	3.8 (0.4)	3.8 (0.4)	3.8 (0.4)
3. Using ICT solutions makes my communication with other health and rehabilitation professionals faster	3.9 (0.5)	3.6 (0.5)	3.8 (0.4)
4. I believe ICT solutions can help us deliver individualized rehabilitation	4.0 (0.2)	3.9 (0.4)	3.9 (0.3)
5. I feel I need more training to use ICT solutions properly	3.9 (0.4)	3.8 (0.4)	3.8 (0.4)
6. I would like to have ongoing training to help me improve skills of using ICT solutions	3.8 (0.4)	3.8 (0.4)	3.8 (0.4)
7. ICT skills are becoming more and more necessary for healthcare and rehabilitation professionals	3.9 (0.3)	3.9 (0.4)	3.9 (0.3)
8. To be successful in my career, I need to be able to work with ICT solutions	3.9 (0.3)	3.9 (0.4)	3.9 (0.3)
9. Using ICT solutions helps to increase professionals' knowledge base	3.9 (0.3)	3.9 (0.4)	3.9 (0.3)
10. I would like to know more about ICT solutions generally	4.0 (0.2)	3.9 (0.4)	3.9 (0.3)
11. I lack confidence in my general ICT skills	2.9 (0.7)	2.3 (0.8)	2.6 (0.8)
12. I generally feel confident working with ICT solutions	3.4 (0.6)	3.5 (0.5)	3.5 (0.6)
13. I am easily able to learn new ICT skills	3.8 (0.4)	3.6 (0.5)	3.7 (0.4)
14. I am often unsure what to do when using the ICT solutions	2.9 (0.5)	2.3 (1.1)	2.7 (0.8)
15. Using ICT solutions is more trouble than it's worth	4.0 (0.2)	3.4 (0.5)	3.7 (0.5)
16. Where I work, ICT solutions make staff less productive	3.5 (0.7)	3.4 (0.5)	3.5 (0.6)
17. I feel there are too many ICT solutions around now	1.5 (0.8)	2.1 (0.9)	1.7 (0.9)
18. I think we are in danger of letting ICT solutions take over	3.2 (0.8)	2.7 (1.1)	3.0 (0.9)
19. Time spent on ICT solutions is out of proportion to its benefits	3.5 (0.8)	3.3 (0.5)	3.4 (0.7)

3.4 Qualitative Themes

Interviews with CHWs about their experiences with the Inclusion App generated five overarching themes: (1) perceived benefits of the application, (2) usability and confidence in use, (3) benefits for service users and CHWs, (4) challenges and barriers, and (5) recommendations for improvement. These themes, illustrated with representative quotations for only the Rwandan participants, are presented below.

Perceived benefits of using the application

The CHWs consistently described the application as a valuable and innovative tool that strengthened their ability to support clients in the community. Many emphasized that the application bridged gaps in rehabilitation service provision, which is often limited in local health facilities.

Several participants highlighted its professionalization impact, stating that it enhanced their credibility and standing within their communities:

"When the client sees me using the phone they think that I am well trained. However, when I was writing in the notebook, they saw me as a CHW who might not know what I am doing. This application showed them that we are motivated and we know what we are doing." (CHW204)

"It gives the public confidence in the community health worker. It made people feel at ease with me." (CHW212)

"People are happy to see us and trust us enough when they see that we know to handle what we are doing." (CHW203)

Usability and confidence in use

Most CHWs reported that the application was user-friendly, particularly after initial training. They described being able to navigate the interface, select programs, and demonstrate exercises:

"Before using the application, I had no experience with using technology. Whatever I have learned was taught to us when they gave us the application. Now I can open my phone, look for the application and open it, select a specific program for a person and give it to them." (CHW202)

"When I reach to a new client, I first discuss the issue, then after I search easily the application in my smartphone. I opened it and I choose the exercises that meet the client condition." (CHW207)

Confidence was also reinforced by the community's perception of CHWs as skilled professionals:

"I feel very confident because even the clients, who visit me and see me talking on the phone, see that I am trained and know what to do." (CHW206)

"The trust from the beneficiaries increased more than before because they get well by using the application." (CHW218)

Benefits for service users and CHWs

The application was viewed as delivering important benefits by improving access, reducing costs, and enhancing health outcomes. CHWs emphasized how using the application eliminated the need for frequent hospital visits:

"Digital services are free of charge; there is no need to travel to the hospital which can be costly. It is not time consuming; time is not wasted in line waiting to be treated. You get your treatment at home." (CHW202)

"The persons are helped at their homes without going to hospital." (CHW218)

Participants also reported improved health outcomes, such as reduced pain and medication use:

"The client's experience told me it reduced the lower back pain and diminished the use of painkillers ... most people I helped reduced the number of hospital attendances." (CHW201)

Beyond patient outcomes, CHWs described benefits for themselves, including increased knowledge and empowerment:

"Before using the app, I did not know how to help people who needed rehabilitation; I would just send them to the health center. But today, I can give to them exercises ... I have gained knowledge." (CHW202)

"After using this App, I learned new things at 80% and also I treated myself and my husband." (CHW207)

"I have gained knowledge about technology. I can use apps, I have learnt how to do video calls and help someone who is far from me." (CHW221)

CHWs also perceived broader social impacts, including strengthening family relationships and the potential to reduce overcrowding in hospitals:

"Families applauded us because we helped the family to unite ... we did it by helping them to recover from the back pain."

"Patients will get the service easily because there is no queue but also the healthcare professionals' work will reduce, though in case this App cannot help the client should be referred to the hospital." (CHW204)

Challenges and barriers

Despite its promise, CHWs identified several barriers to optimal use of the application. A key limitation was clients' lack of smartphones and reliable Internet access:
"I open the app, select the appropriate exercise program and show to the person from my smartphone because most people don't have smartphones." (CHW202)
"The disadvantage is that the users don't have enough internet and even buying it is difficult." (CHW208)

Other technical barriers included limited local-language support and small demonstration videos:

"Some videos do not have the Kinyarwanda audio yet, the video images are very small to look at for some people." (CHW202)

Logistical and contextual challenges, such as travel distances and visiting clients in the evening, were also noted:

"People here in the community are free at evening time or early morning, so when I go to reach them at evening time, I can need the torch, boots and also the raincoat that can help us to do our job." (CHW204)

Recommendations for improvement

CHWs proposed several improvements to enhance the application's effectiveness. They specifically requested additional refresher training on the exercise programs in the application to enhance their confidence and overall digital skills. They also wanted further information on sharing the programs and identifying community members in need of rehabilitation:

"I would need constant training to keep reminding and updating us on how to use technology." (CHW203)

Second, participants emphasized the importance of expanding the application's content to include additional conditions:

"Integrating this App into the system, for various health conditions such as persons with prosthesis and orthosis." (CHW201)

"It would be better if we had more exercise programs, for example exercises for people with facial paralysis are not there." (CHW203).

"Please you should add the conditions related to the head." (CHW208)

Third, they suggested alternative formats such as printed materials or larger screens to improve accessibility:

"The service users wanted to print those exercises in application." (CHW204)

"I request to have exercises that are in one video or putting these exercises on flash." (CHW205/207)

Finally, participants recommended adding local language audio and culturally appropriate visuals:

"Some videos do not have the Kinyarwanda audio yet, the video images are very small to look at for some people." (CHW202)

"There are people who don't understand the clothing of people who practice in the application; but we explain it to them so they can see it without any problems." (CHW211)

4 Discussion

This study explored how Rwandan and Kenyan CHWs perceived a digital rehabilitation application, looking at its usability, challenges, and benefits in their work. By combining usability data with qualitative insights from semi-structured interviews, the research aimed to guide the implementation of a digital rehabilitation approach that is contextually relevant and scalable. Our study broadens understanding of the experiences of CHWs and their attitudes towards an innovative digital rehabilitation application targeted at enhancing access to rehabilitation in low-resource settings. The participants stated that using the application helped them develop their skills and basic understanding of technology. The CHWs feedback showed their commitment to the process, interest in learning, and continued development of the application.

The strong ITASH and SUS scores suggest the CHWs have a positive attitude towards ICT in general, and that the application was well received and found to be usable. The ITASH scale ratings echo findings about aspects of efficiency and communication, such as faster communication and enhanced information availability that are generally rated highly. In contrast, items concerning digital technology confidence and workload/overload, tend to receive lower scores [30]. The CPQ-12 scores and the interviews' findings show the need for additional training. Even though CHWs felt more empowered and had better digital skills, knowledge about digital rehabilitation, and understood community rehabilitation needs, they still believed further training was necessary.

The findings also show that CHWs' social status within their communities improved. They reported feeling more valued by their clients, who in turn perceived them as well-trained. Especially as they had smartphones instead of notebooks as they did earlier. Research has highlighted positive associations between training and digital tool use and the belief in digital impact [19, 36]. The CHWs who are optimistic about digital solutions, find great value in their work and believe digital tools can help them have a greater impact [19, 22, 36]. Whereas the lack of basic digital knowledge and skills may contribute to poor attitudes and behavior [22]. Thus, validated instruments such as CPQ-12 and ITASH which enhance understanding of CHWs' computer proficiency and attitudes towards ICT in healthcare and rehabilitation contexts are important in designing and providing appropriate training which considers the use of the technology for the CHWs [28].

Findings of this study related to the usability of the application are consistent with previous research. Prior studies have highlighted that system familiarity (technical skills gained as a result of training), ease of use and perceived usefulness are important facilitators to the implementation of telerehabilitation and have a significant effect on intention to use, acceptance of technology and successful adoption of digital solutions by CHWs [13, 15, 34, 37]. Their recommendations included further personalization of the application, adding to its content library, improving local language support and additional options for sharing the exercise programs with their clients.

Despite the growing demand for rehabilitation services [1–3, 15], access through the traditional model is often expensive and out of reach for many people especially in LMICs [15]. This study demonstrates that integrating digital rehabilitation into primary care settings is beneficial in low resource settings. Key findings from this study of the challenges in access are consistent with existing research. Common issues identified by

Rwandan CHWs were the lack of mobile phones, reliable Internet access and logistical and contextual challenges such as travel. These resemble barriers reported in similar contexts, such as cost, literacy, language, connectivity, and availability or accessibility issues [6, 7, 13, 15, 20, 22]. Despite these challenges, the findings also indicated potential savings in both cost and time. Solutions to cost constraints of technological access will benefit from further exploration of, for example, reimbursement models [19].

CHWs believe that the application can help them have more impact in their communities regardless of the barriers. Digital rehabilitation can increase their capacity and shape the future of community health work [19]. Investing in task sharing, which involves CHWs in rehabilitation service delivery at the primary care level, enhances service availability and accessibility, particularly in rural areas that have a shortage of rehabilitation professionals [4]. Overall, the results also suggest that CHWs' training and knowledge can address issues of uncertainty with digital interventions, while wider deployment and adoption can resolve challenges with distance, travel time, and transportation expenses [15, 16, 19, 37].

Limitations

Bilingual members of the local research team translated the questionnaires into Kinyarwanda, prioritizing linguistic clarity and relevance for Rwandan CHWs. However, a comprehensive cultural adaptation, including back-translation, review, or pilot testing, was not undertaken. While local collaborators reviewed the translated items for face validity, a formal assessment of conceptual equivalence was not done, potentially leading to differences in interpretation. This could affect the reliability and validity of the responses, as certain attitudinal terms may carry different connotations in the Rwandan and Kenyan context.

As noted by Lee and Clarke [28] when referring to application of ITASH in their study on student nurses, adapting ITASH, originally designed to assess the attitudes of qualified nurses, to the attitudes of CHWs raises some important issues as they often lack formal health education. The results cannot be generalized to all CHWs in LMICs. It is recommended to test the ITASH in different contexts with different samples as some question wordings may affect the face and content validity [31]. As well as more research in LMICs on CHWs' attitudes towards digital technologies.

The SUS was administered to participants only once. Therefore, it is reasonable to assume that if the survey is readministered for the second version of the application – which addresses the identified usability issues and adds more interactive features – the SUS scores will improve.

5 Conclusion

The study highlights the potential of digitization and mobile devices as a path for strengthening community-based rehabilitation. As well as the potential facilitators and barriers to implementation of digital rehabilitation solutions in related settings in sub-Saharan African and other LMICs. Additional training and ensuring equitable access to technology and rehabilitation services are priorities as digital rehabilitation solutions evolve.

Digital rehabilitation has the potential to partly compensate for availability and accessibility issues and the lack of specialists with targeted deployment and scaling. Strengthening service delivery contributes to reducing inequality in access to rehabilitation in LMICs. Sustained support is necessary across all levels of the health system when implementing community-based digital interventions. Future research should further investigate how digital rehabilitation solutions can support scalable service delivery and strengthen support for CHWs to advance progress toward equitable health care.

Acknowledgments. We extend our gratitude to Mr. Jean Damascene Bigirimana for overseeing data collection in Rwanda. We also thank Flora Munezero for her support with data collection and for training all the community health workers. Finally, we acknowledge the Kenyan research team from JKUAT for their coordination of data collection in Kenya.

Funding. This study was part of the project Co-innovation for Digital Rehabilitation in the Global Marketplace, funded by Business Finland (grant 6169/31/2021).

References

1. Cieza, A., Causey, K., Kamenov, K., Hanson, S.W., Chatterji, S., Vos, T.: Global estimates of the need for rehabilitation based on the global burden of disease study 2019: a systematic analysis for the global burden of disease study 2019. Lancet. **396**(10267), 2006–2017 (2020). https://doi.org/10.1016/S0140-6736(20)32340-0
2. Chimatiro, G.L., Rhoda, A.J.: Scoping review of acute stroke care management and rehabilitation in low and middle-income countries. BMC Health Serv. Res. **19**(1), 789 (2019). https://doi.org/10.1186/s12913-019-4654-4
3. Kamenov, K., Mills, J.-A., Chatterji, S., Cieza, A.: Needs and unmet needs for rehabilitation services: a scoping review. Disabil. Rehabil. **41**(10), 1227–1237 (2019). https://doi.org/10.1080/09638288.2017.1422036
4. Dukuzimana, M.J., et al.: Rehabilitation needs at rural primary health care settings: perspectives of health center nurses in Burera district of Rwanda. BMC Prim Care. **26**(1), 224 (2025). https://doi.org/10.1186/s12875-025-02921-y
5. Kumurenzi, A., Richardson, J., Thabane, L., Kagwiza, J., Musabyemariya, I., Bosch, J.: Provision and use of physical rehabilitation services for adults with disabilities in Rwanda: a descriptive study. Afr. J. Disabil. **11** (2022). https://doi.org/10.4102/ajod.v11i0.1004
6. Oduor, M.: Rehabilitation Professionals' Attitudes Towards Technology Use and their Perspectives on Rehabilitation Services. Jamk Arena Public. Accessed 28 Feb 2024. https://urn.fi/urn:nbn:fi:jamk-issn-2984-0791-26
7. Jokinen, K., et al.: Professionals' perspectives on the challenges of implementing digital solutions in rehabilitation settings in Rwanda. Front. Digital Health. **7** (2025) https://www.frontiersin.org/journals/digital-health/articles/10.3389/fdgth.2025.1489288
8. Snyman, S., et al.: The ICanFunction mHealth solution (mICF): a project bringing equity to health and social care within a person-centered approach. J. Interprofessional Work. Res. Dev. **2**(1), 1–17 (2019)
9. Stucki, G.: Advancing the rehabilitation sciences. Front. Rehabilit. Sci. **1**, 617749 (2021). https://doi.org/10.3389/fresc.2020.617749
10. Bakibinga-Gaswaga, E., Bakibinga, S., Bakibinga, D.B.M., Bakibinga, P.: Digital technologies in the COVID-19 responses in sub-Saharan Africa: policies, problems and promises. Pan Afr. Med. J. **35**(Suppl 2), 38–38 (2020). https://doi.org/10.11604/pamj.supp.2020.35.2.23456

11. Balikuddembe, J.K., Reinhardt, J.D.: Can digitization of health care help low-resourced countries provide better community-based rehabilitation services? Phys. Ther. **100**(2), 217–224 (2020). https://doi.org/10.1093/ptj/pzz162

12. World Health Organization: WHO Guideline: Recommendations on Digital Interventions for Health System Strengthening. World Health Organization, Geneva (2019) Accessed 05 Jan 2024. https://iris.who.int/handle/10665/311941

13. Soehnchen, C., Weirauch, V., Schmook, R., Henningsen, M., Meister, S.: An acceptance analysis of a sexual health education digital tool in resource-poor regions of Kenya: an UTAUT based survey study. BMC Womens Health. **23**(1), 676 (2023). https://doi.org/10.1186/s12905-023-02839-6

14. Richardson, J., et al.: Using a web-based app to deliver rehabilitation strategies to persons with chronic conditions: development and usability study. JMIR Rehabil Assist. Technol. **8**(1), e19519 (2021). https://doi.org/10.2196/19519

15. Nizeyimana, E., Joseph, C., Louw, Q.: A scoping review of feasibility, cost-effectiveness, access to quality rehabilitation services and impact of telerehabilitation: a review protocol. Digit. Health. **8** (2022). https://doi.org/10.1177/20552076211066708

16. Ebrahim, H., et al.: Experiences and effects of telerehabilitation services for physiotherapy outpatients in a resource-constrained public health set-up in the backdrop of the COVID-19 pandemic: a proposal. S. Afr. J. Physiother. **77**(1) (2021). https://doi.org/10.4102/sajp.v77i1.1528

17. Oliver, M., Geniets, A., Winters, N., Rega, I., Mbae, S.M.: What do community health workers have to say about their work, and how can this inform improved programme design? A case study with CHWs within Kenya. Glob. Health Action. **8**(1), 27168 (2015). https://doi.org/10.3402/gha.v8.27168

18. World Health Organization, PEPFAR, and UNAIDS, Task Shifting : Rational Redistribution of Tasks among Health Workforce Teams : Global Recommendations and Guidelines," 2007. https://iris.who.int/handle/10665/43821

19. Blondino, C.T., Knoepflmacher, A., Johnson, I., Fox, C., Friedman, L.: The use and potential impact of digital health tools at the community level: results from a multi-country survey of community health workers. BMC Public Health. **24**(1), 650 (2024). https://doi.org/10.1186/s12889-024-18062-3

20. Wilson, E., Lee, L., Klas, R., Nesbit, K.C.: Technology and rehabilitation training for community health workers: strengthening health systems in Malawi. Health Soc. Care Community. **28**(3), 833–841 (2020). https://doi.org/10.1111/hsc.12914

21. Baine, S.O., Kasangaki, A., Baine, E.M.M.: Task shifting in health service delivery from a decision and policy makers' perspective: a case of Uganda. Hum. Resour. Health. **16**(1), 20 (2018). https://doi.org/10.1186/s12960-018-0282-z

22. Bakibinga, P., Kamande, E., Kisia, L., Omuya, M., Matanda, D.J., Kyobutungi, C.: Challenges and prospects for implementation of community health volunteers' digital health solutions in Kenya: a qualitative study. BMC Health Serv. Res. **20**(1), 888 (2020). https://doi.org/10.1186/s12913-020-05711-7

23. Oduor, M., Aartolahti, E.: Community Health Workers and Service Users' Experiences of a Community-Based Digital Rehabilitation Application. Jamk-arena. Accessed 30 Sep 2024. https://urn.fi/urn:nbn:fi:jamk-issn-2984-0791-74

24. Murtonen, K.-P., Korniloff, K., Aartolahti, E., Oduor, M.: Co-innovation of digital rehabilitation in the global marketplace. Zenodo. (2025). https://doi.org/10.5281/ZENODO.15745645

25. Orkin, A.M., et al.: Conceptual framework for task shifting and task sharing: an international Delphi study. Hum. Resour. Health. **19**(1), 61 (2021). https://doi.org/10.1186/s12960-021-00605-z

26. Physitrack®—the world leader in remote patient engagement and Telehealth. Accessed 13 Dec 2024. https://www.physitrack.com/en-gb
27. Boot, W.R., et al.: Computer proficiency questionnaire: assessing low and high computer proficient seniors. The Gerontologist. **55**(3), 404–411 (2015). https://doi.org/10.1093/geront/gnt117
28. Lee, J.J., Clarke, C.L.: Nursing students' attitudes towards information and communication technology: an exploratory and confirmatory factor analytic approach. J. Adv. Nurs. **71**(5), 1181–1193 (2015). https://doi.org/10.1111/jan.12611
29. Ward, R., Pollard, K., Glogowska, M., Moule, P.: Developing information technology attitude scales for health (ITASH). Stud. Health Technol. Inform. **129**(Pt 1), 177–181 (2007)
30. Leonardsen, A.-C.L., et al.: Nursing students' attitudes towards the use of digital technology in the healthcare of older adults-a cross-sectional study in Norway and Sweden. BMC Nurs. **22**(1), 428 (2023). https://doi.org/10.1186/s12912-023-01600-6
31. Ota, Y., Nishimura, A., Adachi, Y., Kasahara, Y., Yokoyama, M.: Japanese translation of the shortened information technology attitude scale for health: evaluation of the reliability and validity of the translated version. JINR. **3**(2), e2023–0033-e2023-0033 (2024). https://doi.org/10.53044/jinr.2023-0033
32. Brooke, J.: SUS: a 'quick and dirty´ usability scale. Usability evaluation in industry, 189–194 (1996)
33. Brooke, J.: SUS: a retrospective. J. Usability Studies. **8**(2), 29–40 (2013)
34. de Oliveira, R.S.C., Sasso, G.T.M.D., Iyengar, M.S., Oinas-Kukkonen, H.: A persuasive mHealth application for postoperative cardiac procedures: prototype design and UsabilityStudy. In: Digital Health and Wireless Solutions—First Nordic Conference, NCDHWS 2024, Oulu, Finland, May 7–8, 2024, Proceedings, Part II, pp. 83–100 (2024). https://doi.org/10.1007/978-3-031-59091-7_6
35. Bangor, A., Kortum, P., Miller, J.: Determining what individual SUS scores mean: adding an adjective rating scale. J. Usability Stud. **4**, 114–123 (2009)
36. Lällä, K., Oduor, M., Aartolahti, E., Tumusiime, D., Korniloff, K.: The relationship between attitudes, emotions and the intention to use the digital rehabilitation solution: insights from Rwandan rehabilitation professionals. FinJeHeW. **17**(1) (2025). https://doi.org/10.23996/fjhw.153484
37. Epalte, K., Grjadovojs, A., Bērziņa, G.: Use of the digital assistant Vigo in the home environment for stroke recovery: focus group discussion with specialists working in Neurorehabilitation. JMIR Rehabil Assist. Technol. **10**, e44285 (2023). https://doi.org/10.2196/44285

Surveying Nurses' Experiences of the National Patient Portal

Tuulikki Vehko[1]([✉]) [iD], Kaija Saranto[2] [iD], Marko Elovainio[1,3] [iD],
Vesa Jormanainen[4] [iD], and Ulla-Mari Kinnunen[2,5] [iD]

[1] Welfare State Research Unit, Finnish Institute for Health and Welfare (THL), Helsinki,
Finland
`tuulikki.vehko@thl.fi`
[2] Department of Health and Social Management, University of Eastern Finland, Kuopio,
Finland
[3] University of Helsinki, Faculty of Medicine, Department of Psychology, Helsinki, Finland
[4] Ministry of Social Affairs and Health, Service System Unit, Helsinki, Finland
[5] Research Center for Nursing Science and Social and Health Management, Wellbeing Services
County of North Savo, Kuopio, Finland

Abstract. The patient portal 'Kanta Services' was implemented in the healthcare
to offer secure exchange of patient data among all healthcare service providers
in Finland. This study examines how nurses experience using it and whether
there are differences by nurse status and work context. A cross-sectional study
included registered nurses and licensed practical nurses. The inclusion criteria
were based on the respondents' answers regarding their professional role and use
of a primary data system, either an electronic health record or a clinical information
system. Responses were received from 2970 registered nurses and from 2341
licensed practical nurses. The associations of nurse status and work context with
positive experiences of Kanta Service use were analyzed using a binary logistic
regression model. Registered nurses' experiences of Kanta Services were more
positive than those of licensed practical nurses. Those who worked in public
healthcare experienced Kanta Services more positively than those who worked
in public social services. Respondents' good competence in using the primary
system was associated with agreement with all five positive statements related to
Kanta Services' use. Kanta Services play a key role in Finland's digital healthcare
infrastructure and are becoming increasingly important in social services, but the
experiences of nurses' use of these services need attention. Specifically, accessing
and retrieving information from Kanta Services through the primary data system
requires improvements to meet the expectations of both nursing groups and to
support their daily work more effectively.

Keywords: Health Information Management · National Patient Portals · Nurses

1 Introduction

Electronic health record systems (EHRs) are integral to modern nursing practice, facilitating the accurate documentation of patient care to enhance both quality and continuity of care [1–5]. Many countries have implemented national patient portals [6], including

M. Särestöniemi et al. (Eds.): NCDHWS 2026, CCIS 3009, pp. 250–270, 2026.
https://doi.org/10.1007/978-3-032-28812-7_19

all Nordic countries [7–11]. In the Nordic countries, the most common functions in these nationwide information systems are electronic prescription and patient data repository services [10–12].

The online access to personal health information for all inhabitants has been a game-changer in healthcare, addressing challenges associated with an aging population [6, 8, 9]. Earlier, it had met resistance from physicians, specifically concerning patient care with mental health problems [13]. However, information availability has been seen to increase patient safety and patient empowerment in many situations [1, 11, 14]. Safe care relies on effective information exchange [2, 15, 16], which is one of the aims of the national patient portals. Emerging evidence shows that patients' access to EHRs can promote patient-centred care [17]. This digital access has been shown to encourage new practices such as reviewing personal health data before medical appointments [13].

Research indicates that patient-accessible EHRs may affect the work of different health care professionals differently [18, 19]. In Uppsala, Sweden, 70% of oncology personnel reported that patient documentation became more restrictive following the implementation of patient accessible EHRs, particularly concerning mental health and addiction documentation. Still, in many aspects, their documentation practices remained unchanged [18].

Finland introduced its national information system for healthcare in 2010, when the Prescription Center was established as a crucial part of Kanta Services [20]. Prescribing medication electronically has been mandatory in Finland since 2017 [7, 12]. In general, Kanta Services provides online access to one's health data via the MyKanta webpages, allows the submission of a prescription renewal request, and enables the management of consents [10, 21]. For those who need services from different service providers [22], the Patient Data Repository of Kanta Services preserves health information. It provides visibility to all service providers in the public and private sectors. Currently, Kanta Services is being introduced to social services, and most of the public social service providers use Kanta Services for data storage [23].

Finnish studies focused on electronic prescription experiences among pharmacists [24], pharmacy customers [25], and the use of real-world data to investigate electronic prescriptions and drug safety [26]. In addition, Kanta Services, as a source of secondary data, has been explored [27]. From the inhabitants' perspective, non-use of Kanta Services has been investigated [21]. Moreover, the different implementation and adoption phases of Kanta Services have been examined [7, 23, 28]. Although studies have explored the Finnish national patient portal, the specific issue of nurses' experiences with Kanta Services remains under-researched.

Registered nurses' work includes coordination of multi-professional teams and planning patient care [29]. The primary focus of licensed practical nurses' work is to deliver basic care together with the patient or client, encouraging their own participation. Both professional groups document patient data into EHRs and social welfare client data into client information systems (CISs) [4, 5]. Finnish legislation makes an essential difference in patient and client data. As a result, nurses' documentation practices differ depending on whether they work in a healthcare or a social care organization.

In healthcare services, the use of EHRs is obligatory, as is the use of CISs in public social services; in private social services, small service providers may not yet use CISs

[20, 23]. The Kanta Services should support the work of all professionals (information sharing) and be easy to use, regardless of different primary data systems or different work responsibilities. In this study, we examine nurses' experiences with Kanta Services and identify where they differ.

2   Methods

2.1   Context

Since the beginning of 2023, twenty-one wellbeing services counties (WSCs) and the capital city of Helsinki have been responsible for organizing public healthcare, public social services, and rescue services in Finland. Organizing responsibility shifted from three hundred municipalities to the WSCs and the city of Helsinki, which are financed by the state budget, and to a smaller part by user fees [30].

In Finland, healthcare and social services are organized under a multi-provider model that involves both public and private service providers. Service providers have used several EHR brands, and only a few WSCs and the city of Helsinki use a single solution at the beginning of their operations. Kanta Services provides information infrastructure that enables the transmission of information between different organizational solutions in the public sector and between public-and private-sector healthcare service providers. Kanta Services is provided and maintained by the Social Insurance Institution of Finland (Kela).

Kanta Services provides several information services, and the length of time each service has been in use varies according to the implementation and adoption dates of the service provider organizations. For example, during data collection in 2023–2024, the Kanta Patient Data Repository has been in regular use since its public and private healthcare availability in late 2013. However, the accession period for Kanta Services' client data repository is ongoing, so public and private social service providers can modify their CISs, be certified, connect to Kanta Services, and start production in due time. A significant proportion (80%) of public social service providers use Kanta Services. The rest of the public and private social service providers are in a transition period in which organizations increasingly use CISs and must begin recording documents by law on September 1, 2026 [23]. Patient or client documentation is entered into the primary data system (EHR or CIS) by professionals, and certain standardized records, such as nursing and medical discharge summaries and laboratory results, are transmitted to Kanta Services [7, 28, 31].

2.2   Sample

The data was collected using an online survey in 2023 (registered nurses) and in 2024 (licensed practical nurses) based on previous studies on digitalization in Finnish healthcare and social services [4, 32–37].

In April 2023, two organizations (The Union of Health and Social Care Professionals 'Tehy' and Finnish Nurses Association 'Sairaanhoitajat ry') forwarded our online survey to their members who had a registered nurse qualification. In March 2024, three trade unions (Trade Union for the Public and Welfare Sectors 'JHL', The Finnish Union of Practical Nurses 'SuPer', and Tehy) sent our online survey to their members who had a licensed practical nurse or equivalent upper secondary education. The survey emails were distributed to members aged 18–65, and one reminder was sent in 2023 and two in 2024. Survey participation was voluntary. The surveys were available in Finnish, Swedish, and English. The inclusion criteria for participation were based on respondents' answers: working as a registered nurse or a licensed practical nurse and using electronic health records or client information systems. The Finnish education of these professionals is described in Appendix 1. The study was conducted in accordance with the ethical principles for research involving human participants as set out by the Finnish National Board on Research Integrity [38].

2.3 Variables

The dependent variables related to the experiences of the national patient portal presented in this study were measured for the first time in 2023 for registered nurses. The statements were operationalized to capture four key aspects: the system's findability, the accessibility of information, the system's ability to facilitate easy discovery, and the availability of a summary of key information. Additionally, one statement presents an overall assessment of the service use. Pilot versions of the surveys were tested by 22 registered nurses and 17 licensed practical nurses. The pilot responses were reviewed, and the researchers were assured that the new parts of the questionnaires were understandable. The five statements have a prologue 'How do you feel about the following statements about Kanta Services? Assess the statements from the perspective of your own work.' a) Kanta Services are easy to open through the electronic health records/client information system I use. b) The client/patient information I need is available through the Kanta Services. c) I can easily find the client/patient information I am looking for in the Kanta Services. d) In Kanta Services, summaries of key health information help to create an overall picture of the patient. e) The Kanta Services concept is easy to use. The response format was 1 = Fully agree, 2 = Somewhat agree, 3 = Neither agree nor disagree, 4 = Somewhat disagree, 5 = Fully disagree, 6 = Not applicable to my work. These responses were further classified into 1 = Fully agree or somewhat agree and 0 = Neither agree nor disagree or Somewhat disagree or Fully disagree. Those who answered that these were not applicable were dropped from the sample.

The independent variables contained contextual factors related to nurses' characteristics and the organizational context. The survey asked respondents for their year of birth, which was used to calculate their age. The nurse status is based on the survey round and recorded as 1 = licensed practical nurses and 2 = registered nurses. The competence of EHR/CIS use was asked 'How experienced do you consider yourself as a user of electronic health record/ client information system?' The respondents rated their competence on a scale of 1 to 5, with 1 indicating a beginner and 5 indicating highly experienced. In the binary logistic regression model, the variable was used as a continuous variable. Work environment was indicated by two questions: 'Which sector pays your salary?' with response options 'Public sector', 'Private sector', 'Third sector', and 'Do you work in: Social services, Healthcare, Neither of these, or I cannot say'. These were further classified as 'Public healthcare', 'Public social care', 'Private healthcare', and 'Private social care'. Those who answered 'Third sector', 'Neither of these', or 'I cannot say', were dropped from the sample.

The number of daily logins referred to the ease of login environment, and was asked, 'How many information systems do you log in to daily when working with clients/patients? (This refers to separate logins using a username or an ID card to systems, which are used to record client or patient data)' with response options 0, 1, 2, 3, 4, 5 or more, and 'I do not work with clients/patients'. These responses were further classified into two categories: 0, indicating two or more, and 1, indicating one. Those who answered that the number of logins was zero or that they do not work with clients/patients were dropped from the sample.

The length of use of the same brand of EHR/CIS was asked 'For how long have you used the X system? The electronic form displayed the brand name chosen in the previous answer. The response options were 1 = Less than six months, 2 = Six months – less than one year, 3 = One year – less than three years, 4 = Three years – six years, 5 = More than six years. These were further classified into 0 = Three years or less, 1 = More than three years. Descriptive statistics were used to summarize the experience of Kanta Services use and nurse status. The differences in experiences of Kanta Services use between registered nurses and licensed practical nurses were analyzed using a two-proportion z-test. The threshold for statistical significance was set at $p < 0.05$. Due to missing responses to some statements, the number of observations varied across these descriptive analyses.

2.4 Data Analysis

To further examine whether the association between nurse status and experiences with Kanta Services varies across different working environments, the analysis was restricted to respondents who answered all statements related to the national patient portal. The binary logistic regression was used to investigate the relationship between nurse status, work environment, number of daily logins, length of use of the same brand of EHR/CIS, competence in EHR/CIS use, and the binary outcome variable, experiences with the national patient portal. Multicollinearity was assessed using variance inflation factors (VIFs). In all models, the VIFs ranged from 1.00 to 1.11, which is below the commonly accepted threshold of 5, indicating that multicollinearity was not a concern. After the main effects were entered, an interaction term (nurse status × work environment) was added to evaluate whether the association between nurse status and the outcome was moderated by work environment. Odds ratios (OR) with 95% confidence intervals (CI) were reported to express the strength of associations. Model fit was evaluated using the Hosmer–Lemeshow test, and model performance was assessed with Nagelkerke's R^2. All analyses were conducted using SPSS 29.02 and Microsoft Excel.

2.5 Ethical Considerations

Respondents received information that the online survey was part of 'Monitoring and evaluation of digital healthcare and social welfare' that took place in Finnish institute for health and welfare (THL). This information emphasizes that participation in the study was completely voluntary. The respondents did not receive any compensation for participation in the study. Ethics approval for conducting the survey for registered nurses from the Institutional Review Board of the Finnish institute for health and welfare (THL) (THL/634/6.02.01/2023) and to survey for licensed practical nurses (THL/620/6.02.01/2024 §963). The study was conducted following the ethical principles of research with human participants by Finnish National Board on Research Integrity [38].

3   Results

A total of 2970 registered nurses responded to the survey, and the mean age was 47 years (SD 10.5). For the descriptive analysis, data were limited to those who were working in healthcare or social services (n = 2878), and further to those who stated that Kanta Services applied to their work (n = 2109–2275), which means that 71–76% of the responses were included in the analyses. A total of 2341 licensed practical nurses responded to the survey, with a mean age of 50 years (SD 10.9). For the descriptive analysis, data were restricted to those who were working in healthcare or social services (n = 2001) and, further, to responses in which Kanta Services applied to respondents' work (n = 960–1051), which means that 41–45% of the responses were included in the analyses. Licensed practical nurses perceived the answer option that Kanta Services does not apply to their work more often than registered nurses.

Figure 1 shows the proportions of respondents who agreed with the five statements related to the national patient portal Kanta Services. Less than half (42.5%) of the registered nurses agreed that Kanta Services is easy to open through their primary data system. Of the registered nurses, 40.2% agreed that the client/patient information they need is available through Kanta Services. Among registered nurses, one out of four (25.3%) agreed that information is found easily in Kanta Services. Some 23.4% agreed that the summaries in the Kanta Services help to create an overall picture of the patient. One out of four (25.3%) registered nurses assessed that Kanta Service concept is easy to use.

Among licensed practical nurses, one fourth (25.7%) agreed that Kanta Services is easy to open in their primary data system (Fig. 1), and one out of four (24.9%) agreed that the client/patient information they need is available through Kanta Services. About 20.9% of licensed practical nurses reported that information is easy to find in Kanta Services. Some 28.3% of licensed practical nurses agreed that the summaries in Kanta Services help to create an overall picture of the patient. Every fifth (20.9%) licensed practical nurse assessed that the Kanta Service concept is easy to use. (Fig. 1)

Table 1 presents a two-proportion z-test between registered nurses and licensed practical nurses, the two independent samples. The proportions present those who agree with the statements related to the national patient portal. Results showed that the proportion of statements that Kanta Services are easy to open in the registered nurses' group (0.43) was significantly higher than in the licensed practical nurses' group (0.26), with a difference of 0.17 (Z = 9.31, p = .000) at the .05 significance level. For the statement 'The client/patient information I need is available through the Kanta Service', the proportion in the registered nurses' group (0.40) was significantly higher than in the licensed practical

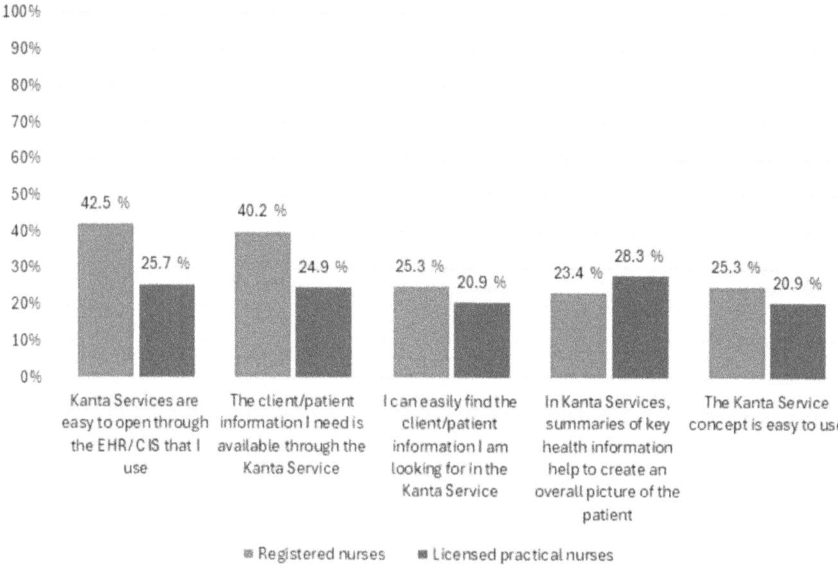

Fig. 1. Agreeing to the statements related to the national patient portal 'Kanta Services' by registered nurses and licensed practical nurses in Finland. Kanta Services are used through primary data systems, electronic health record (EHR), or client information system (CIS). Because the survey statements were not mandatory, the number of responses varied slightly among registered nurses (n = 2109–2275) and licensed practical nurses (n = 960–1051).

nurses' group (0.25) (Z = 8.40, p = .007). The proportions were lower for the following two statements, which present information on findability (registered nurses, 0.25; licensed practical nurses, 0.21) and summary views (registered nurses, 023; licensed practical nurses, 0.28), and a statistically significant difference between the nurses' groups was found. There was no statistically significant difference in the experiences of professional groups regarding the ease of use of the Kanta Service solution.

For binary logistic regression analysis, data were limited to only those who answered all five statements related to the use of the national patient portal Kanta Services. In these analyses, the data contained 875 licensed practical nurses and 2034 registered nurses, totaling 2909 responses. Table 2 presents contextual factors.

The results of the binary logistic regression analyses, considering the experience of Kanta Services use by nurse status and work environment, are presented in Table 3 in five parts (Table 3a, Table 3b, Table 3c, Table 3d, Table 3e) at the end of the article. Licensed practical nurses have lower odds of agreeing in three of the five statements compared to registered nurses (Table 3a, Table 3b, Table 3c and Table 3e). Nurses working in public or private social care settings have lower odds of agreeing that opening the Kanta Services is easy and that patient information is readily available. They also find it more difficult to access patient information in Kanta Services compared to those working in public healthcare. Nurses with good competence in EHR/CIS use have higher odds of agreeing with the statements related to the Kanta Services use than those with lower competence.

Neither the length of the same EHR/CIS use nor the respondent's age have statistically significant association with the experience of Kanta Services use. The nurses who logged to two or more EHR/CIS each day had lower odds for agreeing that summaries of key health information in Kanta Services help to create an overall picture of the patient, and lower overall assessment that the Kanta Services concept is easier to use than for nurses who logged to only one system each day. The interaction effect between nurse status and work environment was not significant.

Table 1. Comparison of the agreement proportions to perception of the national patient portal 'Kanta Services' between registered nurses and licensed practical nurses in Finland. Difference in agreement proportions between groups, z-value and its' p-value.

Statement related to the national patient portal	Registered nurses (n)	Registered nurses' agree proportion	Licensed practical nurses (n)	Licensed practical nurses' agree proportion	Difference (Δ)	Z-value	p-value
Kanta Services are easy to open through the electronic health record/ client information system that I use	2275	0.425	1051	0.257	0.168	9.31	**0.000**
The client/patient information I need is available through the Kanta Service	2226	0.402	1011	0.249	0.152	8.40	**0.007**
I can easily find the client/patient information I am looking for in the Kanta Service	2194	0.253	963	0.209	0.044	2.68	**0.004**

(continued)

Table 1. (*continued*)

Statement related to the national patient portal	Registered nurses (n)	Registered nurses' agree proportion	Licensed practical nurses (n)	Licensed practical nurses' agree proportion	Difference (Δ)	Z-value	p-value
In Kanta Services. summaries of key health information help to create an overall picture of the patient	2109	0.234	960	0.283	−0.049	−2.91	**0.006**
The Kanta Service concept is easy to use	2203	0.253	1022	0.209	0.044	2.74	1.000

4 Discussion

This cross-sectional study aimed to describe the national patient portal Kanta Services' use among registered nurses and licensed practical nurses. Furthermore, the study explains how the association between both nursing status and the experience of Kanta Services use differs across various working environments. The data collection was conducted simultaneously with a massive healthcare and social welfare reform launched in Finland in 2023. One goal of the reform is to ensure the seamless exchange of client and patient information across different service providers [16, 39]. To support the exchange of patent and client information, national solutions like the Kanta Services were already introduced before the reform [10, 20, 21, 28].

Our study results show that respondents who agreed to the use of Kanta Services were more common among registered nurses than among licensed practical nurses. Two out of five registered nurses find the opening of Kanta Services through their primary data system easy, whereas among licensed practical nurses, the proportion is lower. In clinical work, registered nurses often coordinate activities of multi-professional teams and plan patient care [29]. To effectively perform these duties, they need access to shared information on test results, treatments conducted in other organizations, or nursing discharge summaries [40]. To ensure seamless patient data exchange, it is crucial that registered nurses can utilize Kanta Services. Licensed practical nurses also have responsibilities that include documentation and the creation of patient care plans. However, their primary focus is more hands on. This means they are mainly involved in implementing the treatment plan and providing direct patient care [41].

Our results indicate that fewer than half of the registered nurses believe the information they require about patients or clients is readily available through Kanta Services. It is important to note that some of the standardized documentation within primary data systems – such as EHRs or CISs – is transmitted to Kanta Services as part of a standardized health information exchange process. If the data are not entered and recorded correctly, often requiring structured documentation [4, 29, 34], it will not be accepted, and thus, will not be visible through Kanta Services. Improving documentation is a crucial way to promote patient safety and quality of care. Implementing electronic nursing documentation has been shown to reduce documentation errors, falls, and infections,

Table 2. Proportions (%) and means of experiences with Kanta Services by contextual factors (n = 2909). (EHR = Electronic health record, CIS = client information system).

	Kanta Services are easy to open through the electronic health records / client information system I use.		The client/patient information I need is available through the Kanta Services.		I can easily find the client/ patient information I am looking for in the Kanta Services.		In Kanta Services, summaries of key health information help to create an overall picture of the patient.		The Kanta Services concept is easy to use.	
Nurse status	**No** (n = 1798)	**Yes** (n = 1111)	**No** (n = 1845)	**Yes** (n = 1064)	**No** (n = 2205)	**Yes** (n = 704)	**No** (n = 2180)	**Yes** (n = 729)	**No** (n = 2193)	**Yes** (n = 716)
Registered nurse	56.8	43.2	74.2	25.8	78.2	21.8	76.5	23.5	76.5	23.5
Licensed practical nurse	73.5	26.5	58.8	41.2	74.8	25.2	71.3	28.7	72.8	27.2
Working environment										
Public healthcare	58.6	41.4	60.5	39.5	74.0	26.0	74.4	25.6	75.3	24.7
Public social care	75.8	24.2	77.7	22.3	81.6	18.4	79.0	21.0	76.6	23.4
Private healthcare	53.8	46.2	55.4	44.6	76.9	23.1	73.3	26.7	72.9	27.1
Private social care	85.5	14.5	82.9	17.1	84.2	15.8	75.7	24.3	77.6	22.4
Number of daily logins to EHR/CIS										
One	60.3	39.7	62.5	37.5	75.1	24.9	73.6	26.4	73.9	26.1
Two or more	64.5	35.5	65.1	34.9	77.0	23.0	77.4	22.6	78.1	21.9
Length of the same EHR/CIS use										
Three years or less	64.5	35.5	65.4	34.6	76.8	23.2	74.9	25.1	75.6	24.4
Moore than three years	60.1	39.9	62.1	37.9	75.1	24.9	74.9	25.1	75.2	24.8

(continued)

Table 2. (*continued*)

Kanta Services are easy to open through the electronic health records / client information system I use.			The client/patient information I need is available through the Kanta Services.		I can easily find the client/ patient information I am looking for in the Kanta Services.		In Kanta Services, summaries of key health information help to create an overall picture of the patient.		The Kanta Services concept is easy to use.	
Nurse status	**No** (n = 1798)	**Yes** (n = 1111)	**No** (n = 1845)	**Yes** (n = 1064)	**No** (n = 2205)	**Yes** (n = 704)	**No** (n = 2180)	**Yes** (n = 729)	**No** (n = 2193)	**Yes** (n = 716)
Age, mean (std. deviation)	48.7 (10.76)	48.2 (10.57)	48.9 (10.70)	47.9 (10.64)	48.5 (10.62)	48.7 (10.92)	48.5 (10.62)	48.7 (10.92)	48.5 (10.62)	48.7 (10.92)
Competence as EHR/CIS use*, mean (std. deviation)	3.8 (0.89)	4.1 (0.82)	3.9 (0.86)	4.1 (0.84)	3.9 (0.89)	4.1 (0.84)	3.9 (0.88)	4.0 (0.86)	3.9 (0.88)	4.1 (0.85)

a 1 (beginner) - 5 (highly experienced)

which directly impacts patient safety [1, 3, 15]. In Sweden, patients' open access to read their health data influenced professional documentation practices in oncology, where therapeutic relationships can be long term [19]. Ensuring accurate and complete documentation is essential for maintaining patient safety in healthcare [1, 3, 15], and equally important for ensuring client safety in social services. Structured documentation and standardization will also play an important role when the European Health Data Space is introduced [11]. Kanta Services data standards are already applied to cross-border patient data exchange in Finland.

According to our results, the working environment plays a role in the experiences of Kanta Services users. Agreement was more common among nurses working in public healthcare services than among those in social services, which may reflect the ongoing implementation phase of Kanta Services among private social service providers [8, 23]. Besides, during the preparation and implementation phases of Kanta Services for social services, clients' information is stored in social care organizations' data systems unless the organizations have started using the Client Data Repository of Kanta Services. During the surveys' data collection, social welfare data were accessible only to the service provider organizations' professionals, and there was yet no exchange of social welfare data between organizations. Users also had only limited access to their social welfare data, depending on the organization. Thus, social care professionals could access only a restricted amount of information through Kanta Services. In contrast, a substantial portion of a patient's health data is already available in Kanta Services, making it worthwhile to search there for relevant information.

Respondents who have two or more daily logins to EHR or CIS agreed less often with statements that assumed summaries of key health information help create an overall picture of the patient, or that the Kanta Services concept is easy to use. Simplifying the login environment for EHR or CIS end-users would be a practical development sugges-tion for organizations to enhance nurses' work, especially when nurses are providing care to patients who need services from multiple providers [22].

The respondents' chosen answer option was also likely influenced by learning and familiarization factors that were not directly asked in this study. Regarding the statement "In Kanta Services, summaries of key health information help to create an overall picture of the patient," the primary data system often dictates the types of summary views available to the end-user. Regarding the statement "I can easily find the client/patient information I am looking for in the Kanta Service," the assessment is partly related to familiarization; if professionals often use the Kanta Services, they find information more easily. The length and complexity of a patient's medical history also affect how easily the information can be accessed. Overall, it is evident that both the interfaces of primary data systems and Kanta Services require further development.

4.1 Limitations

Our study has limitations that should be acknowledged. Our sample was based on whether the professionals have a membership in trade unions or nursing associations, and although many nurses belong to these, the sample is not fully representative.

Piloting both professionals' surveys is essential to ensure the suitability of the new statements related to Kanta Services. Both surveys were introduced at a time when the private social services were not entirely using the Kanta Services. Therefore, the answer option 'Not applicable to my work' was important. Moreover, in some working environments, the need to use the Kanta Services is relatively rare, for example, when nurses know their customers for an extended period, which may sometimes be the case in service housing.

In the regression models, the independent variables were selected based on contextual importance. The model included typical individual level covariates such as age and competence of EHR/CIS use, and organizational level covariates like number of daily logins, and length of use of the same brand of EHR/CIS to reduce potential bias and account for background differences between participants. As in any observational study, we, however, cannot rule out residual or missing confounding.

5 Conclusion

The results showed that among registered nurses, endorsing the statements related to the Kanta Service use was more common than among licensed practical nurses. Registered nurses regularly coordinate activities of multi-professional teams and plan patient care, while licensed practical nurses' work is more hands-on, hence the results may be related to the familiarity effect among registered nurses who use the Kanta Services more often in their work.

Among both nurse groups nurses, endorsing the Kanta Service was more prevalent in public healthcare services than in social services, which may reflect the unfinished implementation phase of Kanta Services among private social services. Users reported that the client or patient information they needed was not fully available in Kanta Services. This may be due to several factors, such as incomplete documentation during the care process, resulting in missing data in the primary data system, or difficulties locating information within Kanta Services. When introducing infrastructure for cross-border healthcare within the European Health Data Space, proper documentation practices will be paramount to creating summaries that provide the necessary information for safe patient and client care.

Our findings suggest that among nurses, nationwide use of Kanta Services has not yet reached its full potential. In the future, it will be necessary to monitor nurses' as well as other professionals' perceptions of Kanta Services as part of a multi-provider model of Finnish healthcare and social care.

Acknowledgments. The authors acknowledged Finnish trade unions TEHY, JHL, SuPer, and Finnish Nurses Association, which sent the email of the online survey, and all respondents for their contributions. We would like to acknowledge researcher Maiju Kyytsönen (THL) the contributions to developing the statements on Kanta Services during the design phase of the information systems survey for registered nurses. We are grateful to the information officer Pia Pörtfors (THL) for conducting literature searches of national patient portals used in Nordic-Baltic countries.

Disclosure of Interests. The authors declare no conflicts of interest.

Appendix 1

Background information of nurses' education and working opportunities in Finland.

Registered nurses and licensed practical nurses can work in both public and private healthcare and social services in Finland. Registered nurses have 210 competence points in their University of Applied Sciences education and holding a broad scope of responsibilities in clinical work [29, 40]. Public health nurses, midwives, and paramedics are also qualified registered nurses. Licensed practical nurses' upper secondary education at vocational institutions includes theoretical and vocational education up to 180 competence points, and in work-life, licensed practical nurses' responsibilities are tailored to employment's needs [41].

Table 3a. The results of binary logistic regression analyses for positive experience of Kanta Services use among nurses (n = 2909) in Finland. Initially, a basic model including contextual variables was conducted 'Model 1', and subsequently added an interaction term (nurse status × working environment) in 'Model 2'. (EHR = electronic health record, CIS = client information system).

Predictor	**a)** Kanta Services are easy to open through the electronic health records / client information system I use. OR (95% CI) **Model 1**	p value	OR (95% CI) **Model** 2	p value
Nurse status				
Registered nurse	ref.		ref.	
Licensed practical nurse	**0.58 (0.48–0.69)**	**0.00**	**0.49 (0.33–0.72)**	**0.00**
Working environment				
Public healthcare	ref.		ref.	
Public social care	**0.58 (0.48–0.76)**	**0.00**	0.69 (0.44–1.08)	0.11
Private healthcare	1.24 (0.95–1.62)	0.12	1.82 (0.79–4.14)	0.15
Private social care	**0.31 (0.20–0.50)**	**0.00**	0.51 (0.17–1.47)	0.21
Number of daily logins to EHR/CIS				
One	ref.		ref.	
Two or more	0.86 (0.74–1.02)	0.08	0.86 (0.73–1.01)	0.07
Length of the same EHR/CIS use				
Moore than three years	ref.		ref.	
Three years or less	1.07 (0.91–1.26)	0.43	1.07 (0.91–1.26)	0.43
Competence as EHR/CIS use	**1.36 (1.24–1.50)**	**0.00**	**1.37 (1.25–1.5)**	**0.00**
Age	1.00 (0.99–1.01)	0.59	1.00 (0.99–1.01)	0.574
Interaction (nurse status × working environ ment)	–	–	0.90 (0.72–1.12)	0.33

Table 3b. The results of binary logistic regression analyses for positive experience of Kanta Services use among nurses (n = 2909) in Finland. Initially, a basic model including contextual variables was conducted 'Model 1', and subsequently added an interaction term (nurse status × working environment) in 'Model 2'. (EHR = electronic health record, CIS = client information system).

Predictor	b) The client/patient information I need is available through the Kanta Services. OR (95% CI) **Model 1**	p value	OR (95% CI) **Model 2**	p value
Nurse status				
Registered nurse	ref.		ref.	
Licensed practical nurse	**0.61 (0.51–0.74)**	**0.00**	0.71 (0.49–1.04)	0.079
Working environment				
Public healthcare	ref.		ref.	
Public social care	**0.56 (0.43–0.73)**	**0.00**	**0.48 (0.31–0.74)**	**0.00**
Private healthcare	1.24 (0.95–1.63)	0.12	0.87 (0.39–0.74)	0.74
Private social care	**0.41 (0.26–0.64)**	**0.00**	**0.26 (0.09–0.76)**	**0.01**
Number of daily logins to EHR/CIS				
One	ref.		ref.	
Two or more	0.92 (0.78–1.08)	0.34	0.93 (0.79–1.09)	0.36
Length of the same EHR/CIS use				
Moore than three years	ref.		ref.	
Three years or less	1.02 (0.87–1.20)	0.82	1.02 (0.86–1.20)	0.82
Competence as EHR/CIS use	**1.41 (1.28–1.55)**	**0.00**	**1.40 (1.28–1.54)**	**0.00**
Age	0.99 (0.99–1.01)	0.46	1.00 (0.99–1.00)	0.45
Interaction (nurse status × working environ ment)	–	–	1.11 (0.89–1.38)	0.37

Table 3c. The results of binary logistic regression analyses for positive experience of Kanta Services use among nurses (n = 2909) in Finland. Initially, a basic model including contextual variables was conducted 'Model 1', and subsequently added an interaction term (nurse status × working environment) in 'Model 2'. (EHR = electronic health record, CIS = client information system).

Predictor	c) I can easily find the client/patient information I am looking for in the Kanta Services. OR (95% CI) **Model 1**	p value	OR (95% CI) **Model 2**	p value
Nurse status				
Registered nurse	ref.		ref.	
Licensed practical nurse	0.95 (0.77–1.17)	0.63	0.74 (0.49–1.12)	0.16
Working environment				
Public healthcare	ref.		ref.	
Public social care	**0.66 (0.49–0.89)**	**0.01**	0.87 (0.53–1.40)	0.56
Private healthcare	0.84 (0.61–1.14)	0.26	1.50 (0.61–3.67)	0.371
Private social care	**0.56 (0.35–0.88)**	**0.01**	1.12 (0.38–3.32)	0.84
Number of daily logins to EHR/CIS				
One	ref.		ref.	
Two or more	0.92 (0.77–1.10)	0.35	0.91 (0.76–1.09)	0.32
Length of the same EHR/CIS use				
Moore than three years	ref.		ref.	
Three years or less	0.97 (0.81–1.16)	0.73	0.97 (0.81–1.16)	0.74
Competence as EHR/CIS use	**1.32 (1.19–1.46)**	**0.00**	1.32 (1.19–1.46)	**0.00**
Age	1.00 (1.00–1.01)	0.27	1.00 (1.00–1.01)	0.26
Interaction (nurse status ×working environment)	–	–	0.84 (0.66–1.08)	0.17

Table 3d. The results of binary logistic regression analyses for positive experience of Kanta Services use among nurses (n = 2909) in Finland. Initially, a basic model including contextual variables was conducted, 'Model 1', and subsequently added an interaction term (nurse status × working environment) in 'Model 2'. (EHR = electronic health record, CIS = client information system).

Predictor	d) In Kanta Services, summaries of key health information help to create an overall picture of the patient. OR (95% CI) **Model 1**	p value	OR (95% CI) **Model 2**	p value
Nurse status				
Registered nurse	ref.		ref.	
Licensed practical nurse	**1.47 (1.21–1.79)**	**0.00**	1.16 (0.79–1.72)	0.45
Working environment				
Public healthcare	ref.		ref.	
Public social care	**0.64 (0.49–0.86)**	**0.00**	0.82 (0.53–1.29)	0.39
Private healthcare	1.01 (0.75–1.37)	0.93	1.73 (0.76–3.90)	0.19
Private social care	0.79 (0.53–1.17)	0.24	1.48 (0.56–3.94)	0.43
Number of daily logins to EHR/CIS				
One	ref.		ref.	
Two or more	**0.80 (0.67–0.96)**	**0.02**	**0.80 (0.67–0.96)**	**0.01**
Length of the same EHR/CIS use				
Moore than three years	ref.		ref.	
Three years or less	0.90 (0.75–1.08)	0.26	0.90 (0.75–1.08)	0.26
Competence as EHR/CIS use	**1.18 (1.07–1.31)**	**0.00**	**1.18 (1.07–1.31)**	**0.00**
Age	1.01 (1.00–1.01)	0.16	1.001 (1.00–1.01)	0.15
Interaction (nurse status × working environ ment)	–	–	0.85 (0.68–1.07)	0.17

Table 3e   The results of binary logistic regression analyses for positive experience of Kanta Services use among nurses (n = 2909) in Finland. Initially, a basic model including contextual variables was conducted, 'Model 1', and subsequently added an interaction term (nurse status × working environment) in 'Model 2'. (EHR = electronic health record, CIS = client information system).

Predictor	e) The Kanta Services concept is easy to use. OR (95% CI) **Model 1**	p value	OR (95% CI) **Model 2**	p value
Nurse status				
Registered nurse	ref.		ref.	
Licensed practical nurse	**1.32 (1.08–1.61)**	**0.00**	1.03 (0.69–1.53)	0.89
Working environment				
Public healthcare	ref.		ref.	
Public social care	0.84 (0.64–1.10)	0.21	1.08 (0.69–1.69)	0.73
Private healthcare	1.09 (0.81–1.47)	0.57	1.91 (0.83–4.36)	0.13
Private social care	0.80 (0.53–1.20)	0.27	1.55 (0.57–4.19)	0.39
Number of daily logins to EHR/CIS				
One	ref.		ref.	
Two or more	**0.79 (0.66–0.94)**	**0.01**	**0.78 (0.65–0.94)**	**0.01**
Length of the same EHR/CIS use				
Moore than three years	ref.		ref.	
Three years or less	0.91 (0.76–1.09)	0.31	0.91 (0.76–1.09)	0.31
Competence as EHR/CIS use	**1.26 (1.13–1.39)**	**0.00**	**1.26 (1.14–1.40)**	**0.00**
Age	1.00 (0.99–1.01)	0.61	1.00 (0.99–1.01)	0.58
Interaction (nurse status × working environment)	–	–	0.85 (0.68–1.07)	0.16

References

1. McCarthy, B., Fitzgerald, S., O'Shea, M., Condon, C., Hartnett-Collins, G., Clancy, M., et al.: Electronic nursing documentation interventions to promote or improve patient safety and quality care: a systematic review. J. Nurs. Manag. 27(3), 491–501 (2019)
2. Chan, K.S., et al.: Effects of continuity of care on health outcomes among patients with diabetes mellitus and/or hypertension: a systematic review. BMC Fam. Pract. 22(1), 145 (2021)

3. Kinnunen, U.M., Kivekäs, E., Palojoki, S., Saranto, K.: Register-based research of adverse events revealing incomplete records threatening patient safety. Stud. Health Technol. Inform. **270**, 771–775 (2020)
4. Kinnunen, U.-M., et al.: Nurses' informatics competency assessment of health information system usage: a cross-sectional survey. CIN: Comput. Inform. Nurs., **41**(11), 869–876. (2023)
5. Saranto, K., Ikonen, J., Koponen, S., Kyytsönen, M., Kinnunen, U.-M., Vehko, T.: Practical nurses' experiences of client and patient information systems support for performance - cross-sectional study. Finnish Journal of EHealth and EWelfare. **15**(2), 174–198 (2023)
6. Antonio, M., Petrovskaya, O., Lau, F.: The state of evidence in patient portals: umbrella review. J. Med. Internet Res. **22**(11), e23851 (2020)
7. Jormanainen, V.: Large-scale implementation and adoption of the Finnish national Kanta services in 2010–2017: a prospective, longitudinal, indicator-based study. Finnish Journal of EHealth and EWelfare. **10**(4), 381–395 (2018)
8. Jormanainen, V., Parhiala, K., Niemi, A., Erhola, M., Keskimäki, I., Kaila, M.: Half of the Finnish population accessed their own data: comprehensive access to personal health information online is a corner-stone of digital revolution in Finnish health and social care. Finnish Journal of EHealth and EWelfare. **11**(4), 298–310 (2019)
9. Huvila, I., Cajander, Å., Moll, J., Enwald, H., Eriksson-Backa, K., Rexhepi, H.: Technological and informational frames: explaining age-related variation in the use of patient accessible electronic health records as technology and information. Inf. Technol. People. **35**(8), 1–22 (2022)
10. Kujala, S., et al.: A.: benchmarking usability of patient portals in Estonia, Finland, Norway, and Sweden. International journal of. Med. Inf. **181**, 105302 (2024)
11. Hägglund, M., et al.: A Nordic perspective on patient online record access and the European health data space. J. Med. Internet Res. **26**, e49084 (2024)
12. Bruthans, J., et al.: Comparison of electronic prescription systems in the European Union: benchmarking development, use, and future trends. IEEE J. Biomed. Health Inform. **29**(5), 3712–3722 (2025)
13. Kariotis, T.C., Prictor, M., Chang, S., Gray, K.: Impact of electronic health records on Information practices in mental health contexts: scoping review. J. Med. Internet Res. **24**(5), e30405 (2022)
14. Wass, S., Vimarlund, V.: Same, same but different: perceptions of patients' online access to electronic health records among healthcare professionals. Health Informatics J. **25**(4), 1538–1548 (2018)
15. Jylhä, V., Mikkonen, S., Saranto, K., Bates, D.: W.: the impact of information culture on patient safety outcomes: development of a structural equation model. Methods Inf. Med. **56**(S 01), e30–e38 (2017)
16. Koivisto, J., Tiirinki, H., Liukko, E.: Identifying individuals for integrated multidisciplinary care: lessons from Finland. Int. J. Integr. Care. **22**(3), 8 (2022)
17. Benjamins, J., Haveman-Nies, A., Gunnink, M., Goudkuil, A., de Vet, E.: How the use of a patient-accessible health record contributes to patient-centered care: scoping review. J. Med. Internet Res. **23**(1), e17655 (2021)
18. Moll, J., Cajander, Å.: Oncology health-care professionals' perceived effects of patient accessible electronic health records 6 years after launch: a survey study at a major university hospital in Sweden. Health Informatics J. **26**(2), 1392–1403 (2019)
19. Cajander, Å., Huvila, I., Salminen-Karlsson, M., Barimani, M., Bratt, S., Koch, S.: Effects of patient accessible electronic health records on nurses' work environment: a survey study on expectations in Sweden. BMJ Open. **12**, e059188 (2022)
20. Jormanainen, V., Hämäläinen, P., Reponen, J.: The Finnish healthcare and social care system and ICT-policies. In: Vehko, T. (ed.) E-Health and e-Welfare of Finland. Check Point 2022.

Pp. 22–60. Finnish Institute for Health and Welfare (THL). Report 6/2022. Helsinki, Finland. (2022)

21. Kainiemi, E., et al.: The factors associated with nonuse of and dissatisfaction with the national patient portal in Finland in the era of COVID-19: population-based cross-sectional survey. JMIR Med. Inform. **10**(4), e37500 (2022)

22. Hietapakka, L., Sinervo, T., Väisänen, V., Niemi, R., Gutvilig, M., Linnaranta, O., et al.: Patient-sharing networks among Finnish primary healthcare professionals taking care of patients with mental health or substance use problems: a register study. BMJ Open. **15**(1), e089111 (2025)

23. Hujanen, K., Ailio, E., Laukkanen, H.: Introduction of Kanta services in social welfare is the key for utilising information. Finnish Journal of EHealth and EWelfare. **16**(2), 175–180 (2024)

24. Lämsä, E., Timonen, J., Mäntyselkä, P., Ahonen, R.: Pharmacy customers' experiences with the national online service for viewing electronic prescriptions in Finland. Int. J. Med. Inform. **97**, 221–228 (2017)

25. Sääskilahti, M., Ojanen, A., Ahonen, R., Timonen, J.: Benefits, problems, and potential improvements in a nationwide patient portal: cross-sectional survey of pharmacy customers' experiences. J. Med. Internet Res. **23**(11), e31483 (2021)

26. Männikkö, V., Förger, K., Kujanen, H., Tikkanen, J., Antikainen, S., Munukka, J.: Overview of Finnish national patient data repository for research on medical risk assessment. Finnish Journal of EHealth and EWelfare. **16**(3), 254–268 (2024)

27. Frondelius, A., Kinnunen, U.M., Jormanainen, V.: The significance of information quality for the secondary use of the information in the national health care quality registers in Finland. Methods Inf. Med. **63**(3–04), 66–76 (2024)

28. Jormanainen, V., Reponen, J.: CAF and CAMM analyses on the first 10 years of national Kanta services in Finland. Finnish Journal of EHealth and EWelfare. **12**(4), 302–315 (2020)

29. Mykkänen, M., Kinnunen, U-M., Liljamo, P., Ahonen, O., Kuusisto, A., Saranto, K.: Using standardized nursing data for knowledge generation – Ward level analysis of point of care nursing documentation. Int. J. Med. Inform. **167**, 104879 (2022)

30. Karanikolos, M., Tynkkynen, LK., Keskimäki, I. Finland: Health system summary, 2024. In: Observatory on Health Systems and Policies, WHO Regional Office for Europe, pp. 25 Copenhagen, European. ISBN 9789289014410 (PDF) (2024)

31. Nissinen, S.P., Soini, S., Leino, T., Hakulinen, H., Saranto, K.: Kanta-arkiston käyttökokemuksia työterveyshuollossa. Finnish Journal of EHealth and EWelfare. **10**(1), 102–112 (2018)

32. Viitanen, J., Hyppönen, H., Lääveri, T., Vänskä, J., Reponen, J., Winblad, I.: National questionnaire study on clinical ICT systems proofs: physicians suffer from poor usability. Int. J. Med. Inform. **80**(10), 708–725 (2011)

33. Kainiemi, E., Kaihlanen, A.-M., Virtanen, L., Vehko, T., Heponiemi, T.: Registered nurses' digital client work and associating factors: a cross-sectional study. J. Adv. Nurs. (2024)

34. Kinnunen, U.M., Heponiemi, T., Rajalahti, E., Ahonen, O., Korhonen, T., Hyppönen, H.: Factors related to health informatics competencies for nurses—results of a National Electronic Health Record Survey. CIN. Comput. Inform. Nurs. **37**(8), 420–429 (2019)

35. Kinnunen, U.M., Ikonen, J., Koponen, S., Kyytsönen, M., Saranto, K., Vehko, T.: Licensed Practical nurses' perceptions of the benefits of information Systems in Social and Healthcare Services. Stud. Health Technol. Inform. **24**(315), 347–351 (2024)

36. Vehko, T., Kyytsönen, M., Kaihlanen, A.-M., Saranto, K., Kinnunen, U.-M.: Registered nurses' experiences of information systems at the beginning of wellbeing services counties in Finland. Finnish Journal of EHealth and EWelfare. **16**(3), 269–295 (2024)

37. Vehko T. (ed).: E-health and e-welfare of Finland: Check Point 2022. Finnish institute for health and welfare (THL). Report 6/2022, p. 192 (2022)

38. Kohonen, I., Kuula-Luumi, A., Spoof, S.: The ethical principles of research with human participants and ethical review in the human sciences in Finland. (Finnish National Board on Research Integrity TENK guidelines) (2019).
39. Ministry of Social Affairs and Health. Strategy for digitalisation and information management in healthcare and social welfare. Publications of the Ministry of Social Affairs and Health 2024:1. Helsinki, Finland. (2024)
40. Kuusisto, A., Asikainen, P., Saranto, K.: Medication documentation in nursing discharge summaries at patient discharge from special care to primary care. J. Nurs. Care. (2014)
41. Roos, M., Kopra, J., Tevameri, T., Viinikainen, S., Kuosmanen, L.: Licensed practical nurses' (LPNs') evaluations of the attractiveness of work and wellbeing at work: a cross-sectional nationwide study. J. Nurs. Manag. (2024)

Nurses' Experiences Regarding the Impact of the Implementation of Digital Health and Social Center on their Work and Other Practices: A Qualitative Interview Study

Egne Annala[1], Taina Pellikka[1], Hilkka Korpi[1] (iD), Janna Nadav[2] (iD), Anu Kaihlanen[3] (iD), Paulus Torkki[4] (iD), and Elina Laukka[5]([✉]) (iD)

[1] School of Wellbeing and Culture, Oulu University of Applied Sciences, Oulu, Finland
[2] University of Tampere, Tampere, Finland
[3] Finnish Institute for Health and Welfare, Helsinki, Finland
[4] Department of Public Health, Faculty of Medicine, University of Helsinki, Helsinki, Finland
[5] Institute of Health, School of Health and Social Studies, Jamk University of Applied Sciences, Piippukatu 2, 40100 Jyväskylä, Finland
elina.laukka@jamk.fi

Abstract. The aim of the study was to describe how the implementation of a digital health and social care center affected registered nurses' work. The study was conducted as a qualitative descriptive study in primary care, and the data were collected through semi structured remote interviews with 12 nurses. The data were analyzed using inductive content analysis. A total of three impacts and main categories were recognized, namely 1) impacts on patient care work, 2) impacts on interprofessional communication and work processes, and 3) impacts on nurses' and other professionals' work, workload, and wellbeing. Regarding the impacts on patient care, the digital health and social center increased the availability of digital services but also generated failure demand originating from patients. Interprofessional communication and work processes improved due to enhanced information flow, yet this simultaneously led to a substantial increase in both the volume and speed of information. While some processes and operations became more efficient, interviewees also reported instances of incompleteness. Finally, the digital health and social center affected professionals' work and wellbeing by enabling remote work and reshaping work tasks, but it also contributed to an increased workload. In conclusion, the digital health and social care center was found to provide significant benefits for patient service accessibility and professional collaboration. However, its successful implementation requires clear operational practices, sufficient onboarding, standardized processes, and close collaboration between system developers and end users. Poor organizational preparedness and multichannel service use may increase nurses' workload and hinder work-flow efficiency.

Keywords: Digitalization · healthcare · nurse · telemedicine

M. Särestöniemi et al. (Eds.): NCDHWS 2026, CCIS 3009, pp. 271–285, 2026.
https://doi.org/10.1007/978-3-032-28812-7_20

1 Introduction

The importance of digitalization in healthcare and social welfare has increased rapidly in recent years due to several factors, including COVID-19, the rapidly aging population, and the rise in non-communicable diseases [1, 2]. This transformation has not only changed how patients access services but also how healthcare professionals perform their work [3, 4]. As digital solutions have become an integral part of healthcare and social welfare, it is essential to understand how these changes are experienced by those at the frontline, especially registered nurses, who play a central role in the delivery and coordination of digital health services.

Digital health services, such as telemedicine interventions, mobile health applications, and remote monitoring devices, have been proposed as solutions to enhance healthcare accessibility, availability, and cost-effectiveness [5, 6]. One significant approach to delivering digital health services is the establishment of digital health and social centers or digital clinics, which offer various digital health services under one roof [7–9]. Digital health and social centers typically offer various digital health services, which are primarily managed and utilized by registered nurses. These services have enabled new processes and ways of working, and nurses may nowadays either work solely as digital nurses, or they can combine work thus that they work both on digital platforms and traditional face-to-face services [3].

Earlier Kaihlanen et al., [3] noted that digitalization has changed professionals' workload and pace, the field and nature of work, work communication and interaction and information flow and security. As their interviews were conducted in 2020, during the rapid expansion of digital services caused by the COVID-19 pandemic. In contrast, our study examines this phenomenon at a later stage, when Finland has begun implementing comprehensive digital clinics rather than the isolated digital health services used during the COVID-19 pandemic to ensure the service provision. In Finland, digital clinics have expanded rapidly and now serve over 80% of the population [10].

Earlier studies have proposed that digital health services and their implementation may increase the stress experienced by healthcare professionals if they are not properly conducted [11, 12]. Additionally, concerns have been raised about the potential erosion of patient-provider boundaries and the perception that technology may diminish clinical skills and increase workload [13]. The experiences and satisfaction of healthcare professionals can significantly influence the success of digital services [14–16] and should therefore be considered in their implementation and development [2, 11]. Nurses need to develop new skills to coordinate care, solve digital literacy issues, and maintain an empathetic approach in increasingly digital healthcare [17]. However, as digital health and social centers are still relatively new in Finland and have transformed established practices, it is important to examine whether they generate similar impacts to digital services in general. Digital services are often more fragmented, whereas digital health and social centers aim to integrate all digital services within a single, unified system.

As the experience and satisfaction of healthcare professionals is important regarding the use of digital health services, we concentrated on registered nurses' experiences of digital health and social centers. This focus is particularly relevant because nurses represent the largest professional group in the healthcare sector and are often the primary users and implementers of digital health centers. They are responsible for most patient contacts and play a key role in coordinating services. If nurses perceive digital services as burdensome or impractical, this can critically affect the quality of care, the success of digital service adoption, and ultimately patient satisfaction [16]. Therefore, it is essential to gain up-to-date insights into nurses' experiences, especially now that digital health services have become established practices beyond the crisis-driven implementations of recent years. Thus, the aim of the study was to describe nurses' experiences on how the implementation of a digital health and social center has impacted on nurses' work and other practices.

2 Materials and Methods

This study was conducted as a qualitative descriptive study. The chosen method allows for an in-depth examination of the phenomenon in its authentic environment and highlights the voices of professionals in a new situation [18].

2.1 Context

The study was conducted in Finland within primary care services in a wellbeing services county that provides services to over 400,000 residents and employs a total of 18,000 personnel. In Finland, digital social and health centers were first implemented in 2021, with their adoption accelerating significantly following the health and social care reform in 2023 [19]. This reform transferred the responsibility for organizing health, social, and rescue services from municipalities to 21 wellbeing services counties, centralizing governance and financing at the national level to improve equality, access, and cost-effectiveness [20].

In 2025, 3.5 million residents in Finland had access to a digital health and social center. The wellbeing services county examined in this study has operated its own digital center since 2024. Digital services have been implemented across several health and social care centers, of which eleven were selected for this study because they have provided digital services for more than six months. Health and social centers are organized so that some registered nurses work exclusively as digital nurses, while others combine digital duties with traditional face-to-face appointments.

2.2 Interviewees

We solely focused on the experiences of nurses working at the reception and excluded doctors and other staff from the study. One or two nurses from each included health and social center were recruited for interviews. The interviewees were required to have worked at the reception before the digital health and social center was established to ensure they could compare practices before and after the implementation, as only participants with firsthand experience of the change can provide meaningful insights into its impact [21].

2.3 Data Collection

Data collection was conducted through semi-structured remote interviews using Microsoft Teams in spring 2025. The interviews were recorded and transcribed. Interviews were chosen as the data collection method to capture rich, individual insights into the interviewees' experiences regarding changes in their daily work, workload and pace, communication, the nature and content of their tasks, and the skills required following the implementation of the digital social and healthcare centre. The interview framework was developed within the research group, and based on previous scientific research [3]. The interview explored how the digital social and health center has affected employees' work practices, including changes in workload and pace, job tasks and the nature of work, communication and interaction within the work community, information flow and data security, overall satisfaction with the digital service implementation, and any additional reflections the participant wished to share. The number of questions was kept moderate to allow for in-depth and open discussion, as well as clarifications during the interviews.

The interviewees were recruited with the assistance of unit managers. Motivational information material and research information sheet were sent to the unit managers of the selected units, who were then asked to provide contact information about voluntary participants. To be eligible, respondents needed to have work experience at the reception before the digital health and social center started operating in the area. The study included both nurses working solely on-site and those working partially in the digital health and social center but excluded nurses working exclusively in the digital health and social center. Previous study suggests that the parallel use of digital and traditional presence-based work environments without seamless integration can fragment workflows and increase the risk of rejecting digital services in daily routines [22].

The interviews were mostly conducted as individual interviews, with one pair interview also included. A total of 11 units were included in the study, but we were unable to get an interviewee from one unit. Thus, in total 10 units were included and twelve registered nurses. The transcriptions were manually corrected, and the names of the respondents, as well as the initial and final discussions, were removed from the data.

2.4 Inductive Content Analysis

Qualitative content analysis was chosen because it provides a systematic yet flexible approach for interpreting participants' subjective experiences and identifying meaningful patterns within the interview data [23]. Qualitative content analysis consists of three phases: first, the data is prepared for analysis, then it is organized using codes or categories, and finally, the results of the analysis are reported [23]. The content analysis was conducted by two researchers (EA, TP) using an inductive method, and two other researchers commented on the analysis (HK, EL). In the inductive approach, the data guides the analysis [23]. The resulting anonymous 133-page (font: Aptos, line spacing: 1,25) data was transferred to the web-based Taguette system Taguette. (https://www. taguette.org). Essential background information, answers to the research question, and specific development suggestions from the nurses were extracted from the data using Taguette.

Next, these extracts were transferred to an Excel spreadsheet, where the answers were condensed using sentences as the unit of condensation (Table 1). To maintain the integrity of the responses, clarifying additions were sometimes included in the sentences. The simplifications (n = 216) were categorized into subcategories, upper categories, and finally main categories using content analysis (Table 2).

Table 1. Examples of reductions.

Original expression	Reduction
"Adding one more channel can lead to situations where a patient is sitting in acute care, has left a call request, and is also writing in the chat out of frustration because nothing is happening. It is not very efficient to be active in all three channels simultaneously. Patients end up in multiple queues at the same time and become frustrated."	Patients are in multiple queues simultaneously and become frustrated
"Something that might not sound very dangerous over the phone can be directed to the chat. Send a picture of it there, and it might be resolved with that image and consultation, without needing to use appointment time. It's very difficult to say over the phone that it's a harmless fatty mole and doesn't need to be shown, especially when the customer thinks it's terrible, has grown, and looks awful."	Over the phone, you can ask the customer to send a picture to the digital health platform, so it may not be necessary to ask the patient to come in person; the assessment can be made from the picture.
"Digital health services have provided a good route for quick consultations, which previously burdened our own doctors. Now, our nurse consultant doctors can focus more on the consultation needs of nurses, so their lists are not excessively long. This includes urgent prescription renewals or reviewing lab results."	Digital health services have enabled quick consultations for tasks like prescription renewals and reviewing lab results.

3 Results

A total of 12 registered nurses attended from ten different units. All interviewees were women, working either on-site (n = 7) or in a hybrid arrangement (n = 5). A total of three impacts and main categories were recognized, namely 1) impacts on patient care work, 2) impacts on work processes and communication, and 3) impacts on nurses' and other professionals' work (Table 2).

Table 2. Subcategories, upper categories, and main categories answering to research aim.

Subcategory	Upper category	Main category
Awareness of digital health services	Availability of digital services	Impacts on patient care work
Extended hours of operation		
Virtual communication with patients		
Requirement of strong authentication	Digital services causing failure demand	
Several service channels		
Enabling quick consultation	Increased interprofessional communication	Impacts on interprofessional communication and work processes
Interprofessional communication		
Volume and speed of information		
Documentation	Transformed processes and operations	
Forms		
Visual materials		
Instructions and directives		
Incompleteness		
Login to the digital systems		
Remote work	Change in work tasks and the way or working	Impacts on nurses' and other profes-sionals' work, workload, and wellbeing
Reformed work tasks		
Increased workload	Digital services impacting on professionals' wellbeing	
Interprofessional support		
Attitudes towards digital work		

3.1 Impacts on Patient Care Work

The impact on patient care work can be examined from two distinct perspectives: *availability of digital services* and *digital services causing failure demand*.

Regarding the availability, the interviewed nurses recognized variation among patients in *awareness of digital health services*. According to nurses, the *extended hours of operation* of the digital health and social center have brought significant benefits to those patients who were familiar with them. Patients can inquire about laboratory test results and receive medication and treatment based on the results in the evenings and on weekends. Urinary tract infection patients, who previously had to wait over the weekend for their test results, were frequently mentioned as an example. Now, they can receive their results and treatment even on weekends through digital health services. Nurses' ethical stress is reduced when they don't have to leave patients waiting overnight or at the weekend. Patients can be directed to ask about their results and receive assistance also in the evenings and on weekends.

"It's been a relief to be able to say, 'Hey, why not check your answers from DigiSote over the weekend?' so patients don't always have to wait until Monday or the next weekday." RN1

Nurses can also use the platform to stay in contact with their own patients and using to platform for *virtual communication*. Clinic nurses have their own patients for various reasons. Through the digital platform, a nurse can allow messaging from a patient for a certain period, enabling them to communicate about changes in the patient's condition, such as after starting new medication, until the matter is resolved.

However, digital health and social center may cause failure demand when patients communicate with professionals using different service channels. The nurses highlighted two groups responsible for this. Parents of children over 12 years old are often directed to the digital health services. However, they cannot proceed without the child's own bank credentials and *strong authentication*, so they end up returning to physical locations, causing frustration as they cannot manage their child's affairs, and nurses have to face this frustration. The second issue is patients using *several service channels* simultaneously. This problem is exacerbated by longer waiting times. Patients may leave multiple callback requests on different lines, wait in physical queues, and queue in the digital health center's chat via their mobile phones. When an issue is resolved or being handled in one channel, the other channels are not notified. Thus, it might be that several nurses are working with the same issue at the same time without knowing it.

"It might be that you're waiting for a response from the chat, and then you get a message saying that the patient was just on the phone with the health center. It's clear that they are contacting from everywhere. If there's even a slight queue, they manage to send multiple callback requests, chats, and use the online service and everything possible. They might already be sitting in the waiting room by the time you call back." RN3

3.2 Impacts on Interprofessional Communication and Work Processes

The interviewed nurses recognized *increased interprofessional communication* and *transformed processes and operations* having an impact on their work.

Digital physician resources have significantly reduced time pressure on physical clinic doctors, and eased nurses' workload by *enabling quick consultations* for tasks such as prescription renewals and reviewing lab results. Patient matters have progressed more quickly thanks to having a physician whose list can be used to mark items for review. In many units, physical clinic nurses can now forward patient matters directly to digital physicians, which has eased the consultation load for on-site doctors. Although some units still prefer consulting physical clinic physicians to maintain continuity of care, the digital center has created an efficient channel for quick consultations that previously burdened in-house physicians. Having a dedicated consultant physician has improved responsiveness to nurses' needs, and physicians' lists are no longer crowded with urgent prescription renewals or lab result reviews, allowing time-sensitive matters to be handled more efficiently.

"I personally use the DigiSote center [digital clinic] a lot for consulting doctors, renewing prescriptions, and similar tasks. In a way, it has brought real relief. There's a place to send these requests when our reception doctors don't necessarily have the time." RN8A

According to the interviewees, interprofessional communication and information flow between professionals is increasingly carried out remotely. Microsoft Teams is a very popular communication platform, and a new addition is the digital health and social center platform, where professionals can exchange messages with one another. The digital health and social center has led to an increase in multidisciplinary communication, especially with other internal units and other service providers. A few respondents felt that communication had remained unchanged.

"The multidisciplinary approach has really strengthened, and of course, through the digital platform, the opportunities have grown... it's truly a low-threshold way for patients to get help digitally." RN10A

Nurses highlighted an increased *volume and speed of information*, which leads to reduced responsiveness to incoming messages. Challenges in *virtual communication* include the susceptibility of written communication to misunderstandings, as well as individual employees becoming the general messengers of negative feedback within their unit. General busyness also slows down the flow of information. In nearly every unit, respondents noted differences in service providers' practices and policies, which sometimes led to cases being reprocessed in physical clinics. Wellbeing services county's on-call nurses assess patients with broad training backgrounds and often request prescriptions or follow-up care from consultant physicians when home remedies have proven insufficient. Nurses have found it frustrating when some service provider physicians disregard their documentation and assessments, responding with home care instructions and advising patients to visit the clinic if symptoms persist. These cases have occurred with upper respiratory infections, sinusitis, ear infections, and eye infections.

"The patient had already called us once and received home care instructions: use nasal spray, saline rinses, and other measures. These had been followed for a sufficient time, but symptoms persisted, so the patient came to the clinic... At that point, the doctor could simply note continued use of nasal spray and rinses and, if symptoms don't spread, refer to in-person care. In practice, this often bypasses the nurse's entire effort." RN10B

Documentation of patient information was occasionally seen as a challenge. From the perspective of the interviewed nurses, the documentation was described as sluggish, slower, and more difficult than before. Messages written by patients in the digital health and social center's chat are not saved if the professional does not open the message thread during the service hours. Patients are not always aware of this and may assume their message has already been recorded. Texts written in the chat also disappear if the patient closes the chat window before the professional joins the conversation. Some issues have also arisen due to missing entries in the Kanta service. Additionally, when patients interact simultaneously through several different channels, which has led to duplicate entries from different units. The electronic patient record reform was criticized amongst interviewed nurses because it no longer shows whether a patient's records are open simultaneously by multiple professionals. A few respondents reported that the flow and documentation of patient information had remained unchanged.

"From the customer's perspective, it can feel frustrating. You've put effort into uploading images, describing symptoms, and providing detailed background information, only for it to be left hanging, and then you have to start over the next day." RN10A

In some units, the platform was utilized extensively. In addition to digital nurses, even those working solely in physical clinics made use of its features. The platform has offered a secure way to quickly deliver *forms* to patients, such as blood pressure monitoring sheets and sick leave certificates. Patients can even send *visual materials*, such as images, which facilitates the assessment of care needs during phone consultations. Evaluating moles, eye infections, and skin changes becomes easier with images for the healthcare professionals, reducing the need for patients to visit the clinic in person.

"Tasks like filling in blood pressure forms or sending sick leave certificates work much faster through the digital system. The same goes for skin changes, patients can upload a photo, or even request eye drop prescriptions by sending an image of their eyes. For these kinds of issues, the digital service is really effective." RN3

All nurses have been provided with credentials to *log into* the platform. Each unit should have at least one professional logged in to respond to messages and inquiries from other professionals via the platform.

"Everyone has login credentials, but not everyone has necessarily visited the platform or made use of it yet." RN2

However, a major issue with the DigiSote platform has been the *incompleteness* and lack of proper onboarding, which has made it a burden in daily work. In some units, it has been agreed upon who is responsible for logging in and responding to professional inquiries. Yet in many units, this responsibility remains unclear, and in a significant number of units, logging in is currently not being done at all. Another central theme concerned the numerous discrepancies and unclear instructions related to managing appointment lists and handling patient referrals.

"That digital... or the DigiSote platform, yeah. I mean, I get the point of it, but the thing is, it was just announced to us like, 'Here are your credentials, go log in,' and that was it. But then the actual onboarding and training—well, we had absolutely no idea what we were supposed to do." RN8B

3.3 Impacts on Nurses' and Other Professionals' Work, Workload, and Wellbeing

The implementation of digital health and social center caused *changes in work tasks and transformed the way of working* as well as had an impact on *nurses' wellbeing* according to the interviewees.

Partial work as a digital nurse emerged both as an opportunity and a challenge. *Remote work* was seen positively, offering variety and a calmer work environment. However, challenges included adapting to new work methods and the fact that not all situations can be resolved digitally. Peer support among digital nurses was highlighted as essential, especially during the integration of the new model into daily routines.

"Personally, I feel that being somewhat introverted, I really appreciate having the chance to work from home in peace every now and then." RN7

Integration with physical clinics and its impact on *reformed work tasks* varied among respondents. Some felt there were still areas for improvement and confusion about which tasks belong to which role. Some reported only minor changes, while others said there had been no changes at all.

Several comments mentioned *increased workload* caused by wellbeing services county's stricter guidelines for assessing care needs. Non-urgent patients have been directed to emergency appointments. There have also been cases of patients being booked into incorrect appointment lists or directed to the wrong buildings, and even confusion between town names. Some respondents suspected this was due to overfilled appointment schedules, leading to patients being placed wherever space was available. A few respondents described situations where final responsibility for resolving a case was unnecessarily shifted to physical clinic nurses.

The workload and pace in physical clinics were generally described as more burdensome after the digital center's launch. Many responses noted that digital contacts had not reduced the number of cases directed to physical clinics. Instead, some matters ended up in both service channels, increasing the workload. In some responses, it was noted that the digital center has enabled certain cases to be handled directly through digital channels, slightly easing the burden in physical clinics. Some felt the workload remained unchanged, while others reported a slight decrease.

"This is a really big shift in our mindset too—like, oh, things can be handled this way. It clearly brings remote communication into our work and opens up new possibilities." RN10B

Attitudes toward the digital center among nurses were divided. Some respondents viewed the change positively and saw the digital center as an opportunity to improve services and enhance customer experience. Others reported negative experiences related to increased workload, unclear roles, and technical challenges.

4 Discussion

This study demonstrates that the implementation of a digital health and social care center reshapes nursing work, professional roles, and interprofessional collaboration in ways that both enhance and challenge existing practices. The findings align with earlier research showing that digitalization can increase service accessibility, accelerate care processes, strengthen communication pathways, and alleviate pressure on physical appointments, particularly when digital tools are well integrated into everyday workflows [3, 24]. In this study, the ability to provide patient support outside traditional office hours, obtain medical advice quickly, and use visual materials for remote assessment exemplified the added value of digital services. However, because digital health and social centers consolidate digital services in one place, it becomes easier for nurses to notice when patients are simultaneously using several different digital channels along with face-to-face appointments. This fragmentation and overlapping demand have not been as clearly visible in previous studies.

However, the benefits of digitalization do not materialize uniformly. Nurses reported varied patients' readiness to use digital services and inconsistent adoption of the platform across units. These findings mirror earlier studies emphasizing that digitalization does not automatically reduce workloads; rather, its impact depends on implementation quality, onboarding, and the degree to which digital workflows align with existing processes [11, 16]. Similarly, Laukka et al. [25] note that digital services can simultaneously generate value and "value co-destruction" if poorly integrated, creating additional work or confusion instead of streamlining tasks.

The implementation of a digital health and social center has had several significant impacts on nurses' work. One key mechanism through which these centers influence nursing practice or work involves patient-related issues. Although digital health services enable patients to receive test results and access care during weekends, this has not alleviated the traditional Monday rush, as many issues still accumulate and require attention at the start of the week. This suggests that while digital solutions may improve accessibility, they do not necessarily address underlying workflow bottlenecks and may even contribute to fragmentation and duplication of work. Based on our results, nurses reported that they often handle the same patient issues across multiple channels, which can lead to increased workload, time pressure, and frustration, as well as a sense of fragmented responsibilities. Similarly, previous studies have also suggested that digital services may increase the risk of patients contacting professionals through several different platforms [3], which in practice can lead to additional workload for on-site nurses. Failure demand not only poses challenges for nurses' work but also adds strain to already overburdened health and social care systems. These experiences highlight the need to design digital systems that genuinely support nurses' work rather than inadvertently increasing complexity. Comparable challenges have been noted in research on multi-channel healthcare environments, where fragmented information flows or slow response times prompt service users to contact multiple channels at once [26]. This highlights that technological solutions must be accompanied by clear communication processes and integrated information systems to genuinely reduce workload.

Moreover, nurses' perspectives should be more carefully considered when developing digital services [11, 16]. Although written communication is suggested as a way to ease documentation and consultation was seen better in our study, our findings also indicate that nurses perceived digital communication especially with patients as sluggish, slower, and more difficult than before, increasing the risk of duplicate entries in some cases. We suggest that the system developers should address these challenges prior to implementation and co-create solutions with nurses and other end-users to ensure maximum value. Furthermore, our findings suggest that digital communication methods risk diminishing the value experienced by nurses rather than creating it. Therefore, approaching the development, implementation, and use of digital health and social centers from a value co-creation perspective may lead to better outcomes [25].

The present study highlights the complex realities of digital transformation in nursing work, particularly related to communication with the patients and documentation. While digital platforms are often introduced with the promise of increased efficiency and improved information flow [27], our findings suggest that these benefits are not always realized in practice. Instead, nurses may experience digital communication with patients as sluggish, slower, and more difficult than before, increasing the risk of duplicate entries. Previous studies, such as those by Kaihlanen et al. [3] and Konttila et al.

[15], have similarly noted that digitalization can increase workload and introduce new challenges, particularly when systems are not fully aligned with the realities of clinical practice. Whereas consultation and communication with other professionals was found to be beneficial based on our findings. Tools such as Microsoft Teams and the DigiSote platform strengthened collaboration and facilitated faster information exchange, consistent with prior research showing that digital systems can support effective multidisciplinary teamwork [28].

What was highlighted in our study was the complex understanding it provides of how insufficient implementation, unclear responsibilities, and the proliferation of communication channels can undermine the intended value of digital solutions. These findings reinforce the argument that successful digital health service implementation requires more than technical deployment, it demands genuine co-creation with end-users and ongoing organizational support, also supported in earlier studies [11, 16]. If nurses are not actively involved in the development and adaptation of digital systems, there is a risk that these tools may diminish, rather than enhance, the value and meaning of their work. This underscores the importance of a user-centered approach and continuous dialogue between staff and system developers to ensure that digital innovations truly support professional wellbeing and high-quality care.

Our study found that the use of the digital health and social platform supports on-site work in many ways. Sending forms, messages, and images can be done securely and quickly. However, in practice, familiarization with the platform has often remained incomplete, and there has been little time for learning. Professionals are required to have motivation and willingness to develop their digital competence at work, making collegial and organizational support essential for enabling positive experiences and smooth digital workflows [15].

In many units, the digital social and health center has significantly alleviated the shortage of physicians having also an impact on nurses' work. Utilizing digital doctors as part of the on-site reception workflow frees up time for in-person physicians to focus on consultations and appointments that require clinical examination, as well as cases demanding continuity of care. However, guidelines and practices still need to be clarified and standardized to avoid finalizing or even redoing tasks at the physical site, highlighting the need for clearer role definitions and process alignment.

Despite some perceived benefits, the introduction of new digital services can pose significant challenges, such as increased workload, slower work processes, new competence requirements, and exacerbated time constraints due to the need for system training [3, 29]. In our study, nurses commonly reported that their workload, tasks, and overall strain had increased, sometimes beyond tolerable limits. Some even felt that the digital social and health center had only added to their burden, mainly due to increased work. Even in units where the digital center was perceived as helpful in supporting on-site nurses and reducing workload, overall strain often remained alarmingly high. These results underscore the importance of continuous dialogue between staff and management to build a shared understanding of changes in work and workload. Such dialogue is essential for supporting nurses' wellbeing and ensuring the delivery of high-quality social and healthcare services during ongoing digital transformation [3].

4.1 Trustworthiness, Limitations, and Ethical Considerations

In assessing the trustworthiness of qualitative research, this study draws on Lincoln & Guba's [30] framework, which outlines credibility, transferability, dependability, and confirmability as core criteria. Credibility was strengthened by prolonged engagement with the material and iterative analysis that allowed emerging interpretations to be continuously compared against the data. Transferability was supported by providing a sufficiently detailed description of the research context, enabling readers to judge the applicability of the findings to other settings. To ensure dependability, the analytical process was documented systematically, including decision trails that make the progression from raw data to interpretations transparent. Finally, confirmability was enhanced by reflexive consideration of the researchers' assumptions and by maintaining an audit trail that demonstrates how the findings are grounded in the participants' accounts rather than in researcher bias.

This study has certain limitations. The sample consisted of registered nurses from one wellbeing services county in Finland, which may limit the transferability of the findings to other regions or internationally. Although the interviews provided rich insights, the number of participants was relatively small, and those who volunteered may have been particularly motivated or interested in digital service changes. Additionally, the rapid organizational changes occurring during data collection may have influenced participants' perceptions, making some experiences time bound.

Research permission was obtained from the wellbeing services county, and all participants received an information sheet and a data protection notice prior to their involvement in the study. In addition, the study adhered to the ethical principles for research involving human participants as outlined in the Declaration of Helsinki [31]. No ethics committee approval was required, as the study does not constitute medical research involving intervention in the integrity of a person under the Finnish Medical Research Act [32].

5 Conclusions

To conclude, digital health and social centers have expanded service availability for patients, but as new processes, they are still developing. They have generated some positive impacts on nurses and workflow efficiency. However, there remains a risk that they may also increase nurses' workload. The successful integration of digital services requires consistent operational practices, effective onboarding, strong technological support, and leadership that prioritizes both user experience and workflow alignment. Digitalization should be understood as an organizational, not merely technical transformation. When executed thoughtfully, digital health services can enhance care quality, strengthen collaboration, and improve patient experiences. When implementation is fragmented, digitalization risks increasing workload and reducing system efficiency.

Future research should investigate the long-term effects of digitalization on nursing work, continuity of care, patient safety, and organizational structures across wellbeing services counties from different perspectives.

Disclosure of Interests. The authors have no competing interests to declare that are relevant to the content of this article.

References

1. Golinelli, D., Boetto, E., Carullo, G., Nuzzolese, A.G., Landini, M.P., Fantini, M.P.: Adoption of digital Technologies in Health Care during the COVID-19 pandemic: systematic review of early scientific literature. J. Med. Internet Res. **22**(11), e22280 (2020)
2. Härkönen, H. et al.: Impact of digital services on healthcare and social welfare: an umbrella review. Int. J. Nurs. Stud. **152**, 104692 (2024)
3. Kaihlanen, A-M., Laukka, E., Nadav, J., Närvänen, J., Saukkonen, P., Koivisto, J., Heponiemi, T.: The effects of digitalisation on health and social care work: a qualitative descriptive study of the perceptions of professionals and managers. BMC Health Serv. Res. **23**(1), 714 (2023)
4. Strange, M., Zdravkovic, S., Gustafsson, H., Mangrio, E.: Everyday digitalization of health care: the experiences of dental healthcare Workers in a Diverse Swedish Region. Int. J. Health Wellness Soc. **15**(1), 39–59 (2025)
5. Shigekawa, E., Fix, M., Corbett, G., Dylan, H.R., Coffman, J.: The current state of telehealth evidence: a rapid review. Health Aff. **37**(12), 1975–1982 (2018)
6. Laukka, E. et al.: Effectiveness of interactive digital health services in non-communicable diseases: an umbrella review and evidence synthesis from 26 meta-analyses. Int. J. Nurs. Stud. **174**, 105277 (2026)
7. Rodriguez-Villa, E., Rauseo-Ricupero, N., Camacho, E., Wisniewski, H., Keshavan, M., Torous, J.: The digital clinic: implementing technology and augmenting care for mental health. Gen. Hosp. Psychiatry. **66**, 59–66 (2020)
8. Rauseo-Ricupero, N., Henson, P., Agate-Mays, M., Torous, J.: Case studies from the digital clinic: integrating digital phenotyping and clinical practice into today's world. Int. Rev. Psychiatry. **33**(4), 394–403 (2021)
9. Macrynikola, N., et al.: Testing the feasibility, acceptability, and potential efficacy of an innovative digital mental health care delivery model designed to increase access to care: open trial of the digital clinic, JMIR mental. Health. **12**, e65222 (2025)
10. Sotedatalab. https://sotedatalab.fi/en/uutinen/julkisten-digiklinikoiden-vaestokattavuus-nousi-toukokuussa-2025-jo-yli-43-miljoonaan/. Assessed 28 Jan 2026
11. Nadav, J. Kaihlanen, A-M., et al.. : Factors contributing to successful information system implementation and employee Well-being in health care and social welfare professionals: comparative cross-sectional study. JMIR Med. Inform. **12**, e52817–e52817 (2024)
12. Wirkkala, M., Wjik, K., Larsson, A.C., Engström, M.: Technology frustration in healthcare – does it matter in staff ratings of stress, emotional exhaustion, and satisfaction with care? A cross-sectional correlational study using the job demands-resources theory. BMC Health Serv. Res. **24**(1), 1557 (2024)
13. Odendaal, W.A., et al.: Health workers' perceptions and experiences of using mHealth technologies to deliver primary healthcare services: a qualitative evidence synthesis. Cochrane Database Syst. Rev. **26**(3), CD011942 (2020)
14. Henry, B.W., Block, D.E., Ciesla, J.R., McGowan, B.A., Vozenilek, J.A.: Clinician behaviors in telehealth care delivery: a systematic review. Adv. Health Sci. Educ. **22**(4), 869–888 (2016)
15. Konttila, J., et al.: Healthcare professionals' competence in digitalisation: a systematic review. J. Clin. Nurs. **28**(5–6), 745–761 (2019)
16. Nadav, J., et al.: How to implement digital Services in a way that They Integrate into routine work: qualitative interview study among health and social care professionals. J. Med. Internet Res. **23**(12), e31668 (2021)

17. Isidori, V., et al.: Digital technologies and the role of health care professionals: scoping review exploring nurses' skills in the digital era and in the light of the COVID-19 pandemic. JMIR nursing. **5**, e37631 (2022)
18. Sandelowski, M.: Focus on research methods: whatever happened to qualitative description? Res. Nurs. Health. **23**, 334–340 (2000)
19. Kihlström, L., Keskimäki, I., Paananen, H., Paatela, S., Satokangas, M., Tynkkynen, L.: How is a large-scale reform perceived by citizens in Finnish primary health care? Soc. Sci. Med. **387**, 118688 (2025)
20. Tynkkynen, L.-K., Karanikolos, M., Litvinova, Y.: Finland: Health System Summary. World Health Organization. Regional Office for Europe, WHO IRIS (2023)
21. Negrin, K.A., Slaughter, S.E., Dahlke, S., Olson, J.: Successful recruitment to qualitative research: a critical reflection. Int J Qual Methods. **21**, 1–12 (2022)
22. Greenhalgh, T., et al.: Beyond adoption: a new framework for theorizing and evaluating nonadoption, abandonment, and challenges to the scale-up, spread, and sustainability of health and care technologies. J. Med. Internet Res. **19**(11) (2017)
23. Elo, S., Kajula, O., Tohmola, A., Kääriäinen, M.: Laadullisen sisällönanalyysin vaiheet ja eteneminen. Hoitotiede. **34**(4), 215–225 (2022)
24. Németh, G.: Impact of digital tools on patient assessment and documentation accuracy in nursing practice. Journal of Patient Care and Nursing Practice. **2**(1), 40–44 (2025)
25. Laukka, E., et al.: Value Cocreation and Codestruction in digital health services: protocol for a systematic review. JMIR Research Protocols. **14**, e63015 (2025)
26. Moreira, A., Duarte, J., Santos, M.F.: Case study of multichannel interaction in healthcare services. Information. **14**(1), 37 (2023)
27. Laukka, E., et al.: Health care professionals' experiences of patient-professional communication over patient portals: systematic review of qualitative studies. J. Med. Internet Res. **22**(12), e21623 (2020)
28. Williams, V., Peachey, L.: Digital health systems may not fully incorporate the nursing process, thus posing a risk to effective clinical decision-making. Evid. Based Nurs. **27**(4), 129 (2023)
29. Al Shammasi, G.M., Bafaraj, A.M.: The impact of digital transformation on enhancing nursing experience and medical reporting efficiency. International Journal of Innovative Research in Medical Science. **8**(1), 1–4 (2020)
30. Lincoln, Y.S., Guba, E.G.: Naturalistic Inquiry. SAGE Publications, Newbury Park (1985)
31. Declaration of Helsinki. https://www.wma.net/policies-post/wma-declaration-of-helsinki/. Accessed 28 Jan 2026
32. Medical Research Act (488/1999). https://finlex.fi/en/legislation/translations/1999/eng/488. Accessed 28 Jan 2026

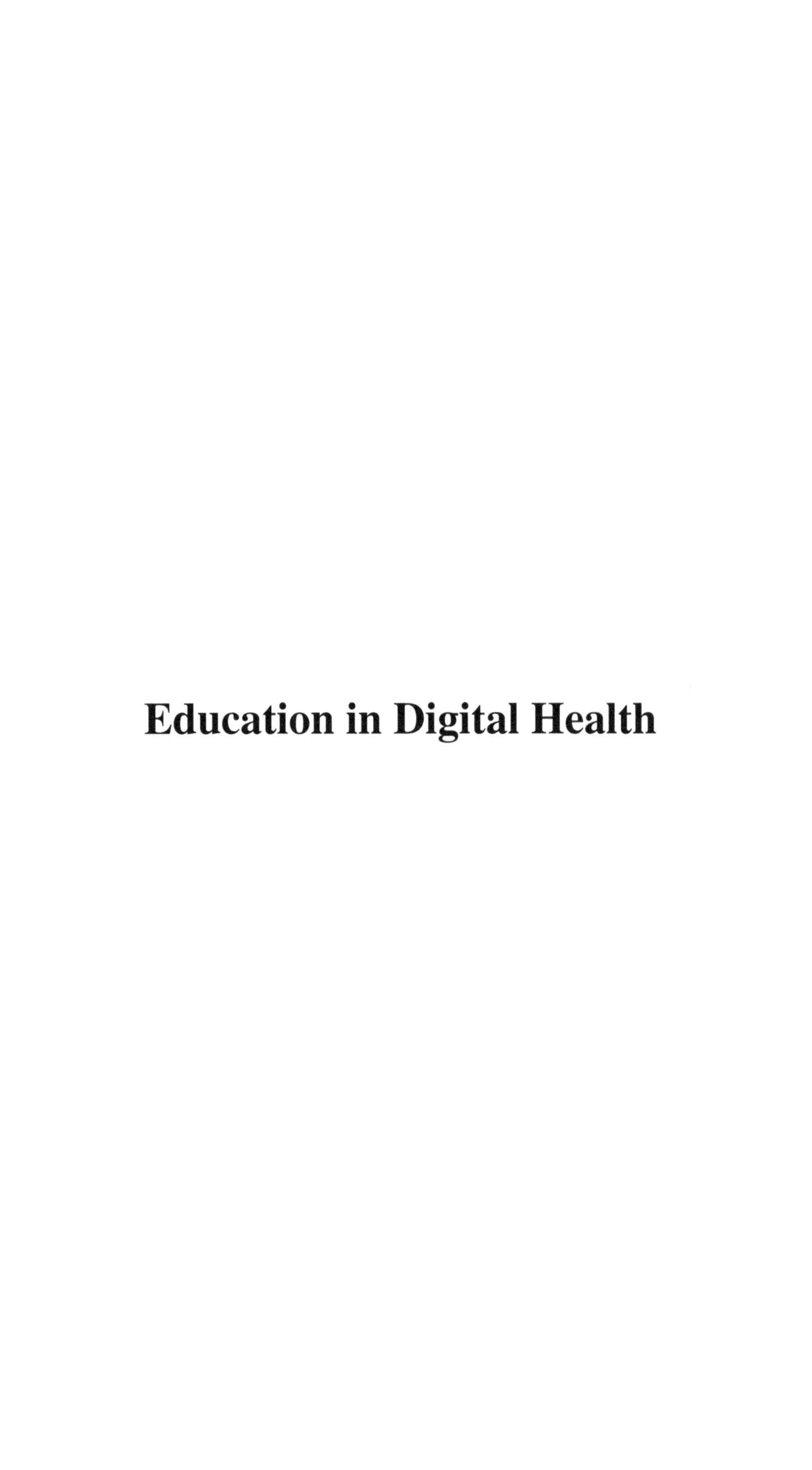

Education in Digital Health

Designing Safe Hybrid AI–XR Simulations for Healthcare Communication and Interaction Training

Kristina Mikkonen[1,2]([✉]) [iD], Egle Butkeviciute[3] [iD], Patrikas Armalis[3] [iD],
Evelina Aluzaite[1] [iD], Rita Baranauskaite[1], Lukas Paulauskas[3] [iD], Lina Spirgiene[1] [iD],
Andrejus Subocius[1] [iD], Tomas Blazauskas[3] [iD], and Olga Riklikiene[1] [iD]

[1] Lithuanian University of Health Sciences, Kaunas, Lithuania
kristina.mikkonen@oulu.fi
[2] University of Oulu, Oulu, Finland
[3] Kaunas University of Technology, Kaunas, Lithuania

Abstract. Effective healthcare education must address not only clinical knowledge but also communication, teamwork, and decision-making under pressure. Extended Reality (XR) combined with artificial intelligence (AI) offers new opportunities for immersive, scalable communication training, yet raises critical concerns related to safety, reliability, and learner trust. This paper presents the design rationale and early insights from VirtualHealEd, a human-centred hybrid AI–XR simulation for healthcare communication and interaction training. The platform integrates conversational AI, speech recognition, and immersive XR while employing a hybrid architecture that combines generative AI with deterministic system components to ensure safety in life-critical scenarios. In parallel, multimodal data, including speech transcripts, performance indicators, and physiological signals—are collected to explore stress and cognitive load during AI-mediated interactions with healthcare students (n = 52). Early observations suggest that AI-driven dialogue increases learners' workload, with substantial inter-individual variability, highlighting the need for adaptive, stress-aware learning designs. The paper contributes design principles for safe hybrid intelligence in healthcare XR education and outlines challenges and future directions for stress-aware adaptive simulations.

Keywords: Extended reality · Hybrid intelligence · Conversational AI · Healthcare education · Stress-aware learning

1 Introduction

Healthcare education has traditionally focused on discipline-specific clinical knowledge and technical skills [1]. However, modern healthcare environments demand strong non-technical competences, including communication, teamwork, situation awareness, and decision-making under stress. Communication failures remain a significant contributor to adverse events, underscoring the need for structured and scalable communication training solutions.

© The Author(s) 2026
M. Särestöniemi et al. (Eds.): NCDHWS 2026, CCIS 3009, pp. 289–299, 2026.
https://doi.org/10.1007/978-3-032-28812-7_21

Extended Reality (XR) technologies have emerged as promising tools for immersive healthcare education, enabling learners to engage with realistic clinical scenarios in a safe environment [2]. This is consistent with broader evidence from higher education, where immersive virtual reality has been shown to enhance experiential learning and skill acquisition across disciplines [3]. When combined with artificial intelligence (AI), XR simulations can move beyond scripted scenarios toward adaptive, interactive learning experiences. Conversational AI, in particular, enables natural language interaction with virtual patients and team members, increasing realism and learner engagement.

While prior AI-driven XR training systems have demonstrated benefits in simulation realism and learner engagement, many remain limited to pre-scripted dialogue trees or constrained interaction models, reducing their adaptability and ecological validity. In contrast, recent advances in large language models enable more open-ended communication, but introduce new challenges related to reliability, controllability, and pedagogical alignment.

Despite this potential, the use of AI in healthcare education introduces critical challenges [4]. Large language models may generate inconsistent or incorrect information, posing risks when simulations involve medical instructions or treatment decisions. Such limitations are widely discussed in AI safety research, particularly regarding hallucinations, lack of grounding, and risks in high-stakes contexts [5]. Additionally, immersive AI-driven interactions may increase cognitive load and stress, potentially affecting learning outcomes. These risks are well-documented in broader AI safety literature, including concerns related to hallucinations, alignment, and robustness in high-stakes domains. These challenges highlight the importance of hybrid intelligence approaches that balance AI flexibility with human-centred design, transparency, and safety [6]. Hybrid intelligence emphasises the complementary strengths of human and artificial cognition, enabling more reliable and context-aware decision-making in complex environments [7].

This paper presents VirtualHealEd, an AI-powered XR simulation designed for healthcare communication and interaction training. The novelty of this work lies in its integration of a hybrid intelligence architecture that constrains generative AI through safety-aware design mechanisms, while preserving conversational flexibility within XR-based clinical scenarios, operationalising hybrid intelligence principles in an immersive learning context [7]. Rather than focusing solely on system implementation, the paper emphasises (1) the design rationale behind a hybrid AI–XR architecture, (2) safety-driven decisions that constrain AI behaviour in critical contexts, and (3) early observations from multimodal data, including physiological indicators of stress. In doing so, the study bridges healthcare education research with emerging technical and ethical frameworks in AI and XR systems design. The goal is to contribute design insights for the responsible and effective use of hybrid intelligence in healthcare education. VirtualHealEd has been approved by Kaunas Regional Biomedical Research Ethics Committee (Nr. 2025-BE10–0011).

2 Related Work

XR-based simulations are increasingly used in healthcare education to support clinical skills, teamwork, and communication training. Prior studies have shown that immersive simulations can enhance learner engagement and improve transfer of skills to clinical practice [1, 3]. Virtual patients, in particular, have been used to train communication skills in nursing and medicine [2].

Recent advances in conversational AI have enabled more dynamic virtual patient interactions. Large language models allow simulations to respond flexibly to learner input, supporting unscripted dialogue and personalised learning paths. However, concerns have been raised regarding the reliability, explainability, and safety of AI-generated content in medical contexts [4, 5, 8].

In parallel, research on stress and cognitive load in simulation-based learning has highlighted the importance of physiological measures such as heart rate variability and EEG-derived metrics. These measures provide insights into learner states that may not be captured through performance metrics alone. Integrating such data into XR environments remains challenging due to sensor noise, synchronisation issues, and individual variability.

While prior work has explored XR, conversational AI, and stress measurement separately, fewer studies have addressed how these components can be combined within a unified, safety-aware hybrid intelligence framework. This paper contributes to this gap by presenting design choices and early insights from an integrated AI–XR healthcare education platform.

3 Hybrid AI–XR Design Rationale

3.1 Human-Centred Hybrid Intelligence

The design of VirtualHealEd is grounded in the principles of hybrid intelligence, where human pedagogical intent and system constraints guide the use of AI. Rather than maximising AI autonomy, the system emphasises transparency, controllability, and alignment with educational objectives. AI is used to enhance realism and feedback, while critical decisions remain bounded by deterministic logic.

This approach reflects a core assumption: in healthcare education, realism must never come at the expense of safety or correctness. Consequently, AI-generated content is selectively constrained based on the educational and ethical implications of each interaction.

3.2 Two-Mode Communication Training Design

VirtualHealEd implements two complementary learning modes that support progressive skill development. The VR was developed for anaphylactic shock management, clinical reasoning and decision making in urgent situations, with the focus of communication among professionals and patients (NPC) themselves, including students in a clinical practice context. The first mode focuses on AI-assisted scripted communication practice[5]. Learners read from a teleprompter while local speech recognition transcribes their utterances in real time. Recognised phrases are compared against an expected script, and successfully completed segments are visually marked. This mode supports the acquisition of correct medical terminology and structured communication sequences, particularly for novice learners.

The second mode enables unscripted conversational interaction with virtual patients and healthcare professionals. In this mode, learners engage in natural dialogue, asking questions and responding to dynamic character behaviour (Fig. 1). This design supports higher-level communication skills, such as empathy, clarification, and adaptive questioning, which are difficult to train through scripted approaches alone.

Together, these modes provide pedagogical scaffolding, allowing learners to transition from structured practice to realistic, open-ended interaction.

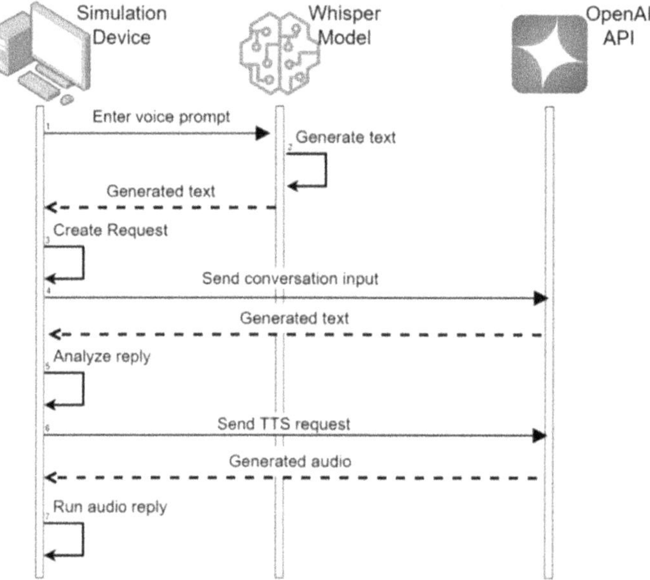

Fig. 1. Simplified AI conversation sequence diagram.

3.3 Safety-Critical Hybrid Architecture

A defining feature of the system is its hybrid AI architecture. While conversational AI is used for patient and nurse interactions, scenarios involving life-critical medical instructions—such as medication dosages or emergency protocols—are handled through deterministic dialogue paths with pre-recorded audio.

This design decision addresses the well-documented risk of AI hallucinations. Even minor inaccuracies in medication information could reinforce unsafe practices. By isolating AI-generated dialogue from safety-critical content, the system ensures absolute correctness while preserving conversational flow.

The architecture separates speech recognition, language generation, response analysis, and speech synthesis into modular components. This modularity supports future upgrades and allows AI components to be replaced or constrained without redesigning the entire system.

4 Stress-Aware Data Collection and Early Observations

A total of 52 fourth-year healthcare students participated in the study, the majority of whom were female (96.2%), with a mean age of 23.1 years (SD = 5.28; median = 22; range 21–51). More than half of the participants (55.8%) reported having work experience in healthcare settings ranging from 2 to 72 months. Among those who specified their experience, the average duration was 16.8 months (SD = 15.61), with a median of 12 months.

To support stress-aware analysis of AI-mediated XR learning, VirtualHealEd implements a multimodal data processing pipeline, illustrated in Fig. 2. The process begins with the learner engaging in an XR-based clinical scenario (scripted or AI-powered), during which multimodal data are captured, including wearable physiological signals (EEG, ECG, PPG), audio for speech recognition, VR and screen recordings, optional room video, and self-report questionnaires. These heterogeneous data streams are ingested through a validation and synchronisation layer that ensures data integrity, metadata extraction, and temporal alignment across devices and modalities. Signal processing is then applied to each stream, including filtering and feature extraction for cardiovascular and neurophysiological signals, speech and task-related metrics, and optional video-based event analysis. The processed data are subsequently analysed using descriptive statistics, robust inferential tests, and offline machine learning models to explore stress and workload patterns at both state and subject levels. Finally, results are visualised through dashboards and research reports, with a forward-looking design that supports future real-time adaptation of XR scenarios and feedback based on learner state.

4.1 Multimodal Data Sources

In addition to conversational interaction, VirtualHealEd collects multiple data streams to explore learner workload and stress during immersive XR training. These include speech-to-text transcripts, task and interaction events, and physiological signals recorded via wearable sensors. Neurophysiological and cardiovascular data—specifically EEG, ECG, and PPG—are collected during XR-based clinical simulations and synchronised with interaction timestamps and scenario states.

At the current stage, physiological signals are processed offline using standard preprocessing, filtering, and feature extraction procedures, followed by within-subject normalisation to account for individual baseline differences. Extracted features include heart rate and heart rate variability measures (e.g., RMSSD, SDNN), EEG spectral power indices, and speech- and task-related temporal metrics. The primary aim of this multimodal data collection is to examine how different interaction modes—resting baseline, scripted non-AI interaction, and AI-powered conversational XR—relate to physiological responses indicative of cognitive workload and stress.

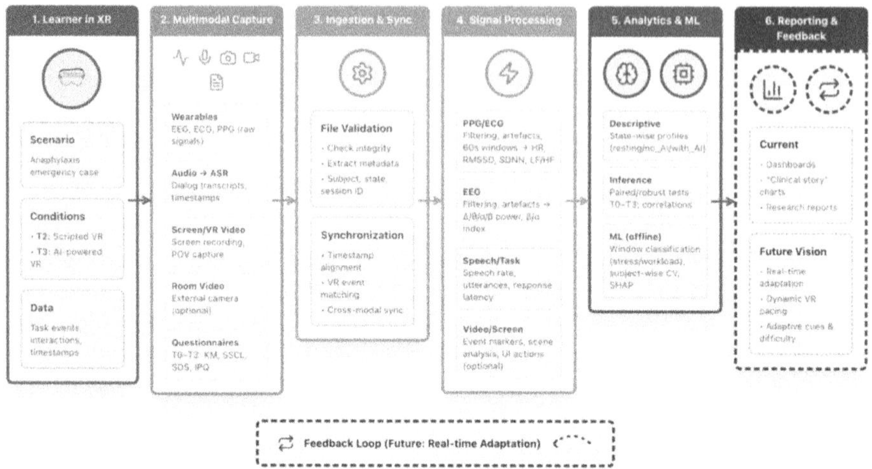

Fig. 2. Multimodal stress-aware learning pipeline in VirtualHealEd.

Integrating these heterogeneous data sources presents several challenges, including sensor noise and motion artefacts in immersive XR environments, temporal synchronisation across devices, and substantial inter-individual variability in physiological responses. These challenges motivate the use of within-subject analytical approaches and cautious interpretation of group-level trends.

4.2 Early Observations

Preliminary physiological analyses reveal systematic differences between learning conditions, with AI-driven conversational XR interaction emerging as the most demanding state.

Table 1. Within-participant differences in PPG-derived heart rate and HRV across states: Friedman test statistics and effect sizes (Kendall's W).

Parameter	Friedman's chi-square	p value	Kendall's W
HR (PPG)	35.70	**<0.001**	0.54
RMSSD (PPG)	6.73	**0.03**	0.10
SDNN (PPG)	2.62	0.27	0.04

Repeated-measures comparisons across resting, scripted, and AI-powered conditions indicate a significant increase in heart rate during the AI condition ($p < 0.05$), accompanied by a significant reduction in heart rate variability (RMSSD, $p < 0.05$), reflecting increased sympathetic activation and reduced parasympathetic regulation.

In contrast, EEG-derived measures, including relative theta power, were analysed using Friedman test, with statistical significance defined as $p < 0.05$, and did not show statistically significant differences across conditions. Visual inspection (see Fig. 3) suggested substantial inter-individual variability, with widely scattered values across participants, which limits the interpretation of group-level EEG trends in the present sample.

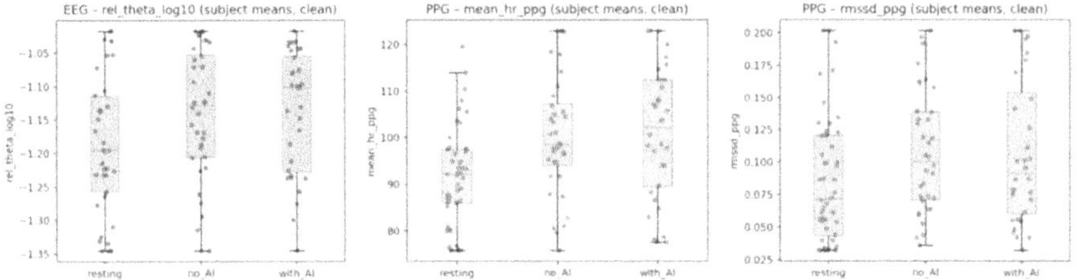

Fig. 3. Subject-level distributions of physiological markers across learning conditions. Boxplots show mean relative EEG theta power (log10-transformed), mean heart rate derived from PPG, and RMSSD derived from PPG for resting baseline, scripted non-AI interaction and AI-powered conversational XR conditions. Individual data points represent subject means. The AI-powered condition exhibits higher heart rate, reduced heart rate variability, and elevated theta power relative to resting and scripted conditions, indicating increased cognitive and physiological workload, with substantial inter-individual variability.

$$\text{Load} = z(HR) - z(\log(\text{RMSSD})) - z(\log(\text{SDNN}))$$

Cardiovascular responses were compared across conditions using PPG-derived heart rate and HRV indices(with z denoting standardisation) Load index was constructed from HR, RMSSD, and SDNN to reflect complementary aspects of cardiovascular regulation rather than to retain only individually significant markers. HR captures overall cardio-vascular activation, RMSSD primarily reflects short-term parasympathetic modulation, and SDNN reflects overall beat-to-beat variability across the recording window [9]. Although SDNN did not show a significant condition effect (see Table 1) in the present sample, it was retained in the composite as a theory-informed component of global auto-nomic variability and to avoid over-representing a single HRV facet. This is particularly relevant in exploratory multimodal studies with substantial inter-individual variability, where some markers may contribute more clearly at the composite or subject-specific level than in group-level univariate tests. In future analyses with larger samples, the relative contribution of SDNN will be re-evaluated and may become more informative as statistical power increases. As shown in Fig. 3, the AI-powered condition was associ-ated with higher heart rate and lower RMSSD than the resting and scripted conditions, although substantial inter-individual variability remained evident.

Effect magnitude for the Friedman test was quantified using Kendall's W, where values closer to 0 indicate weak agreement (small effects) and values closer to 1 indicate strong agreement (large effects) across repeated measures. Heart rate showed a large effect (W $\approx$ 0.54), whereas RMSSD showed a small effect (W $\approx$ 0.10) and SDNN showed a negligible effect (W $\approx$ 0.04) (see Table 1).

Post-hoc comparisons indicate higher load values during AI-powered interaction relative to both resting and scripted conditions, with small-to-moderate within-subject effect sizes. These trends align with participant self-reports, although considerable inter-individual variability is observed. To summarise these cardiovascular changes at the subject level, a composite physiological load index was calculated (Fig. 4).

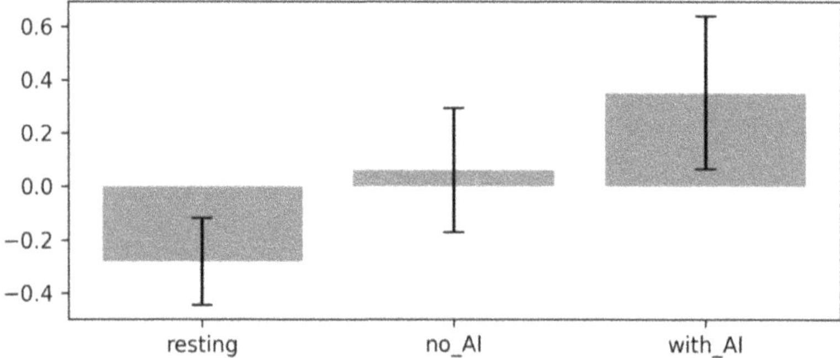

Fig. 4. Composite physiological load index across resting, scripted non-AI, and AI-powered XR conditions. Bars represent condition means and error bars indicate inter-individual variability. The right panel presents the corresponding confusion matrix for three stress classes (no stress, low stress, high stress), illustrating above-chance classification performance with notable overlap between adjacent stress levels.

Complementing the physiological analyses, offline machine learning models trained on multimodal physiological features demonstrate the feasibility of classifying stress states above chance level. A tuned Random Forest classifier identifies cardiovascular features, particularly PPG-derived heart rate and variability measures, as the most informative predictors. However, confusion matrix analysis reveals substantial overlap between low- and high-stress classes, indicating graded physiological transitions rather than clearly separable stress states. The feasibility of stress-state classification based on multimodal physiological features is illustrated in Fig. 5.

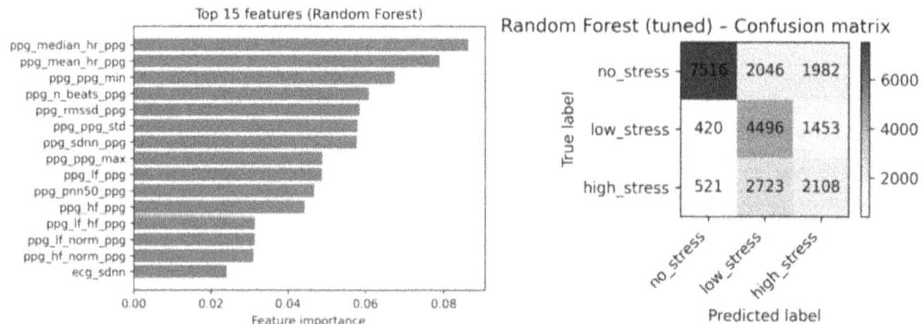

Fig. 5. Offline machine learning results for physiological stress classification. The left panel shows the top 15 feature importances from a tuned Random Forest model, highlighting the dominance of PPG-derived heart rate and heart rate variability features. The right figure demonstrates the performance of the Random Forest classifier within three states (resting, low_stress, high_stress) with up to 70% accuracy.

Overall, these findings should be interpreted as exploratory. The observed variability underscores the limitations of group-level averages and highlights the importance of within-subject analysis in stress-aware learning research. Rather than supporting causal claims regarding learning effectiveness, the results motivate future work toward real-time, individualised adaptation of XR learning environments based on multimodal stress indicators.

5   Design Implications for AI-Driven Healthcare Education

Based on the design experience and early observations, several implications emerge for the development of AI-driven XR healthcare education systems. First, AI realism must be balanced with pedagogical and ethical safety. Fully generative systems may enhance immersion but require strict constraints in medical contexts. Second, hybrid architectures that combine AI-driven flexibility with deterministic safety mechanisms provide a practical pathway for responsible deployment in healthcare education. Third, stress and workload are integral aspects of immersive learning and should be considered design parameters rather than unintended side effects. Multimodal sensing offers valuable insights but must be interpreted cautiously.

Finally, language and cultural context significantly shape AI feasibility. Implementing conversational AI in less-resourced languages requires careful model selection and prompt engineering, influencing system performance and latency.

6   Limitations and Future Work

The current work has several limitations. Data collection is ongoing, and the physiological analyses should therefore be considered exploratory in nature. Stress indicators are analysed offline, and adaptive mechanisms are not yet implemented. Additionally, latency in AI response generation affects conversational flow.

Future work will focus on larger-scale studies, improved signal synchronisation, and the development of real-time adaptive mechanisms that adjust scenario complexity or feedback based on learner state. Advances in locally executable language models may further enhance privacy and performance.

7   Conclusion

This paper presented the design rationale and early insights from VirtualHealEd, a hybrid AI–XR simulation for healthcare communication training. By combining conversational AI with deterministic safety mechanisms and stress-aware data collection, the system illustrates how hybrid intelligence can support realistic yet responsible healthcare education. The findings highlight both the promise and the challenges of AI-driven immersive learning and provide design principles for future stress-aware, human-centred XR training environments.

Acknowledgements. Project"EnhancingHealthcareEducationwithHuman-
CentredExtendedVirtualReality–VirtualHealEd"hasreceived-
fundingfromtheResearchCouncilofLithuania (LMTLT) underGrantNo.S-MIP-24-132. We would
like to acknowledge the support of The University of Oulu & The Academy of Finland Profi 7
(352788) for also supporting this study. Finally, we gratefully acknowledge the collaboration with
FrostBit Software Lab at Lapland University of Applied Sciences, whose expertise in emerging
technologies and extended reality contributed valuable insights and support to this work.

Disclosure of Interests ChatGPT (version 5.3, OpenAI) was used to support linguistic revision
of the manuscript. The authors take full responsibility for the content.

References

1. Ropponen, P., Tomietto, M., Pramila-Savukoski, S., Kuivila, H., Koskenranta, M., Liaw, S.Y., et al.: Impacts of virtual reality simulation on nursing students' competence, confidence, and satisfaction: a systematic review and meta-analysis of randomised controlled trials. Nurse Educ. Today. **152**, 106756 (2025). https://doi.org/10.1016/j.nedt.2025.106756
2. Mikkonen, K. et al.: Multidimensional pedagogical framework for interprofessional education: blending classroom, high fidelity and extended reality simulation. Nurse Educ. Today. (2025). https://doi.org/10.1016/j.nedt.2025.106838
3. Radianti, J., Majchrzak, T.A., Fromm, J., Wohlgenannt, I.: A systematic review of immersive virtual reality applications for higher education: design elements, lessons learned, and research agenda. Comput. Educ. **147**, 103778 (2020)
4. Graham, A., Hökkä, M., Tomietto, M., Mikkonen, K.: The use of digital gamification, extended reality, artificial intelligence, and other digital learning tools in palliative care education of undergraduate nurses: a systematic review of mixed-methods. Nurse Educ. Today. (2026). https://doi.org/10.1016/j.nedt.2026.106982
5. Bender, E.M., Gebru, T., McMillan-Major, A., Shmitchell, S.: On the dangers of stochastic parrots: can language models be too big? In: Proceedings of the 2021 ACM Conference on Fairness, Accountability, and Transparency (FAccT), pp. 610–623 (2021)
6. Kovalainen, T. et al.: Utilising artificial intelligence in developing education of health sciences higher education: an umbrella review of reviews. Nurse Educ. Today. **147**, 106600 (2025). https://doi.org/10.1016/j.nedt.2025.106600
7. Dellermann, D., Ebel, P., Söllner, M., Leimeister, J.M.: Hybrid intelligence. Bus. Inf. Syst. Eng. **61**, 637–643 (2019)
8. Mikkonen, K. et al.: How does human-centred extended reality support healthcare students' learning in clinical conditions? In: Särestöniemi, M. et al. (eds.) Digital Health and Wireless Solutions (NCDHWS 2024). Commun. Comput. Inf. Sci., vol. 2083, pp. 169–184. Springer, Cham (2024). https://doi.org/10.1007/978-3-031-59080-1_13
9. Wang, B.X., Brennand, E.E., Le Page, P., Mitchell, A.R.J.: Heart rate variability in cardio-vascular disease diagnosis, prognosis and management. Front. Cardiovasc. Med. **12**, 1680783 (2025). https://doi.org/10.3389/fcvm.2025.1680783

Examining Nursing Students' Perceptions of Virtual Reality for Language Learning and Culture Immersion: A Mixed-Methods Study

Agostinho A. C. Araújo[1,2](✉) , Paula Ropponen[2] , Sari Pramila-Savukoski[2,3] , Lucas Gardim[1,4] , Isabel Amélia Costa Mendes[1] , and Kristina Mikkonen[2,5,6,7]

[1] Ribeirão Preto College of Nursing, University of São Paulo, Ribeirão Preto 14040902, Brazil
agostinhoaraujo@usp.br
[2] Research Unit of Health Sciences and Technology, Faculty of Medicine, University of Oulu, Oulu 90220, Finland
[3] Lapland University of Applied Sciences, Kemi 98400, Finland
[4] Faculty of Nursing, College of Health Sciences, University of Alberta, Edmonton, AB T6G 1C9, Canada
[5] Medical Research Center Oulu, Oulu University Hospital and University of Oulu, Oulu 90220, Finland
[6] MRC Department of Nursing, Midwifery and Health, Faculty of Health and Life Sciences, Northumbria University, Newcastle Upon Tyne, NE7 7XA, UK
[7] Department of Evidence-Based Clinical Nursing, Division of Health Sciences, Graduate School of Medicine, University of Osaka, Osaka 565-0871, Japan

Abstract. Virtual reality (VR) can potentially support immersive language learning and cultural immersion in the context of growing global migration of patients and professionals. For this reason, we aimed to examine nursing students' perceptions of a VR simulation and explore their understanding of its usability in supporting language learning and cultural immersion. This is a mixed-methods study conducted between Autumn 2023 and Spring 2024. A purposive sampling was used to recruit 16 students from culturally and linguistically diverse backgrounds (CALD) enrolled in an English language degree nursing undergraduate program from two universities of applied sciences in Finland. Quantitative and qualitative results were integrated following a convergent parallel design. Our findings demonstrate that native country significantly influenced perceptions of simulation fidelity, with African and European nursing students rating realism higher than Asian students. Cultural familiarity and engagement enhanced the learning experience, while motivation and cultural connection enhanced the effectiveness of VR-based learning. Motivation, cultural immersion, and task interest play a critical role in shaping students' perceptions with VR-based education, underscoring the need to integrate these factors into design and implementation of VR-based education to enhance learning outcomes.

Keywords: Cultural diversity · Immersive learning · Linguistic diversity · Nursing students · Virtual reality

M. Särestöniemi et al. (Eds.): NCDHWS 2026, CCIS 3009, pp. 300–320, 2026.
https://doi.org/10.1007/978-3-032-28812-7_22

1 Introduction

In the context of increasing global migration of patients and professionals, healthcare systems are facing growing cultural and linguistic diversity [1, 2]. The International Council of Nurses (ICN) shows that the mobility of health workers across borders has intensified, reshaping workforce dynamics and clinical environments worldwide [3]. The International Organisation for Migration (IOM) also highlights that international migration is projected to rise in the coming years due to factors such as geopolitical instability, climate change, and economic disparity [4]. This evolving landscape underscores the urgent need for healthcare systems to adapt through the development of inclusive policies and intercultural competencies, particularly in nursing education and practice, to enhance equity in diverse societies.

For this reason, communication and cultural competence have become essential components of safe and ethical nursing practice [5, 6]. Ensuring nursing student readiness to interact with diverse patient populations is critical, not only in terms of language, but also in understanding cultural nuances that influence health beliefs, behaviours, and care expectations in the healthcare organisations [7]. Exploring the use of virtual reality (VR) as a tool for language learning [8] and cultural immersion [9, 10] is beneficial, as it can simulate real-life scenarios and foster the competencies necessary for culturally responsive care.

Traditional teaching methods often lack the immersive, real-world relevance needed in clinical education, whereas simulations and interactive games yield greater cognitive gains and more positive learning attitudes [11, 12]. VR technology offers immersive, interactive environments where nursing students can practice language skills and engage with culturally specific situations in a safe and controlled setting [9, 10, 13]. This approach can improve language fluency, enhance communication confidence, and foster a deeper understanding of cross-cultural care dynamics, addressing a gap identified in the literature by a systematic review and meta-analysis of randomised controlled trials [14].

There is limited empirical evidence on how VR-based, culturally contextualised language training impacts clinical performance, long-term language retention, and cultural communication competence among nursing students. When issues such as limited trust in their capabilities, experiences of marginalisation, and persistent language barriers remain unaddressed, the quality of their educational experience is significantly diminished. Beyond individual implications, these barriers reflect broader structural shortcomings that impede the development of a culturally responsive healthcare workforce [15]. As such, fostering inclusive and supportive clinical learning environments is not merely an educational imperative; it is a critical step toward advancing health equity and improving care for diverse populations. To address these challenges, immersive VR headset-based simulation was used to enhance presence, contextual realism, and interactive communication. The headset-enabled 3D environments, voice-based interaction, and responsive avatars allowed learners to engage in situated language use and culturally nuanced communication that would be difficult to replicate in lower-dimension desktop or mobile formats. For this reason, we aimed to: (1) explore nursing students' perceptions of a VR simulation to support language learning and cultural immersion; and (2) examine how nursing students evaluate the design elements of a VR simulation to support language learning and cultural immersion.

The study was guided by the research questions:

– Quantitative research question: "How do nursing students evaluate the design elements of a VR simulation to support language learning and cultural immersion?"
– Qualitative research question: "What are the perceptions of nursing students regarding a VR simulation to support language learning and cultural immersion?"
– Mixed-methods research question: "In what ways do nursing students' quantitative evaluations of the design elements of a VR simulation converge with, diverge from, or expand upon their qualitative perceptions of its role in supporting language learning and cultural immersion?"

2 Background

Caring for Culturally and Linguistically Diverse (CALD) populations has become increasingly important in the healthcare setting. Language barriers and cultural differences can significantly affect the quality of care and health outcomes [16, 17]. Delivering care to patients involves more than clinical skills; it requires essential intercultural competences such as self-awareness and adaptability, the strategic use of language support tools, and a nuanced understanding of within-group diversity to prevent stereotyping and better align with individual health beliefs and expectations [18]. These elements help avoid stereotypes and ensure that care is responsive to each patient's unique values and expectations.

A systematic review of qualitative studies identified three barriers that hinder the learning of CALD students in clinical placements: the lack of recognition and trust in their motivation and capabilities, the emotional burden of being perceived as different, which undermines their sense of dignity and belonging, and persistent language barriers that impede effective communication and participation in learning opportunities [19]. Therefore, integrating VR-based learning environments that simulate linguistically and culturally diverse interactions with avatar patients offers a powerful pedagogical strategy to enhance cultural competence and communication skills, both of which are critical for fostering equitable, person-centred care in the education of CALD nursing students. These challenges are particularly pronounced within clinical placements, where CALD students frequently face compounded barriers that hinder their learning and integration [10, 20, 21].

3 Methods

3.1 Design

This is a mixed-methods convergent parallel study. An exploratory approach was used for the quantitative component (QUAN), and these findings were further explored in the qualitative component (QUAL). The mixed-methods study was reported following the Mixed Methods Appraisal Tool (MMAT) [22]. Data were obtained through secondary analysis of both datasets from Autumn 2023 to Spring 2024.

3.2 Setting, Population and Recruitment

This study was conducted in an English language degree nursing undergraduate program at two universities of applied sciences in Finland. The program integrates theoretical instruction and clinical practice to support the development of competencies needed for various roles in the Finnish Social and Health Care System. Purposive sampling was used to recruit CALD nursing students for both quantitative and qualitative phases of the study. The eligibility criteria were that nursing students volunteered to participate in the VR learning experience, either assessing a patient to go home after the knee surgery or evaluating and treating a patient in anaphylactic shock [14]. Students went through VR experiences, and straight after, they were interviewed. All invited students consented to participate, resulting in a sample composed of 30 participants. This secondary data analysis focused on a subset of 16 randomly selected CALD nursing students. Only those 16 students contributed complete datasets that allowed the examination of nursing students' perceptions of a VR simulation and explored their understanding of its usability in supporting language learning and cultural immersion.

3.3 VR Learning Experience

The first VR simulation focused on the safe and comprehensive discharge of a patient from a healthcare facility to home. Learners were guided through best practices in patient education, medication reconciliation, follow-up planning, and identification of social or environmental risk factors. This scenario underscored the importance of patient-centred communication, interdisciplinary collaboration, and ensuring continuity of care to reduce readmission risk and promote recovery at home. The second VR simulation immersed healthcare learners in a high-stakes scenario where a patient receives IV medication and, as a result, receives anaphylactic shock. The learner had to rapidly recognise symptoms, initiate emergency interventions, conduct ABCDE evaluation, and coordinate with the interprofessional team, including intramuscular epinephrine administration. The case emphasised clinical decision-making under pressure, adherence to acute care protocols, and effective communication to stabilise the patient in a realistic, time-sensitive environment [23, 24]. This VR learning experience is now further used in several countries, at over 7 universities to educate CALD and national nursing students.

Both VR cases were designed to offer a highly immersive and pedagogically learning experience, each case taking approximately 20–30 min to complete. They were developed by the institution's software engineering laboratory, which adopted a user-centred and co-design approach. A multidisciplinary team (e.g., nurses, health pedagogists, educational scientists, engineers, graphic designers and XR experts) collaborated through the development of the VR simulation, which is experienced through VR headsets and incorporates voice-based interaction. We utilised MetaHuman avatars to represent patients and healthcare team members with high-fidelity facial expressions and body movements, enhancing realism and emotional engagement. Communication within the scenarios was enabled through natural language processing (AI) powered by Google technologies (Local Language Model-LLMs), allowing learners to interact with VR content. To support reflective learning and formative assessment, intermediate evaluations were embedded throughout each case. These checkpoints assessed the learner's understanding of clinical decisions and communication effectiveness in real-time, offering tailored feedback to guide improvement. The combination of responsive avatars, intuitive verbal interaction, and immersive 3D environments provided learners with a deep sense of presence, mirroring real-world complexity and fostering the development of both clinical reasoning and professional competences [23, 24]. Fig. 1 provides examples of both cases.

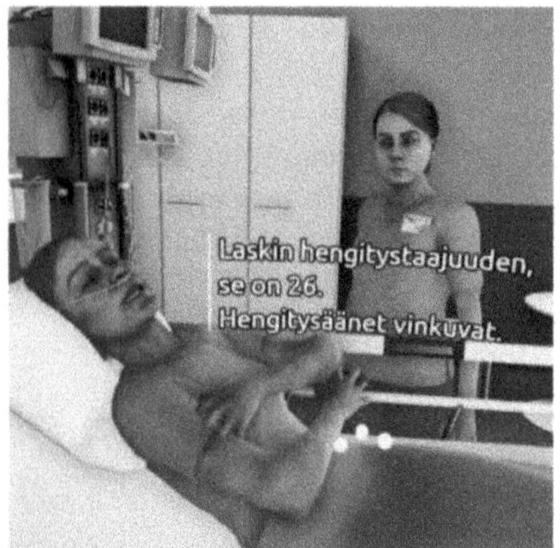

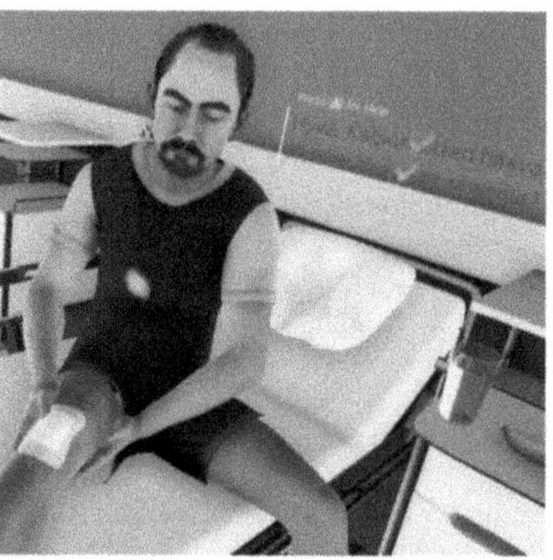

Fig. 1. Examples of VR simulation scenarios

3.4 Data Collection

The sociodemographic questionnaire gathered information on participants' age, native country, linguistic background, time living in Finland, self-assessed Finnish language skills, highest level of education, year of nursing degree studies, overall work experience (not limited to healthcare), and work experience (limited to healthcare). The background information was collected prior to the VR simulation at T0 baseline.

3.5 Quantitative Component

The Simulation Design Scale (Student English Version) [25] was used to evaluate the design elements of a VR simulation to support language learning and cultural immersion. Specifically, to measure if the best simulation design elements were implemented in the simulation and were collected after the VR simulation at T1 measurement. This is a 20-item instrument designed to assess the quality of simulation design across five key domains: objectives/information, support, problem solving, feedback, and fidelity. Each item is rated twice using a five-point Likert scale: once to evaluate the presence of each feature in the simulation (ranging from strongly disagree to strongly agree, with a not applicable option when the statement does not pertain to the specific simulation) and once to assess its importance to the learner (ranging from not important to very important). Additionally, at T1 measurement, task interest was measured using 1–10

Likert scale, ranging from not interesting (1) to highly interesting (10). In this study, Cronbach's alpha for the Simulation Design Scale was 0.88.

3.6   Qualitative Component

In the second phase, qualitative data were gathered through individual interviews conducted by two researchers with expertise in qualitative research. Interviews took place either online via Microsoft Teams or in a classroom setting, depending on the participant's preference. No other individuals were present during the interviews. Each interview lasted approximately 20 min and was audio recorded, transcribed, and supported by field notes. Interviews were not repeated, and participants did not have access to the transcripts for comments or corrections.

Data collection continued until thematic saturation was reached, meaning that the information provided by participants began to repeat and no new themes, insights, or experiences emerged regarding the topic [26].

3.7   Data Analysis

Quantitative data were analysed with IBM SPSS Statistics (31.0.0). Descriptive statistics were used to summarise frequencies and percentages for each item. To explore associations between variables and background information, one-way ANOVA was performed. A significance level of $p < .05$ was adopted. Qualitative data from interviews were transcribed using NVivo software. An inductive content analysis approach was used to analyse the qualitative data [26]. This method allowed themes to emerge directly from the participants' responses without imposing preconceived categories. The analysis involved open coding, categorisation, and abstraction. Transcripts were read multiple times to ensure immersion in the data, and meaningful units were identified and labelled with codes ($n = 64$). These codes were then grouped into subcategories ($n = 6$) and broader categories ($n = 3$) based on recurring patterns. To enhance analytical rigour, the researchers collaboratively reviewed and refined the categories to ensure they accurately reflected the participants' perspectives. Mixed-methods integration occurred during the data analysis phase, when quantitative and qualitative findings were merged and interpreted to generate meta-inferences [27]. Quantitative and qualitative results were integrated following a convergent parallel approach by O'Cathain, Murphy, and Nicholl (2008) [28]. Quantitative and qualitative data were analysed simultaneously and independently, and were merged to identify convergences, divergences and complementary insights through meta-inferences [29].

3.8   Ethical Aspects

The study was approved by the University of Oulu Ethics Committee of Human Sciences in August 2023 (ID7/2023). Anonymity was maintained for all participants, who were identified by random letters of the alphabet (e.g., A, B, C…) and numbers (e.g., 1, 2, 3…). No prior relationship was established between the researchers and the participants. However, participants were informed about the purpose of the study before data collection. All participants provided informed consent in accordance with the EU's General

Data Protection Regulation (GDPR). Research data were treated confidentially, stored securely, and will be destroyed after ten years [30].

4 Results

A total of 16 CALD nursing students were selected for the secondary analysis of this study. Their ages ranged from 19 to 43 years, with a mean age of 31 years. One participant did not provide age information. Participants represented diverse native countries. The most frequently represented country was Nigeria (n = 3), followed by Finland (n = 2) and Nepal (n = 2). The remaining participants (n = 1 each) were from Bangladesh, Ghana, Indonesia, Kenya, Pakistan, the Philippines, the United States of America (USA), Zambia, and Zimbabwe. Linguistic backgrounds were equally diverse. Three participants reported speaking English alongside another language (e.g., Filipino, Swahili, or Twi), while two identified English as their native language. Other native languages included Finnish, Igbo, and Nepali (n = 2 each), as well as Bahasa Indonesia, Bemba, Bengali, Shona, and Urdu (n = 1 each). In terms of residence in Finland, three participants had lived in the country for up to one year, two for 1–2 years, four for 2–5 years, five for 5–10 years, and two for more than 10 years. See Table 1 for the descriptive characteristics of the sample.

4.1 Quantitative Data

One-way ANOVA was conducted to examine whether participants' native country had a statistically significant effect on five dimensions of the simulation-based learning experience: Objectives Support (F1), Support (F2), Problem-Solving (F3), Feedback and Guided Reflection (F4), and Fidelity (F5). The results revealed a statistically significant difference in Fidelity (F5) scores across native country groups (F (2, 13) = 14.91, p < .001), indicating that perceptions of simulation fidelity varied significantly depending on participants' native country. Participants from Africa (M = 4.60, SD = 0.45) and Europe (M = 4.60, SD = 0.34) reported the highest mean for Fidelity, indicating complete agreement on the realism of the simulation. In comparison, participants from Asia (M = 3.90, SD = 0.34) scored lower. Additionally, results for Objectives Support (T1F1) (F (2, 13) = 3.57, p = .058) and Feedback and Guided Reflection (T1F4) (F (2, 13) = 3.70, p = .054) approached significance, suggesting potential group differences that may warrant further investigation with a larger sample. No significant differences were found in Support (T1F2) or Problem-Solving (T1F3) scores (p = .340 and .779, respectively). The effect size (eta squared) for Fidelity (T1F5) was large, indicating a substantial impact of native country on perceptions of simulation fidelity (Table 2).

Table 1. Descriptive characteristics

Variables	n
Self-assessment of Finnish language skills	
Beginner	10
Intermediate	4
Advanced	2
Highest level of education	
High School	4
Vocational Education	1
Bachelor's Degree	8
Master's Degree	3
Doctoral Degree	0
Year of nursing degree studies	
1	11
2	4
3	1
4	0
Work experience (not limited to healthcare work experience)	
Yes, under a year	4
Yes, year or more	7
No	5
Work experience in nursing/healthcare	
Yes, under a year	5
Yes, year or more	2
No	9

Additionally, a one-way ANOVA was performed to assess whether task interest influenced perceptions of five dimensions of simulation-based learning on the same five factors. The analysis revealed a statistically significant effect of task interest on Objective Support (T1F1) $F (4, 11) = 5.73$, $p = .010$), suggesting that participants' interest in the task significantly affected how well they perceived the simulation objectives were supported. However, no significant differences were found in the remaining dimensions: Support (T1F2) $F (4, 11) = 1.71$, $p = .218$; Problem-Solving (T1F3) $F (4, 11) = 1.36$, $p = .310$; Feedback and Guided Reflection (T1F4) $F (4, 11) = 1.74$, $p = .211$. These results indicate that task interest is associated with perceived support for objectives, but does not significantly influence self-evaluation of support, problem-solving, or feedback processes within the simulation perceptions. The effect size (eta squared) for Objectives Support (T1F1) was substantial, indicating that task interest had a meaningful influence on students' perceptions in this dimension (Table 3).

Table 2. ANOVA results examining the effect of participants' native country on five dimensions of simulation-based learning

		Sum of squares	df	Mean square	F	Sig.
T1F1SDS	Between groups	1.700	2	0.850	3.569	0.058
	Within groups	3.097	13	0.238		
	Total	4.798	15			
T1F2SDS	Between groups	0.568	2	0.284	1.172	.340
	Within groups	3.147	13	0.242		
	Total	3.715	15			
T1F3SDS	Between groups	0.194	2	0.097	.255	.779
	Within groups	4.944	13	.380		
	Total	5.137	15			
T1F4SDS	Between groups	1.313	2	.657	3.698	.054
	Within groups	2.308	13	0.178		
	Total	3.621	15			
T1F5SDS	Between groups	2.786	2	1.393	14.912	<.001
	Within groups	1.214	13	0.093		
	Total	4.000	15			

T1F1SDS = objectives/information; T1F2SDS = support; T1F3SDS = problem solving; T1F4SDS = feedback; T1F5SDS = fidelity; Significance level of $p < .05$

Table 3. ANOVA results assessing the influence of task interest on five dimensions of simulation-based learning

		Sum of squares	df	Mean square	F	Sig.
T1F1SDS	Between groups	3.241	4	.810	5.729	.010
	Within groups	1.556	11	.141		
	Total	4.797	15			
T1F2SDS	Between groups	1.423	4	.356	1.708	.218
	Within groups	2.292	11	.208		
	Total	3.715	15			
T1F3SDS	Between groups	1.699	4	.425	1.359	.310
	Within groups	3.439	11	.313		
	Total	5.138	15			
T1F4SDS	Between groups	1.404	4	.351	1.742	.211
	Within groups	2.217	11	.202		
	Total	3.621	15			
T1F5SDS	Between groups	1.308	4	.327	1.337	.317
	Within groups	2.692	11	.245		
	Total	4.000	15			

T1F1SDS = objectives/information; T1F2SDS = support; T1F3SDS = problem solving; T1F4SDS = feedback; T1F5SDS = fidelity; Significance level of $p < .05$

4.2 Qualitative Data

Table 4 outlines the findings derived from an inductive content analysis of the interview data. Three main categories emerged as follows: (1) VR for Language Learning and Cultural Immersion; (2) Challenges and Limitations of VR in Language Learning; and (3) Motivation and Satisfaction with VR Learning Experience. Each category encompasses subcategories and illustrative codes reflecting the participants' perceptions. The analysis revealed that students recognised VR as a useful educational tool to enhance Finnish language learning and cultural understanding. However, participants also reported technical difficulties and emotional challenges such as frustration.

Table 4. Content analysis

Code	Sub-category	Category
– VR as a strategy to improve communication with the patient; – VR as a potential strategy for learning Finnish language; – VR helps language learning; – VR is good for preparing for clinical practice; – VR as a potential strategy for immigrant education; – Boosting language learning through technology; – Language learning through repetition; – Feeling like a real experience through VR; – Improvement in pronunciation of the language; Recognition of the role of language in VR.	Language learning	VR for language learning and cultural immersion

(continued)

Table 4. (*continued*)

Code	Sub-category	Category
– Language Barriers; – Language Barriers in Immigration to Finland; – Prediction of clinical practice; – Predictions of practice based on cultural aspects; – Immersion in Finnish culture; – Recognition of the importance of self-confidence for professional development; – Recognition of the need for language improvement; – Learning related to professional development; – Cultural differences in patient care; – Finnish people converse less, and a careful choice of words is needed in the dialogue; – Difficulties in interpersonal relationships in the Finnish context; – Lack of practice due to an immigrant background.	Cultural immersion within professional practice	VR for language learning and cultural immersion
– System failed to respond; – Difficulty in pronouncing Finnish words; – Difficulty in forming correct sentences in Finnish; – Difficulty in being recognized by the VR system; – Lack of understanding of the situation presented in the VR; – VR is good for visual learning, but might not be for everyone; – Repetition of words made the process difficult; – Limited time for the proposed activity.	Technical and system limitations	Challenges and limitations of VR in language learning

(continued)

Table 4. (*continued*)

Code	Sub-category	Category
– Uncertainty in making decision through the system; – No learning through VR; – No new learning; – Frustration caused by the repetition of words; – Unanticipated questions arise; – Stress related to repetition – The Finnish language is challenging for CALD students; – The Finnish language as the biggest challenge in VR; – Perceiving VR as a game; – Fear of making mistakes when learning a new language; – Negative reactions associated with VR limitations; – Frustration in learning Finnish language through VR; – Lack of knowledge about Finnish culture.	Uncertainty and frustration in the learning process	Challenges and limitations of VR in language learning
– Motivation to learn Finnish language; – Confidence and motivation for learning; – VR as a strategy that aligns imagination and learning; – Satisfaction with VR; – VR as a creative and enjoyable tool; – VR seems a creative strategy; – VR as an interactive environment; – Fun through VR; – VR increases motivation since it eliminates the feeling of nervousness; – VR is a motivating strategy.	Motivational factors and engagement with VR	Motivation and satisfaction with VR learning experience

(*continued*)

Table 4. (*continued*)

Code	Sub-category	Category
– Satisfaction with the VR experience; – Feeling encouraged by having a complete conversation; – Feeling more confident through the VR experience; – Satisfaction with the use of VR; – Satisfaction with VR; – Feeling like a real-life experience through VR; – Persistence to achieve good results in patient care; – VR as a strategy to improve self-confidence, especially for shy people; – Recognition of how to meet the patient's unique needs; – VR as a strategy for the future of universities; – Feeling like a real experience through VR.	Satisfaction and personal growth through VR	Motivation and satisfaction with VR learning experience

4.3 VR for Language Learning and Cultural Immersion

VR is changing how students learn language and immerse themselves in different cultures. By simulating real-world experiences, VR enhances language learning and enables culture immersion, making it especially beneficial for individuals that came from other cultural realities. However, despite its advantages, VR technology also faces some challenges including technical and system limitations and the uncertainty that some students experience when adapting to a virtual learning experience. Nevertheless, its potential to boost motivation and engagement aligns with the satisfaction derived from interactive and dynamic learning experiences, positioning VR as a promising tool for fostering language learning and providing cultural competence.

VR provides a dynamic platform for language learning, especially for CALD students who often face challenges in practising the local language due to limited opportunities for conversation. This method enhances vocabulary, improves grammar retention, boosts confidence in speaking, and inspires students to explore additional ways to develop their language skills. Several participants highlighted its value. For example, Student H explained that VR provided "[…] a perfect platform to talk to someone". Student M noted that "[…] every letter is read separately. I could practice. Also, we do not have enough lessons to practice Finnish, so I find that some things which I have learnt I tend to forget because we only have it like once a week that we can practice conversation with new words we learned at school but not more [...]. Similarly, student 17, who had lived in Finland for over eight years, emphasized that motivation is "[...] one of the best tools to learn any language, not only Finnish, or any things [...].

Incorporating VR into nursing education allows students to immerse themselves in cultural aspects through realistic scenarios, helping them better understand the needs and preferences of patients. This immersive approach is particularly valuable for future healthcare professionals working in multicultural environments, where cultural competence is essential to providing patient-centered care. Participants reflected on how VR supported their adaptation to Finnish culture and healthcare practices. As student G noted, "[...] It helped me a lot in understanding how things are going to happen here in Finland. You are in the technology world now [...]". Student C appreciated the cultural insight, explaining that "we all don't know what to expect from Finnish people and culture. So, if you like, give us that impression in Virtual reality – it's nice! (Student C). Similarly, Student M emphasized that, upon moving to Finland "[...] you have to interact with people in Finnish, so the simulation would help you to start learning the language so you can then learn about other things like culture." These reflections show how VR supports students' adaptation to Finland by easing cultural immersion, fostering language learning, and providing practical insights into local social and technological contexts.

4.4 Challenges and Limitations of VR in Language Learning

VR's effectiveness can be limited by challenges related to voice recognition and communication, as highlighted by student feedback. For instance, some students noted that the system struggled to understand their words, even when spoken clearly, causing frustration and interrupting the learning flow. Student C noted, "we had this problem and it didn't understand my words," while Student 21 added that despite speaking clearly, "sometimes it didn't understand me either... for those who don't speak Finnish clearly, it could get in the way." Similarly, Student G described "a lot of difficulties in communication," explaining that they had to pronounce words "exactly correctly" to receive a response from virtual patients, making the experience "quite challenging." These accounts highlight the importance of improving voice recognition technology to ensure smoother, more intuitive, and inclusive VR interactions.

Adapting to VR-based learning can be challenging for some students, leading to feelings of uncertainty or frustration. This may stem from difficulties in navigating the virtual environment, sensory overload, or the lack of clear instructions, which can affect their confidence and motivation to learn. As Student M shared, "sometimes you have to repeat the word... three times in the simulation... to pronounce it correctly," which could become discouraging. Similarly, Student A explained, "I had to ask what to say or do constantly from our supervisor... I could not use it unfortunately," highlighting how the lack of independence in the simulation hindered their learning experience. These accounts highlight how challenges and limitations of VR, especially difficulties with pronunciation and reliance on supervision, restricted students' autonomy and, at times, diminished their learning motivation and satisfaction.

4.5 Motivation and Satisfaction with VR Learning Experience

VR's interactive and gamified nature increases learner engagement, as it transforms traditional, passive learning into an active and enjoyable experience. Features like role-playing, instant feedback, and virtual rewards motivate users to practice more frequently, making the learning process both exciting and rewarding. Student 18 described it as "[…] 200 % interactive […]", highlighting the difference from simply "sitting in a room" to engaging directly with a patient. Student M echoed this, noting the satisfaction of "[…] I was happy about it because I felt like I'm interacting with the real patients in Finnish". Similarly, student 17 admitted expecting the activity to be "a bit more boring", but was surprised to feel a genuine connection, even "cheering"for the virtual patient by the end.

The sense of accomplishment derived from mastering language and cultural skills in VR enhances learners' overall satisfaction. Additionally, the immersive experience promotes personal growth by building confidence, improving adaptability, and fostering a deeper appreciation for cultural diversity. As Student 18 described, understanding more of what patients were saying was highly motivating, leading them to feel, "[…] Yes, I, I'm improving, when I understand what the patient is talking, what the patient is asking. So, this really… It's it's, I think my self, self-estimation really has gone up." Similarly, Student 20 highlighted the value of VR for language acquisition, noting that while reading conversations from a book was sometimes difficult, VR made it "[…] very quickly, very easily, clearly to know what's what situation is in it?". These reflections emphasize the potential of VR to foster motivation and self-confidence by helping students better understand patient interactions and making language learning more accessible than traditional methods.

4.6 Mixed-Methods Results

When viewed from a broader perspective, the quantitative and qualitative findings reinforce one another, with both pointing to VR's potential to foster engagement, cultural immersion, and skill development. Higher perceived realism and immersion, as described qualitatively, were mirrored in the quantitative ratings of fidelity among some participant groups, suggesting that positive experiential impressions aligned with stronger evaluations of authenticity. Similarly, students' narratives about increased motivation and clearer connections between VR and their learning goals were consistent with the higher ratings given by those with greeted task interest, indicating a shared recognition of VR's role in supporting objectives.

While quantitative scores suggested relatively even experiences of support and problem-solving opportunities across groups, qualitative findings added nuance by highlighting how these elements were experienced in practice, often as highly motivating, confidence-building and interactive. Challenges such as technical limitations and frustrations with repetitive processes were present in the qualitative data but absent from the quantitative measures, showing that some aspects influencing learners' experiences were not fully captured by the survey. This interplay suggests the value of integrating both perspectives to gain a fuller understanding of VR's strengths and areas for improvement.

The study was designed as a convergent mixed-methods study. The integration of quantitative and qualitative findings occurred during interpretation. The quantitative findings evaluated the quality of simulation design elements (e.g., objectives, support, feedback, fidelity). In parallel, the qualitative findings report technical difficulties, pronunciation challenges and frustration, which helped explain why no clear differences were observed in quantitative measures of support and problem-solving. These findings informed the meta-inferences, suggesting that while VR was generally experienced as immersive and motivating, technical and contextual factors have also been considered.

5 Discussion

This mixed-methods study aimed to examine nursing students' perceptions of a VR simulation and explore their understanding of its usability in supporting language learning and cultural immersion. Participants described VR as an engaging and interactive environment for practising communication and reflecting on the cultural aspects of care, with reported benefits in motivation, engagement, and personal growth, despite some technical challenges.

VR can be used as a complementary tool in nursing education, enhancing skill acquisition by simulating realistic clinical scenarios in a safe environment, especially when access to real patients is limited [31]. As nursing education continues to evolve [32–35], VR should keep pace with emerging trends such as Artificial Intelligence (AI), ensuring that technological advancements are integrated thoughtfully to meet the future needs of healthcare training. AI can be leveraged to address students' individual needs, making it possible to offer personalised learning experiences [36] and further strengthening the effectiveness of technological strategies in nursing education [37]. High-fidelity simulation, when embedded within a multidimensional pedagogical framework, can be purposefully integrated with classroom learning and high-fidelity simulation to align theory with immersive, scenario-based practice. Grounded in socio-constructivist, experiential, and self-regulated learning theories, this integration enhances critical thinking, adaptability, digital competence, and collaborative decision-making, ensuring technological tools are used to meet the evolving needs of healthcare training [12].

Although students from Africa and Europe demonstrated higher perceptions of simulation fidelity, overall, all students, including those from Asia, demonstrated strong scores in this domain. Perceived fidelity is a key element in simulation-based learning, as emphasised in Jeffries' Simulation Framework, which identifies realism as essential for promoting student engagement, satisfaction, and the effective transfer of knowledge to clinical practice [38]. High-fidelity simulation enhances the authenticity of the learning experience, thereby supporting deeper learning and the development of clinical competence [39, 40]. Our findings suggest that VR may support learners' perceived understanding of cultural nuances and healthcare practice, particularly for students encountering unfamiliar clinical norms or patient expectations.

Task interest appears to play an important role in how students engage with and perceive the value of simulation-based learning. Prior students have highlighted that when learners find the experience meaningful and interactive, their motivation and perceived learning outcomes tend to improve [41, 42]. This perspective aligns with the idea that engagement enhances not only satisfaction but also the depth of learning in simulation environments. The sense of "interacting with real patients" expressed by some participants reflects how immersive scenarios can create authentic learning experiences that support both skill development and confidence. This reinforces the importance of designing simulations that go beyond technical realism to also consider student interest and emotional involvement, thereby maximising their educational potential.

Based on our findings, it is essential to make adjustments in the VR simulation to ensure alignment with learners' needs. Although the simulation integrates LLMs to support language-based interactions, some challenges, such as technical limitations and learner adaptation, need to be addressed to maximise its effectiveness [23, 24]. While LLMs are designed to adapt to individual needs by providing personalised, interactive, and responsive language support, their effectiveness depends on the broader pedagogical and technological context in which they are embedded [43, 44]. While VR provides enhanced realism and presence, lower-immersion alternatives (e.g., desktop simulations) are more cost-effective, scalable and easier to implement with larger groups [45]. Potential drawbacks of high immersion, such as cybersickness and accessibility barriers, must also be considered [46]. These challenges were reflected in the present study, where some participants reported stress and frustration associated with the limitations of the VR experience. Therefore, further refinement of the VR simulation is needed to improve technical stability, better support learner engagement, and embed LLM-based interactions within a clear and coherent instructional framework. These adjustments are essential to ensure that the technology supports language learning, cultural immersion, and active student engagement, rather than functioning as an isolated technical feature.

Although our findings indicate that VR has been beneficial in addressing both language and cultural barriers, the existing literature remains limited on that. For example, a multimethod study aimed to develop and evaluate the feasibility of a VR simulation to enhance cross-cultural communication skills in nursing education. The simulation scenarios were designed with the assumption that communication between nurses and patients was linguistically accessible, thereby positioning cultural differences as the primary challenge to be navigated [9]. This highlights a gap in the literature and suggests that linguistic aspects related to VR-based training warrant further research.

Investigating CALD nursing students' perceptions of VR-based learning experiences is crucial for evaluating the accessibility and acceptability of this innovative educational tool. Their insights can inform curriculum development and help educators tailor immersive experiences to meet specific learning needs. By centring students' voices, the study also aligns with learner-centred pedagogies, ensuring that technological advancements in nursing education are both meaningful and responsive to the challenges of preparing globally competent healthcare professionals. As this study focused on participants' perceptions rather than objective outcomes, findings related to the effectiveness of VR for language learning or educational outcomes are limited. Future research should incorporate measures of language proficiency, communication performance, and cultural competence to better evaluate these outcomes.

This study has some strengths and limitations that should be considered. Although the data were collected in the Finnish context, the mixed-method analysis was led by an international research team member. While it could highlight important cultural aspects, the brief experience in the Finnish educational context could overshadow key data.

The multicultural research team allowed validation by a Finnish researcher, which supported contextual and methodological cohesion. The quantitative component of this study involved a small sample (n = 16), reflecting the limited size of the cohort available during the implementation period. Accordingly, claims regarding statistical influence or generalizability were intentionally minimised, and the findings are presented as exploratory to inform future research with larger samples. Although purposive sampling and the small sample size of CALD students limit the generalizability of the findings, the study provides in-depth, context-specific findings that can guide future research.

6 Conclusion

Our findings show that motivation and cultural connection can enhance VR-based learning. However, its effectiveness in terms of learning outcomes was not directly measured and should be examined in future research. Participants' native country and their cultural background significantly influenced experiences and perceptions of simulation fidelity, with African and European nursing students rating realism higher than Asian students. Task interest also shaped perceptions of how well learning objectives were supported. These factors need to be addressed in the design and implementation of VR-based education to enhance learning outcomes. In the future, AI agency could play a pivotal role in supporting and encouraging self-directed learning by fostering cultural diversity and ensuring greater cultural acceptance.

Acknowledgments. We would like to acknowledge the support of The University of Oulu & The Academy of Finland Profi 7 (352788) for supporting this study. This study was funded by the National Council for Scientific and Technological Development (CNPq), Brazil, and the Coordination for the Improvement of Higher Education Personnel (CAPES), Brazil.

Disclosure of Interests. The authors have no competing interests to declare that are relevant to the content of this article.

References

1. Jones, C.B., Sherwood, G.D.: The globalization of the nursing workforce: pulling the pieces together. Nurs. Outlook. **62**(1), 59–63 (2014)
2. Villamin, P., Lopez, V., Thapa, D.K., Cleary, M.: Retaining a multicultural nursing workforce: a self-determination theory perspective. J. Transcult. Nurs. **36**(4), 352–362 (2025)
3. ICN   Homepage.   https://www.icn.ch/sites/default/files/2023-04/PS_C_International%20c areer%20mobility%20and%20ethical%20nurse%20recruitment_En.pdfAccessed   04   Jan 2026
4. IOM Homepage. https://publications.iom.int/books/world-migration-report-2022. Accessed 01 Apr 2026
5. Gradellini, C., Gómez-Cantarino, S., Dominguez-Isabel, P., Molina-Gallego, B., Mecugni, D., Ugarte-Gurrutxaga, M.I.: Cultural competence and cultural sensitivity education in university nursing courses. A scoping review. Front. Psychol. **12**, 682920 (2021)
6. Ličen, S., Prosen, M.: The development of cultural competences in nursing students and their significance in shaping the future work environment: a pilot study. BMC Med. Educ. **23**(1), 819 (2023)

7. Sharifi, N., Adib-Hajbaghery, M., Najafi, M.: Cultural competence in nursing: a concept analysis. Int. J. Nurs. Stud. **99**, 103386 (2019)
8. Hua, C., Wang, J.: Virtual reality-assisted language learning: a follow-up review (2018-2022). Front. Psychol. **14**, 1153642 (2023)
9. Chae, D., Kim, J., Kim, K., Ryu, J., Asami, K., Doorenbos, A.Z.: An immersive virtual reality simulation for cross-cultural communication skills: development and feasibility. Clin. Simul. Nurs. **77**, 13–22 (2023)
10. Ropponen, P. et al.: Culturally and linguistically diverse nursing students' experiences of integration into the working environment: a qualitative study. Nurse Educ. Today. **120**, 105654 (2023)
11. Vogel, J.J., Vogel, D.S., Cannon-Bowers, J., Bowers, C.A., Muse, K., Wright, M.: Computer gaming and interactive simulation for learning: a meta-analysis. J. Educ. Comput. Res. **34**(3), 229–243 (2006)
12. Mikkonen, K. et al.: Multidimensional pedagogical framework for interprofessional education: blending classroom, high fidelity and extended reality simulation. Nurse Educ. Today. **154**, 106838 (2025)
13. Wu, J.G., Miller, L., Huang, Q., Wang, M.: Learning with immersive virtual reality: an exploratory study of Chinese college nursing students. RELC J. **54**(3), 697–713 (2021)
14. Ropponen, P. et al.: Impacts of VR simulation on nursing students' competence, confidence, and satisfaction: a systematic review and meta-analysis of randomised controlled trials. Nurse Educ. Today. **152**, 106756 (2025)
15. Suleiman, K. et al.: Factors associated with the integration of culturally and linguistically diverse nurses into healthcare Organisations: a systematic review of quantitative studies. J. Nurs. Manag. **5887450** (2024)
16. Harrison, R. et al.: Beyond translation: engaging with culturally and linguistically diverse consumers. Health Expect. **23**(1), 159–168 (2020)
17. Khatri, R.B., Assefa, Y.: Access to health services among culturally and linguistically diverse populations in the Australian universal health care system: issues and challenges. BMC Public Health. **22**(1), 880 (2022)
18. Schouten, B.C., Manthey, L., Scarvaglieri, C.: Teaching intercultural communication skills in healthcare to improve care for culturally and linguistically diverse patients. Patient Educ. Couns. **115**, 107890 (2023)
19. Mikkonen, K., Elo, S., Kuivila, H.M., Tuomikoski, A.M., Kääriäinen, M.: Culturally and linguistically diverse healthcare students' experiences of learning in a clinical environment: a systematic review of qualitative studies. Int. J. Nurs. Stud. **54**, 173–187 (2016)
20. Jeong, S.Y. et al.: Understanding and enhancing the learning experiences of culturally and linguistically diverse nursing students in an Australian bachelor of nursing program. Nurse Educ. Today. **31**(3), 238–244 (2011)
21. Ivziku, D. et al.: International nursing students and clinical learning environments: a convergent mixed-methods study. Nurse Educ. Pract. **80**, 104144 (2024)
22. Hong, Q.N. et al.: The mixed methods appraisal tool (MMAT) version 2018 for information professionals and researchers. Educ. Inf. **34**(4), 285–291 (2018)
23. Koutonen, J., Partanen, R., Taikina-aho, Juha-Matti. https://kulttuuriosaaja.blogspot.com/2022/10/. last accessed 2026/01/04
24. Mikkonen, K. et al.: How does human-Centred extended reality support healthcare students' learning in clinical conditions? In: Sarestoniemi, M., Keikhosrokiani, P., Singh, D., Harjula, E., Tiulpin, A., Jansson, M., Isomursu, M., van Gils, M., Saarakkala, S., Reponen, J. (eds.) Digital Health and Wireless Solutions. NCDHWS 2024. Communications in Computer and Information Science. Springer, Cham (2024)
25. National League for Nursing. Simulation Design Scale© (Student Version) (2005)

26. Kyngäs, H., Kääriäinen, M., Elo, S.: The trustworthiness of content analysis. In: Kyngäs, H., Mikkonen, K., Kääriäinen, M. (eds.) The Application of Content Analysis in Nursing Science Research. Springer, Cham (2020)
27. McCrudden, M.T., Marchand, G., Schutz, P.A.: Joint displays for mixed methods research in psychology. Methods Psychol. **5**, 100067 (2021)
28. O'Cathain, A., Murphy, E., Nicholl, J.: The quality of mixed methods studies in health services research. J. Health Serv. Res. Policy. **13**(2), 92–98 (2008)
29. Creswell, J., Plano-Clark, V.: Designing and conducting mixed methods research. Chapter 3. Sage. Los Angeles. (2011)
30. General Data Protection Regulation Homepage, http://data.europa.eu/eli/reg/2016/679/oj. Accessed 01 Apr 2026
31. Jallad, S.T., Işık, B.: The effectiveness of immersive virtual reality simulation as an innovative learning strategy for Acquisition of Clinical Skills in nursing education: experimental design. Games Health J. **14**(2), 110–118 (2025)
32. Risling, T.: Educating the nurses of 2025: technology trends of the next decade. Nurse Educ. Pract. **22**, 89–92 (2017)
33. Poindexter, K.: The future of nursing education: reimagined. Nurs. Educ. Perspect. **42**(6), 335–336 (2021)
34. Sumpter, D., Blodgett, N., Beard, K., & Howard, V. Transforming nursing education in response to the future of nursing 2020-2030 report. Nurs. Outlook, 70(6) Suppl 1, S20-S31 (2022)
35. Araújo, A.A.C., Gardim, L., Bernardes, A., Mendes, I.A.C., Mikkonen, I.: Embracing artificial intelligence (AI) in nursing education through wearable technology: innovation-driven teaching. Investigación y Educación en Enfermería. **43**(2), 1 (2025)
36. Araújo, A.A.C., Gardim, L., Pramila-Savukoski, S., Mendes, I.A.C., Mikkonen, I.: Artificial intelligence (AI) in nursing education: an evolutionary concept analysis. Nurse Education Today [under analysis]. (2026)
37. Ma, J. et al.: The role of artificial intelligence in shaping nursing education: a comprehensive systematic review. Nurse Educ. Pract. **84**, 104345 (2025)
38. Jeffries, P.R., Rodgers, B., Adamson, K.: NLN Jeffries simulation theory: brief narrative description. Nurs. Educ. Perspect. **36**(5), 292–293 (2015)
39. Nair, M.A., Muthu, P., Abuijlan, I.A.M.: The effectiveness of high-Fidelity simulation on clinical competence among nursing students. SAGE Open Nurs. **10**, 23779608241249357 (2024)
40. Casallas-Hernández, N., Castillo-Daza, C.A., González-Guzmán, V.A.: Acceptance and effectiveness of high-fidelity simulation in nursing education: application of the technology acceptance model (TAM). Clin. Simul. Nurs. **105**, 101765 (2025)
41. Kong, Y.: The role of experiential learning on students' motivation and classroom engagement. Front. Psychol. **12**, 771272 (2021)
42. Lo, K.W.K., Ngai, G., Chan, S.C.F., Kwan, K.P.: How students' motivation and learning experience affect their service-learning outcomes: a structural equation modeling analysis. Front. Psychol. **13**, 825902 (2022)
43. Rodrigues, D., Cruz-Correia, R.: Large language models in nursing education: state-of-the-art. Stud. Health Technol. Inform. **316**, 1024–1028 (2024)
44. Harrington, J., Booth, R.G., Jackson, K.T.: Large language models in nursing education: concept analysis. JMIR Nurs. **8**, e77948 (2025)

45. Liaw, S.Y. et al.: Desktop virtual reality versus face-to-face simulation for team-training on stress levels and performance in clinical deterioration: a randomised controlled trial. J. Gen. Intern. Med. **38**(1), 67–73 (2023)
46. Baniasadi, T., Ayyoubzadeh, S.M., Mohammadzadeh, N.: Challenges and practical considerations in applying virtual reality in medical education and treatment. Oman Med. J. **35**(3), e125 (2020)

Paramedic and Nursing Students' Experiences of Developing Pre-hospital Emergency Care Competence Using Mobile Game - A Qualitative Study

Sari Pramila-Savukoski[1,2]([envelope]) [iD], Sofia Jaakkola[1] [iD], Heli-Maria Kuivila[1] [iD], Petri Roivainen[3] [iD], Erika Jarva[1] [iD], Hanna-Mari Ylitalo[1] [iD], and Kristina Mikkonen[1,4] [iD]

[1] Research Unit of Health Sciences and Technology (HST), University of Oulu, Oulu, Finland
`sari.pramila-savukoski@oulu.fi`
[2] Lapland University of Applied Sciences, Rovaniemi, Finland
[3] Oulu University of Applied Sciences, Oulu, Finland
[4] Medical Research Center Oulu, Oulu University Hospital, Oulu, Finland

Abstract. The use of mobile games in nursing education is increasing. More research is needed on mobile games designed for pre-hospital emergency care education. Aim of this study was to describe paramedic and nursing students' experiences of developing pre-hospital emergency care competence through BREATHe: Paramedic – mobile game. A total of 14 paramedic and nursing students from Finland were interviewed. Data was collected using individual semi-structured interviews during the summer of 2024 and analysed using inductive content analysis. Students found that the BREATHe: paramedic mobile game enhanced their theoretical knowledge, systematic assessment, and decision-making skills. Its flexibility, feedback, structured tasks, and unlimited practice opportunities increased motivation and competence. However, while it complemented face-to-face simulations, it could not replace them for practical skills and did not engage all students. As a conclusion, The BREATHe: Paramedic mobile game is a flexible educational tool that supports competence development. Its integration into higher and continuing education could enhance versatility through diverse patient scenarios and AI-driven interactivity, e.g. part of mixed reality intervention.

Keywords: Competence · Education · Learning · Mobile game · Paramedic · Pre-hospital emergency care

1 Introduction

Emergency medical service workers provide pre-hospital emergency care to the suddenly ill and injured, and their competence is crucial for patient safety [1, 2]. Pre-hospital emergency care means providing critical care and stabilisation to patients at the scene of an

---

S. Pramila-Savukoski and S. Jaakkola—equal contribution.

M. Särestöniemi et al. (Eds.): NCDHWS 2026, CCIS 3009, pp. 321–336, 2026.
https://doi.org/10.1007/978-3-032-28812-7_23

emergency and during transport to healthcare facilities. That requires knowing about emergency care, the ability to perform demanding care procedures independently, skills in using technical equipment, collaboration and communication, systematic assessment and decision-making, among others. [1–4]. In Finland, there are statutory educational requirements for those working in emergency medical services. A basic-level emergency care unit must be staffed by at least a licensed practical nurse specialised in emergency care (level 4 of the European Qualification Framework), while an advanced-level emergency care unit requires at least a paramedic with a Bachelor's degree in paramedicine or a registered nurse (EQF 6) with 30 ECTS (European Credit Transfer and Accumulation System) credits in emergency care studies (EQF 6) [5–7].

Mobile games are a promising and increasingly used method in nursing education [8–11]. The benefits of mobile games include flexibility, immediate feedback and unlimited repetition [8, 12, 13]. However, there is little research on mobile games designed for pre-hospital emergency care education. In one mobile game, the urgency of a stroke patient was assessed by students with the same accuracy but at a faster rate compared to simulation teaching [14]. Another mobile game showed promise for training in trauma patient care, although some challenges were noted due to the small screen size [15].

In Finland, the mobile game BREATHe: paramedic (Fig. 1) has been developed to enhance pre-hospital emergency care competence (PR, JU, JH). PR has supported developing the mobile game from pedagogical point of view in 2020. The mobile game consists of virtual simulations that can be followed and played on a smartphone or tablet screen (websites in English) [16]. BREATHe: Paramedic is a commercial mobile game that has been validated for use before being released to the market [16]. It is available for paramedic and nursing students nationally on Campusonline online platform [17]. Students played the mobile game with their own mobile devices. The student can choose whether they want to play the game at a basic (EQF 4) or advanced level (EQF 6), and the mobile game requires them to act according to their level. The app includes more than 170 different games about emergency care patient situations. Students performed all the tasks. The treatment guidelines required by the game are based on national and international evidence-based treatment recommendations about different diseases and care guidelines [16, 18].

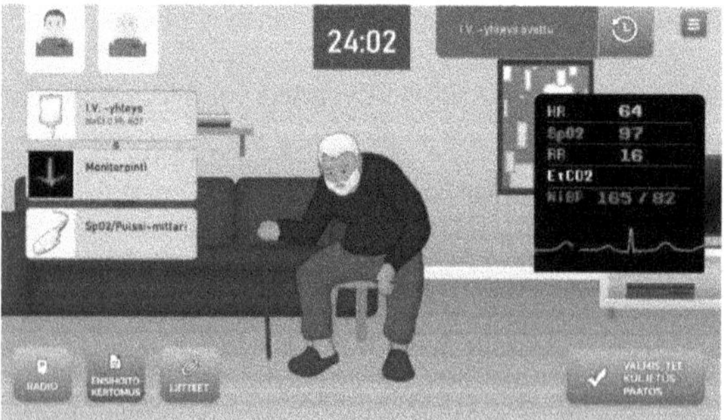

Fig. 1. BREATHe: Paramedic mobile game view on screen.

The areas evaluated in the game include systematic examination, medication treatment, emergency care measures, electrocardiography (ECG) interpretation, vital signs assessment, use of status measures, consultation and transport decision [16]. These competence areas are essential in pre-hospital emergency care [e.g. 1–4]. When the players have made a transport decision regarding the virtual patient's treatment location and urgency, they receive feedback on their performance. The mobile game has simplified graphics, and the patient is visually almost unchanged. However, the patient's position can be changed, and the patient can be transferred to an ambulance. The values on the defibrillator monitor, which measure vital functions, change as the simulation progresses. Although the target group of the mobile game was primarily paramedic students, it is also used in the workplace to train paramedics. The game is used in the workplace primarily as a supplementary learning tool. Rather than serving as initial skills training, it is employed to reinforce clinical reasoning, situational awareness, and decision-making in pre-hospital emergency care that is important for paramedics and registered nurses [16]. Ylitalo et al. [11] have found that BREATHe: Paramedic – mobile game has improved nursing and paramedic students subjective, self-assessed competence and objectively especially medication management. The mobile game for developing pre-hospital emergency care competence is unique nationally and internationally.

This study aims to describe paramedic and nursing students' experiences of developing pre-hospital emergency care competence using BREATHe: Paramedic –mobile game. Research results can be used for the development of evidence-based education as well as continuing education. Understanding experiences with mobile games is needed to develop flexible paramedic and nursing training and innovative solutions in supporting the individual learning process and competence in rural areas. The research question was: What were the experiences of paramedic and nursing students in developing their pre-hospital emergency care competence through a mobile game?

2   Methods

2.1   Study Design

The research was conducted as a qualitative descriptive study using inductive content analysis [19]. The research was based on critical realism, which acknowledges the existence of objective reality and that our perceptions of reality are socially constructed and change [20]. The study was informed by a critical realist perspective, which guided the analysis beyond surface-level descriptions towards identifying underlying mechanisms and contextual factors influencing participants' experiences. This perspective was also reflected in the interpretation and discussion of findings, where individual accounts were considered in relation to broader structural and social conditions.

2.2   Participants

A total of 14 paramedic (n = 9) and nursing (n = 5) students around Finland were involved in the study. In the Finnish context, registered nurses are eligible to work in emergency medical services, including pre-hospital emergency care. Consequently, core competencies related to assessment, decision-making, and emergency interventions in pre-hospital settings overlap substantially between paramedic and nursing education. The students played the mobile game between 8 January 2024 and 12 May 2024 via the Campusonline online platform. Students were recruited by purposive sampling by asking about willingness at the time the student started the course. The inclusion criteria for participation in the study were: 1) the participant was paramedic or nursing student; 2) the student had played the BREATHe: Paramedic mobile game from start to the end; and 3) wanted to participate in a voluntary interview in the end of the course 4) was studying in a university of applied sciences where the ethical permission was granted.

Students were recruited by posting information on the course about participation in the study in the end of the course. Students who met the inclusion criteria enrolled for the interview through the online survey and reporting platform, Webropol. The Webropol link was integrated into the course and included contact information with the researcher. Also, the effect of playing BREATHEe: Paramedic mobile game on pre-hospital emergency care competence has been studied and will be published in a separate publication.

2.3 Data Collection

The data was collected through video and mobile phone interviews lasting approximately half an hour (24–36 min) in the summer of 2024. The interviewer was a researcher (SJ) with a paramedic background but had no relation or connection with the participants. Semi-structured, individual thematic interviews were used, and the students were free to talk about their experiences concerning the themes [21] (Table 1). The themes were "Developing pre-hospital emergency care competence by playing the BREATHEe: Paramedic mobile game" and "Mobile game experience and usability". The themes were developed based on theoretical evidence about mobile games [12, 22] and pre-hospital emergency care competence development [4]. We conducted a focused mapping of literature on competence development in pre-hospital emergency care and learning with mobile/serious games to identify recurring constructs relevant to our context. Also, literature about serious games was utilised in generating questions [23, 24]. The themes were made as open as possible because there was no clear prior understanding of the topic. Background information about the students was collected (e.g., year of study and attitude toward gaming), but the mobile game did not provide data on how many times a student completed different tasks. The pilot interview was conducted and included in the data analysis, as no changes were made to the questions. The interviews were recorded. Data was anonymised during transcription. The data was analysed by the first authors (SPS, SJ) and the analysis was discussed with several researchers (H-MK, KM). After 14 interviews, it was noticed that no new information emerged from the interviews, and the data started to repeat itself, i.e. the data was saturated. According to Elo et al. [25], saturation occurs when additional data ceases to contribute new information relevant to the content categories, and the researcher can confirm that the data are sufficiently rich and comprehensive for the purposes of inductive content analysis. Therefore, no additional students were interviewed.

Table 1. Themes and questions of the interviews.

Theme: Developing pre-hospital emergency care competence by playing the BREATHe: Paramedic mobile game	1.From your experience, how did playing the BREATHe: Paramedic mobile game changed your pre-hospital emergency care competence? 2. How would you describe developing pre-hospital emergency care competence through playing the BREATHe: Paramedic mobile game?
Theme: Experiences about BREATHe: Paramedic mobile game	1.What kind of experiences do you have with the BREATHe: Paramedic mobile game as a game? 2. How would you describe the influence of the BREATHe: Paramedic mobile game as a method to develop pre-hospital emergency care competence? 3. From your experience, what kind of role is appropriate for the BREATHe: Paramedic mobile game in paramedic studies or development as a registered nurse? 4. From your experience, what kind of timing is appropriate for BREATHe: Paramedic mobile game in paramedic studies or your development as a registered nurse? 5. Would you like to share more on the BREATHe: Paramedic mobile game in the context of developing your pre-hospital emergency care competence?

2.4 Data Analysis

The data was analysed using inductive content analysis, as the aim was to explore students' experiences and to gain understanding of a phenomenon on which there was limited research data [19]. The data was transcribed in the Microsoft Office Word file and read several times. A word or phrase that addressed the research question was selected as the unit of analysis. The transcribed interviews were systematically reviewed with the research question. Relevant expressions were extracted from the data, coded (n = 1286), and codes were grouped into subcategories (n = 175), subcategories into categories (n = 32) and categories into main categories (n = 5) to answer the research question.

2.5 Trustworthiness

The reliability of the research was assessed by paying attention to credibility, confirmability, transferability and reflexivity [26]. Credibility was ensured by truthfully reporting the students' experiences and the conduct of the study. Confirmability was enhanced by reporting direct quotes from the data. The participants, their backgrounds and the phenomenon being studied were described to enable the reader to assess the transferability of the results. The researchers sought to be aware of their preconceptions and analysed the data as objectively as possible by several researchers to increase reflexivity. From a critical realist perspective, objectivity is understood as an ideal rather than an absolute, as knowledge is always interpretive. In this study, reflexivity was used to critically examine researchers' assumptions and their potential influence on the analysis. Thus, reflexivity was not seen as conflicting with objectivity but as a means to enhance the credibility and transparency of the interpretive process. To increase credibility, the SRQR (Standards for Reporting Qualitative Research) checklist for reporting qualitative research, developed by O'Brien and colleagues [27], was used to report the study.

2.6 Ethical Considerations

At all stages of the research, the study followed the principles of good scientific practice recognised by the scientific community, which are based on reliability, integrity, respect and accountability [28, 29]. The data were processed following the European Union and national data protection laws and regulations [30, 31]. Ethical statement of ethical committee was not required according to Finnish data protraction act [32]. Also, the study did not violate the integrity of the participants, didn't cause emotional or social harm to the participants and the participants were not under the age of 18 years. That's why the ethical approval of university of applied sciences was sufficient [33].

The Declaration of Helsinki [28] and Finnish Research Integrity Advisory Board principles [29] were followed to guide the participants' privacy, humanity and voluntariness during the entire study process. Each student gave their written consent about participation and could withdraw at any phase. Playing the game was part of the course, but students had the option to withdraw from the course. ECTS credits were awarded based on course requirements, and students could complete the course without participating in the research component. The data was protected according to the regulations of the Data Protection Act [30]. The game was free for students, and they played it on their own mobile devices. The device requirements (the mobile device must be Android or iOS-based) were informed before the course. The course grade was based on the game's content and task completion. The principal researcher (SJ) has recruited the students independently, and the co-owner (PR) who is also co-author has not been involved in the practical research or the recruitment of students. The study has not produced any financial benefit for the co-owner, nor has he/she been able to influence the students' responses. This person has also not participated in data collection or analysis but has contributed to the manuscript by describing expertise in pre-hospital emergency care competence.

3   Results

The participating students had an average age of 27 years (20–46, 11 female and 3 male), and they were both paramedic (P) and registered nursing (RN) students. Their backgrounds are described in Table 2. The experiences of the mobile game were described using five main categories: 1) The influence of mobile gaming on developing pre-hospital emergency care competence; 2) Pedagogical structures in the mobile game that influence learning; 3) Mobile gaming as a learning method compared to traditional approaches; 4) Applicability and usability of mobile gaming in paramedic and nursing education; 5) Development needs and future potential of mobile gaming in education (Table 3).

Table 2. Backgrounds of the participants (n = 14)

Background	Participants
Gender, n (%)	
Female	11 (78.6)
Male	3 (21.4)
Degree program, n (%)	
Paramedic	9 (64.3)
Registered nurse	5 (35.7)
Year of study, n (%)	
First	3 (21.4)
Second	4 (28.6)
Third	3 (21.4)
Fourth	4 (28.6)
Work experience in the social and health sector	
No	3 (21.4)
Less than 1 year	8 (57.1)
1–5 years	2 (14.3)
More than 5 years	1 (7.1)
Attitude towards mobile learning games[a] mean, standard deviation	8.9 (1.7)

[a]Likert scale 1–10 (1−extremely negative, 10−extremely positive)

Table 3. Paramedic and nursing students' experiences of developing paramedic competence using BREATHe: Paramedic –mobile game

Main category	Category
The influence of mobile gaming on developing pre-hospital emergency care competence	The mobile game enhances theoretical knowledge of emergency care The mobile game improves systematic assessment and treatment competence The mobile game supports evaluation and decision-making competence The mobile game builds practical readiness Playing the mobile game fosters pre-hospital emergency care competence Challenges in developing practical skills through the mobile game Challenges in developing interaction and teamwork competence through the mobile game Challenges in improving real patient observation with the mobile game
Pedagogical structures in the mobile game that influence learning	Pedagogical methods from the mobile game enhanced learning The mobile game's flexibility supported learning Practicing challenging patient cases in the mobile game advanced learning The mobile game's structured tasks and timetables fostered learning Safe environment to practice The feedback of mobile game increased motivation to develop pre-hospital emergency care competence Difficulty progressing in the game can lower motivation Motivating all learners is a challenge in game-based learning
Mobile gaming as a learning method compared to traditional approaches	Mobile gaming is seen as a better learning method than reading books The mobile game offers more flexibility than traditional simulations The mobile game cannot replace traditional simulations for practical skill development

(continued)

Table 3. (*continued*)

Main category	Category
Applicability and usability of mobile gaming in paramedic and nursing education	Satisfaction with the mobile game's usability
	The mobile game can introduce users to paramedicine
	The mobile game suits those with a theoretical foundation in paramedicine
	The mobile game supports paramedic degree studies
	The mobile game enhances competence development during clinical training
	The mobile game strengthens existing emergency care competence
	The mobile game improved competence development in traditional simulations
Development needs and future potential of mobile gaming in education	The need to improve the functionality of the mobile game
	The need to introduce more variety to the mobile game
	The need to increase the challenge level in the mobile game
	The need to make the mobile game more realistic
	The need to improve the feedback provided by the mobile game
	A desire to broaden the use of gamification in education

3.1 The Influence of Mobile Gaming on Developing Pre-hospital Emergency Care Competence

The students experienced playing the mobile game can develop theoretical knowledge of emergency care, systematic assessment and treatment competence, as well as decision-making competence and practical readiness. One nursing student described this as follows: "It teaches you really well about the systematic examination and treatment of the patient, the ABCDE [Airway, Breathing, Circulation, Disability, Exposure] protocol. The mobile game can teach you maybe what to examine first, what to treat first, and in what order. It may not serve to know how to do things." (P7, RN). Playing the mobile game fosters pre-hospital emergency care competence based on students' experiences. Still, students experienced that the mobile game challenged developing practical skills: "Then of course... practical skills and these of course are left out." (P7, RN). Although students perceived that practical skills, interaction and cooperation competence were challenged, and the ability to observe a real patient did not develop directly, the theoretical knowledge gained from playing the game provided readiness and confidence for practical worth.

3.2 Pedagogical Structures in the Mobile Game that Influence Learning

The mobile game's pedagogical methods and flexibility contributed to learning. The pedagogical methods from the mobile game helped students identify strengths and weaknesses in their skills and enhance confidence. The flexibility, unlimited number of repetitions, the large number of different patient cases and the possibility to study independently of time and place at a pace that suits the student were perceived as fostering learning: *"You can do it when it suits you, at a time when you're awake and alert and can concentrate on it. And the fact that you have unlimited possibilities to do those repetitions."* (P4, RN). It was also possible to practice challenging patient cases. The immediacy, objectivity, visuality and seeing your success rate of structured tasks and timetables supported learning and competence development. Learning was also supported by, for example, systematic examination and treatment, decision-making, and consideration of patient care pathways required by the mobile game. The mobile game was perceived as a safe environment to practice demanding situations and make mistakes without harming the patient.

The students felt that the mobile game motivated them to develop pre-hospital emergency care competence by playing independently and reading theory from the book and emergency care guidelines. Feedback from the game and seeing progress motivates students: *"When you get the feedback right after the task, it motivates you to do more, which I think is really good. I think it also increases the motivation to keep playing and develop yourself through the game and reading."* (P4, RN). The ease of starting to play and the flexibility of playing were found to be enjoyable and inspiring but still, the game didn't engage everyone. An appropriate level of difficulty in the mobile game was perceived as motivating, while tasks that were too difficult or stopped progressing were perceived as demotivating. The suitability of gamification for every student was also questioned: *"I don't think this is necessarily an effective learning method for everyone, or that you need to approach the game in a certain way for it (…) to actually improve your competence."* (P9, P)

3.3 Mobile Gaming as a Learning Method Compared to Traditional Approaches

Students perceived mobile game as a better, more valuable, meaningful and activating teaching method than traditional ways of learning, such as reading a textbook or attending a lecture. It allowed students to test their own competence independently. They received more direct feedback on personal competence compared to traditional learning that motivated them: *"That was the nice thing about it, you get to be in every case and make all the decisions yourself (…) it's much more efficient in that sense than traditional teaching."* (P10, P). The mobile game differed from the traditional face-to-face simulation in that it is flexible, independent from time and place, has unlimited repetitions, and is autonomous. Students felt that playing the mobile game contributed to the development of competence in traditional simulations, but the mobile game cannot replace a traditional simulation in developing practical skills: *"The game is not a substitute for simulations, that's not what it replaces. (…) It gives you the tools to run a simulation. You'll be more confident to start a simulation once you've played through it with the game."* (P14, P)

3.4 Applicability and Usability of Mobile Gaming in Paramedic and Nursing Education

After the initial tutorials and learning how to play, the students were satisfied with the usability of the game. The students considered the mobile game suitable as an introduction to paramedicine, to support their paramedic studies, emergency care simulations and clinical training, and to strengthen existing emergency care competence. Students perceived that the mobile game improved competence development both in their studies and potentially in the workplace: *"This required some basic knowledge, perhaps not for students at the very beginning. I guess it depends a bit on what you want to use it for. For example, is the game used to hone existing skills, or is it a way to prepare the skills before practical training?"* (P6, P). The students felt that the mobile game is suitable for a wide range of timing in paramedic studies, but that a sufficient theoretical background before playing the game will contribute to the development of competence.

3.5 Development Needs and Future Potential of Mobile Gaming in Education

Students perceived that the functionality and usability of the mobile game should be improved, for example, to reduce the time needed to learn the game initially. More variety and different challenge levels were requested for the mobile game's tasks, patients and interpretable ECGs. Students also hope that the mobile game could be developed to be more realistic, for example, in terms of examining the patient, increasing interaction and the flexibility of systematic examination. One paramedic student described: *"It would be good, even basic rough neurology: to look at the pupils, facial mimicry, mouth drooping and limb movements, to get a kind of overall picture."* (P8, P). Students felt they could not develop the observation of a real patient and interaction by playing the game. They felt that the mobile game's feedback should also be made clearer, and any inconsistencies identified should be corrected. Mobile game-based learning was seen as the teaching method of the future. There was a desire to see more use of gamification in teaching and to develop similar games for different specialities: *"It would be nice if every speciality could have a kind of... "BREATHe obstetrics" or "BREATHe occupational health" or whatever. The possibilities are probably endless."* (P5, P)

4 Discussion

The results of our study provide insights into the experiences of paramedic and nursing students in developing pre-hospital emergency care competence through mobile gaming. The students' experience was promising, but there were also some areas for improvement in the mobile game.

Regarding the influence of a mobile game on the development of pre-hospital emergency care competence, students perceived that the mobile game develops theoretical knowledge but not practical skills. This is in line with earlier evidence that pointed to the restrictions regarding training practical skills through mobile games [8, 34, 35]. As evidence is controversial whether playing a mobile game enhances decision-making skills [8] there is a need to evaluate each mobile game used in education separately [22]. According to our research, students perceived their decision-making skills to have improved through playing a mobile game, which was in line with the results of Kolcun et al. [36] and Sim et al. [37].

In our study, students' experiences with facilitating competence development through mobile gaming were confirmed by previous research evidence. Students described many benefits which are in line with previous studies: flexibility [35], immediate feedback [12, 13], and the ability to practice independently until the required skills are achieved [8]. In our study, safe practice without the risk of harm to the patient was perceived as beneficial. Regarding motivational aspects of mobile gaming in learning, Harring and colleagues [14] pointed out in their study that students felt that mobile games motivated them to play and increased their simulation time. In our study, the students also perceived that the mobile game was not necessarily motivating all students in the same way. This motivational challenge has been identified earlier, the students may spend less time playing than expected [38]. A mobile game may support the development of some students' competences very well, but game-based learning may not be equally suitable for all students.

As a learning method, mobile gaming was perceived as more efficient than traditional approaches by students. These experiences are in line with previous research, e.g. Cheng et al. [39] and Hu et al. [40] have pointed out that students will get better learning outcomes with mobile apps than with lecture-based instruction or using traditional written cases. Still, playing mobile games, students won't get better outcomes compared to traditional face-to-face simulation [8]. In our study, students recommended mobile games to support competence development in face-to-face simulations and practical training. Still, they did not see the possibility of replacing traditional simulations with mobile games. Similar findings have been found earlier [8, 15, 39]. The advantage of a mobile game would thus be to reinforce the confidence in the simulation and competencies of paramedics and registered nurses.

Regarding the applicability and usability of mobile games, students experienced some frustrating technical problems, as reported in previous studies [8, 15, 36]. Still, students felt that the game was usable. Students' experiences of the applicability and usability of mobile games in pre-hospital emergency care are novel since evidence is scarce in the field. In our study, students expressed their wish to see mobile gaming developed and used more in education. Students had suggestions for developing more interactive mobile games that included a variety of specialities and more diverse patient groups, such as more pediatric patients of different ages. Could the game be developed as a multi-professional game, where, for example, medical students could receive consultations in real-time, which would also make the game more realistic? The results of our study can be used to develop paramedic and nursing education by optimising the use of mobile games in pre-hospital emergency care education. Also, artificial intelligence systems could be utilised to enhance interaction between students and virtual patients and reporting and speaking aloud may make gaming more fluent.

5   Limitations

The limitation was that only students who completed the mobile game were interviewed. Another limitation is that if only paramedic students had been included in the study, the findings might have differed. In addition, the study did not collect detailed information about the participants' work experience, which may have influenced the analysis. Students with limited or no prehospital work experience, as well as those in their first year of study, may have found it more difficult to evaluate the game's impact on their competence; this variation could not be fully examined. It would also have been valuable to explore the experiences of students who didn't complete the mobile game.

Although the sample size was relatively small (n = 14), data saturation was achieved; however, the limited number of participants may restrict the range of perspectives captured. In addition, the use of interviews as the sole data collection method may have influenced the findings, as they are based on self-reported experiences. Furthermore, the critical realist perspective guided the interpretation towards identifying underlying mechanisms and contextual influences, which may have shaped how the findings were understood. Thus, the results of the study cannot be generalised.

6   Conclusion

Based on students' experiences, a mobile game is an effective tool for developing prehospital emergency care competence, offering several advantages over traditional learning methods. Students found the game more engaging than reading textbooks, more flexible than conventional simulations, and particularly beneficial for self-assessment. Therefore, mobile games hold a strong potential for education. To maximise their influence, we recommend further development of mobile games to enhance realism and interactivity, for example, through artificial intelligence. Additionally, expanding the game to cover various specialisations and interprofessional collaboration could strengthen multiprofessional skill development. The mobile game could be used or developed further to become part of a mixed reality intervention, which is growing in popularity. This would help overcome the design flaws mentioned by the student players who are trying to develop their practical skills.

Future research should explore the experiences of students who discontinued gameplay, the use of mobile games for competence development in the workplace, and empirical evaluations of the game's effectiveness. Furthermore, investigating the perspectives of educators on integrating mobile games into paramedic education could provide valuable insights.

References

1. Tanninen, A., Kouvonen, A., Nordquist, H.: Advanced-level paramedics' support needs for developing and utilising competence. Int. Emerg. Nurs. **66**, 101233 (2023)

2. Vähäkangas, P., Nordquist, H., Terkamo-Moisio, A.: Urgent hospital transfers – The experiences and required skills of paramedics. Int. Emerg. Nurs. **67**, 101269 (2023)
3. Strandås, M., Vizcaya-Moreno, M.F., Ingstad, K., Sepp, J., Linnik, L., Vaismoradi, M.: An integrative systematic review of promoting patient safety within prehospital emergency medical services by paramedics: a role theory perspective. J. Multidiscip. Healthc. **17**, 1385–1400 (2024)
4. Weber, A., Devenish, S., Lam, L.: Exploring the alignment between paramedicine's professional capabilities and competency frameworks for current and evolving scopes of practice: a literature review. BMC Med. Educ. **24**(1), 31 (2024)
5. Act on Health Care Professionals. 28.6.1994/559. https://www.finlex.fi/en/laki/kaannokset/1994/en19940559_20110312.pdf. Accessed 27 Nov 2025
6. Decree of the Ministry of Social Affairs and Health on emergency medical services 6.4.2011/340. (in Finnish). https://finlex.fi/fi/laki/smur/2017/20170585. Accessed 17 Oct 2025
7. Europass. Description of the eight EQF levels. https://europass.europa.eu/en/description-eight-eqf-levels. Accessed 17 Oct 2025
8. Cant, R., Ryan, C., Kelly, M.A.: Use and effectiveness of virtual simulations in nursing student education: an umbrella review. CIN: Comput. Inform. Nurs. **41**(1), 31–38 (2023)
9. Celik, F., Turan, R., Bektas, H.: The effect of game-based interventions on the nursing students' level of knowledge: a systematic review and meta-analysis of randomized controlled trials. Nurse Educ. Today **151**, 106746 (2025)
10. Demircan, B., Kıyak, Y., Kaya, H.: The effectiveness of serious games in nursing education: a meta-analysis of randomized controlled studies. Nurse Educ. Today **142**, 106330 (2024)
11. Ylitalo, H.M., Roivainen, P., Kuivila, H.M., Juntunen, J., Mikkonen, K., Pramila-Savukoski, S.: The effect of the BREATHe paramedic - paramedic mobile game on nursing and paramedic students' competence development - a quasi-experimental study. Int. Emergency Nurs. 41762863 (2026)
12. Killam, L.A., Silva, A., Gordon, R., Tyerman, J., Luctkar-Flude, M.: Virtual screen-based clinical simulation: an integrative review of student experiences. Teach. Learn. Nurs. (2024)
13. Liu, Z., Yu, R., Yao, X., Yan, Q.: The impact of feedback elements in serious games on nursing learning outcomes: a systematic review and meta-analysis. Nurse Educ. Today **150**, 106689 (2025)
14. Harring, A.K.V., et al.: Gamification of the National Institutes of Health Stroke Scale (NIHSS) for simulation training-a feasibility study. Adv. Simul. (Lond. Engl.) **8**(1), 4 (2023)
15. Bauchwitz, B., et al.: The use of smartphone-based highly realistic MCI training as an adjunct to traditional training methods. Mil. Med. **189**(Supplement 3), 775–783 (2024)
16. Breath Mobile Solutions. Mobile simulators/eLearning games. https://breathe-mobile.com/en/. Accessed 26 Mar 2026
17. Campusonline. Basic level prehospital emergency care as a virtual simulation – learn emergency care with a mobile game (in Finnish). https://campusonline.fi/course/perustason-ens ihoito-virtuaalisimulaatioina-opi-ensihoitoa-mobiilipelin-avulla-4/. Accessed 17 Oct 2025
18. Current Care guidelines (2025). https://www.kaypahoito.fi/en/. Accessed 17 Oct 2025
19. Kyngäs, H.: Qualitative research and content analysis. In: Kyngäs, H., Mikkonen, K., Kääriäinen, M. (eds.) The Application of Content Analysis in Nursing Science Research, pp. 3–12 Springer, Cham (2020). https://doi.org/10.1007/978-3-030-30199-6_1
20. Koopmans, E., Schiller, D.C.: Understanding causation in Healthcare: an introduction to critical realism. Qual. Health Res. **32**(8–9), 1207–1214 (2022)
21. Polit, D.F.K., Beck, C.T.: Nursing Research: Generating and Assessing Evidence For Nursing Practice, 10th edn. Wolters Kluwer Health (2017)
22. Min, A., Min, H., Kim, S.: Effectiveness of serious games in nurse education: a systematic review. Nurse Educ. Today **108**, 105178 (2022)

23. Archuby, F., Sanz, C., Manresa-Yee, C.: DIJS: methodology for the design and development of digital educational serious games. IEEE Trans. Games **15**(2), 273–284 (2023)
24. Silva, F.G.M.: Practical methodology for the design of educational serious games. Information (Basel) **11**(1) (2020)
25. Elo, S., Kääriäinen, M., Kanste, O., Pölkki, T., Utriainen, K., Kyngäs, H.: Qualitative content analysis: a focus on trustworthiness. SAGE Open **4**(1), 2158244014522633 (2014)
26. Lincoln, Y.S., Guba, E.G.: Naturalistic inquiry (1985)
27. O'Brien, B.C., Harris, I.B., Beckman, T.J., Reed, D.A., Cook, D.A.: Standards for reporting qualitative research: a synthesis of recommendations. Assoc. Am. Med. Coll. **89**(9), 1245–1251 (2014)
28. Declaration of Helsinki: Ethical principles for medical research involving human subjects. JAMA **310**(20), 2191–2194 (2013)
29. Finnish National Board on Research Integrity. The Finnish Code of Conduct for Research Integrity and Procedures for Handling Alleged Violations of Research Integrity in Finland 2023. https://tenk.fi/sites/default/files/2023-05/RI_Guidelines_2023.pdf. Accessed 27 Nov 2025
30. Data Protection Act 1050/2018. https://www.finlex.fi/en/laki/kaannokset/2018/en20181050.pdf. Accessed 27 Nov 2025
31. General Data Protection Regulation 2016/679. Regulation (EU) 2016/679 of the European Parliament and of the Council on the protection of natural persons with regard to the processing of personal data and on the free movement of such data, and repealing Directive 95/46/EC (General Data Protection Regulation). https://eur-lex.europa.eu/legal-content/EN/TXT/?uri=CELEX:31995L0046. Accessed 17 Oct 2025
32. Finnish data protraction act. https://www.oulu.fi/en/university/faculties-and-units/eudaimonia-institute/ethics-committee-human-sciences. Accessed 17 Oct 2025
33. Medical Research Act 488/1999. Ministry of Social Affairs and Health, Finland (1999). https://www.finlex.fi/api/media/statute-foreign-language-translation/235096/mainPdf/main.pdf?timestamp=1999-04-09T00%3A00%3A00.000Z
34. Fijačko, N., et al.: Effects of a serious smartphone game on nursing students' theoretical knowledge and practical skills in adult basic life support: randomized wait list-controlled trial. JMIR Serious Games **12**(1), e56037 (2024)
35. Yalcinkaya, T., Cinar Yucel, S.: Mobile learning in nursing education: a bibliometric analysis and visualization. Nurse Educ. Pract. **71**, 103714 (2023)
36. Kolcun, K., et al.: Identifying best practices for virtual nursing clinical education: a scoping review. J. Prof. Nurs. **48**, 128–146 (2023)
37. Sim, J.J.M., Rusli, K.D.B., Seah, B., Levett-Jones, T., Lau, Y., Liaw, S.Y.: Virtual simulation to enhance clinical reasoning in nursing: a systematic review and meta-analysis. Clin. Simul. Nurs. **69**, 26–39 (2022)
38. Maheu-Cadotte, M.A., et al.: Efficacy of serious games in healthcare professions education: a systematic review and meta-analysis. Simul. Healthc. **16**(3), 199–212 (2021)
39. Cheng, P., et al.: The effects of serious games on cardiopulmonary resuscitation training and education: systematic review with meta-analysis of randomized controlled trials. JMIR Serious Games **12**, e52990 (2024)
40. Hu, H., Lai, X., Li, H., Nyland, J.: Teaching disaster evacuation management education to nursing students using virtual reality mobile game-based learning. CIN: Comput. Inform. Nurs. **40**(10), 705–710 (2022)

Temporal Stress Patterns in Virtual Reality Based Trauma Care Training: A Multimodal Study of Nursing Students' Physiological and Interactional Responses

Laura Kohonen-Aho[1]([✉]) [iD], Delfin Tursin[1] [iD], Joonas Ojanen[1], Matti Pouke[2] [iD], and Kristina Mikkonen[1] [iD]

[1] Research Unit of Health Sciences and Technology, University of Oulu, Oulu, Finland
`laura.kohonen-aho@oulu.fi`
[2] Research Unit of Computer Science and Engineering, University of Oulu, Oulu, Finland

Abstract. Healthcare education must prepare students for complex, high-pressure clinical environments such as emergency and trauma care. While simulation-based education and extended reality (XR) technologies have shown promise in supporting clinical skill development, little is known about how learners experience and regulate stress during immersive trauma simulations. This exploratory study investigates nursing students' physiological stress responses and interactional behaviours during three trauma-related learning tasks within a virtual reality (VR) emergency care simulation: wound care, auscultation, and chest tube insertion. Six nursing students participated in individual VR sessions, during which electrocardiogram data were collected to assess heart rate variability (HRV), alongside synchronised video recordings of participants' verbal and embodied conduct. Results indicate distinct stress patterns across tasks. The wound care task showed the greatest inter-individual variability in HRV, reflecting differences in task familiarity and coping strategies. Auscultation elicited moderate physiological engagement, while chest tube insertion was associated with consistently lower HRV, indicating higher task demand but adaptive engagement rather than excessive stress. Video analysis revealed visible signs of confusion and coping efforts, particularly during the initial wound task, aligning with physiological findings. Together, the results highlight the value of multimodal approaches for understanding stress regulation in XR-based trauma education and inform the design of pedagogically supportive and psychologically safe simulations.

Keywords: Virtual reality · Healthcare education · Simulation-based learning · Psychophysiology · Multimodal analysis · Conversation analysis

1 Introduction

Healthcare education is facing increasing pressure to prepare future professionals for complex, unpredictable, and interprofessional clinical environments. Rising patient acuity, workforce shortages, and rapid digital transformation demand educational

M. Särestöniemi et al. (Eds.): NCDHWS 2026, CCIS 3009, pp. 337–357, 2026.
https://doi.org/10.1007/978-3-032-28812-7_24

approaches that go beyond traditional, discipline-specific teaching methods. In particular, acute and emergency care settings require learners to integrate theoretical knowledge, technical skills, clinical reasoning, communication, and emotional regulation under pressure–competences that cannot be developed through a single pedagogical modality alone [1, 2].

Simulation-based education has emerged as a key strategy for bridging the gap between theory and practice. High-fidelity simulation (HFS) provides controlled, realistic environments that support experiential learning, critical thinking, teamwork, and reflective practice [3, 4]. More recently, extended reality (XR, i.e., a spectrum of immersive display technologies ranging from Augmented to Virtual and Mixed Reality) technologies have expanded the pedagogical toolkit by offering immersive, repeatable, and adaptive learning environments that foster self-regulation, digital competence, and situated cognition [5, 6]. Evidence suggests that XR can effectively support the development of knowledge and technical skills, particularly when opportunities for clinical exposure are limited, while also enhancing learner engagement and confidence [2, 6].

However, evidence remains limited regarding how learners experience and manage the intense cognitive and emotional demands inherent in trauma-focused simulations, particularly within immersive XR environments [6]. Trauma care scenarios are characterised by time pressure, uncertainty, high emotional salience, and the need for rapid prioritisation, all of which can evoke substantial stress responses that directly influence learning, decision-making, and performance. XR is known for its capacity to invoke realistic emotional, physiological, and behavioural reactions in its users, even though the users understand neither the virtual locations nor the events and characters simulated within are real [7, 8]. For example, simulating difficult human encounters through digital characters in a clinical consultation setting has been shown to elicit pressure in medical trainees and professionals [9]. This makes XR a promising tool to simulate stressful scenarios taking place in trauma care. While prior studies have demonstrated the effectiveness of simulation and XR for skill acquisition, far fewer have examined the processes of stress regulation and learner support during trauma simulations, or how students transition from guided practice to independent performance under pressure. Existing research has also largely relied on post hoc self-reports, offering limited insight into learners' real-time behavioural and physiological responses during high-stakes scenarios. Consequently, there is a need for multimodal research approaches that capture the dynamic interplay between cognitive load, emotional stress, instructional scaffolding, and learner agency in XR-based trauma education. Addressing this gap is essential for designing trauma simulations that are not only technically realistic but also pedagogically supportive and psychologically safe, enabling learners to develop both clinical competence and resilience in preparation for real-world emergency care.

In this exploratory study, we examine nursing students' temporal stress patterns and their visible interactional indicators during three critical learning tasks in a VR simulation featuring emergency trauma care: 1) wound care, 2) auscultation and 3) chest tube insertion. We ask the following research questions:

RQ1. How do nursing students' physiological stress responses differ across the three trauma care tasks in a VR-based simulation?

RQ2. What temporal stress patterns emerge within and across the three trauma care tasks?

RQ3. How are these stress patterns associated with the participants' verbal and multimodal conduct captured in video recordings?

2 Materials and Methods

2.1 Research Setting and Participants

The studied Virtual Reality (VR) simulation was developed by VRTrauma (https://vrt rauma.com/). This company has developed several VR scenarios for medical and health-care students and personnel to rehearse the recognition of injuries, selection of appropriate tools, and enactment of basic procedural steps in different types of emergency trauma care situations.

The study was conducted in a simulation laboratory at the premises of Oulu University of Applied Sciences. Permissions for the study have been granted by the University of Oulu ethical board and the Oulu University of Applied Sciences. The experiment room was arranged in a simulation laboratory and equipped specifically for research data collection. The setup included a head-mounted display (VR headset) and hand-held controllers for participating in the VR scenario, two video cameras, and external microphones to capture participants' behaviour and communication during the sessions. Several laptops were used for camera operation, administration of questionnaires, recording of VR gameplay, and collection of physiological sensor data. Physiological measurements were recorded using a PLUX biosignal acquisition system kit, enabling synchronised acquisition of biosignals during the VR training scenarios.

Six nursing students participated in the study and were recruited from a course on teamwork and leadership in emergency situations. All participants were second- or third-year nursing students (half-and-half), their age ranged from 20 to 30 (Mdn = 20.5) and all but one identified as women. The participants' experience in clinical training ranged between 12–50 ECTS (Mdn = 17.5). All participants had normal (n = 4) or corrected-to-normal vision (n = 2).

The participants had very little previous experience with VR systems; four participants had never tried VR, whereas one had tried it once or twice, and the last one was using VR roughly once per year. None of the participants reported susceptibility to motion sickness; however, all but one participant reported some initial discomfort or sickness already before the exposure to the VR application (ranging from 1–8 in a scale of 0–20). During the simulation, it was also revealed that the participants did not have previous experience with two of the specific tasks required in this scenario: insertion of a foley catheter balloon tamponade for haemorrhage control, as well as a chest tube.

Data collection was conducted in individual sessions with these students. Participation in the study compensated for one of the course pre-assignments. A researcher was present throughout each session to ensure participants' safety and to provide guidance on how to proceed in the scenario, as well as technical support. The total duration of each session was approximately 1.5 h.

The study included a rehearsal scenario where the participants learned to use the VR controllers to move in the virtual emergency room, examine the patient (e.g., measuring pulse, turning the patient) and use the medical tools (e.g., stethoscope, pulse oximeter). In this rehearsal, each step of examining and treating the patient was guided with written instructions visible in the environment.

After the rehearsal scenario, the participants conducted the actual learning scenario, where they needed to proceed without written instructions. In the selected scenario for this study, the participants took care of a patient who was brought to an emergency care unit after being assaulted with a knife. The patient had a bleeding wound in their neck due to stabbing and his left lung was also filled with fluid. At the beginning of the scenario, the participants were provided with a description of the situation and the patient's condition using the ISBAR communication tool in healthcare (Identify, Situation, Background, Assessment, Recommendation), after which they proceeded to take care of the patient. In this scenario, the three main learning tasks were 1) the treatment of the external injury (wound) by inserting a foley catheter balloon tamponade for hemorrhage control in the wound, 2) auscultating the patient's lungs to find an internal injury: breathing was not audible on the left side, and 3) inserting a chest tube to the patient to aid their breathing. The medical equipment for conducting these tasks were visible for the participants on the tables in the virtual room. Although the participants were not provided with written instructions anymore, they were allowed to ask for help from the researcher on how to proceed. In addition, if the participants otherwise expressed difficulties with proceeding in the scenario, the researcher also provided help, first by asking open questions (e.g., can you see anything that could be used to treat the wound? What else could be done to examine the patient?), and if necessary, explicitly guiding the participants on what to do. The VR scenarios were mirrored from the headset to a laptop, enabling the researcher to follow the participants' actions in VR.

2.2 Data Collection

Each participant first signed an informed consent form and then completed a background questionnaire. Following this, the physiological sensor system (PLUX kit) was attached to the participant by a researcher, and baseline physiological measurements were recorded. Participants then entered the VR environment using the head-mounted display and proceeded to complete both the rehearsal scenario and the main trauma scenario, focusing on the stabbing injury. After completing the VR scenarios, the physiological sensors were removed. Participants subsequently completed post-research questionnaires and participated in a short thematic interview reflecting on their experiences during the scenario. Participation in the VR scenarios and the thematic interviews were video-recorded.

The completed questionnaires included a background questionnaire about demographic information, simulation sickness assessment, the STAI-Y2 scale (trait anxiety), and the Nurses Clinical Reasoning Scale (NCRS; clinical reasoning ability). In addition, a post-session questionnaire was administered, including items about simulation sickness, the STAI-Y1 scale (state anxiety), Nurses Clinical Reasoning Scale (NCRS; clinical reasoning ability), the Simulation Design Scale (perceived quality of the simulation), the NASA Task Load Index (NASA-TLX; perceived workload), and a measure of satisfaction and self-confidence in the learning situation. In the present study, only demographic variables from the background questionnaire were included in the analysis. All other questionnaires were collected for broader research purposes but were not analysed, as they fall outside the scope of this study.

For the physiological data, electrocardiogram (ECG) data were collected during a VR-based trauma training session using the PLUX biosignal acquisition system (sampling rate: 1000 Hz). R peaks (the peaks corresponding to individual heartbeats in the ECG signal) detected from band-pass filtered ECG signals, and RR (the peaks corresponding to individual heartbeats in the ECG signal) intervals were derived. Heart rate variability was identified using RMSSD (Root Mean Square of Successive Differences), calculated for the full session within 15-s time windows. RMSSD values were averaged following each learning task, including wound, auscultation, and chest tube. ECG data were recorded continuously during the VR-based trauma training session using the PLUX system.

The collected video data includes screen recordings from the participants' first-person perspective in VR, as well as recordings of participants and the instructing researcher in the physical space. For this study, we analyse data from the background questionnaires, physiological measurements, and the video-recorded stabbing scenario.

2.3 Data Analysis

This study employs a multi-method design that integrates physiological measurements with Conversation Analysis (CA) to investigate how participants experience, display, and manage stress during the three learning tasks in the stabbing scenario. Heart-rate variability (HRV) is used to track fluctuations in autonomic arousal across tasks, providing continuous physiological indicators of stress. In parallel, video-based CA is used to examine how participants publicly display and manage these moments in interaction, for example, how they show confusion, hesitation, or nervousness, and how such displays are responded to and organized sequentially. While CA does not infer participants' internal psychological states, it enables a fine-grained analysis of how orientations to stress or difficulty are made observable and consequential in the participants' conduct. Together, these methods offer a complementary view on how stress is experienced and managed during the three learning tasks.

ECG data were analysed offline in MATLAB. ECG signals were visually inspected and band-pass filtered (5–15 Hz) to reduce baseline drift and high-frequency noise. R-peaks were detected using an automated peak detection algorithm based on amplitude, prominence, and minimum inter-beat interval criteria. To reduce artefacts, RR intervals shorter than 0.30 s or longer than 2.00 s were excluded as non-physiological. Heart rate (HR) was calculated as 60 divided by the RR interval (beats per minute), where the RR interval is the time (in seconds) between two successive R-wave peaks. Heart rate variability (HRV) was quantified using the root mean square of successive differences between RR intervals (RMSSD), which is a standard time-domain index of short-term HRV, suggesting parasympathetic nervous system modulation. RMSSD was computed in 15-s time windows to capture rapid changes in autonomic activity during dynamic VR learning tasks. For each subject, RMSSD was averaged within specific task learning following the wound, auscultation, and chest tube, which were determined using synchronised VR video recordings. Due to signal dropouts, not all subjects could provide usable ECG data for all learning tasks. Therefore, HRV analyses were conducted descriptively and reported as exploratory.

Participants' interactions, captured in video recordings, were analysed using Conversation Analysis [10, 11] to identify how participants publicly display their orientation to the tasks and their ways of proceeding with them through their talk and multimodal conduct. CA focuses on how people jointly accomplish social actions during their unfolding talk-in-interaction [13] and by using multimodal resources such as gestures, gaze, body movements, and objects [14]. Video recordings are used as materials for investigating this practical achievement of social order in micro-level detail. The analyses are validated via a close examination of how the participants display their own understanding of and orientation to the unfolding turns and actions, which becomes visible to the analyst in the participants' turn design and the use of embodiment, space and virtual objects.

Conversation analytic data analysis process typically begins with an "unmotivated looking" [15] of the research data, meaning that first the data is viewed without preconceptions so that the phenomena meaningful to the participants themselves can be recognised. Within our aim to connect the analysis of participants' interactions with the physiological measurements, we viewed all participants' recordings of the three learning tasks, and started to identify moments of participants expressing confusion, nervousness, and not knowing how to proceed with the task. According to the further analytic principles of CA, these repetitive expressions were gathered into a collection of cases (N = 60) that were targeted to a more detailed analysis [11]. We transcribed all cases according to the CA transcription principles [16], which are used to depict what is being said or done, how, and when. This was followed by a detailed analysis of the sequential and temporal unfolding of the interactions for each case. Here we noticed that 41 of the expressions emerged during the first learning task: wound treatment, whereas 3 occurred during the auscultation task and 16 during the chest tube task.

3   Results

3.1   Physiological Measurements in the Learning Tasks

To address our first research question, we examined differences in physiological responses across the three learning tasks (wound, auscultation, and chest tube) using heart rate variability (HRV), indexed by RMSSD, as a measure of short-term autonomic regulation.

3.1.1   Wound Learning Task

During the wound learning task, RMSSD values showed a wide range across participants, from 15.56 to 263.23 ms. The mean RMSSD was 105.89 ± 92.50 ms, with a median of 86.18 ms (N = 6). Compared to the auscultation and chest tube tasks, RMSSD values were higher on average and showed substantial inter-individual variability. This pattern suggests greater autonomic flexibility during the wound task, with participants differing markedly in their physiological responses. The large variability indicates that some participants experienced the task as relatively manageable, while others showed increased physiological engagement or effort, potentially reflecting differences in prior experience, confidence, or emotional responses.

3.1.2   Auscultation Learning Task

During the auscultation learning task, RMSSD values ranged from 17.12 to 121.18 ms across participants. The mean RMSSD was 69.44 ± 43.30 ms, with a median of 69.72 ms (N = 4). Compared to the chest tube task, RMSSD values were higher on average and showed greater inter-individual variability. This pattern suggests moderate autonomic engagement with preserved physiological flexibility during the auscultation task. The variability in RMSSD values indicates individual differences in cognitive load and task familiarity, with some participants showing higher physiological regulation while others exhibited lower variability consistent with increased attentional demand.

3.1.3   Chest Tube Learning Task

During the chest tube learning task, heart rate variability (HRV) indexed by RMSSD ranged from 23.24 to 44.52 ms across subjects. The mean RMSSD Was 30.55 ± 8.78, with a median of 27.91 ms (N = 5). These results indicate likely low short-term HRV during the task compared to the other learning tasks. The reduced RMSSD suggested increased physiological load, consistent with the higher complexity of chest tube learning tasks. Despite reduced variability, RMSSD values remained within a range of indicative of adaptive task engagement, rather than excessive physiological stress or autonomic dysregulation. This pattern suggests increased task demand while participants remained physiologically engaged (Fig. 1).

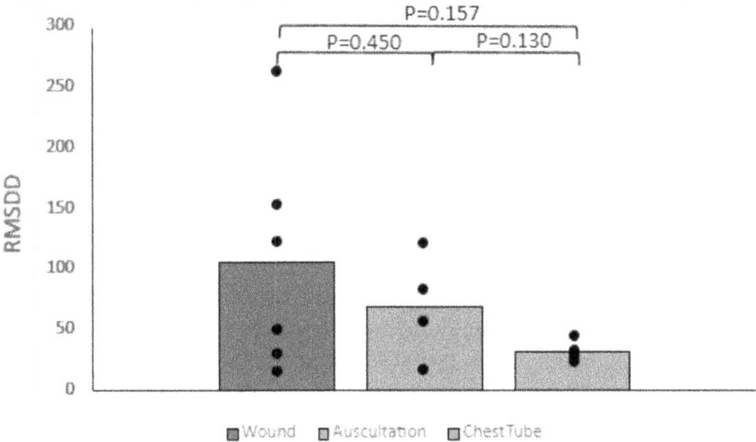

Fig. 1. Mean $\pm$ SD RMSSD (ms) across VR learning tasks.

Preliminary paired two-tailed t-tests did not show statistically significant differences in RMSSD between tasks (wound vs lungs: p = 0.450; lungs vs chest tube: p = 0.130; wound vs chest tube: p = 0.157). However, descriptive results suggested higher RMSSD during the wound task and lower RMSSD during the chest tube task, indicating a potential trend toward increased physiological load with higher task demands. The between-task differences were not statistically significant, likely due to the small sample size.

3.2 Temporal Patterns of Physiological Responses Across Tasks

To address our second research question, we examined how physiological responses varied over time within and across the three learning tasks (wound, auscultation, and chest tube). Across the learning tasks, distinct temporal patterns in physiological responses were observed. The wound task, which was typically the first task, showed the greatest inter-individual variability in RMSSD, suggesting differences in how participants initially responded to the unfamiliar scenario. In contrast, the auscultation task showed more moderate and relatively stable RMSSD values, indicating a more consistent level of physiological engagement across participants. The chest tube task was associated with lower RMSSD values overall, reflecting increased task demands and reduced physiological variability during this more complex procedure. These patterns suggest that physiological responses varied not only between tasks but also across the progression of the scenario, with initial variability during early task engagement followed by more stable or constrained responses as task demands increased.

3.3 Video-Based Observations of the Participants' Behaviour During the Wound Learning Task

In this section, we address our final research question: how stress patterns are associated with the participants' verbal and multimodal conduct captured in the video recordings.

3.3.1 Overview of Verbal and Multimodal Expressions

The video recordings revealed the novelty of this VR scenario to the participants, as evidenced in their verbal and multimodal (non-lexical, embodied) expressions of confusion and nervousness. Most of these expressions (n = 41) emerged during the first learning task: wound treatment, which is why we focus on presenting findings of the participants' interactions during this task. Central to this observation is that all participants had trouble identifying a correct device to stop the bleeding in the patient's neck: a foley catheter balloon tamponade for haemorrhage control. This became evident in the participants' behaviour as five types of expressions reflecting their aim to navigate and cope in an unfamiliar situation. These behavioural observations can also be considered alongside the physiological findings, as RMSSD during the wound task showed substantial inter-individual variability. This suggests that participants differed in their physiological responses during this initial and unfamiliar task, although no direct one-to-one interpretation between behavioural and physiological measures is assumed.

We present the five expression types in Table 1. We observed that the majority of participants (5/6) engaged in two types of expressions: 1) direct verbalisations of trouble, confusion, or uncertainty in how to proceed, and 2) trouble-marking laughter. In addition, two participants engaged in 3) code-switching (i.e., as a Finn, starting to speak English) and one participant in uttering 4) non-lexical vocalisations while treating the patient, which also act as displays of coping in an unfamiliar or confusing situation. Finally, one participant engaged in 5) a non-serious embodied move while treating the patient, that is, throwing an object towards the patient as a reaction to struggling in the task.

Table 1. Expressions indicating trouble, confusion, and/or nervousness during the wound task.

Expression type	Example/participant (English translations*)
Direct verbalization	"I forget here all the time what I am even supposed to do because I'm kind of anxious here" (P1)
	"Well I don't really know what I'm supposed to do" (P2)
	"Now I'm somehow completely lost" (P3)
	"I have a first day at work" (P4)
	"I don't even know what one has here, this is not logical at all"(P6)
Trouble-marking laughter	"I don't know if you can see what I'm trying to do here he he" (P1)
	"He he he I'm somehow completely in shock here in this task" (P2)
	"So difficult hh hh hh" (P3)
	"Well this hh hh this requires action here (P4)
	"I will now examine what can be found here ha ha ha" (P6)
Code-switching from Finnish to English	"I'm trying to help you, I can't" (P4)
	"He's dying" / "Don't die" / "Don't you die" (P4)
	"I'm so sorry guy" (P4)
	"This is really confusing" (P6)
Non-lexical vocalisations	"Swoosh swoosh" (while moving patient's arm up and down) (P6)
	"Ti-di-di-di" (when lifting equipment from the table and when trying to place the foley catheter into the patient's neck) (P6)
Non-serious embodied move	Throwing an object at the patient (P4)

* Except the code-switching utterances, which are originally spoken in English.

In the following sub-sections, we illustrate each expression type with a short excerpt from the video data.

3.3.2 Direct Verbalisations of Trouble, Confusion and/or Nervousness

The most visible expression of trouble or confusion was observed when a participant directly verbalised it. We illustrate this in Excerpt 1. The excerpt begins with the participant (PAR) gazing at the medical equipment in the room and then asking the instructor (INS) about band-aids to stop the bleeding (Line 1).

Data excerpt 1

01 PAR: onko täällä jossai semmosia ihan haavalappuja?
does one have any band-aids somewhere here?
02   (1.0)
03 PAR: tai jotain?
or something?
04 INS: ei oo haavalappua mutta tos olis esimerkiks
one does not have a band-aid but there is for example
05   katetri pöydällä, voisko sitä käyttää?
a catheter on the table, could one use that?
06   (7.0) ((PAR gazes towards equipment on the table))
07 PAR: **nyt mä oon jotenki iha hukassa.**
now I am somehow completely lost.
08 INS: se on se mis on se pallo.
it is the one with the balloon.

Following PAR's question, a 1.0-s pause follows (line 2). This pause becomes consequential for the interaction as it indicates a problem in PAR's question. Indeed, as a response to the lack of reply from INS, PAR adds *or something* (line 3) to repair their question, which shows that PAR now orients to the initially requested equipment (band-aid) not being the right one to request for treating this wound. Now INS replies and directs PAR's attention to the foley catheter (lines 4–5). PAR gazes around the equipment for seven seconds (line 6), which is followed by their direct verbalisation of confusion: *now I am somehow completely lost* (line 7). INS replies by providing a specific characterization of the appearance of the catheter: *it is the one with the balloon* (line 8).

Prior research shows that such verbalisations can be interpreted as publicly addressed coping strategies (e.g., scaffolding thinking aloud under pressure) in challenging, high-arousal environments [17–19]. Such verbalizations become interactionally relevant, because they make the participant's lack of knowledge *observable* through talk [20, 21]. Thus, when the participant verbalizes confusion, they are producing an interactionally recognizable display of trouble that organises the situation as one requiring clarification or assistance from the instructor. This is indeed what can be seen to happen after the trouble display, as the instructor responds immediately with a turn providing assistance.

3.3.3 Trouble-Marking Laughter

Laughter was also frequently present during the wound treatment task, and it occurred during moments of trouble with proceeding in the task. In the second excerpt, PAR approaches the patient and places their fingers on the bleeding wound (Line 1, Fig. 2).

Data excerpt 2

01   (7.0)
            ((PAR approaches patient, then places fingers on the wound#fig2))
02 PAR: pystyykö tän jotenki tukkimaan?
            can one block this somehow?
03   (1.0)
04 INS: kyllä siinä pitäis käyttää jotain välineitä.
            yes one should use some equipment for that.
05   (2.0) ((PAR gazes to the equipment))
06 INS: mitää ideaa mitä vois lähtee kokeilemaa?
            any idea what one could start to test?
07 PAR: no painesidettä. Mietin tota hemostaasii.
            well a pressure bandage. I'm thinking about that haemostasis
08 INS: tuleeko jotain muuta mieleen ku paineside?
            does anything else come to mind besides a pressure bandage?
09 PAR: e::h hh hh ((laughter))
10 INS: onko siinä mitään tuttuja välineitä pöydillä.
            are there any familiar equipment on the tables?

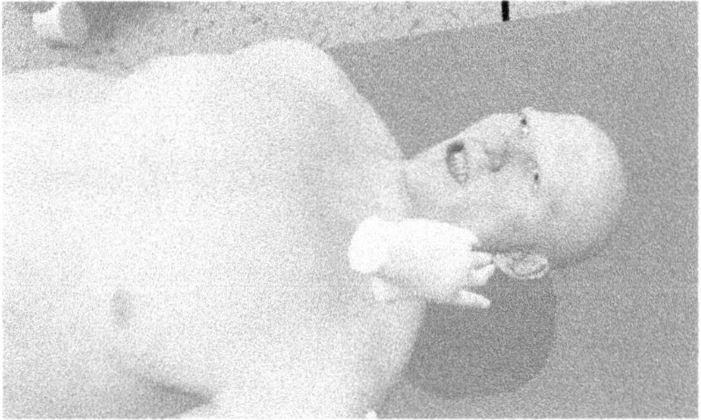

Fig. 2. PAR places their fingers on the wound

PAR asks if the bleeding in the wound can be blocked (line 2). The turn design of this question interestingly reflects the novelty of this VR situation for the participant: inquiring if (and how) an action can be conducted in this environment. INS replies by confirming the problem PAR has noticed (bleeding wound) and initiates knowledge retrieval (line 4): instead of directly telling what to do, INS encourages PAR to retrieve existing knowledge, which creates a pedagogical preference for the learner to produce the knowledge, not the instructor. A pause of 2.0 s follows, during which PAR gazes at the equipment. INS orients to the pause (or PAR's gazing) by asking another knowledge eliciting question: *any idea what one could start to test?* (line 6). Now PAR offers a candidate solution: a pressure bandage. INS rejects the answer by pushing for additional options: *Does anything else come to mind?* (line 8). Instead of providing an answer to this question, PAR now produces a laughter utterance (line 9).

In the field of Conversation Analysis, laughter as a response to a question has been recognized as a display of uncertainty or a marker of epistemic trouble [22–24]. These studies show that speakers often laugh when responding to delicate questions, especially in medical consultations. Here, laughter has been shown to index uncertainty or difficulty in producing an answer, trouble with the epistemic implications of the question, or embarrassment. Similarly in Excerpt 2, laughter indexes that PAR either does not know an alternative answer to the pressure bandage or is still searching for the answer. Either way, INS orients to the laughter as marking trouble since he now changes his strategy and offers a gentler prompt: directing PAR's attention to look for familiar items on the table (line 10).

3.3.4 Code-Switching

Two participants in our data engaged in *code-switching*, which means that, as native Finns in a Finnish-speaking simulation, they occasionally started to speak english. Code-switching has previously been identified as playing a role in interpersonal stance and identity management, both of which are relevant to stress mitigation in a new situation [25, 26]. let us examine an example below.

Data excerpt 3

01 PAR: onko mulla kaikki tämä pöydillä mitä minulla on
         do I have everything on the tables that I have
02   käytettävissä?
         in use?
03 INS: juu.
         yup.
04 PAR: kiva. Don't die.
         nice.
05   (2.0) ((PAR takes a cervical collar))
06 PAR: emmä tiä=
         I don't know
07 INS: =tuleeko mitää muuta mitä käytetää veren tyrehdytyk-see
         does anything else come to mind that is used to stop bleeding?
08   (1.0) ((puts cervical collar to the patient's neck))
09 PAR: he he he. I'm so sorry guy.

The sequence begins with PAR's resource-check question in lines 1–2: *Do I have everything available on the tables?,* which INS confirms minimally in line 3 (*yup*). This closes the information-seeking sequence and shifts the participant into a phase of performing the actual task. What happens now is that PAR immediately engages in code-switching: *don't die* (Line 4). This appears as a playful, humorous utterance directed to the virtual patient, and it can be seen to play different functions. First, it can act as a distancing device where PAR creates an ironic or playful distance from the seriousness of the task that they now need to perform: the use of English signals informality compared to Finnish. Code-switching changes the current 'activity frame' [27] of the simulation into something less "high-stakes", which can be a result of the simulation taking place in a game-like VR environment. Second, code-switching can be used to mitigate uncertainty about not knowing what the upcoming action should be or simply help PAR to transition from thinking to doing.

Next, PAR grabs a cervical collar as a candidate solution to treating the wound, but produces a self-disclosure of uncertainty: *I don't know* (lines 5–6). This confirms the epistemic trouble which was already incipient when engaging in code-switching. As a response, INS initiates a pedagogical prompt: *Does anything else come to mind that is used to stop bleeding?* (line 7), which also reveals that he treats PAR taking the collar as an incorrect solution for treating the wound.

Now, a pause follows, after which in line 9 PAR starts with nervous laughter (*he he he*), which, similarly to Excerpt 2, signals the presence of epistemic trouble, even embarrassment. Then, switching to English again right after the laughter makes the turn explicitly non-serious, or at least less formal and less accountable if it were in Finnish. It is noteworthy that this turn *I'm so sorry guy* is, although projecting affiliation towards the patient, typically not something a healthcare worker would say to a patient (even in a simulation). The turn itself mitigates responsibility (*sorry*) and frames the moment as humorous, which seems to be uttered to relieve the pressure of INS' previous question.

To summarise, code-switching indexes a change in frame. In the excerpt, it appears at similar moments: when needing to take action after the instructor's reply (after line 3) and following the instructor's inquiry about naming a correct device to stop bleeding (after line 7). Using English serves not only as a coping mechanism in the pedagogical activity when the participant lacks epistemic certainty, but also as a way to frame the utterance as less serious, in order to relieve the interpersonal and emotional weight of the moment.

3.3.5 Non-Lexical Vocalisations

One of the participants produced *non-lexical vocalisations* during the wound task, a term commonly used in conversation analytic research to capture vocal behaviours such as sound effects, rhythmic noises, or playfully mimetic sound sequences that stand in for verbal commentary [28, 29]. In the excerpt, the participant is confronted with an unfamiliar equipment in the VR scenario: the foley catheter balloon tamponade, to which INS Has directed PAR's attention to.

Data excerpt 4

```
01 PAR:  kysymys on, miksi mä tän ottaisin?
         the question is, why would I take this?
02       (5.0)#fig3 ((holds the catheter))
03 INS:  kyl sitä voi koittaa.
         one can certainly try it.
04       (2.0)
05 PAR:  ti-di-di-di#fig4((flickers the catheter through
         patient's neck))
06       (5.0)#fig5 ((places the catheter in the wound, bleeding stops))
07 PAR:  no eipä olla käytetty virtsakatetria verenvuotoon.
         well one certainly has not used a urinary catheter to stop bleeding.
```

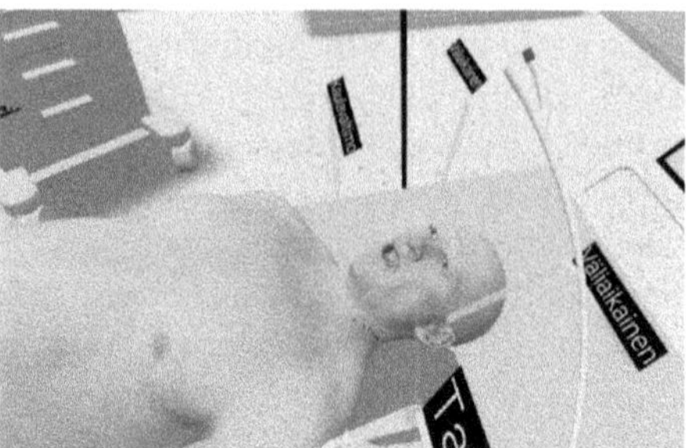

Fig. 3. PAR holds the catheter.

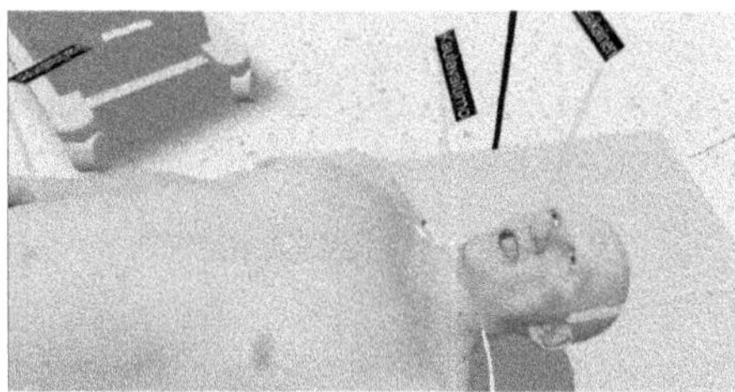

Fig. 4. PAR flickers the catheter fast through the patient's neck.

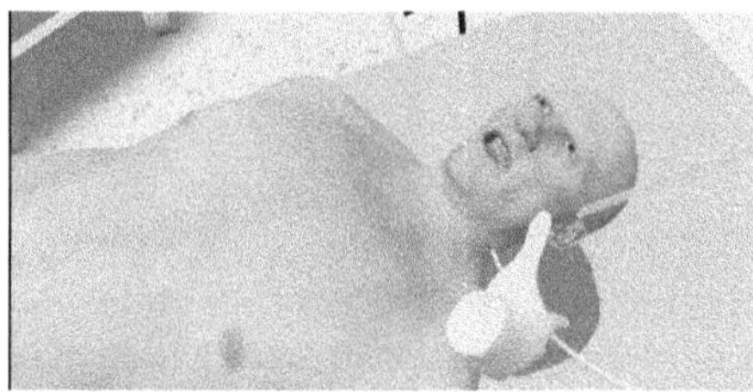

Fig. 5. PAR places the catheter in the wound, bleeding stops.

In line 1, PAR formulates a problem with choosing this object: *the question is, why would I take this?* The turn reveals both an epistemic gap and an orientation to the unfamiliarity of using a catheter for treating a bleeding wound. The 5-second silence that follows, during which PAR just holds up the object (Fig. 3), highlights PAR's hesitancy and need for justifying the selection of this particular tool. INS' reply, *one can certainly try it* (line 3) offers conditional permission without authoritative guidance, maintaining the pedagogical preference for PAR to lead the problem-solving.

During this moment of needing to decide, PAR produces the vocalisation *ti-di-di-di* (line 5) while flickering the catheter through the patient's neck (Fig. 4). These sounds do not constitute lexical content, nor are they attempts at speech. The vocalisation functions as a multimodal accompaniment to the fast, experimental manipulation of the object and, as such, lightens this moment of using a tool that one is not familiar with. The flickering movement also allows PAR to tone down the risk of making an incorrect move when placing the catheter. Producing the playful sound also provides awareness of the oddity of the manoeuvre and a humorous detachment from a potential error.

The situation is resolved after the successful placement of the catheter and the cessation of bleeding (line 6, Fig. 5). Now, PAR produces a meta-commentary on the unfamiliarity of the procedure: *well, one certainly has not used a urinary catheter to stop bleeding* (line 7). The turn displays retrospective orientation to the strangeness of the action, marking PAR's earlier behaviour, including the non-lexical vocalisation, as part of navigating an unfamiliar task. It also works to justify or excuse the tentative and playful experimentation that preceded it, reframing the experimental flickering as a reasonable response to an uncommon situation.

This excerpt shows how a non-lexical vocalisation emerged at the moment of uncertainty and helped the participant to momentarily step outside the seriousness of the clinical frame. Similarly to the earlier examples of laughter and code-switching, these sound-based expressions function as socially shared coping practices that allow the participant to proceed in spite of insufficient knowledge and unfamiliar tools.

3.3.6 Non-Serious Embodied Move: Throwing an Object Towards the Patient

In the final example, we show how one participant engages in what we call a non-serious embodied move in the context of treating a bleeding patient: they throw an object towards the patient as a response to struggling in the task. Before the excerpt begins, the participant has placed objects randomly on the bleeding patient for several seconds, including a cervical collar. Then, the instructor suggests the use of the foley catheter to stop the bleeding.

This example again shows how the participant is navigating an unfamiliar situation. The excerpt begins when PAR tries to remove the cervical collar from the patient's neck for eight seconds, without success (line 1). This struggle with the collar as well as the audible exhalation *hh* together with the participant's gaze shifting toward the equipment (line 2) further reveal a moment of trouble, searching, and/or indecision.

Data excerpt 5

01   (8.0) ((tries to remove collar))
02 PAR: hh. ((gazes towards equipment))
03   (5.0)#fig6
            ((takes a chest tube and throws it towards patient))
04 PAR: v(h)oiko m(h)ä v(h)aa nak(h)ella sit(h)ä n(h)äillä
            can I just throw it (patient) with these
05   ha ha asioilla.
            ha ha things
06 INS: [tos on noi]
            there are those
07 PAR: [ää mä tapan sen]
            argh I'll kill it
08 INS: kaks samanlaista niin se toinen vois toimia
            two similar so the other one could work
09   siihen katetrina...
            there as a catheter...

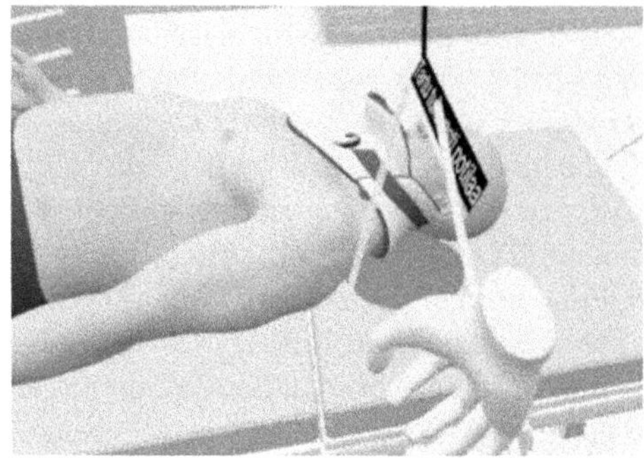

Fig. 6. PAR throws a chest tube towards the patient.

PAR's subsequent act, picking up a chest tube and throwing it toward the patient (line 3, Fig. 6), constitutes what might be described as *a non-serious embodied move.* This action departs from an expected clinical frame and can be characterised as a playful disalignment of the activity, where PAR temporarily suspends the seriousness of the task through exaggerated, humorous, or incongruous embodied conduct.

The participant's question, accompanied with laughter tokens *v(h)oiko mä v(h)aa nak(h)ella sit(h)ä n(h)äillä ha ha asioilla / can I just throw it (patient) with these ha ha things* (lines 4–5) explicitly frames the throw as non-serious or a "norm breach", revealing also self-awareness of the breach. The laughter particles also frame the preceding throwing action as play rather than as literal aggression [see, e.g., 12]. Indeed, PAR seems to be using humour and embodied exaggeration to cope with not knowing what to do. When INS begins to respond, their turn is partially overlapped by PAR's next utterance, *argh, I'll kill it* (lines 6–7), which is another humour-marked exaggeration. Again, this exaggeration is not to be treated as literal, but allows PAR to relieve the pressure of performing a correct clinical action. Then, INS's response reorients the interaction back to the task by referring to available equipment (lines 8–9), thereby re-establishing the clinical frame and providing a path back to task progression.

Across the sequence, the throwing gesture and the laughter-embedded turn function together as a socially shared multimodal coping mechanism, similar in logic to the code-switching and non-lexical vocalisations observed in the earlier examples. The participant uses humour, bodily exaggeration, and non-seriousness to temporarily reduce the weight of the task they need to complete. The embodied move allows the participant to cope with the unfamiliarity of the task and/or VR simulation. In sum, the embodied move aligns with the understanding that participants can manipulate the seriousness of an activity through embodied and vocal means, using humour or exaggeration to manage discomfort or reduce task pressure.

4   Discussion

The aim of this study was to explore how nursing students' physiological stress responses differed across three trauma care tasks conducted in a virtual reality simulation and what temporal stress patterns emerged within and across these tasks. We also investigated the association between these stress patterns and participants' verbal and multimodal behaviour during the tasks. The study employed a multi-method design that integrated psychophysiological measurements with video-based Conversation Analysis.

The results of this exploratory study highlight the complex and individualised nature of learners' stress responses during immersive VR-trauma simulations, particularly in the absence of prior experience with emergency trauma care. Previous studies have demonstrated that VR can elicit genuine responses in its users appearing both at the behavioural level (e.g. [9]) and as physiological responses [30]. In this study, both physiological data and participants' behaviours captured in video recordings suggest that participants experienced and displayed some level of stress and confusion when conducting the tasks, although these observations are exploratory and drawn from a small sample. From a healthcare perspective, such stress and confusion are highly relevant, as elevated cognitive and emotional load during clinical procedures may impair decision-making, technical performance, and communication, all of which are critical determinants of patient safety in trauma care [31]. Furthermore, these reactions appeared to stem from clinical tasks themselves instead of emotional reactions towards the virtual patient, unlike in the study of [9], for example (i.e. if the participants felt genuine stress, it was most likely related to the pressure of displaying their nursing skills instead of reacting to the virtual patient as if they were a real person). This type of performance-related stress closely reflects the pressures experienced by novice clinicians in real-world trauma situations, where task execution rather than emotional response to patients often drives stress [32].

Physiological data suggested a trend toward increased physiological load as task complexity increased, with higher RMSSD values during the wound task and lower values during the chest tube task. Although between-task differences were not statistically significant, likely due to the small sample size, the descriptive patterns indicate that more demanding procedures may constrain autonomic flexibility, reflecting heightened cognitive and emotional load. In clinical contexts, such increased load may correspond to situations where learners are at greater risk of performance degradation, particularly during complex or unfamiliar procedures. Importantly, RMSSD values remained within a range consistent with adaptive engagement rather than excessive stress, suggesting that participants were challenged but not overwhelmed.

It is important to note that heart rate (HR) and heart rate variability (HRV) should not be interpreted as a direct indicator of stress. Besides, HRV demonstrates autonomic nervous system regulation, particularly the balance between sympathetic and parasympathetic activity. For instance, changes in HRV may be influenced by multiple factors, including task complexity, novelty, cognitive demand, and situational context. Therefore, the observed physiological patterns are interpreted as indicators of physiological engagement and task-related demand rather than as direct measures of stress. In addition, individual differences in baseline physiological activity may further contribute to variability across participants.

The findings suggest that the physiological patterns were somewhat mirrored in the video-based behavioural data, especially during the first learning task. This wound treatment task, which elicited the greatest inter-individual variability in RMSSD, was also characterised by the most frequent verbal and multimodal expressions of uncertainty, confusion, and nervousness. Direct verbalisations of trouble, trouble-marking laughter, code-switching, non-lexical vocalisations, and a non-serious embodied move functioned as observable coping strategies through which participants navigated the unfamiliar situation. From a healthcare perspective, these behaviours may be interpreted as early-stage coping and regulation strategies that novice clinicians use to manage clinical uncertainty and maintain task progression under pressure. These utterances also function as examples of interactionally meaningful ways of softening the accountability of the participants' actions when they do not yet know what to do. These behaviours temporarily reframed the activity from a serious clinical frame into a lighter, less consequential one, allowing participants to relieve immediate pressure while still remaining engaged in the task. Rather than being disruptive, such actions seem to constitute systematic coping practices: they buy time, signal uncertainty without fully stalling progress, and enable participants to continue experimenting with tools, objects, and bodily manoeuvres when completing the scenario. Such behaviours may also be linked to non-technical skills, particularly emotional regulation, communication, and maintenance of situational awareness [6], which are essential competencies for safe clinical practice. These multimodal practices also illustrate how learners actively recruit support and maintain interactional flow and task engagement during moments of heightened challenge and pressure, and how their help-seeking was then also immediately responded to.

Together, the findings suggest that VR-based trauma simulations can elicit substantial regulatory demands on learners, particularly when clinical procedures are novel. This has important implications for simulation-based healthcare education, as unmanaged cognitive and emotional load during early training may negatively affect skill acquisition and subsequent clinical performance. This reinforces the pedagogical importance of providing adaptive instructional and human support during early exposure to high-stakes VR scenarios, as well as the value of multimodal methodologies for capturing the interplay between physiological stress, observable behaviour, and learning processes in trauma education [33]. In practice, this may involve scaffolded simulation design, gradual increases in task complexity, and structured debriefing sessions that explicitly address stress recognition and regulation as part of clinical competence.

This study has limitations that should be considered. First, the physiological measures used, particularly HRV, do not provide a direct indicator of psychological stress, but rather reflect autonomic regulation that may be influenced by task demands and individual differences. In addition, the relatively small sample size limits the robustness and generalizability of the findings.

Second, while the multimodal approach combining physiological data and interactional video analysis offers valuable complementary perspectives, the integration of these data sources remains exploratory in the present study. The alignment between physiological signals and specific interactional events was not systematically modelled, and therefore, interpretations should be considered indicative rather than conclusive. While Conversation Analysis provides detailed insight into participants' observable behaviour, it does not allow direct access to internal psychological states such as stress or anxiety. In a previous study, physiological measures were used to complement such observations by capturing features of autonomic activity during task performance [34]. These signals are not interpreted as direct indicators of specific psychological states, however, they provide an additional layer of information about physiological engagement that can be considered alongside behavioural data. By combining these perspectives, the multimodal approach supports a more nuanced and cautious interpretation of participants' responses to complex and unfamiliar tasks. Such integrated approaches are particularly valuable in healthcare research, where understanding both observable performance and underlying physiological processes can inform more effective training interventions.

Third, the simulation context does not fully replicate real clinical environments, where additional factors such as team dynamics, time pressure, and responsibility for patient outcomes may significantly influence stress responses and behaviour.

In sum, combining physiological measures with the synchronised video recordings allowed us to start exploring *when* physiological stress responses occur and *how* participants socially manage those moments in real time. Our approach invites conducting further research to reach a situated understanding of stress as both a bodily and an interactional phenomenon. Ultimately, these findings highlight the importance of supporting learners in managing stress during training, with the goal of enhancing clinical performance and contributing to patient safety in high-stakes healthcare environments.

Acknowledgments. We thank Jussi Kosola from VRTrauma for allowing the use and examination of their VR scenario. We also thank Philip Lê for assistance during data collection. This work is co-funded by the European Union's Digital Europe Programme (DIGITAL) under grant agreement No. 101083544, and partly funded by Business Finland (No. 765/31/2023) and the University of Oulu. This work is also supported by the University of Oulu and the Research Council of Finland (PROFI7, decision no. 352788).

Disclosure of Interests. The authors report there are no competing interests to declare.

Appendix: Transcript Conventions

Conventions for transcribing audible interaction based on [16].

hh.   Audible exhale.
ha ha   laughter.
wo(h)rd   laughter within talk.
[beginning of overlap in speech.
]   end of overlap in speech.
(0.5)   pause in seconds.
=   no pause between speakers.
:   sound lenghtening.
(())   comment by transcriber.
screenshot of that moment in the video (figure).

References

1. Liaw, S.Y., Tan, K.K., Wu, L.T., Tan, S.C., Choo, H., Yap, J., Lim, S.M., Wong, L., Ignacio, J.: Finding the right blend of technologically enhanced learning environments: randomized con-trolled study of the effect of instructional sequences on Interprofessional learning. J. Med. Internet. Res. **21**(5), e12537 (2019). https://doi.org/10.2196/12537. PMID: 31140432. PMCID: PMC6658293

2. Radianti, J., Majchrzak, T.A., Fromm, J., Wohlgenannt, I.: A systematic review of immersive virtual reality applications for higher education: design elements, lessons learned, and research agenda. Comput. Educ. **147**, 103778 (2020). https://doi.org/10.1016/j.compedu.2019.103778

3. Kolb, D.A.: Experiential learning: experience as the source of learning and development. Prentice Hall, Englewood Cliffs (NJ) (1984)

4. Liaw, S.Y., Rusli, K.D.B., Schmidt, L.T., Siah, C.J.R., McKenna, L., Wee, H.N.C., et al.: Multimodal simulation to prepare final year nursing students for transition to clinical practice: a mixed methods study. Clin. Simul. Nurs. **93**, 101559 (2024). https://doi.org/10.1016/j.ecns.2024.101559

5. Johnson-Glenberg, M.C.: Immersive VR and education: Embodied design principles that include gesture and hand controls. Front Robot AI Jul 24;5:81 (2018). https://doi.org/10.3389/frobt.2018.00081. PMID: 33500960; PMCID: PMC7805662

6. Ropponen, P., Tomietto, M., Pramila-Savukoski, S., Kuivila, H., Koskenranta, M., Liaw, S.Y., et al.: Impacts of virtual reality simulation on nursing students' competence, confidence, and satisfaction: a systematic review and meta-analysis of randomised controlled trials. Nurse Educ. Today **152**, 106756 (2025). https://doi.org/10.1016/j.nedt.2025.106756

7. Slater, M.: Place illusion and plausibility can lead to realistic behaviour in immersive virtual environments. Philos. Transact. Royal Soc. B: Bio. Sci. **364**(1535), 3549–3557 (2009).

8. Gonzalez-Franco, M., Lanier, J.: Model of illusions and virtual reality. Front. Psychol. **8**, 1125 (2017). https://doi.org/10.3389/fpsyg.2017.01125

9. Pan, X., Slater, M., Beacco, A., Navarro, X., Bellido Rivas, A. I., Swapp, D., Delacroix, S.: The responses of medical general practitioners to unreasonable patient demand for antibiotics-a study of medical ethics using immersive virtual reality. PloS one **11**(2), e0146837 (2016). https://doi.org/10.1371/journal.pone.0146837

10. Sacks, H., Schegloff, E.A., Jefferson, G.: A simplest systematics for the organization of turn-taking for conversation. Language **50**(4), 696–735 (1974). https://doi.org/10.2307/412243

11. Sidnell, J., Stivers, T. eds.: The Handbook of Conversation Analysis. Blackwell Publishing (2013)

12. Glenn, P.: Laughter in interaction. Cambridge University Press (2003)

13. Sacks, H.: Lectures on conversation, volumes I and II. Blackwell (1992)

14. Mondada, L.: Contemporary issues in conversation analysis: Embodiment and materiality, multimodality and multisensoriality in social interaction. J. Pragmat. **145**, 47–62 (2019). https://doi.org/10.1016/j.pragma.2019.01.016

15. Sacks, H.: Notes on methodology. In: Structures of Social Action (1st ed.), J. Maxwell Atkinson (Ed.), Cambridge University Press, Cambridge, UK, 21–27 (1985). https://doi.org/10.1017/CBO9780511665868.005

16. Jefferson, G.: Glossary of transcript symbols with an introduction. In G. Lerner (ed.), Conversation Analysis: Studies from the first generation, pp. 13–31. John Benjamins (2004)

17. LeBlanc, V.R., Brazil, V., Posner, G.D.: More than a feeling: Emotional regulation strategies for simulation-based education. Adv. Simul. **9**(1), 53 (2024). https://doi.org/10.1186/s41077-024-00325-z

18. Orvell, A., et al.: Does distanced self-talk facilitate emotion regulation across a range of emotionally intense experiences? Clinical Psychological Sci **9**(1), 68–78 (2021). https://doi.org/10.1177/2167702620951539

19. Theodoratou, M., Argyrides, M.: Neuropsychological insights into coping strategies: integrating theory and practice in clinical and therapeutic contexts. Psychiatry International **5**(1), 53–73 (2024). https://doi.org/10.3390/psychiatryint5010005

20. Heritage, J.: Epistemics in Conversation. In: Sidnell, J., Stivers, T. (eds.) Handbook of Conversation Analysis, pp. 370–394. Blackwell, Oxford (2013)

21. Melander, H.: Transformations of knowledge within a peer group. Knowing and learning in interaction. Learning, Culture & Social Interaction **1**(3–4), 232–248 (2012). https://doi.org/10.1016/j.lcsi.2012.09.003
22. Haakana, M.: Laughing matters: a conversation analytical study of laughter in doctor–patient interaction. Doctoral dissertation, University of Helsinki (1999)
23. Haakana, M.: Laughter as a patient's resource: dealing with delicate aspects of medical interaction. Text & Talk **21**(1–2), 187–219 (2001). https://doi.org/10.1515/text.1.21.1-2.187
24. Haakana, M.: Laughter in medical interaction: from quantification to analysis, and back. J. Socioling. **6**(2), 207–235 (2002). https://doi.org/10.1111/1467-9481.00185
25. Almelhi, A.M.: Understanding code-switching from a sociolinguistic perspective: a meta-analysis. Internat J Lang Ling **8**(1), 34–45 (2020). https://doi.org/10.11648/j.ijll.20200801.15
26. Auer, P.: Code-switching in conversation: Language, interaction and identity. Routledge (2002)
27. Goffman, E.: Frame Analysis. Harper & Row (1974)
28. Albert, S., vom Lehn, D.: Non-lexical vocalizations help novices learn joint embodied actions. Lang. Commun. **88**, 1–13 (2023). https://doi.org/10.1016/j.langcom.2022.10.001
29. Keevallik, L., Ogden, R.: Sounds on the margins of language at the heart of interaction. Res. Lang. Soc. Interact. **53**(1), 1–18 (2020). https://doi.org/10.1080/08351813.2020.171296129
30. Meehan, M., Insko, B., Whitton, M., Brooks, F.P., Jr.: Physiological measures of presence in stressful virtual environments. ACM Transact. Graphics (tog) **21**(3), 645–652 (2002). https://doi.org/10.1145/566654.566630
31. Young, J.Q., Thakker, K., John, M., Friedman, K., Sugarman, R., van Merriënboer, J.J., O'Sullivan, P.S.: Exploring the relationship between emotion and cognitive load types during patient handovers. Adv Health Sci Educat **26**(5), 1463–1489 (2021). https://doi.org/10.1007/s10459-021-10053-y
32. Anton, N.E., Huffman, E.M., Ahmed, R.A., Cooper, D.D., Athanasiadis, D.I., Cha, J., Lee, N.K.: Stress and resident interdisciplinary team performance: results of a pilot trauma simulation program. Surgery **170**(4), 1074–1079 (2021). https://doi.org/10.1016/j.surg.2021.03.010
33. Mikkonen, K., Liaw, S.Y., Spirgienė, L., Subočiūtė, A., Ignatavičius, P., Blažauskas, T., et al.: Multidimensional pedagogical framework for interprofessional education: blending classroom, high-fidelity and extended reality simulation. Nurse Educ. Today **154**, 106838 (2025). https://doi.org/10.1016/j.nedt.2025.106838
34. Fairclough, S.H.: Fundamentals of physiological computing. Interact. Comput. **21**(1–2), 133–145 (2009). https://doi.org/10.1016/j.intcom.2008.10.011

Induction of Empathic Concern and Cognitive Empathy with Experts and Adults in an Immersive Virtual Reality Magnetic Resonance Imaging (MRI) Experience with Child's Perspective

Iresh Jayasundara[1]([✉])[iD], Paula Alavesa[1][iD], Severi Pitkänen[1][iD], Eemeli Häyrynen[1][iD], Nirasha Thennakoon[1][iD], Katherine J. Mimnaugh[1][iD], Sirpa Kekäläinen[2][iD], and Tarja Pölkki[2][iD]

[1] Center for Applied Computing, Faculty of ITEE, University of Oulu, Oulu, Finland
`Iresh.JayasundaraMudiyanselage@oulu.fi`
[2] Research Unit of Health Sciences and Technology, Faculty of Medicine, University of Oulu, Oulu, Finland

Abstract. Children frequently experience anxiety during magnetic resonance imaging (MRI), where confined space, loud acoustic noise, and the requirement to remain still can make the procedure difficult to complete and may contribute to the use of sedation or general anaesthesia. Digital health preparation tools, including immersive approaches, have been proposed to support familiarisation and coping. However, many existing experiences emphasize distraction or strongly gamified metaphors, which may create unrealistic expectations of the clinical pathway and its sensory cues. This paper presents a realism-first immersive Virtual Reality (VR) experience co-designed with medical imaging professionals to simulate the procedural journey surrounding paediatric MRI. The experience is delivered from a child-height perspective and guides users through key steps of the visit culminating in a stillness-focused interaction. A mixed-method pilot study with an a priori qualitative focus was conducted with parents and MRI domain experts due to ethical and practical constraints for paediatric testing in this phase (N = 6; 3 parents and 3 MRI experts). Validated questionnaires (System Usability Scale (SUS) and User Experience Questionnaire (UEQ)) and semi-structured interviews were used to assess usability, perceived realism, and empathy-related responses. These were analysed with distinction between empathic concern and cognitive empathy; qualitative results highlight perceived procedural clarity and realism, especially for environmental cues and scanner audio. An additional emergent theme was reported by adult participants: experiencing the pathway from a child's perspective supported empathy, specifically empathic concern more than cognitive empathy. These results provide feasibility and acceptability evidence to support further translation and a staged paediatric evaluation with objective outcomes (e.g., child anxiety measures and scan-related metrics).

© The Author(s) 2026
M. Särestöniemi et al. (Eds.): NCDHWS 2026, CCIS 3009, pp. 358–371, 2026.
https://doi.org/10.1007/978-3-032-28812-7_25

Keywords: Virtual reality · paediatric MRI · Patient preparation ·
User experience · Inducing Empathy

1   Introduction

Children frequently experience anxiety during magnetic resonance imaging
(MRI), where the confined bore, loud acoustic noise, and the requirement to
remain still can make the procedure difficult to complete [14,15]. Elevated anxiety may lead to motion during scanning, which can degrade image quality and
increase the likelihood of repeated acquisitions [15]. In paediatric settings, these
challenges can also contribute to the use of sedation or general anaesthesia,
introducing additional risks, costs, and scheduling complexity [8].

To improve readiness and reduce uncertainty, a range of preparation
approaches has been employed, including informational materials, mock-scanner
programs, and structured familiarisation [8,15]. More recently, digital health
interventions have explored interactive and immersive preparation, where experiential familiarisation can be delivered in a controlled and repeatable manner
[6,17,23,27]. While promising outcomes have been reported, the design space
remains open regarding how preparation is framed. Some interventions prioritize distraction or strongly gamified metaphors, which may be beneficial for
engagement but can underrepresent procedural steps and salient sensory cues,
potentially shaping unrealistic expectations of the clinical pathway [18,21].

In this paper, a realism-first immersive VR preparation experience for paediatric MRI is presented. The experience was iteratively developed via user-centric
approach with medical imaging professionals to reflect an end-to-end pathway,
from arrival and waiting to preparation and scanner familiarisation. A child-
height viewpoint was used to support perspective-taking and caregiver understanding. Locomotion and interaction were designed to balance engagement with
comfort, informed by prior discussions on VR safety and cybersickness considerations [29].

This study aims for the following contributions:

– A realism-first immersive VR preparation experience that simulates key steps
  of a paediatric MRI pathway, co-designed with medical imaging professionals
  to emphasize procedural clarity and salient sensory cues.
– Formative evidence of usability, user experience, and stakeholder acceptability from a mixed-method pilot with parents and MRI domain experts using
  standardised instruments (SUS and UEQ) and semi-structured interviews
  [7,24].
– Implications for digital health translation of immersive preparation tools,
  including the observed caregiver perspective-taking effect and practical refinements to induce empathic concern and cognitive empathy in experts and
  adults preparing them and their children for MRI [17,18].

2   Related Work

Preparation for paediatric MRI has been approached through informational materials, mock-scanner programs, and structured familiarisation, aiming to reduce uncertainty and improve cooperation [8,15]. Prior work highlights that anxiety is shaped not only by the scanner itself but also by the broader clinical pathway, including waiting, unfamiliar staff, medical equipment, and uncertainty about what will happen next [15]. These observations motivate preparation approaches that support anticipatory coping by making key steps predictable and understandable.

2.1   Immersive Preparation as a Digital Health Intervention

Immersive VR has been investigated as a preparation and education tool in healthcare because it can provide experiential familiarisation in a controlled, repeatable, and engaging way [6,23,27]. In imaging-related contexts, VR preparation has been reported to improve perceived readiness and may reduce anxiety-related responses, although evaluation designs and outcome measures vary across studies [17]. A recurring design question concerns whether an intervention primarily supports distraction (diverting attention away from stressors) or familiarisation (helping users understand and anticipate stressors). familiarisation-oriented designs may be particularly relevant for MRI, where sensory cues such as scanner noise can be intense and unfamiliar [15].

2.2   Realism-First versus Gamified Preparation

A number of immersive and interactive experiences for paediatric healthcare emphasise playful metaphors and game mechanics to increase engagement [18,21]. While gamification can support motivation, a strong departure from clinical reality may create mismatched expectations of the procedure. By contrast, realism-first preparation aims to represent the environment, procedure flow, and salient sensory cues with higher fidelity, potentially supporting anticipatory coping and increasing trust in the intervention. In the context of paediatric MRI, procedural clarity and sensory realism can also facilitate caregiver communication, as caregivers often explain the procedure and support the child's coping strategies [17].

2.3   Inducing Empathy and VR

Empathy is commonly described as multi-component. Cognitive empathy refers to understanding another person's perspective or mental state (perspective taking), whereas empathic concern refers to other-oriented feelings of compassion and care for another's welfare [10].

VR has been dubbed as "empathy machine" by some scholars due to its potential in inducing empathy related responses. VR's ability to allow perspective-taking through embodiment has been used in empathy training, however, the outcomes are sometimes unintended, which suggest that we still have lot to learn on how perspective-taking, body ownership and embodiment in VR influence human empathy [16,25,28]. VR seems to enhance prosocial characteristics which support empathy. Despite this there is little direct evidence of positive outcomes in VR mediated empathy training, in fact VR can also produce negative effects and enhance stress. It is, still, undeniable that VR influences empathy, or can induce other reaction where empathy is the underlying mechanism, but there is still a lot we do not know about the underlying mechanisms; the social, collective and individual factors that would allow facilitation of better empathic resonance [9,20,25,28]

2.4   Comfort and Safety Considerations for Child-Focused VR

For VR applications intended for children, comfort and cybersickness risk require careful attention. Locomotion methods, visual motion cues, and session length can influence discomfort, and conservative interaction choices are commonly recommended when designing for younger users [2,29]. These constraints motivate designs that preserve immersion while reducing motion-related discomfort, for example by using teleportation, guided movement, and accessibility supports such as subtitles and adjustable audio.

3   Design and Implementation

The VR game was designed to simulate an MRI procedure in the University of Oulu Hospital. The full MRI procedure was observed in detail during a hospital visit in November 2023, where radiographers and a radiologist were interviewed on process details. Due to access limitations to the location and experts working on the MRI device, a scenario-based design method was selected for initialisation. This was followed with a user centric approach [1], where the scenario, script, and dialogue were written first based on the hospital visit and later adapted based on an additional round of feedback from radiographers [5,11].

The overall narrative of the experience was divided into the following steps:

1. **Home preparation:** Parents inform the child about the scan, the hospital visit, and provide comfort by explaining that the procedure is safe.
2. **Arrival and waiting room:** The child arrives at the hospital, registers, and waits until a nurse guides them to the next stage.
3. **Cannulation room:** Cannulation is a necessity in some MRI procedures, and the experience includes this step while aiming to avoid unnecessarily frightening details.
4. **Transition and waiting:** The child is guided between rooms and waits until being called in.
5. **Dressing room:** The child is reminded about suitable clothing and removing metal items.

6. **Radiographer dialogue:** The child can ask questions about the procedure via on-screen prompts and can choose from a few options of what to listen to during the scan.
7. **MRI scan minigame:** The scan itself is represented as a minigame where the goal is to stay still.
8. **Positive closure:** After the scan, the radiographer encourages the child and the child receives a small reward.

The original target group for the game are 7–12-year-old children. However, due to the size limitations of current HMDs, the final intervention may target children slightly older than seven due to the HMDs sizing. To reduce the chance of cybersickness during frequent room-to-room transitions, locomotion was implemented with teleportation. Teleportation locomotion was selected to reduce cybersickness risk, consistent with common VR comfort guidance [29]. Cybersickness symptoms were not formally measured in this pilot. The original plan aimed at realistic character visuals, but a more caricature style was selected to avoid the uncanny valley effect. Voice acting was conducted by one expert in medical imaging procedures and the development team.

Meta Quest 2 was selected as the platform since it can be used as a standalone device, allowing children and parents to use it at home before a hospital visit. The game was developed with Unity 3D. The player camera was set low to enhance the sense of looking at the experience through the eyes of a child. After play testing, the avatar hands were adjusted to be smaller than standard avatar hands based on received feedback (Fig. 1).

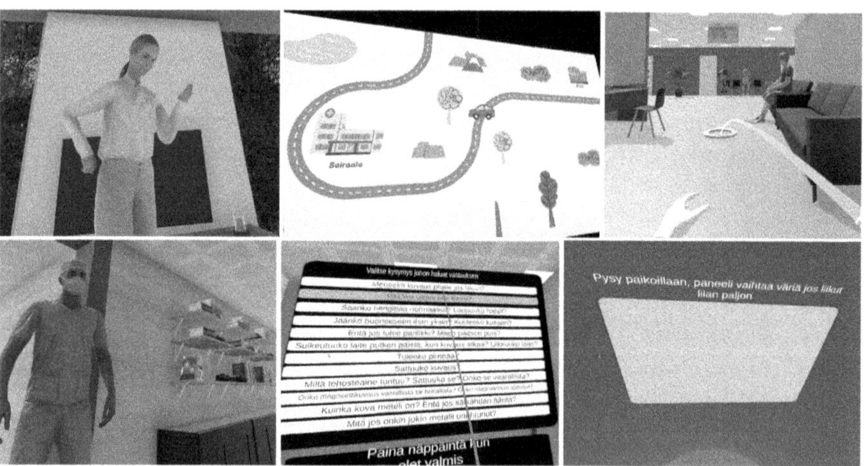

Fig. 1. Collage of screenshots showing few steps in the game: The game starts at home with a child's perspective on player camera(top, left). The travel between home and hospital is depicted by a 2D animation (top, middle). The hospital scene has been designed to resemble a hospital, and there are other children there as non player characters (NPC) (top, right) along other NPCs (bottom, left). In addition to spoken instruction the player can ask about the procedure (bottom, middle). Inside the MRI machine there is a minigame where the purpose is to stay still.

4   Materials and Methods

A user study (N = 6) was conducted to evaluate the MRI simulation. The participants were experts in MRI or parents. Prior user evaluation the testing consisted of internal tests and play testing [12].

Technical Testing. VR user experience is dependent on a consistent frame rate, and even momentarily going below certain thresholds may influence user experience or cause cybersickness. To assess performance and address issues, a technical evaluation was carried out by logging frames per second (fps). Meta Quest has a ceiling fps of 72, which was set as the highest reachable. Benchmarking was conducted with three running cycles using Oculus Tray Tool [4]. The application was running at a ceiling fps of 72 for 96.78% of the running time. The lowest reported fps drop was 41 in the hallway scene. Overall, fps was consistent, supporting a good user experience, and allowed continuing with a user study.

The User Study

Participants. A mixed-method pilot evaluation with parents ($N = 3$) and medical imaging domain experts ($N = 3$) was conducted. Participants had children aged between 6 to 13, and domain experts had prior knowledge of MRI and imaging procedures, while also being parents themselves. Out of the parents, some reported prior MRI experience for their children. Participants were adults between 27 to 44 years old and had varying levels of prior VR experience.

Procedure. Participants first completed consent forms and a pre-questionnaire about demographics and prior experiences in VR and MRI. Each participant wore a Meta Quest 2 device and navigated the VR application by following inbuilt instructions and intuition to avoid biasing the experience. The total study duration ranged approximately from 31 to 46 min, including gameplay and a post-experience interview. Participants experienced the game in the sequence of events described above.

Data Collection and Analysis. All participants took part in a recorded semi-structured interview to gather qualitative and descriptive feedback. Interviews were conducted in Finnish for native Finnish speakers and in English for non-Finnish speakers. Audio transcripts were used for analysis. A post-study questionnaire containing the User Experience Questionnaire (UEQ) and System Usability Scale (SUS) was administered to all participants [7,24]. Informed written consent was obtained before the evaluation, The ethical principles of research with human participants and ethical review in the human sciences in the Finnish National Board on Research Integrity TENK guidelines 2019 and EU legislation were followed [22]. No formal ethics board approval was required for this study under the host organisation's policy for this type of human-participant research.

5   Results

In this section the results from the basic usability and user experience evaluation are described first followed with analysis results from the semi-structured interviews.

5.1   Usability and User Experience (SUS/UEQ)

Overall usability was assessed with SUS. Scores ranged from 57.5 to 80.0 with a mean of 72.1 (SD = 10.4), indicating a generally good level of usability in this pilot, although one participant scored below 60. Table 1 and Fig. 2 reports participant-level SUS values. User experience was assessed with UEQ. The UEQ benchmark comparison suggested an above-average overall user experience across attributes. Given the pilot sample size (N = 6), SUS and UEQ results are reported descriptively and should be interpreted with caution.

Table 1. SUS scores by participant

Participant	1	2	3	4	5	6
SUS score	77.5	57.5	60.0	80.0	77.5	80.0

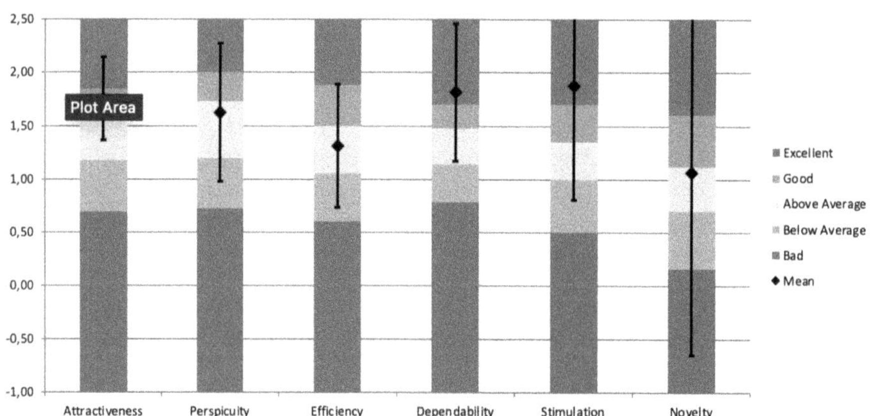

Fig. 2. UEQ benchmark, where means are set in relation to values in a benchmark data set that contains data from over 21000 participants in 468 studies [24]. The lines depicting the confidence intervals of the scale scores and show quite high unreliability especially in Novelty.

5.2   Qualitative Findings

Interview data were analysed using thematic analysis with a combination of inductive (for clinical utility and technological fidelity) and deductive coding (for empathy related themes). The coding framework retained the following five subcategories, consistent with the original analysis: *Technological Fidelity, Clinical Utility, Cognitive Empathy, Empathic Concern*, and *Miscellaneous Observations*. The *Technological Fidelity* and *Clinical Utility* categories were applied particularly for expert participants. Empathy-related content was coded as *Cognitive Empathy* (recognising the child's possible mental state) and *Empathic Concern* (a sympathetic, tender emotional response towards the child). Agreement testing was conducted, resulting in a Cohen's Kappa of 0.801, indicating excellent agreement. Across a total of 205 coded items, 177 agreements were observed (86.34%).

Technological Fidelity: Realism and Interaction. Two of the domain experts were radiographers. There was a common consensus that the path of going from home to the hospital, cannulation and finally MRI room was well done as stated by one of them

> "Really accurately, it was an impressive experience, I have been in a lot of MRI imaging." (P2)

The Audio was praised as very realistic as well as the MRI machine. They liked that the nurses tell the player what can be taken into the room. The list of questions for the player can select were also praised.

The experts found the nurse NPCs to be a bit unnatural and stated that they were moving around "uncanny" and without purpose at times. MRI imaging audio and the dialogue from the mother was too quiet in their opinion. For four participants, the mother's voice was too low as mentioned by one of them "Mother's speech was very low at first". The hospital environment itself gained some praise for being realistic but one participant mentioned that "The hospital seemed more open and peaceful than a real hospital". This is a known issue with VR scenes, which tend to be less cluttered and messy than actual locations, apparently even hospitals.

The experts were not that used to using VR so some of them needed more help than others while playing the game. Teleporting turned out to be difficult at the beginning. But after they got used to the few controls, they handled the game easily. Participants stated that allowing free navigation with a greater degree of freedom to the child within the virtual environment would be beneficial. This, however, would contradict best practices that prefer teleportation since free locomotion causes vection and cyber sickness.

> "At first, I struggled with teleporting, but once I got used to it, the experience felt seamless. I think allowing more movement could help make the experience more engaging" (P1)

Clinical Utility: Perceived Usefulness in Care Pathways. Experts perceived the application as potentially useful for preparation and for easing workload while preparing children to procedures. One of them stated:

> "Yes, I believe that when you really come to the imaging its easier. Videos already help, but this is more realistic." (P3)

One expert noted that while videos can already help, the VR experience was perceived as more realistic. Another participant emphasised potential efficiency benefits for staff time during preparation. These observations were framed as perceived clinical utility from stakeholders rather than demonstrated clinical efficacy, given the staged evaluation.

> "I hope these are introduced for support; it will shorten the work time for nurses." (P5)

Cognitive Empathy. During coding, *cognitive empathy* was applied when participants described perspective taking or inferring the child's feelings or thoughts. *Empathic concern* was applied when participants expressed compassion, sympathy, or protective concern for the child's wellbeing [10]. A recurrent qualitative finding was that the child-height perspective supported adult perspective-taking. Participants described how experiencing the pathway as a child could benefit parents as well as children, and one expert who was also a parent stated that they would encourage other parents to use the experience as well.

> "Other parents who still were not prepared for MRI. I would totally encourage to use, but not only the kids, but also them." (P1)

It was expected the game might help parents to see the child's perspective, but it was, also, encouraging to notice that the parent's participating in the study sensed this. One participant recommended the experience to just anyone who is afraid of tight spaces and medical examinations.

All participants came to the conclusion that the MRI game would help children, especially small children combat their anxiety and fears before MRI imaging. One of them (P2) was happy that the user is told that they can do the imaging with their parent but then the user cannot see or hear the mother even though the mother is close by.

A specific design implication raised by one participant concerned caregiver presence during scanning: the experience informs the player that a parent can be present, but the parent character is not seen or heard during the scan scene. Participants suggested that aligning this moment more closely with real practices could strengthen reassurance:

> "It was good that the user is told they can do the imaging with their parent, but then the user cannot see or hear the mother, even though she is close by." (P2)

Empathic Concern. Participants commonly stated that familiarisation could reduce fear of the unknown and that the experience could reduce anxiety by making the procedure predictable. In particular, the inclusion of loud MRI sounds in-context was described as a mechanism for making the real experience less frightening.

"The device itself is not as scary if you know where you are going." (P3)

Another participant shared a similar perspective:

"Children are often afraid of the unknown, so just seeing the whole process in VR-especially hearing those loud MRI sounds can make it much less frightening when they experience it for real." (P6)

Miscellaneous Observations. Participants suggested that the same realism-first preparation logic could be adapted for other stressful paediatric medical procedures (e.g., blood tests or dental treatments). This was coded as an outlier but meaningful observation indicating possible generalisability of the results beyond MRI.

"This kind of VR game could be useful beyond MRI. It could help prepare children for other medical exams or treatments too." (P6)

6   Discussion

This study contributes a realism-first VR preparation experience that simulates the procedural pathway of paediatric MRI and reports formative findings from parents and MRI domain experts. The pilot results should be interpreted as feasibility-oriented evidence: SUS scores indicated generally good usability (M = 72.1), UEQ results suggested a positive overall user experience, and interview feedback emphasised procedural clarity and perceived realism-especially scanner audio-as key design strengths. Given the staged evaluation and small sample size, these findings are best understood as early indicators that the application is usable and experienceable in its current form, rather than evidence of clinical efficacy or broad adoption. The most encouraging insights from the study came from the interviews, where both parents and experts expressed empathy for the child's perspective during the game. This suggests that the VR application could benefit not only children but also adults-helping them prepare emotionally and mentally for the MRI process, whether for themselves or for their child. This dual benefit indicates the potential for the game to serve as a valuable tool in both clinical and preparatory settings.

6.1   Practical Relevance

The present approach prioritised a faithful end-to-end journey, co-designed with medical imaging professionals. Participants' feedback suggests that this realism-first emphasis can be valuable both for children (preparation) and for caregivers (understanding and communication), which is relevant for translation into clinical preparation packages that often combine multiple modalities (printed instructions, videos, and interactive tools).

6.2 Design Implications and Iterative Improvements

Several practical refinements were identified. Audio mixing and speech volume should be adjusted to ensure intelligibility while preserving realism. NPC movement and behavioural cues should be refined to reduce "uncanny" impressions. Additionally, the child-height camera calibration should be revisited to better match the intended age range and to avoid exaggerated height differences in social scenes. Finally, while teleportation supports comfort and aligns with best practices to mitigate cybersickness in VR, onboarding should be improved for novice users to reduce early interaction friction.

6.3 User Experience, Acceptability, and Adoption in Digital Health

Adoption of digital health systems depends not only on technical feasibility but also on perceived usefulness, ease of use, and fit with the healthcare context [3,13,19,26]. In early-stage development, evaluations commonly rely on known usability and user experience tools, including standardised instruments such as SUS and UEQ [7,24]. This perspective is especially relevant for paediatric interventions where staged validation with caregivers and domain experts may be required before direct evaluation with children. Accordingly, the present work is positioned as feasibility study.

6.4 Limitations and Future Work

The main limitations identified in the earlier IEEE VR review are directly acknowledged here. First, the pilot sample size was small (N = 6), and the participants were not the final target population (children). However, expert and parent users allowed us to observe new potential for medical imaging simulations in inducing empathy and educating parents as well as children. Overall, the present findings should be interpreted as formative evidence of usability, acceptability, and perceived suitability rather than clinical efficacy. Extending the sample size might, also, provide new details on types of empathy induced by immersive VR, in addition to allowing to observe further the learning outcomes and benefits these types of simulations could provide for parents preparing for their children's MRI.

Objective anxiety outcomes were not measured in this phase as the target at this stage were not children. Future evaluation should therefore include child-appropriate anxiety measures and imaging-related outcomes (e.g., ability to remain still, scan repetitions, and sedation/GA-related metrics) to quantify impact beyond stakeholder perceptions.

Considering the interpretability of the results from the qualitative analysis, after agreement testing [27] between two coders the calculated Kappa value was 0.801, indicating substantial agreement across the five subcategories: Technological Fidelity, Clinical Utility, Cognitive Empathy, Empathic Concern, and Miscellaneous Observations. Out of a total of 205 items, the number of observed agreements was 177 (86.34%).

6.5   Next Steps Toward Clinical Translation

A staged evaluation with paediatric participants remains the next critical step. Based on the current feasibility evidence, the system is considered mature enough for a paediatric study where usability and comfort can be monitored alongside objective outcomes. In parallel, integration considerations can be explored (e.g., home use prior to visits versus in-hospital preparation), including how the VR experience complements existing preparation materials and vendor-provided solutions.

7   Conclusions

In this study an immersive VR simulation for MRI was designed and implemented for children in collaboration with experts. The resulting simulation was then tested in a mixed-method user study (N = 6) with qualitative priori, as the main contribution was distilled from semi-structured interviews. Our findings show induction of two types of empathic responses in the adults towards children preparing for MRI: empathic concern and cognitive empathy. The results overall highlight potential that immersive VR simulation targeted at children has in educating and preparing parents for their children's medical imaging.

Acknowledgments. The first and the second author have received funding from the Research Council of Finland (former Academy of Finland) 6Genesis Flagship (318927) and 6G Flagship Program (Grant Number: 346208) funded EMETA (8719/31/2022) and Business Finland funded (4135/31/2024) Resilient Enterprise ITEA (23046).

Disclosure of Interests. The authors have no competing interests to declare that are relevant to the content of this article.

References

1. ISO 9241-210:2019 ergonomics of human-system interaction—part 210: Human-centred design for interactive systems (2019)
2. Ahmadpour, N., Keep, M., Janssen, A., Rouf, A.S., Marthick, M.: Design strategies for virtual reality interventions for managing pain and anxiety in children and adolescents: scoping review. JMIR Serious Games **8**(1), e14565 (2020)
3. AlQudah, A.A., et al.: Technology acceptance in healthcare: a systematic review. Appl. Sci. **11**(22), 10537 (2021)
4. ApollyonVR: Oculus tray tool | apollyonvr (n.d.). https://www.apollyonvr.com/oculus-tray-tool. Accessed 16 May 2025

5. Årsand, E., Demiris, G.: User-centered methods for designing patient-centric self-help tools. Inform. Health Soc. Care **33**(3), 158–169 (2008)
6. Ashmore, J., et al.: A free virtual reality experience to prepare pediatric patients for magnetic resonance imaging: cross-sectional questionnaire study. JMIR Pediatr Parent **2**(1), e11684 (2019). https://doi.org/10.2196/11684
7. Brooke, J.: SUS: a quick and dirty usability scale. Usabil. Eval. Ind. **189** (1995)
8. Carter, A.J., Greer, M.L.C., Gray, S.E., Ware, R.S.: Mock MRI: reducing the need for anaesthesia in children. Pediatr. Radiol. **40**, 1368–1374 (2010)
9. Crone, C.L., Kallen, R.W.: Interview with an avatar: comparing online and virtual reality perspective taking for gender bias in stem hiring decisions. PLoS ONE **17**(6), e0269430 (2022)
10. Davis, M.H.: Measuring individual differences in empathy: evidence for a multidimensional approach. J. Pers. Soc. Psychol. **44**(1), 113–126 (1983)
11. Ermi, L., Mäyrä, F.: Player-centred game design: experiences in using scenario study to inform mobile game design. Game Stud. **5**(1), 1–10 (2005)
12. Fullerton, T., Swain, C., Hoffman, S.: Game Design Workshop: Designing, Prototyping, & Playtesting Games. CRC Press (2004)
13. Greenhalgh, T., et al.: Beyond adoption: a new framework for theorizing and evaluating nonadoption, abandonment, and challenges to the scale-up, spread, and sustainability of health and care technologies. J. Med. Internet Res. **19**(11), e367 (2017)
14. Grey, S.J., Price, G., Mathews, A.: Reduction of anxiety during MR imaging: a controlled trial. Magn. Reson. Imaging **18**(3), 351–355 (2000) . https://doi.org/10.1016/S0730-725X(00)00112-0, https://www.sciencedirect.com/science/article/pii/S0730725X00001120
15. Hallowell, L.M., Stewart, S.E., de Amorim e Silva, C.T., Ditchfield, M.R.: Reviewing the process of preparing children for MRI. Pediatric Radiology **38**(3), 271–279 (2008). https://doi.org/10.1007/s00247-007-0704-x
16. Hassan, R.: Digitality, virtual reality and the 'empathy machine.' Digit. Journal. **8**(2), 195–212 (2020)
17. Hudson, D., Heales, C., Vine, S.: Scoping review: how is virtual reality being used as a tool to support the experience of undergoing magnetic resonance imaging? Radiography **28**(1), 199–207 (2022). https://doi.org/10.1016/j.radi.2021.07.008, https://www.sciencedirect.com/science/article/pii/S1078817421000882
18. Knop, M., Reßing, C., Mueller, M., Weber, S., Freude, H., Niehaves, B.: Virtual reality technologies in health care: a literature review of theoretical foundations (2022). https://doi.org/10.24251/HICSS.2022.223
19. Lee, A.T.: A review of tam (technology acceptance model) and unified theory of acceptance and use of technology (utaut) frameworks in healthcare. Healthcare (2025)
20. Maister, L., Slater, M., Sanchez-Vives, M.V., Tsakiris, M.: Changing bodies changes minds: owning another body affects social cognition. Trends Cogn. Sci. **19**(1), 6–12 (2015)
21. Nakarada-Kordic, I., Reay, S., Bennett, G., Kruse, J., Lydon, A.M., Sim, J.: Can virtual reality simulation prepare patients for an MRI experience? Radiography **26**(3), 205–213 (2020) . https://doi.org/10.1016/j.radi.2019.11.004, https://www.sciencedirect.com/science/article/pii/S107881741930166X
22. of Oulu, U.: (2024). https://www.oulu.fi/en/university/faculties-and-units/eudaimonia-institute/ethics-committee-human-sciences

23. Ryu, J.H., et al.: Virtual reality vs. tablet video as an experiential education platform for pediatric patients undergoing chest radiography: a randomized clinical trial. J. Clin. Med. **10**(11), 2486 (2021). https://doi.org/10.3390/jcm10112486, https://www.mdpi.com/2077-0383/10/11/2486
24. Schrepp, M., Hinderks, A., Thomaschewski, J.: Applying the user experience questionnaire (UEQ) in different evaluation scenarios, pp. 383–392 (2014). https://doi.org/10.1007/978-3-319-07668-3_37
25. Sora-Domenjó, C.: Disrupting the "empathy machine": the power and perils of virtual reality in addressing social issues. Front. Psychol. **13**, 814565 (2022)
26. Stoumpos, A.I.: Digital transformation in healthcare: technology acceptance and its determinants. Healthcare (Basel) (2023)
27. Stunden, C., Stratton, K., Zakani, S., Jacob, J.: Comparing a virtual reality–based simulation app (VR-MRI) with a standard preparatory manual and child life program for improving success and reducing anxiety during pediatric medical imaging: randomized clinical trial. J Med Internet **23**(9), e22942 (2021). https://doi.org/10.2196/22942, https://www.jmir.org/2021/9/e22942
28. Trevena, L., Paay, J., McDonald, R.: VR interventions aimed to induce empathy: a scoping review. Virtual Reality **28**(2), 80 (2024)
29. Tychsen, L., Foeller, P.: Effects of immersive virtual reality headset viewing on young children: visuomotor function, postural stability, and motion sickness. Am. J. Ophthalmol. **209**, 151–159 (2020). https://doi.org/10.1016/j.ajo.2019.07.020, https://www.sciencedirect.com/science/article/pii/S0002939419303812

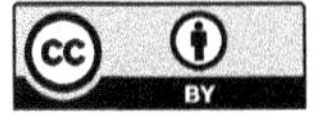

Educators' Perceptions of a National Learning Material Repository in Finnish Medical and Dental Education

Tiina Salmijärvi[1(✉)] [iD], Konsta Parttimaa[1] [iD], Henri Takalo-Kastari,[1] [iD],
Anu Kajamaa[2], Hanni Muukkonen[2] [iD], Petri Kulmala,[1,5] [iD], and Jarmo Reponen[1,3,4] [iD]

[1] Faculty of Medicine, University of Oulu, Oulu, Finland
{tiina.salmijarvi,henri.takalo-kastari,petri.kulmala,
jarmo.reponen}@oulu.fi, konsta.parttimaa@student.oulu.fi
[2] Faculty of Education and Psychology, University of Oulu, Oulu, Finland
{anu.kajamaa,hanni.muukkonen}@oulu.fi
[3] Medical Research Center, Oulu University Hospital, Oulu, Finland
[4] FinnTelemedicum, Research Unit of Health Sciences and Technology, Oulu, Finland
[5] Medical Research Center, Oulu University Hospital, Oulu, Finland

Abstract. This study examines perceived usefulness and adoption-related challenges of a national learning material repository. It also examines the repository as a collaborative pedagogical and organisational process. Data were collected in 2023 from 128 medical and dental teachers. A mixed-methods approach was applied, combining quantitative and qualitative analysis. The study applied technology acceptance model and expansive learning theory. The results show that users were generally satisfied with content and usability, and the repository showed moderate benefits for teaching preparation. Barriers included limited content, time constraints, copyright concerns, and usability issues. Nearly half of respondents had not used the repository. Among users, most supported broader organisational implementation. The findings indicate that repository use is not yet established and requires stronger organisational support. The development process reflects a collaborative interaction between individual agency and organisational structures. Sustained use requires institutional support, clear practices, and cultural change.

Keywords: Medical education · Dental education · National repository · Digital learning material · Educational technology · Expansive learning

1 Introduction

Digitalisation has contributed [1] to learning and teaching processes, as well as services, in higher education. The number of information systems used in higher education institutions has increased significantly in recent years, as has their significance [2, 3]. The wide array of information systems to students enables them to study more versatile than before.

Tiina Salmijärvi and Konsta Parttimaa: These authors have contributed equally to this work.

© The Author(s) 2026
M. Särestöniemi et al. (Eds.): NCDHWS 2026, CCIS 3009, pp. 372–388, 2026.
https://doi.org/10.1007/978-3-032-28812-7_26

The new information systems enable, for example, the production of joint digital learning material for teachers nationally. There is a need to understand how digital education solutions are integrated into everyday teaching practices and how they support teaching and learning. Understanding users' needs and usage patterns is central to developing new processes. This study addresses this challenge. A related question is how educational organisations support and encourage the use of educational information systems. There is limited empirical research on nationally shared, discipline-specific learning material repositories and on how such systems are integrated into everyday teaching practice.

This study examines a national digital learning material repository used in medical and dental education across five Finnish universities. A need to create shareable learning material was identified during the MEDigi project (2018–2021) [4, 5]. At that time, medical and dental teachers lacked a technical platform to distribute learning materials nationally. The repository aims to distribute high-quality, ready-made learning materials nationally. The MEDigi repository has three distinct features: (1) It is maintained collaboratively by five universities. (2) Access is limited to teaching staff. (3) It is specific to medicine and dental education. The repository aims to increase the availability and versatility of teaching materials at the national level while levelling the quality of teaching across universities and faculties. The repository has been developed collaboratively across universities with active involvement of teaching staff. After the active construction phase, the universities have continued to cooperate. As proof of this, universities have, for example, incorporated ideas from a user panel composed of teachers. The implementation of the repository is viewed not only as a technical process but also as a process requiring cultural change.

Previous studies have shown that development work in higher education institutions is often project based and rarely systemically interconnected. The risk is that even meaningful development efforts remain as individual measures or operating models and remain disconnected from the strategy, implementation or basic mission of higher education institutions, resulting in a weak impact [6]. In previous studies that have examined organisational change processes from the perspective of expansive learning, it has been found that change processes are often long-lasting, contain discontinuities and are prone to breaks [7]. This requires long-term development work and the ability to solve challenges and discontinuities building a bridge over them [7].

In this study, a repository is defined as a collection of datasets composed of logically or physically related information compiled for a specific purpose. This is a narrower concept than the open educational resource (OER), which refer to publicly available educational materials [8, 9]. No comparable repository targeting a single scientific field and jointly maintained by multiple universities was identified in the literature review (2023). Globally, various data repositories and their commercial counterparts are in use at the national and international levels in academic education. In Finland, widely used open repositories include the AOE (the Open Educational Resources Library of the Finnish National Agency for Education) and its commercial counterpart repository, Duodecim, alongside its various services, such as Terveysportti (a portal for healthcare professionals) and Oppiportti (a learning portal) [10, 11].

The study has two main objectives. The first is to examine the perceived usefulness and awareness of the MEDigi repository from the perspective of teaching staff. This provides insights into how the repository has been received. The second objective is to analyse the process of developing the repository to support interpretation of the findings. The repository is examined both as a technological solution and as a collaborative pedagogical and organisational process.

In light of the above, the present study addresses the following research questions (RQs):

RQ1: How have teachers experienced the MEDigi repository?

RQ2: What challenges did teachers identify in using the MEDigi repository?

RQ3: How did the learning process evolve during the creation of the MEDigi repository?

These questions address teaching staff's experiences, challenges, and the development process of the repository. The findings inform the development of future educational information systems. The study adressess both individual and organisational levels relevant to implementation. To address these questions, we combined a survey-based approach grounded in the technology acceptance model (TAM) with a process-oriented analysis informed by expansive learning theory.

2 Materials and Methods

2.1 Research Setting and Data Collection

The primary data are based on a survey of medical and dental teachers in Finland. The survey also included open-ended questions. The survey was developed collaboratively by the authors (authors 1, 2, 6 and 7). The data were collected through an anonymous survey using the Webropol survey tool (version 3.0, Webropol Ltd). The survey link was sent to all medical and dental teaching staff nationwide via organisational email lists. Responses were collected from both users and non-users of the repository. This study meets all the national and international research excellence criteria for non-medical research involving human participants, following the Finnish National Board on Research Integrity TENK's guidelines on ethical principles (http://www.tenk.fi/en/ethical-review) and the data protection regulations of the European Union. The voluntary participation was based on informed consent. All data analyses were performed without personal identification data. The survey was open for four weeks in August and September 2023. During this period, two reminder messages were sent to increase the response rate.

A pilot study was conducted before distribution. Four individuals with experience in actively using the repository participated. Based on the pilot, minor linguistic and technical revisions were made to improve clarity.

The survey included multiple-choice questions on experiences, usability, and content. The response format used was a 5-point Likert scale (1 = *strongly disagree* to 5 = *strongly agree*). Additional question formats included yes/no/maybe responses, predefined options, and open-ended questions. Answering all questions was mandatory to submit the survey. The questions were designed to minimise ambiguity. Respondents who had not used or logged in to the repository were directed to a separate response path. This part addressed RQ1. Questions covered experiences of use, barriers, content, and attitudes.

Questions were informed by the technology acceptance model (TAM) (Fig. 1) [12]. TAM is widely used to explain technology acceptance. It describes how perceived usefulness and ease of use influence attitudes and use. *Perceived usefulness* refers to the degree to which a person believes that using a system will improve their work. *Perceived ease of use* refers to how easy a person believes it is to use a system. These factors influence attitudes, intentions, and actual use [12]. TAM was used to analyse perceived usefulness, ease of use, and adoption-related attitudes.

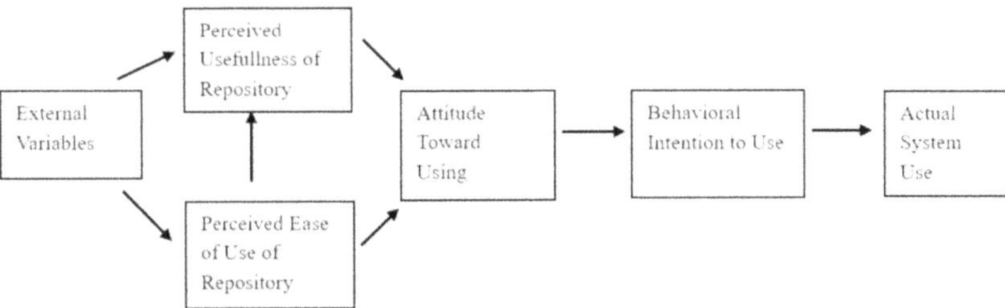

Fig. 1. Technology acceptance model, based on Davis, Bogozzi and Warshaw's model, 1989, p. 985 [12].

A total of 128 open-ended responses were analysed. The units of analysis were single words or longer sentences. Responses were analysed thematically to identify similarities and differences. Five categories were identified (Table 7). The analysis followed a theory-guided, abductive approach, in which expressions emerged from the material and their grouping TAM [12]. This part addressed RQ2. The study applied mixed methods: quantitative data described overall patterns, and qualitative data provided contextual understanding. Together, these provided a more comprehensive view of the phenomenon.

2.2 Expansive Learning as a Theoretical Model for the Process of Creating the MEDigi Repository

RQ3 examined the repository development process using expansive learning theory [13]. The analysis related to RQ3 is based on a theory-informed, reflective case description drawing on the authors' direct involvement in the repository development. This part of the study does not rely on survey data but on a qualitative, theory-guided interpretation of the development process. The theory integrates individual and collective activity and views tensions as drivers of change. The theory integrates individual and collective activity and views tensions as drivers of change [13, 14]. Learning in our study is defined as a collective and cyclical process (Fig. 2). Organisational boundaries may limit shared understanding [15, 16]. The expansive learning cycle improvides a framework for analysing change [14]. The repository development process was analysed through this framework.

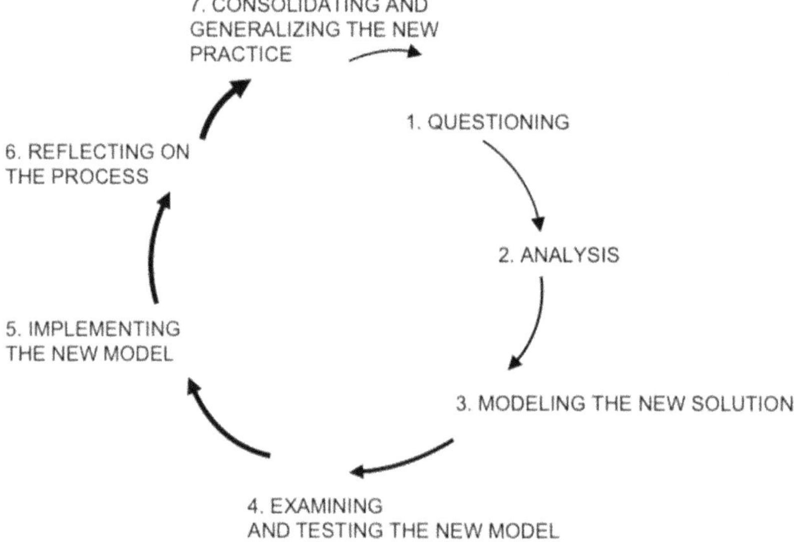

Fig. 2. Sequence of learning actions in an expansive learning cycle (adopted from Engeström & Sannino, 2010: 8 [17]; see also Engeström, 1987: 322) [18].

3   Results

The results follow the structure of the survey, with qualitative findings and process-related analysis presented separately.

3.1   Teachers' Experiences of Using the MEDigi Repository (RQ1)

Of the 149 respondents who started the survey, 128 participated to the extent required of them. However, only 65 respondents answered all the questionnaire items. Accordingly, in the question-specific overviews, the percentage shares are proportionate to the total number of respondents who answered each question. There is no national information available on the size of the target group, but we estimate it exceeds one thousand teachers.

Respondents represented all Finnish medical faculties, with relatively even distribution across universities (Table 1).

Table 1. Organisation represented by survey respondents

Respondents' affiliated university	Number of respondents ($n = 128$)	Percentage of respondents (%)
University of Oulu	43	33.6
University of Helsinki	24	18.8
University of Turku	30	23.4
University of Tampere	5	3.9
University of Eastern Finland	26	20.3

Familiarity and logging in to the repository. Awareness of the repository was high, but use remained limited. Of 128 respondents who answered the first question in this section, eight (6%) had not heard of the repository. The remaining 120 respondents were then asked if they had ever logged into the repository. Fifty-five respondents (46%) had never done so, although they were aware of its existence. The main reasons were lack of time (25%), lack of need (18%), and not knowing how to obtain a username (18%).

Content of the repository. The repository content was generally perceived as high quality, while content availability varied (Table 2). Fourty-nine percent of the respondents partially agreed and 20% strongly agreed this statement. In addition, the answers of the respondents who had themselves uploaded learning materials to the repository were examined separately. No differences were observed between these groups. Regarding speciality-specific content, 39% found it scarce or very scarce. Fourthy-eight percent could not assess the quantity, and 14% found the content of their speciality to be versatile or very versatile. Regarding the general versatility of the repository content, respondents neither agreed nor disagreed. Slightly more than two-fifths (43%) could not assess the versatility. However, based on the response distribution, the content was perceived as somewhat versatile.

Table 2. Items and results concerning the quality of the repository content, the versatility of speciality-specific material and the versatility of general content

Item	1 = Strongly disagree (%), n	2 = Partially disagree (%), n	3 = Neither agree nor disagree (%), n	4 = Partially agree (%), n	5 = Strongly agree (%), n
I feel that the content of the repository is of high quality	0.0, $n = 0$	3.1, $n = 2$	27.7, $n = 18$	49.2, $n = 32$	20.0, $n = 13$

(*continued*)

Table 2. (*continued*)

Item	1 = Strongly disagree (%), n	2 = Partially disagree (%), n	3 = Neither agree nor disagree (%), n	4 = Partially agree (%), n	5 = Strongly agree (%), n
I feel that the repository has versatile learning material for my own speciality	15.4, $n = 10$	23.1, $n = 15$	47.7, $n = 31$	10.8, $n = 7$	3.1, $n = 2$
I feel that the content of the repository is versatile	7.7, $n = 5$	12.3, $n = 8$	43.1, $n = 28$	33.8, $n = 22$	3.1, $n = 2$

Uploading material to the repository. Uploading of learning materials was limited and varied in type. For those who had not uploaded their own learning material to the repository, their reasons and possible inducements were explored. Around one-third of respondents (34%, $n = 22$) uploaded material to the repository. They were asked a follow-up question about the kind of content they had uploaded. Diverse material had been uploaded to the repository: lecture material (32% of these respondents), video material and/or examination questions (20%), and other materials (27%).

Among those who had not uploaded materials (66%, n = 43), several barriers were identified (Table 3). Time constraints were the most common reason (49%). About 42% selected "other reason" and provided additional explanations. User interface problems were reported by 19%, and 33% cited copyright-related reasons.

Respondents also identified factors that could encourage future uploading (Table 3). These included more allocated work time (56%), clearer instructions and operating models (44%), and stronger reciprocity (37%).

Table 3. Barriers to and possible incentives for uploading material reported by respondents who had not uploaded materials

Why haven't you uploaded your own learning material to the repository?	Number of respondents ($n = 43$)	Percentage of respondents
Copyright issues	14	32.6
No time / time management	21	48.8
No interest	2	4.7
I don't have my own teaching material	1	2.3
User interface problems	8	18.6

(continued)

Table 3. (*continued*)

Why haven't you uploaded your own learning material to the repository?	Number of respondents (*n* = 43)	Percentage of respondents
The MEDigi project is still in its early stages	3	7.0
Other similar services in use	2	4.7
Differences in views regarding the content of the material	2	4.7
What would encourage you to upload your own teaching material to the repository in the future?	*Number of respondents (n = 43)*	*Percentage of respondents*
More time during working hours for producing and finalising materials	24	55.8
Realisation of the principle of reciprocity	16	37.2
Clear instructions and operating models for producing material	19	44.2
Uploading material to the repository being more straightforward	14	32.6
I do not see the repository as relevant in my work	2	4.7

Utilising the repository in teaching. Use of the repository in teaching was moderate, and perceived benefits varied. Answers from those who utilised it are in Table 4, and answers from those who did not are in Table 5. Approximately two-fifths (42%, $n = 27$) reported using the repository in their own teaching. Regarding the repository's impact on the efficiency of teaching, respondents leaned slightly towards the positive side (Table 4). Just over half (56%) could not assess the effect, 37% reported improved efficiency, and 7.4% reported a negative impact.

Repository use was also deemed to make teaching preparation more efficient (Table 4). Fourthy-four percent reported improved efficiency in preparation, while 7.4% reported a negative impact.

Among those who had not used repository materials (59%, n = 38), several reasons were identified (Table 5). These included lack of speciality-specific material (34%), lack of time (26%), and lack of suitability for teaching (29%). Open-ended responses highlighted difficulties in using materials created by others and the use of alternative systems.

Table 4. Experiences of respondents who utilised repository materials in teaching regarding the increased efficiency of teaching and teaching preparation ($n = 27$)

Item	1 = Strongly disagree (%), n	2 = Partially disagree (%), n	3 = Neither agree nor disagree (%), n	4 = Partially agree (%), n	5 = Strongly agree (%), n
Using the repository has made my teaching more efficient	0.0, $n = 0$	7.4, $n = 2$	55.6, $n = 15$	14.8, $n = 4$	22.2, $n = 6$
Using the repository has made the preparation of teaching materials more efficient	0.0, $n = 0$	7.4, $n = 2$	48.2, $n = 13$	25.9, $n = 7$	18.5, $n = 5$

Table 5. Follow-up questions for respondents not using the repository material regarding the reason for not using the repository in their own teaching

Why haven't you used the repository in your own teaching?	Number of respondents ($n = 38$)	Percentage of respondents
The repository does not contain material for the speciality I teach	13	34.2
I haven't had time to familiarise myself with the materials already uploaded to the repository	10	26.3
The material found in the repository is not suitable for my teaching	11	28.9
I use another repository (e.g. DigiCampusMoodle)	1	2.6
Materials/images created by others are difficult to utilise	1	2.6

Organisational perspectives on repository use. Nearly 70% of respondents wished for the general implementation of the repository within their own work organisation (see Table 6). Only three respondents (4.6%) opposed this. Reported concerns included limited content, challenges in using materials created by others, and mismatch with teaching practices.

Table 6. Respondents' views on the general implementation of the repository within their own work organisations ($n = 65$)

Item	1 = Strongly Disagree (%), n	2 = Partially Disagree (%), n	3 = Neither Agree nor Disagree (%), n	4 = Partially Agree (%), n	5 = Strongly Agree (%), n
I wish that my work organisation would implement the MEDigi repository for general use	1.5, $n = 1$	3.1, $n = 2$	26.2, $n = 17$	40.0, $n = 26$	29.2, $n = 19$

3.2 Qualitative Results: Challenges in Using the MEDigi Repository (RQ2)

The categories in Table 7 are formed based on the open-answer fields of the entire survey.

Usability and technical functionality of the repository. Respondents raised several issues related to the technical usability of the repository. The user interface was generally perceived as smooth and intuitive. Accuracy and relevance were primarily expected from the search functions. The search function was identified as requiring further development. Weak search functionality reduced willingness to use the repository. The search function was expected to work, as were search engines commonly used for information retrieval. Some respondents raised the issue that repository content should be grouped differently.

The amount of content. Limited content was a key constraint, particularly in the early stage of use. More content was desired. Respondents described the early phase as uncertain and challenging. The system had not yet been systematically integrated into teaching. Use in teaching preparation and planning had not been established. Information about meaningful use cases was also lacking.

Boundary conditions: Time constraints and workload. The repository was perceived as time-consuming, particularly when uploading materials. Issues related to copyright and contracts were perceived as demanding and cited as reasons for not wanting to upload their own material. Lack of time also limited familiarisation with the repository.

Collaboration and sharing practices. Inter-university cooperation was perceived as insufficient, and material sharing was not yet a shared practice. Respondents emphasised the need for stronger reciprocity and a shared culture of material use. Many teachers still preferred to use their own materials rather than shared resources.

Communication, guidance, and orientation. Respondents highlighted the need for more active and continuous communication. There was also a need for training and guidance, particularly related to copyright.

Table 7. Openended response categories

	Category (Qualitative challenge/Theme)	Technology acceptance model dimension
1	Usability and technical functionality of the repository	Perceived ease of use
2	The limited amount of material and the initial phase of use	Perceived usefulness
3	Boundary conditions: More work and takes time	Perceived usefulness
4	The scarcity of cooperation and the need to develop it	Perceived usefulness
5	Information, communication and orientation	Perceived ease of use

3.3 Development of the Repository (RQ3)

This section describes the repository development process as context for interpreting the survey findings (RQ3; see Table 8). The description is based on the authors' direct involvement in the development process. Authors 6 and 7 have been actively involved from the beginning and Author 1 from 2022. These perspectives reflect the roles of three faculty members involved in the process.

The process is interpreted using expansive learning theory [13]. The theory describes a collaborative learning process in which new solutions emerge through iterative development. (e.g. when traditional work processes become inadequate in the digital era). Through different stages, a new solution is constructed. This learning process is typically long-term and cyclical, moving from an abstract idea to a new way of operating. The model reflects the observed development process.

We justify this choice of theory as follows: (1) The MEDigi-repository learning process was highly collaborative, as it involved interactions among actors from five universities, forming an important community of learners. (2) It changed traditional university activity systems by crossing interuniversity boundaries. (3) The aim was broad-based, continuous national development, not just to develop individual teachers' own competence. (4) The goal was to create a new theoretical and practical concept for teachers' practices. The repository introduced a new collaborative model that differs from traditional teacher-centred practices. The work process itself played a crucial role in supporting collaboration between actors. Survey results alone do not fully capture this process.

In the first phase of the expansive learning cycle, the repository idea emerged from a practical need to share medical and dental learning materials nationally (Table 8). There was uncertainty about how this idea would be received, as sharing teaching materials was not a common or self-evident practice. Traditionally, teachers prepare learning materials on their own and use them themselves or, at most, share them within their own faculty.

In phase 2, it became clear that existing systems did not support national distribution of learning materials. The second and third phases focused on analysis, planning and modelling of a new repository within the MEDigi project. The initial plan was to create a broader portal for both teaching staff and students, with the repository as one component. The plan was abandoned due to cost and scheduling constraints.

In the fourth phase, the model was examined, tested and piloted. Feedback was used to refine the repository. Technical, administrative and legal challenges (e.g. legislation, copyright, data protection, accessibility and trade union perspectives) slowed and complicated the process. Developing the repository proved more difficult and labour-intensive than expected. Large-scale use began in 2021 (implementation phase). Teachers perceived system implementation as burdensome. At that time, an agreement between the universities ensured continued use and development beyond the project. Evaluation and reflection took place throughout the process, particularly at the end of the project in 2021. After the project ended and the universities assumed responsibility for development in early 2022, the process began to consolidate.

Table 8. Timeline and key events in the MEDigi-repository project

	Timeline	The MEDigi-repository development process	The cycle of expansive learning	Number of users and materials
1	2019	Identification of the need for a repository	Questioning, analysis	
2	2019–2020	Development of a pilot version of the core idea during the MEDigi project	Modelling the new solution	
3	2020	Pilot of the first version (design phase: operating principles, functionalities, search functions, user interface, user management); development work continues based on feedback, adding legal agreement form and instructions for teaching staff	Examining and testing the new model	
4	2021	Launch of a repository for nationwide use to establish the system; development work continues	Implementing the new model	Users: 130 Materials: 70

(continued)

Table 8. (*continued*)

	Timeline	The MEDigi-repository development process	The cycle of expansive learning	Number of users and materials
5	End of 2021	End of the MEDigi project	Implementing the new model, continuing evaluating and reflecting on the process	Users: 193 Materials: 145
6	2022–	Joint development by universities of the repository with basic funding; development work continues	Consolidating and generalising the new practice	Users: 320 Materials: 160
7	August–September 2023	Quantitative survey of medical and dental teachers in Finland		Users: 380 Materials: 210

4 Discussion

This study examined how medical and dental teaching staff have received the digital learning material repository. It addressed how teachers experienced the MEDigi repository (RQ1) and what challenges they identified (RQ2). It also examined the development process using expansive learning (RQ3). Based on our findings, repository use has not yet become an established part of everyday teaching practice.

Three main findings emerge from the results (RQ1). First, use of the repository had not yet been established in teaching practices. Nearly half of respondents (46%) had not logged into the repository despite being part of an active respondent group.

Second, users perceived the repository content as high quality. However, only 34% had uploaded their own materials. Reported barriers included time constraints, copyright issues, and usability challenges. Perceived usefulness in teaching remained moderate. This may reflect limited content and the lack of established practices for using shared materials.

The third finding relates to organisational culture and integration into everyday teaching practices. Pedagogical development is shaped by organisational culture. The results indicate that changes in established practices occur gradually. Organisational commitment is required to support systematic adoption. This is supported by the finding that nearly 70% of respondents support systematic adoption. These findings are consistent with earlier studies showing that a supportive pedagogical environment and sense of community promote the reflective development of university teaching through a collegial atmosphere [19–24].

These findings highlight the need for structured organisational support in implementing new technologies. Clear organisational decisions may support more consistent use among teachers. Based on our present results, implementation is challenged by unstructured use practices, limited content, and lack of time. At the same time, teachers expect high-quality, easy-to-use materials that support everyday work. In our data, perceived usefulness and ease of use were closely linked to actual use and willingness to adopt the repository. These findings align with TAM, where perceived usefulness and ease of use shape attitudes and use. The results also highlight the need for long-term organisational commitment as in previous studies [7]. Alignment between individual and organisational goals is required.

RQ3 examined how the development process evolved. The analysis of the development process provides context for interpreting the survey findings. From the perspective of expansive learning, the process was gradual and iterative. The main result was that collaboration developed gradually and required sustained effort. Implementation required changes in practices, structures and ways of working. The results indicate progress, but systematic use remains limited. This requires changes in both thinking and practice. More active, consistent and systematic communication is needed. Participation in content production indicates a positive shift. However, initiating and maintaining collaboration requires sustained effort. Organisations and networks can support this through structured support and collaboration. Institutional culture and rules, trust and respect, as well as pedagogical approaches and training [25] are important. Other enhancing factors at the individual level may include shared experiences, new insights, strengthened pedagogical awareness, and community level help in solving problems [26].

The findings highlight the interaction between individual agency and organisational structures [26]. Key elements of a pedagogical community include mutual interaction, respect and cooperation, organisational conditions can support or constrain development [19, 27]. Participation in a supportive learning community benefit both teachers and students and strengthens pedagogical culture [28]. The teaching and pedagogical development of academic communities is also influenced by contextual elements, such as structures [29–31], pedagogical leadership and the alignment of ongoing collaborative academic development projects with current institutional policy [24, 32].

Based on these findings, the following recommendations can be made for educational organisations: 1. Ensure clear organisational commitment to implementing new technology. 2. Support teaching staff through structured measures that promote adoption and collaboration. 3. Ensure that technology supports teaching work and meets user needs. 4. Recognise that pedagogical development is gradual and requires sustained effort and understanding of organisational change. Our recommendations for teaching staff are as follows: new technologies can enrich teaching and learning processes but require time and resources. Initial workload may increase, but long-term benefits are expected. Teachers are encouraged to use shared materials and contribute their own in collaborative processes. Digital solutions should be aligned with existing systems and everyday practices. Other essential questions include the added value of the solution and the involvement of teaching staff in the change.

Out study has several strengths, including a defined respondent population and effective reqruitment. The sample was broadly representative, with one exception. The survey design reduced unreliable responses. Furthermore, the questions were clear and tested in a pilot study. These measures supported the reliability of the data. A key limitation is the relatively small number of respondents. Limited prior research constrains comparison. Further research, such as interviews, could provide additional insights.

.

5   Conclusion

This study shows that implementing digital systems in a higher education requires long-term collaboration, organisational support, and cultural change. The MEDigi repository represents a national model that differs from open OER libraries by targeting a specific user group (teachers) and disciplines (medicine and dentistry). The study applied TAM to examine user acceptance of the repository. The findings highlight the importance of user experience and organisational support in technology adoption. Usability, particularly searchability, influences adoption. Systematic support for teachers is required in implementation. Teachers benefit from allocated time, clear guidance, and support. Educational organisations should commit to systematic use and support of the repository. The study also contributes to understanding collaborative development through expansive learning. Repository development can be understood as a collaborative pedagogical process. The findings highlight the role of trust, collaboration, and organisational culture in enabling shared practices. Overall, implementing a shared digital repository in higher education is not only a technical issue but also a question of organisational alignment and cultural change.

Acknowledgements. The process of building the repository was funded by the Ministry of Education and Culture (grant number OKM/270/523/2017) in 2018–2021.

Disclosure of Interests. Authors 1, 6 and 7 participated in the process of building the repository: Author 1 in the role of coordinator, Author 6 as an executive team expert member, and Author 7 in the roles of project manager and executive team chair. Author 1 has worked since 2022 as a national MEDigi coordinator. In this role, she promotes national cooperation in medical and dental education. This cooperation includes the repository.

References

1. Korkeakoulutus ja tutkimus 2030-luvulle vision tiekartta. 23 Dec 2025. Available from: Korkeakoulutus+ja+tutkimus+2030-luvulle+VISION+TIEKARTTA_V2.pdf
2. Sejati, W., Melinda, V.: Education on the use of IoT technology for energy audit and management within the context of conservation and efficiency. Int Trans Educ Technol. **1**(2), 138–143 (2023)
3. Rahardja, U., Ngadi, M., Budiarto, R., Aini, Q., Hardini, M., Oganda, F.P.: Education exchange storage protocol: transformation into decentralized learning platform. Front Educ. **6**, 782969 (2021). https://doi.org/10.3389/feduc.2021.782969
4. Levy, A., Reponen, J.: Digital leap in medical education: report of the MEDigi project. University of Oulu, Oulu, (2021). https://oulurepo.oulu.fi/handle/10024/36419

5. Salmijärvi, T., Kulmala, P., Takalo-Kastari, H., Reponen, J.: Developing national medical and dental education: from digital leap to digital marathon. In: NCDHWS 2024, Oulu, Finland, May 7–8, 2024, Proceedings, Part I. Springer, pp. 401–403 (2024)
6. Toom, A., Pyhältö, K.: Kestävää korkeakoulutusta ja opiskelijoiden oppimista rakentamassa: Tutkimukseen perustuva selvitys ajankohtaisesta korkeakoulupedagogiikan ja ohjauksen osaamisesta. Opetus-ja kulttuuriministeriön julkaisuja, Nro 2020:1, Valtioneuvoston kanslia, Helsinki. http://urn.fi/URN:ISBN:978-952-263-696-6
7. Engeström, Y., Kerosuo, H., Kajamaa, A.: Beyond discontinuity: expansive organizational learning remembered. Manag. Learn. **38**(3), 319–336 (2007)
8. Zaidi, I., Amir, R., Bhatia, H.K.: Benefits and barriers to open educational resources (OERS): preservice teachers' perception. Int. J. Educ. Dev. **15**(3), 45–62 (2021). https://doi.org/10.1016/j.ijedudev.2021.102345
9. Finto. Suomalainen asiasanasto-ja ontologiapalvelu n.d. Verkkosivu. Viitattu 23 Dec 2025. tietovaranto-TT-Finto
10. Suomen Opetushallitus n.d. Avointen oppimateriaalien kirjasto. Verkkosivu. Viitattu 23. Dec 2025, Avointen oppimateriaalien kirjasto, Opetushallitus
11. Suomalainen lääkäriseura Duodecim n.d. Verkkosivu. Viitattu 9 June 2024. https://www.duodecim.fi/seura/
12. Davis, F.D., Bagozzi, R.P., Warshaw, P.R.: User acceptance of computer technology: a comparison of two theoretical models. Manage. Sci. **35**(8), 982–1003 (1989). https://doi.org/10.1287/mnsc.35.8.982
13. Engeström, Y.: Learning by expanding: an activity-theoretical approach to developmental research. Cambridge University Press, New York (2015)
14. Engeström, Y.: Ekspansiivinen oppiminen ja yhteiskehittely työssä. Vastapaino, (2004)
15. Kajamaa, A., Tuunainen, J., Hyrkkö, S., Cornér, T.: Rajanylitykset ja ekspansiivinen oppiminen asiantuntijaorganisaatioissa: Esimerkkeinä kolme Muutoslaboratoriota. Kasvatus. **54**(3), 206–220 (2023)
16. Kerosuo, H.: Boundaries in action: an activity-theoretical study of development, learning, and change in health care organization for patients with multiple and chronic illnesses. Doctoral dissertation. University of Helsinki, Helsinki (2006)
17. Engeström, Y., Sannino, A.: Studies of expansive learning: Foundations, findings and future challenges. Educat. Res. Rev. **5**(1), 1–24 (2010)
18. Engeström, Y.: Learning by expanding: An activity-theoretical approach to developmental research. Orienta-Konsultit, (1987)
19. Cipriano, R.E., Buller, J.L.: Rating faculty collegiality. Change **44**(2), 45–48 (2012). https://doi.org/10.1080/00091383.2012.655219
20. Kurtts, S.A., Levin, B.B.: Using peer coaching with preservice teachers to develop reflective practice and collegial support. Teach. Educ. **11**(3), 297–310 (2000). https://doi.org/10.1080/713698980
21. Alpay, E., Verschoor, R.: The teaching researcher: faculty attitudes towards the teaching and research roles. Eur. J. Eng. Educ. **39**(4), 365–376 (2014). https://doi.org/10.1080/03043797.2014.895702
22. Boyd, P.: Academic induction for professional educators: supporting the workplace learning of newly appointed lecturers in teacher and nurse education. Int. J. Acad. Dev. **15**(2), 155–165 (2010). https://doi.org/10.1080/13601441003738368
23. Clarke, C., Reid, J.: Foundational academic development: building collegiality across divides? Int. J. Acad. Dev. **18**(4), 318–330 (2013). https://doi.org/10.1080/1360144X.2012.728529
24. Remmik, M., Karm, M.: Novice university teachers' professional learning: to follow traditions or change them? Stud Learn Soc. **2**(2–3), 121–131 (2012)

25. Esterhazy, R., de Lange, T., Bastiansen, S., Wittek, A.L.: Moving beyond peer review of teaching: a conceptual framework for collegial faculty development. Rev. Educ. Res. **91**(2), 237–271 (2021). https://doi.org/10.3102/0034654321990721
26. Myllykoski-Laine, S., Murtonen, M., Postareff, L.: Korkeakoulupedagogiikan kehittäjien käsityksiä yhteisöllisyydestä pedagogisen kehittymisen kontekstissa. Kasvatus. **55**(2), 200–214 (2024). https://doi.org/10.33348/kvt.130705
27. Jääskelä, P., Häkkinen, P., Rasku-Puttonen, H.: Supporting and constraining factors in the development of university teaching experienced by teachers. Teach. High. Educ. **22**(6), 655–671 (2017). https://doi.org/10.1080/13562517.2016.1273206
28. Vescio, V., Ross, D., Adams, A.: A review of research on the impact of professional learning communities on teaching practice and student learning. Teach. Teach. Educ. **24**(1), 80–91 (2008). https://doi.org/10.1016/j.tate.2007.01.004
29. Englund, C., Olofsson, A.D., Price, L.: The influence of sociocultural and structural contexts in academic change and development in higher education. High. Educ. **76**, 1051–1069 (2018). https://doi.org/10.1007/s10734-018-0254-1
30. Katajavuori, N., Virtanen, V., Ruohoniemi, M., Muukkonen, H., Toom, A.: The value of academics' formal and informal interaction in developing life science education. High. Educ. Res. Dev. **38**(4), 793–806 (2019). https://doi.org/10.1080/07294360.2019.1576595
31. McCune, V.: Experienced academics' pedagogical development in higher education: time, technologies, and conversations. Oxf. Rev. Educ. **44**(3), 307–321 (2018). https://doi.org/10.1080/03054985.2017.1389712
32. Leibowitz, B.: Understanding the challenges of the South African higher education landscape. In: Leibowitz, B. (ed.) Community, self and identity: educating South African university students for citizenship, pp. 3–18. HSRC Press (2012)

Defining AI Competence for Health and Social Care Professionals: A Scoping Review of Competence Domains, Practice Requirements and Educational Gaps (2020–2025)

Birgitta Tetri[1,2]([⊠]) [iD] and Outi Ahonen[1] [iD]

[1] Laurea University of Applied Sciences, Vantaa, Finland
`birgitta.tetri@laurea.fi`
[2] University of Helsinki, Helsinki, Finland

Abstract. Artificial intelligence (AI) is rapidly permeating health and social care, creating new competence requirements across professional roles, while existing evidence on AI competence remains fragmented. This scoping review synthesises AI competence domains, practice requirements and educational gaps for health and social care professionals. Structured literature searches in Academic Search Ultimate, CINAHL, MEDIC, and the Cochrane Library identified 19 peer-reviewed studies (2020–2025) addressing AI-related competence, literacy, or skills among health and social care professionals, students, or educators. Studies were screened against predefined inclusion and exclusion criteria, and data were extracted on professional context, AI competence domains, training approaches, training needs, ethical and human-centred competence, and attitudes/readiness, then synthesised using narrative thematic analysis. Five core AI competence domains emerged: foundational AI literacy; data and analytical skills; critical evaluation and decision-making; workflow and contextual integration; and domain-specific AI application competencies, supported by cross-cutting domains of ethical, legal and responsible AI use, communication and interaction skills, and AI self-efficacy and continuous learning. Practice requirements varied by profession, with imaging and pathology demonstrating advanced, task-specific applications and rare examples of empirical competence assessment, whereas nursing, public health, and social work remained largely conceptual. Across contexts, current training appeared fragmented, relying on scattered initiatives and informal learning, with substantial gaps in depth of AI literacy, ethical implementation skills, faculty expertise and validated competence measures. AI competence thus appears as a multi-domain construct combining shared cross-professional capabilities with profession-specific applications, underscoring the need for role-sensitive frameworks, robust assessment tools and ethically grounded, workflow-integrated training in health and social care education and continuing professional development.

Keywords: Artificial intelligence · Digitalisation · Competence · Healthcare education · Social work · Curriculum · Interdisciplinary

© The Author(s) 2026
M. Särestöniemi et al. (Eds.): NCDHWS 2026, CCIS 3009, pp. 389–408, 2026.
https://doi.org/10.1007/978-3-032-28812-7_27

1 Introduction

Artificial intelligence is increasingly embedded in healthcare and social care workflows, from clinical decision-support systems to automated documentation and epidemiological modelling [1–4]. At the same time, large-scale organisational studies indicate that AI adoption in public social and health services is shaped by a systemic network of technological, organisational and environmental challenges, including limited financial resources, insufficient AI expertise and regulatory gaps that constrain meaningful use in practice [5]. These developments create an urgent need for health and social care professionals to develop AI competence that supports safe, ethical and effective use of AI tools in diverse practice contexts. In this paper, we use the term AI competence to refer to an integrated set of knowledge, skills and attitudes that enables professionals to work with AI in ways that maintain patient and client safety, support human-centred care and respect legal and ethical requirements [6–8]. AI competence builds on broader digital competence frameworks in healthcare, which emphasise the ability to navigate digital systems, manage data and critically evaluate digital technologies from a human-centred, ethical perspective. Within this overarching construct, AI literacy and specific AI-related skills are treated as constituent dimensions of AI competence rather than separate concepts [6–8].

Emerging European and national policy frameworks on AI governance, data protection, and professional accountability further shape expectations for AI-related competence, even though explicit, profession-specific AI competence standards remain limited. AI applications in health and social care now span diagnostic support in radiology, pathology and oncology, predictive risk models in public health, digital documentation and triage tools in nursing, and algorithmic decision-support in welfare services [2, 4, 6–10]. Natural language processing and generative AI extend these uses to documentation, education and communication, while introducing new risks related to bias, transparency, accountability, privacy and professional identity [11–14]. Evidence from AI innovation projects in intensive care and other high-stakes settings further shows that many AI initiatives fail already in early ideation and problem-formulation phases, when multidisciplinary teams struggle to identify clinically valuable and technically feasible use cases or to align AI capabilities with real-world workflows, underscoring the need for robust professional AI competence and collaborative skills [15].

Competence to work effectively and safely with AI is not automatic [9, 16, 17]. Surveys and reviews suggest that many professionals recognise AI's growing importance and express generally positive attitudes, yet report limited understanding of how AI systems work, their limitations and appropriate use cases [8, 16, 18, 19]. Finnish health and social service professionals, for example, showed a 59% AI competence deficit overall, with the largest gap in analysing the ethical implications of AI-based applications [19]. Nursing literature similarly documents concerns about patient safety, fairness and erosion of human-centred care, alongside a shortage of concrete training models for ethical implementation and critical appraisal [17].

In Europe, qualification and competence levels are regulated through the European Qualifications Framework (EQF). In the field of health and social care, this corresponds to levels 4–8, which cover vocational qualifications; the bachelor's degree from a university of applied sciences and the bachelor's degree from a university (level 6); the master's degree from a university of applied sciences and a university master's degree (level 7); as well as the doctoral degree (level 8) [20]. In this study, AI-related competence is examined with reference to EQF levels 5–7, which encompass vocational education and training (VET), bachelor's- and master's-level education, and continuing professional development.

Recent international recommendations on biomedical and health informatics education similarly emphasise the need for systematic, competence-based curricula that integrate digital health, data science and AI-related skills across professions and educational levels and describe core and specialised knowledge domains for a digitally capable health workforce [21]. In the Finnish context, national foresight work on lifelong learning has highlighted that future competence increasingly emerges in ecosystems rather than within isolated organisations, calling for networked, data-informed and impact-oriented approaches to competence development across sectors [22].

The aim of this literature review is to gather information on the artificial intelligence competencies of various health and social care professionals and the factors that relate to them. The review addresses two research questions:

What kinds of AI competence domains emerge for health and social care professionals?

What kinds of current training approaches and integration practices for AI competence can be identified in health and social care education and continuous professional development?

2 Methods

This study was designed as a scoping literature review with a structured search and narrative thematic synthesis. The review aimed to map how AI competence is described across different health and social care professions, and to identify current training approaches and educational gaps, rather than to evaluate the effectiveness of specific interventions. The reporting of the review follows the PRISMA 2020 statement, which was used as a reporting guideline to enhance transparency in documenting the search, selection and synthesis processes, rather than as a methodological framework defining the type of review [23]. A review protocol specifying the databases, search strategy, inclusion and exclusion criteria, and data extraction plan was developed a priori for internal use but was not prospectively registered or published.

Literature searches were conducted between September and October 2025 in four electronic databases: Academic Search Ultimate and CINAHL (via EBSCOhost), the Finnish MEDIC healthcare database and the Cochrane Library. The search period was restricted to publications from January 2020 to October 2025 to capture recent developments in AI and its integration into health and social care practice. The search strategy combined controlled vocabulary terms (e.g. MeSH terms and CINAHL Headings) with free text keywords organised into four concept blocks: (1) artificial intelligence; (2) health and social care professionals; (3) competence-related concepts; and (4) education and learning contexts. Within each concept block, terms were combined using the Boolean operator OR, and the four concept blocks were combined using AND. We used broad professional terms such as "healthcare professional", "social care professional", "social worker" and "medical professional" to capture multiple occupational groups, including nurses and physiotherapists, within a manageable search string. To enhance coverage of social care-specific contexts, additional search terms related to social work, social welfare, inclusion, accessibility, vulnerability, and marginalisation were incorporated into the search strategy. Searches were limited to peer-reviewed journal articles and peer-reviewed conference papers published in English and available in full text; studies focusing primarily on business, marketing, engineering, manufacturing or finance were excluded. MEDIC was included to improve coverage of Nordic health and social care contexts, including English-language articles indexed in this database, although the English-language restriction may have led to the omission of relevant local-language studies.

Titles and abstracts were screened against predefined inclusion and exclusion criteria, followed by full-text assessment of potentially eligible studies. Screening and selection were conducted using the AI-assisted tool Elicit in an iterative, dialogic process, with two

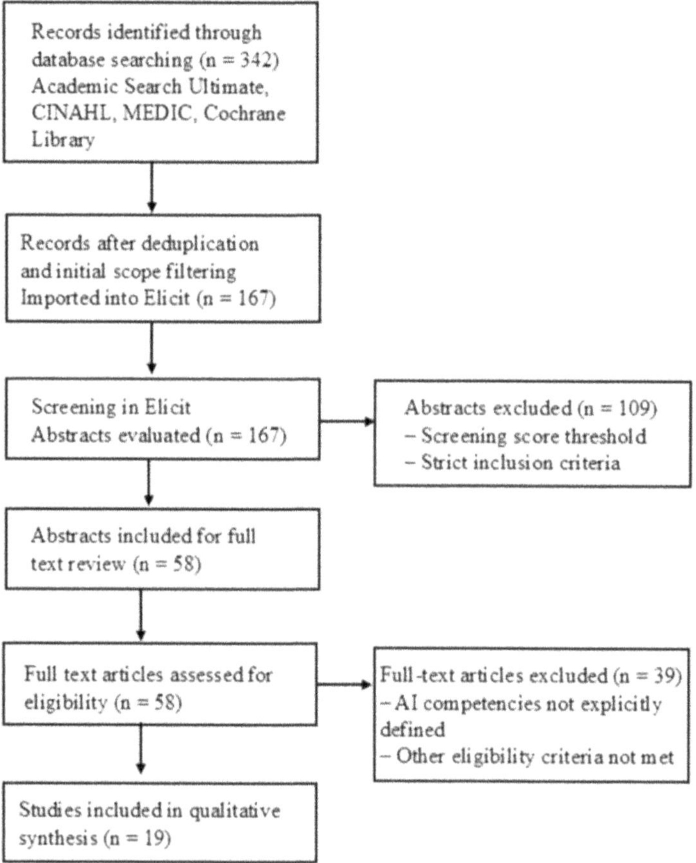

Fig. 1. Flow diagram of study identification, Elicit-supported screening, and inclusion in the qualitative synthesis.

reviewers involved throughout, and any uncertainties or borderline cases were discussed and resolved jointly. Eligible full texts were imported into Elicit to support structured screening, data extraction and thematic synthesis of AI competence domains and educational approaches, as summarised in the flow diagram (Fig. 1). Data were extracted using a structured template covering publication details, country, professional groups, study design, AI competence domains, training approaches and reported educational needs or gaps. Thematic synthesis was performed by combining inductive coding of reported AI competence elements and training practices with deductive grouping into conceptually coherent competence domains and educational themes. A formal appraisal of methodological quality or risk of bias across all included studies was not conducted, and the findings should therefore be interpreted as an indicative synthesis of the available evidence rather than definitive conclusions about effectiveness.

3 Results

The review included 19 studies published between 2021 and 2025, covering a wide range of professions, settings and methodological approaches. Study designs comprised systematic and rapid reviews, Delphi consensus work, expert guidance documents, cross-sectional surveys and perspective or proposal papers.

3.1 Core AI Competence Domains

Across professions, the review identified five core domains of AI competence for health and social care professionals, supported by a set of cross-cutting transversal competencies. The core domains were: foundational AI literacy, data and analytical skills, critical evaluation and decision making, workflow and contextual integration, and domain specific AI application competencies, while ethical, legal and responsible AI use, communication and interaction skills, and AI self-efficacy and continuous learning emerged as cross cutting domains that underpin how the core domains are enacted in practice [16, 24].

Foundational AI literacy refers to a basic conceptual understanding of what AI is, how it works and its core components, capabilities and limitations. Across the studies, this encompassed knowledge of machine learning concepts, data structures and model logic, awareness of the "black box" nature of many systems and the principles of model training, validation, generalisability and explainability [2, 4, 25, 26]. One systematic review reported that 86% of included studies explicitly emphasised AI fundamentals as essential competencies for future health professionals, underscoring the centrality of this domain in the broader competence landscape [16].

Data and analytical skills, critical evaluation, and decision-making together demonstrated the ability to work with, interpret, and appraise AI-generated outputs to support professional judgement. These domains included interpreting AI predictions in clinical or social care decision-making; evaluating validity, accuracy, and reliability; understanding performance metrics such as sensitivity and specificity; and identifying data quality issues and sources of bias [6, 24, 25]. Social work and public health frameworks emphasised the need to judge when AI is appropriate or inappropriate for a given task and to recognise potential harms and unintended consequences, especially for marginalised populations [4, 13].

Workflow and contextual integration focused on how AI tools are embedded into existing professional, organisational and interprofessional processes. Studies highlighted hands-on skills in using decision support systems, operating AI-assisted imaging workflows (e.g. automatic patient positioning, scout image analysis), AI-supported documentation and triage, and mapping AI tools to specific tasks, pathways and information systems [1, 6, 8, 11, 18, 27]. This domain also encompasses recognising safety and governance risks in real-world use, understanding human–AI task division and collaborating in multidisciplinary teams to align AI capabilities with interprofessional practice [3].

Domain-specific AI application competencies reflected profession-tailored uses of AI. Nursing sources described competencies in AI-enhanced assessment, triage, documentation, and patient education, including co-designing AI tools with patients and carers in oncology nursing [6, 8, 11, 12, 17]. Imaging and radiography guidance emphasised AI-enabled workflow optimisation and safety in radiology and radiotherapy [1, 18, 27], while pathology and oncology papers focused on AI-supported diagnostic reasoning and performance evaluation using annotated cases and simulations [2, 7, 28]. Public health frameworks highlighted skills in AI-driven epidemiological modelling, risk prediction and policy analysis [4], whereas social work proposals stressed competencies for integrating generative AI into case management and documentation while maintaining a strong focus on equity and client well-being [13].

Ethical, legal, and responsible AI use; communication and interaction skills; and AI self-efficacy and continuous learning emerged as cross-cutting domains that shape and constrain the core competencies. Ethical and human-centred competence encompassed duty of care, accountability, bias and fairness, privacy and data governance, GDPR compliance, explainability, and shared decision-making, as articulated in pathology, imaging, oncology, and social work sources [1, 2, 13, 19, 28]. Communication competence involved explaining AI-supported decisions transparently to patients, clients and colleagues, addressing concerns and maintaining the human-centred character of care even when technology is pervasive [8, 11]. Self-efficacy and continuous learning were related to confidence in working with AI, motivation to engage with new tools and the ability to update AI-related skills through ongoing education and professional development [4, 16–19, 24]. Table 1 summarises these core and cross-cutting domains and illustrates how they are represented across the included studies.

Table 1. Core AI competence domains for health and social care professionals.

Domain	Definition	Key elements and skills	Illustrative sources
Foundational AI literacy	Basic conceptual understanding of what AI is, how it works, core components, capabilities, and limitations; prerequisite for safe and informed use of AI tools in professional practice.	Understanding basic AI/ML concepts (machine learning, algorithms, automation); recognising types of AI applications in healthcare and social care; understanding data structures and data quality requirements; awareness of model limitations, errors, and biases; understanding how AI systems are trained and validated; recognition of the "black box" nature of many systems; understanding generalisability and explainability.	Schwendicke et al. [25], Acosta [4], Hanna et al. [2], Ossa et al. [26], Ng et al. [24]
Data and analytical skills	Ability to work with, interpret, and critically evaluate data and AI-generated outputs to support professional judgement; includes assessment of validity, accuracy, and reliability of AI predictions and identification of bias.	Interpreting AI outputs in clinical or social care decision making; assessing validity, accuracy, and reliability of AI predictions; evaluating data quality and data fit for AI tools; understanding performance metrics (e.g. sensitivity, specificity, false positives); identifying sources of bias in datasets and algorithms; recognising data quality problems.	Schwendicke et al. [25], O'Connor et al. [9], Ng et al. [24], Rodriguez et al. [15], Acosta [4], Stogiannos et al. [19]
Critical evaluation and decision making	Ability to appraise AI recommendations critically, integrate them with professional expertise, judge when AI should or should not influence decisions, and maintain appropriate human oversight; covers evaluation of appropriateness, detection of risks, and understanding uncertainty.	Evaluating the appropriateness of AI for a given task or situation; detecting inconsistencies or risks in AI recommendations; assessing reliability, accuracy, validity and risk profile of AI outputs; judging where AI is appropriate or inappropriate; combining AI insights with professional reasoning; understanding uncertainty and confidence scores in outputs; identifying when human oversight or override is required; recognising potential harms, biases and unintended consequences, especially for marginalised populations.	Hanna et al. [2], Malamateniou et al. [1], Connolly et al. [3], Rodriguez et al. [15], Acosta [4], Montejo et al. [13]

(continued)

Table 1. (*continued*)

Domain	Definition	Key elements and skills	Illustrative sources
Workflow and contextual integration	Understanding how AI fits into existing professional, organisational, and interprofessional processes; knowing when and where AI is suitable to use within workflows; ability to integrate AI into information systems, documentation, and routines while understanding risks and human–AI task division	Understanding when and where AI is suitable to use within workflows; mapping AI tools to specific tasks and patient/client pathways; integrating AI into clinical or social care workflows, documentation and routines; identifying risks and safety considerations in real world use; understanding human–AI task division and responsibilities; practical operational skills such as using decision support tools, operating AI assisted workflow optimisation tools (e.g. automatic patient positioning, scout image analysis), AI supported documentation and triage; collaborating in multidisciplinary teams to embed AI safely and meaningfully into interprofessional practice.	Malamateniou et al. [1], Crotty et al. (2024), O'Connor et al. [9], Montejo et al. [12], Hobensack et al. (2024), Rodriguez et al. [15], Acosta [4]
Domain-specific AI application competencies	Profession-tailored uses of AI reflecting the specific roles, tasks and contexts of different health and social care professions; includes competencies in AI-enhanced assessment, diagnosis, care planning and documentation	Nursing: AI-enhanced assessment, triage, documentation, patient education and co-design with patients and carers. Imaging/radiography: AI-enabled workflow optimisation and safety in radiology and radiotherapy. Pathology: AI-supported diagnostic reasoning and performance evaluation. Oncology: AI-supported clinical decision making and patient-tailored education. Public health: AI-driven epidemiological modelling, risk prediction and policy analysis. Social work: integrating generative AI into case management and documentation while maintaining a focus on equity and client well-being	Montejo et al. [12], O'Connor et al. [9], Papachristou et al. [28], Malamateniou et al. [1], Rösler et al. [11], Acosta [4], Rodriguez et al. [15]
Cross-cutting, supporting domains			

(*continued*)

Table 1. (*continued*)

Domain	Definition	Key elements and skills	Illustrative sources
Ethical, legal, and responsible AI use	Using AI in ways that respect ethical principles, legal requirements, fairness, transparency, and professional accountability; includes the duty of care, privacy protection, bias and fairness considerations, and maintaining human oversight and shared decision-making.	Identifying ethical risks (bias, fairness, discrimination), including heightened risks for marginalised and vulnerable populations; ensuring data privacy, confidentiality and GDPR compliance; understanding accountability and professional responsibility; recognizing limitations of non-explainable AI systems; maintaining appropriate human oversight and shared decision making; communicating AI supported decisions responsibly to patients, clients and colleagues; analyzing the ethical implications of concrete AI applications in local contexts; managing algorithmic bias and fairness risks; maintaining critical thinking rather than over relying on AI outputs.	Hanna et al. [2], Malamateniou et al. [1], Rösler et al. [11], Papachristou et al. [28], Rodriguez et al. [15], Turja and Ahonen [20]
Communication and interaction skills	How professionals communicate AI-supported information in a clear, responsible, and human-centred way to patients, clients, colleagues, and stakeholders, including explaining results, addressing concerns transparently, and supporting shared decision-making.	Explaining AI-generated results in understandable terms; addressing patient/client concerns about AI use; discussing uncertainty or limitations transparently; supporting shared decision-making with AI as a tool; documenting AI-supported decisions clearly; maintaining the human-centred nature of care even when technology is involved; communicating AI-informed decisions to patients, clients, and colleagues.	Hobensack et al. [13], Montejo et al. [12], Rodriguez et al. [15]

(continued)

Table 1. (continued)

Domain	Definition	Key elements and skills	Illustrative sources
AI self-efficacy, readiness and continuous learning	Psychological and motivational factors that influence professionals' willingness and confidence to use AI tools in practice, combined with their capacity to update AI-related competence over time.	Confidence in interpreting AI outputs; willingness to engage with AI and learn new tools; recognising one's own competence limits and training needs; appropriate skepticism and critical mindset; managing AI related anxiety or uncertainty; positive but cautious attitudes towards AI's impact on work and professional identity; identifying personal training needs related to AI; using hands on and simulated learning opportunities to build competence; engaging in reflective practice; following new guidelines, standards and best practices; integrating AI competence into ongoing professional development and micro credentialing initiatives; staying current with emerging AI models, regulations and working methods; developing an innovative mindset that adapts competence frameworks to different organizational and resource contexts.	Stogiannos et al. [19], El Arab et al. [18], Montejo et al. [12], Ng et al. [24], Gazquez Garcia et al. [6], Acosta [4], Turja and Ahonen [20]

3.2 Professionals' Current Training Approaches and Integration

The 19 studies covered a wide range of professional contexts, including nursing, medicine, dentistry, radiography and medical imaging, pathology, oncology, public health, social work, interprofessional practice and the Finnish social and healthcare sector. Participants ranged from undergraduate and postgraduate students to practising clinicians, educators, managers and policy actors, with settings spanning hospitals, universities, continuing professional development programmes and national-level health and social service systems. Table 2 provides an overview of these professional areas, example foci and typical study types.

Table 2. Examples of included studies and professional contexts.

Professional area	Example focus (illustrative sources)	Typical study types
Nursing	AI applications and competence in nursing education and practice [12–14, 18]	Umbrella and rapid reviews, narrative syntheses
Radiography/imaging	AI guidance and curricula for imaging professionals [1, 19, 27]	Guidance documents, curriculum-oriented reviews, surveys
Dentistry	Core AI education curriculum for oral and dental healthcare [25]	Delphi consensus, curriculum proposals
Pathology/oncology	AI evaluation guidance and oncology-specific competence needs [2, 9, 11, 28]	Concept papers, systematic reviews, expert statements
Public health	Embedding AI literacy in public health education [4]	Perspective frameworks
Social work	Generative AI skills in social work education [15]	Proposal and perspective papers
Interprofessional/Social and healthcare sector	AI in interprofessional practice and Finnish social and healthcare sector [3, 20]	Case studies, surveys, national analyses

Training approaches differed markedly between professions and mirrored the maturity of AI integration in each field. Medical education appeared the most systematically developed, with compulsory or elective modules in AI, clinical data science and biomedical informatics implemented in several universities using case-based and project-based learning, self-directed study and, increasingly, autoML and large language model tools combined with formative and summative assessments [24, 26]. Dentistry and radiography had developed structured AI curricula and guidance through professional bodies, incorporating lectures, workshops, industry-led seminars, and authentic assessments such as critical appraisal of AI research and evaluation of AI-assisted imaging workflows [1, 18, 25, 27].

By contrast, nursing education was characterised by fragmented and largely descriptive evidence: umbrella and rapid reviews and perspective papers consistently advocated integrating AI into undergraduate and postgraduate nursing curricula but provided few empirically evaluated programmes or robust competence assessments [8, 11, 12, 17]. Reported initiatives focused on raising general AI awareness, incorporating AI into digital health or informatics courses and experimenting with AI-supported teaching tools, yet offered limited structured opportunities for hands-on work with deployed AI systems in clinical environments [8, 11]. Public health education remained mostly informal, relying on general AI literacy initiatives and short courses, with calls to embed AI and data science as core elements of public health curricula rather than optional add-ons

[4]. Social work education was at an early stage, with proposals to incorporate genera-tive AI-related competencies into existing modules and accreditation standards, but no evaluated AI-specific curricula or competence assessments were identified [13].

Interprofessional perspectives highlighted emerging initiatives but also substantial variation in scope and depth. In the Finnish social and healthcare context, AI-related topics began to appear through micro-credentials and eHealth-oriented teaching for physicians, dentists, and practical nurses as part of broader digital health education, yet these initiatives remained limited in number and coverage [19]. The same national survey reported that 59% of professionals exhibited an AI competence deficit, with the largest gap concerning the ability to analyse the ethical implications of concrete AI appli-cations, despite generally positive attitudes and willingness to learn [19]. This pattern suggests that motivation and readiness to engage with AI may outpace the availability of structured, ethically grounded training opportunities.

3.3   Gaps, Barriers and Development Needs

Across settings, the synthesis revealed recurring content, structural and assessment-related gaps. Content gaps included limited depth of AI and data literacy, sparse coverage of biostatistics and informatics, and a very small number of comprehensive, standardised AI curricula, particularly in nursing and general health professions education [8, 12, 16, 17]. Many programmes lacked opportunities for real-world or simulated practice with deployed AI tools, leaving workflow and contextual integration skills underdeveloped in nursing, imaging, public health and pathology [2, 4, 6, 11, 27].

Despite strong rhetorical emphasis on ethics across the literature, there was a notable deficit in advanced ethical implementation competence: professionals and students reported difficulties in analysing the ethical implications of specific AI applications, managing bias and fairness risks and maintaining critical thinking rather than over-relying on AI outputs [13, 19, 28]. Structural barriers spanned faculty expertise, time, and institutional support: many educators described limited confidence, resources, and support for designing and delivering AI-related teaching, particularly when combining technical, ethical, and practice-oriented content [4, 16, 24]. The Excel-based synthesis confirmed that, while ethical and human-centred competence was addressed in 18 of the 19 studies, communication and continuous learning were explicitly discussed in fewer than half of them, suggesting that these cross-cutting domains are often assumed rather than systematically embedded as learning outcomes.

Several studies proposed responses to these gaps and barriers. Suggested strategies included multimodal, case-based and experiential learning; alignment of AI learning out-comes with clearly defined competence frameworks such as the domains summarised in Table 1; faculty development and interprofessional collaboration; and staged models that differentiate between AI "consumers", "translators" and "developers" with escalating requirements for technical and analytical skills [4, 16, 24]. In this review, AI "consumers" are understood as professionals who primarily interpret and apply AI outputs within their own practice, without responsibility for developing models or infrastructures; "transla-tors" act as intermediaries between domain experts and technical developers, aligning clinical, social or organisational needs with data science and implementation choices; and "developers" refer to professionals with advanced competencies in computer and data science who design, train and maintain AI systems and therefore require the most extensive technical and analytical skill set.

3.4 Attitudes, Readiness and Role Stratification

Across professions, attitudes towards AI were generally positive but cautious. Professionals and students perceived potential benefits for efficiency, quality and learning, but expressed concerns about reliability, bias, transparency, loss of control and threats to professional identity, particularly in nursing and social work [8, 13, 17]. Self-reported readiness and confidence varied by professional group: imaging professionals reported relatively high readiness to work with AI-assisted tools while simultaneously acknowledging competence gaps, whereas public health educators and students described lower confidence and uncertainty about appropriate pedagogical approaches for AI and data-driven methods [4, 18].

The synthesis of AI self-efficacy findings suggested that many professionals hold positive attitudes and motivation to learn, but do not feel fully competent to use AI responsibly in practice. Confidence increased when participants had opportunities for hands-on or simulated practice, understood basic AI concepts and had clearer guidance on appropriate use, while limited explainability, lack of exposure to AI tools and unclear governance structures reduced perceived capability [17–19]. This pattern aligns with the cross-cutting domain of AI self-efficacy and continuous learning, indicating that psychological and motivational factors are tightly interwoven with the core technical and analytical domains [16, 24].

Finally, several sources pointed to a stratified competence model based on professional roles. Basic AI literacy and awareness of ethical, legal and governance issues were considered sufficient for "consumers" who primarily interpret AI outputs, whereas "translators" were expected to possess intermediate skills that bridge domain expertise, data science and implementation contexts, and "developers" to hold advanced competencies in computer science, data science and algorithm development [16, 24].

The domain structure identified in this review is consistent with such stratification: the five core domains define a shared baseline and profession-specific application areas, while the cross-cutting domains of ethics, communication, self-efficacy and continuous learning shape how these competencies are distributed and applied across consumer, translator and developer roles in different professions.

4 Discussion

This review synthesised evidence on AI competence domains, current training approaches and educational gaps for health and social care professionals across 19 studies published between 2021 and 2025. The findings indicate that AI competence functions as a multi-domain construct that combines five core domains with several cross-cutting, supporting domains, while competence development remains uneven across professions and is still rarely assessed empirically. In the following, the identified domains are related to existing competence frameworks, training patterns for different professional groups are outlined, and directions for curriculum design, assessment and policy are suggested.

One central contribution of this review is the articulation of a structured AI competence framework that distinguishes between core and cross-cutting domains. The five core domains of foundational AI literacy, data and analytical skills, critical evaluation and decision-making, workflow and contextual integration, and domain-specific AI application competencies capture the recurring content of AI competence across nursing, medicine, dentistry, imaging, pathology, oncology, public health, and social work. The cross-cutting domains of ethical, legal and responsible AI use, communication and interaction skills, and AI self-efficacy and continuous learning describe how competence is enacted, sustained and adapted in practice. Together, these domains refine the earlier five-domain models by making explicit the transversal ethical, communicative, and developmental components that were previously implicit or treated as background assumptions [21, 24, 25].

The review also reveals how unevenly AI competence development and training are distributed across professional groups. Imaging and pathology appear particularly advanced in terms of practical exposure to deployed AI tools and the availability of profession-specific guidance on AI-enabled workflows, diagnostic reasoning and performance evaluation [1, 2, 7, 18, 27, 28]. Medical education more broadly has begun to integrate AI, clinical data science and biomedical informatics into curricula, although implementation remains uneven across institutions and countries [4, 24, 26]. In contrast, nursing and social work are characterised by strong conceptual discussion and a widely recognised need for AI competence, but there is little evidence of evaluated curricula, limited opportunities for hands-on training with real AI systems and a tendency for ethical concerns to dominate over practical competence development [8, 11–13, 17].

The Finnish national survey further illustrates how such disparities manifest at the system level: 59% of social and healthcare professionals reported an AI competence deficit, with the largest gap in their ability to analyse the ethical implications of AI-based applications, even though attitudes and willingness to learn were generally positive [19]. This combination of motivation and perceived deficit suggests that readiness to engage with AI may outpace the availability of structured, ethically grounded training, particularly in frontline and community-oriented professions such as nursing and social work. It also underscores that ethical competence cannot be assumed to emerge automatically from technical instruction, but requires explicit, practice-based education that addresses bias, fairness, and accountability in concrete AI use cases.

Another important pattern is the pronounced gap between conceptual competence models and empirical measurement. Most included studies propose AI competence frameworks, curricula or lists of required skills, or assess self-reported readiness and attitudes, but very few provide validated, task-based assessments of actual AI competence. Pathology and imaging form notable exceptions: here, annotated cases, diagnostic simulations and performance metrics are used to evaluate professionals' ability to interpret AI-supported outputs, yet even these measures tend to focus on narrow tasks rather than holistic competence across domains [2, 7, 18]. As long as empirical measurement remains limited, educators and organisations will struggle to monitor competence development systematically, to compare training approaches, or to ensure that AI-related qualifications align with EQF-based expectations across educational levels.

The findings also highlight the relevance of role-stratified AI competence models for health and social care. Building on Ng et al.'s [24] distinction between AI "consumers", "translators" and "developers", the review suggests that basic AI literacy, ethical awareness and the ability to interpret AI outputs are essential for all professionals, whereas more advanced data, workflow and domain-specific competencies may be concentrated in translator and developer roles within each profession [16, 24]. In this framework, consumers are professionals who primarily interpret and apply AI outputs within their own practice; translators act as intermediaries who align clinical, social, or organisational needs with data science and implementation choices; and developers are professionals with advanced competencies in computer and data science who design, train, and maintain AI systems. The domain structure summarised in Table 1 is consistent with this stratification and can support the design of tiered learning outcomes and assessment criteria that reflect differing responsibilities and risk profiles across roles. The role-stratified structure proposed here, however, is based on a limited and heterogeneous set of studies and should be further refined and tested in empirical educational and practice settings.

A further implication of our findings is that required AI competence should be defined primarily by role- and task-specific demands rather than by formal educational level. In practice, highly educated professionals may only need basic AI literacy if their day-to-day work remains largely analogue, while vocationally trained staff can require relatively advanced skills when they routinely interpret AI-generated outputs or coordinate AI-enabled workflows. This points to a "level-as-need" logic, where target proficiency is determined by task complexity, responsibility and risk, and where individual variation in job profiles is explicitly acknowledged. Consequently, AI competence frameworks should not assume a linear relationship between qualification level and AI proficiency but instead specify differentiated expectations for professionals whose roles range from occasional AI consumers to those with sustained responsibility for AI-enabled decision-making.

These role- and task-sensitive requirements also underline the need for explicitly interdisciplinary and interprofessional approaches to AI competence development. Because consumers, translators and developers often collaborate across professional and organisational boundaries, AI-related learning outcomes are best co-designed and delivered in interdisciplinary settings where health and social care professionals, data scientists, educators and managers can jointly negotiate appropriate divisions of labour, oversight and responsibility for AI-supported decisions. Such interdisciplinary arrangements help ensure that no single professional group is expected to cover the full spectrum of AI expertise, while the team's collective competence remains sufficient for the safe, ethical, and context-appropriate use of AI in practice.

These insights have direct implications for curriculum design and faculty development. AI learning outcomes in health and social care education should explicitly cover both core and cross-cutting domains, avoiding an overly narrow focus on technical literacy at the expense of ethical, communicative and self-efficacy-related competencies. Curricula also need to be tailored to professional and role-specific contexts, distinguishing between generic AI literacy for all students and more advanced competencies for those who are likely to assume translator or developer roles in interprofessional teams. Faculty development emerges as a crucial enabling factor: educators require support, time and resources to build their own AI competence, to design experiential learning opportunities involving real or simulated AI tools, and to integrate AI-related content into existing courses in ways that are pedagogically robust and ethically grounded [4, 16, 24].

The fragmented and project-based nature of current AI training suggests that isolated course or programme development is unlikely to close competence gaps on its own. National analyses of lifelong learning in Finland propose an ecosystem-based model in which competence development is coordinated through networked, data-informed collaboration between education providers, employers, regions and policymakers, supported by shared impact goals and iterative, need-driven funding [22, 29]. Applying this ecosystem perspective to AI competence would mean treating curricula, workplace learning, micro-credentials, living labs and sandboxes as parts of a connected skills system rather than separate initiatives, with joint governance and shared competence data guiding where and how AI training is offered.

In health and social care, such an ecosystem-oriented approach could help reduce duplication, improve alignment between national strategies, local service needs and educational provision, and support the scaling of effective AI competence models beyond single institutions or professions. Instead of each organisation designing its own AI training in isolation, regional and national AI education ecosystems could coordinate learning pathways across EQF levels, pool interdisciplinary faculty and infrastructure, and use shared indicators to monitor whether investments in AI competence translate into safer, more equitable, and person-centred digital health and social care.

4.1 Further Research

The review points to several priorities for future research. There is a clear need to move beyond descriptive accounts and conceptual models towards empirical studies that develop and validate AI competence assessment tools, test tiered competence frameworks in diverse educational settings and examine how AI training influences actual practice and patient or client outcomes over time. Under-researched professions such as nursing and social work, as well as the experiences of marginalised and vulnerable populations affected by AI-mediated decisions, warrant particular attention [4, 13, 19]. Addressing these questions would help ensure that AI-related education does not reproduce existing competence and equity gaps in health and social care systems but instead reduces them.

4.2 Limitations

This scoping review has several limitations that should be considered when interpreting its findings. Although the reporting follows the PRISMA 2020 statement to enhance transparency, the review was not conducted as a fully protocol-driven systematic review, and the protocol was not prospectively registered. Screening and selection were conducted using the AI-assisted tool Elicit, with two reviewers involved throughout and jointly resolving any uncertainties or borderline cases, which may still have introduced a risk of missing or misclassifying eligible studies. No formal methodological quality or risk-of-bias appraisal was conducted across all included studies, and the synthesis relied on narrative thematic analysis of heterogeneous study designs; consequently, the results should be interpreted as an indicative synthesis rather than as definitive conclusions about the effectiveness of specific educational interventions or competence models. The review was further limited to peer-reviewed journal articles and peer-reviewed conference papers published in English and indexed in four databases, including MEDIC, so relevant work in other languages, grey literature, and local guidance documents may have been excluded. Finally, the interpretation of AI competence domains and training approaches is constrained by how competence was defined and operationalised in the included studies, many of which remain conceptual and provide limited empirical measurement of AI competence.

5 Conclusions

This review suggests that health and social care professionals require a coherent set of AI competencies spanning foundational AI literacy, data and analytical skills, critical evaluation and decision-making, workflow and contextual integration, and domain-specific applications, complemented by ethical, communicative, and continuous learning capabilities. Across professions, these domains appear to form a shared core that can guide AI-related education and continuing professional development, even though the emphasis on individual competencies necessarily varies by role, context and risk profile. At the same time, AI competence integration into education and training remains uneven, with more advanced developments in medicine, dentistry and imaging than in nursing, public health and social work, and with limited evidence of comprehensive, evaluated curricula. Persistent gaps, particularly in advanced ethical implementation skills, opportunities for real-world or simulated practice and faculty expertise, may risk widening the AI competence deficit already documented among health and social care professionals.

The findings also suggest that required AI competence is best defined by role- and task-specific demands rather than by formal qualification EQF levels, calling for role-sensitive, tiered expectations across consumer, translator, and developer roles rather than assuming a linear correlation between educational level and AI proficiency. Because AI-enabled workflows are inherently interdisciplinary and interprofessional, competence development is likely to be most effective when organised in shared learning environments where health and social care professionals, data experts and educators jointly negotiate the division of labour, oversight and responsibility for AI-supported decisions. Moving beyond fragmented, project-based training towards more coordinated, ecosystem-oriented AI competence development across organisations and educational levels may be essential if investments in AI skills are to translate into safer, more equitable and human-centred digital health and social care.

Acknowledgments. This research was supported by funding from DigiFinland Oy. The authors would like to thank Hanna Rantala for her support in implementing the database searches.

Disclosure of Interests. The authors have no competing interests to declare that are relevant to the content of this article.

References

1. Malamateniou, C., McFadden, S., McQuinlan, Y., England, A., Woznitza, N., Goldsworthy, S., et al.: Artificial intelligence: guidance for clinical imaging and therapeutic radiography professionals, a summary by the Society of Radiographers AI working group. Radiography. **27**, 1192–1202 (2021). https://doi.org/10.1016/j.radi.2021.07.028
2. Hanna, M.G., Olson, N.H., Zarella, M., Dash, R.C., Herrmann, M.D., Furtado, L.V., et al.: Recommendations for performance evaluation of machine learning in pathology: a concept paper from the College of American Pathologists. Arch. Pathol. Lab Med. **148**, e335–e361 (2024). https://doi.org/10.5858/ARPA.2023-0042-CP
3. Connolly, C., Hernon, O., Carr, P., Worlikar, H., McCabe, I., Doran, J., et al.: Artificial intelligence in interprofessional healthcare practice education – insights from the home health project, an exemplar for change. Comput. Sch. **40**, 412–429 (2023). https://doi.org/10.1080/07380569.2023.2247393
4. Zhang, P., Haykal, D., Sallam, M., Acosta, J.: Advancing public health education by embedding AI literacy. Front. Digit. Health. **7**, 1584883 (2025). https://doi.org/10.3389/fdgth.2025.1584883
5. Pulkkinen, J., Huttu, K., Suhonen, M.: Systemic challenges in AI adoption in public social and health organizations in Finland: a technology–organisation–environment perspective. J. Health Organ. Manag. **39**, 435–456 (2024). https://doi.org/10.1108/JHOM-06-2025-0309
6. Gazquez-Garcia, J., Sánchez-Bocanegra, C.L., Sevillano, J.L.: AI in the health sector: systematic review of key skills for future health professionals. JMIR Med. Educ. **11**, e58161 (2025). https://doi.org/10.2196/58161
7. Ng, F.Y.C., Thirunavukarasu, A.J., Cheng, H., Tan, T.F., Gutierrez, L., Lan, Y., et al.: Artificial intelligence education: an evidence-based medicine approach for consumers, translators, and developers. Cell Rep. Med. **4**, 101230 (2023). https://doi.org/10.1016/j.xcrm.2023.101230
8. Mikkonen, K., Tuunainen, S., Oikarinen, A., Jansson, M., Woo, B., Zhou, W., et al.: Artificial intelligence technologies supporting nurses' clinical decision-making: a systematic review. J. Clin. Nurs. (2025). https://doi.org/10.1111/jocn.70156
9. O'Connor, S., Vercell, A., Wong, D., Yorke, J., Fallatah, F.A., Cave, L., et al.: The application and use of artificial intelligence in cancer nursing: a systematic review. Eur. J. Oncol. Nurs. **68**, 102510 (2024). https://doi.org/10.1016/j.ejon.2024.102510
10. Cosgrove, J., Cachia, R.: DigComp 3.0: European Digital Competence Framework, fifth edition [Internet] edn. Publications Office of the European Union, Luxembourg (2025) Available from: https://publications.jrc.ec.europa.eu/repository/handle/JRC144121
11. Rösler, W., Altenbuchinger, M., Baeßler, B., Beissbarth, T., Beutel, G., Bock, R., et al.: An overview and a roadmap for artificial intelligence in hematology and oncology. J. Cancer Res. Clin. Oncol. **149**, 7997–8006 (2023). https://doi.org/10.1007/s00432-023-04667-5
12. Montejo, L., Fenton, A., Davis, G.: Artificial intelligence (AI) applications in healthcare and considerations for nursing education. Nurse Educ. Pract. **80**, 104158 (2024). https://doi.org/10.1016/j.nepr.2024.104158
13. Hobensack, M., von Gerich, H., Vyas, P., Withall, J., Peltonen, L.-M., Block, L.J., et al.: A rapid review on current and potential uses of large language models in nursing. Int. J. Nurs. Stud. **154**, 104753 (2024). https://doi.org/10.1016/j.ijnurstu.2024.104753
14. Gerçek, A., Çiftci, N., Durmuş, M., Sarman, A., Taşcı, Ö., Yıldız, M.: ChatGPT in nursing: applications, advantages, and challenges in education, research, and clinical practice. Ann. Biomed. Eng. **53**, 3202–3207 (2025). https://doi.org/10.1007/s10439-025-03832-w
15. Rodriguez, M.Y., Goldkind, L., Victor, B.G., Hiltz, B., Perron, B.E.: Introducing generative artificial intelligence into the MSW curriculum: a proposal for the 2029 educational policy and accreditation standards. J. Soc. Work. Educ. **60**, 174–182 (2024). https://doi.org/10.1080/10437797.2024.2340931

16. Weaver, B., Gillon, F., Heron, G., Reid, F., Dong, F.: Working with OpenAI: a Guide for Social Workers. University of Strathclyde Social Work Scotland, Glasgow (2025). https://socialworkscotland.org/wp-content/uploads/2025/06/Weaver-and-Gillon-et-al-2025-Working-with-OpenAI_Briefing-Paper.pdf
17. Yildirim, N., Zlotnikov, S., Sayar, D., Kahn, J.M., Bukowski, L.A., Amin, S.S., et al.: Sketching AI concepts with capabilities and examples: AI innovation in the intensive care unit. In: CHI 2024: Proceedings of the CHI Conference on Human Factors in Computing Systems, 1–18 ACM, New York (2024). https://doi.org/10.1145/3613904.3641896
18. El Arab, R.A., Al Moosa, O.A., Abuadas, F.H., Somerville, J.: The role of AI in nursing education and practice: umbrella review. J. Med. Internet Res. **27**, e69881 (2025). https://doi.org/10.2196/69881
19. Stogiannos, N., Litosseliti, L., O'Regan, T., Scurr, E., Barnes, A., Kumar, A., et al.: Black box no more: a cross-sectional multi-disciplinary survey for exploring governance and guiding adoption of AI in medical imaging and radiotherapy in the UK. Int. J. Med. Inform. **186**, 105423 (2024). https://doi.org/10.1016/j.ijmedinf.2024.105423
20. Turja, T., Ahonen, O.: Perceptions of AI competence in social and healthcare services: readiness, reliance and realism. Finnish J. eHealth eWelfare. **17**, 73–83 (2025). https://doi.org/10.23996/fjhw.155017
21. Europass: Description of the eight EQF levels. https://europass.europa.eu/en/description-eight-eqf-levels. (2024). Accessed 29 Jan 2026
22. Bichel-Findlay, J., Koch, S., Mantas, J., Abdul, S.S., Al-Shorbaji, N., Ammenwerth, E., et al.: Recommendations of the international medical informatics association (IMIA) on education in biomedical and health informatics: second revision. Int. J. Med. Inform. **170**, 104908 (2023). https://doi.org/10.1016/j.ijmedinf.2022.104908
23. Arola, M. et al.: Tulevaisuuden osaaminen syntyy ekosysteemeissä [Future competence is created in ecosystems]. Sitran selvityksiä, 204. Sitra, Helsinki, (2021). https://www.sitra.fi/julkaisut/tulevaisuuden-osaaminen-syntyy-ekosysteemeissa/
24. Page, M.J., McKenzie, J.E., Bossuyt, P.M., Boutron, I., Hoffmann, T.C., Mulrow, C.D., et al.: The PRISMA 2020 statement: an updated guideline for reporting systematic reviews. BMJ. **372**, n71 (2021). https://doi.org/10.1136/bmj.n71
25. Schwendicke, F., Chaurasia, A., Wiegand, T., Uribe, S.E., Fontana, M., Akota, I., et al.: Artificial intelligence for oral and dental healthcare: Core education curriculum. J. Dent. **128**, 104363 (2023). https://doi.org/10.1016/j.jdent.2022.104363
26. Ossa, L.A., Rost, M., Lorenzini, G., Shaw, D.M., Elger, B.S.: A smarter perspective: learning with and from AI-cases. Artif. Intell. Med. **135**, 102458 (2023). https://doi.org/10.1016/j.artmed.2022.102458
27. Crotty, E., Singh, A., Neligan, N., Chamunyonga, C., Edwards, C.: Artificial intelligence in medical imaging education: recommendations for undergraduate curriculum development. Radiography. **30**, 67–73 (2024). https://doi.org/10.1016/j.radi.2024.10.008
28. Papachristou, N., Kotronoulas, G., Dikaios, N., Allison, S.J., Eleftherochorinou, H., Rai, T., et al.: Digital transformation of cancer care in the era of big data, artificial intelligence and data-driven interventions: navigating the field. Semin. Oncol. Nurs. **39**, 151433 (2023). https://doi.org/10.1016/j.soncn.2023.151433
29. Tepponen, M., Ahonen, O., Turja, T.: Käsikirja: Digitalisaatiota ja sitä koskevien toimintatapojen, osaamisen ja kulttuurin edistäminen [Handbook: Promoting digitalisation and related practices, competences and culture]. Ministry of Social Affairs and Health, Helsinki (2024) Available from: https://urn.fi/URN:ISBN:978-952-00-8657-2

From Shared Input to Negotiated Comparison and Situated Action: Staging a Transnational Course in Digital and Data-Driven Healthcare

Casper Knudsen[✉][iD], Signe Pedersen[iD], and Ditte Weber[iD]

Department of Sustainability and Planning, Aalborg University, Aalborg, Denmark
casper@plan.aau.dk

Abstract. Digital and data-driven healthcare increasingly depends on workforce development and cross-national learning. Yet transnational continuing professional development (CPD) is often organised around expert input and best-practice inspiration, with less attention to how participants compare experiences across contexts and translate course learning into situated action in their own work context. This paper presents a conceptual and practice-oriented analysis of a transnational CPD course in digital and data-driven healthcare hosted in Denmark. Using Denmark as a reference case, the course combines shared input through e-learning, expert presentations, and site visits; negotiated comparison through a ranking-based negotiation game; and situated action through individual and group action plans. The analysis shows that these elements support different parts of the learning process. Shared input establishes a common empirical and conceptual reference point, the negotiation game makes national priorities explicit and discussable across countries, and the action plans attempt to translate these insights into context-sensitive action. At the same time, the action plans reveal that the movement from comparison to concrete short-term action is the most difficult part of the progression. The paper contributes design knowledge for transnational CPD in digital and data-driven healthcare by showing how learning formats can be staged to support comparison and translation without reducing contextual differences to best-practice transfer.

Keywords: Learning health systems · Digital and data-driven healthcare · Participatory methods

1 Introduction

Digital and data-driven healthcare has become central to contemporary health system development. Across policy and practice, digital infrastructures, registries, data platforms, telehealth, and forms of AI-supported decision-making are increasingly positioned as key enablers of more coordinated, efficient, and responsive healthcare services [1–3]. These ambitions resonate with the concept of the learning health system, in which data, experience, and practice are continuously connected to improve care and support informed action [4, 5]. Yet such ambitions do not depend on technology alone. They also depend on the capabilities of the professionals, managers, and policymakers expected to work with digital and data-driven change in practice [6].

© The Author(s) 2026

M. Särestöniemi et al. (Eds.): NCDHWS 2026, CCIS 3009, pp. 409–422, 2026.
https://doi.org/10.1007/978-3-032-28812-7_28

This places workforce development at the centre of current digital health agendas. There are strong calls to prepare professionals to "deliver the digital future" [7], and training is frequently highlighted as a key enabler of digital health adoption [8]. While substantial attention has been paid to digital competencies and their integration into formal education [9, 10], less attention has been given to short, practice-near continuing professional development (CPD) formats through which professionals build capabilities while already working in complex organisational settings [11]. This matters because digital and data-driven healthcare is not only a technical matter. It also depends on coordination across professional groups [12], on situated interpretation [11], and on work practices that connect infrastructures, data, and care processes in concrete settings [13].

The issue becomes more complex in transnational learning settings. Digital health is increasingly shaped by cross-national interdependence, shared standards, and ambitions to make interventions, infrastructures, and forms of implementation knowledge reusable across settings [14–16]. However, such reusability cannot be assumed. It requires practical learning arrangements that connect people, experiences, and problem framings across countries—so that similarities and differences can be articulated, compared, and translated into feasible action rather than reduced to superficial replication. This points to the value of learning programmes that are both inter-professional and international, enabling participants to negotiate priorities, meanings, and constraints across roles and contexts. In practice, transnational learning is often organised around expert input, examples, and forms of best-practice inspiration. While these formats may expose participants to relevant models and experiences, they do not necessarily create the conditions under which participants can compare priorities across contexts or translate shared learning into feasible action in their own healthcare settings.

This points to a central but underexplored challenge in transnational CPD: how to move participants from shared input to meaningful comparison across heterogeneous contexts, and further towards situated forms of action. Shared exposure to examples is not the same as mutual learning. Likewise, recognising similarities and differences across countries does not automatically make action possible once participants return to their own institutional environments. What is needed is not only expert-led teaching but learning formats that actively stage comparison and translation.

This paper addresses that challenge through a conceptual and practice-oriented analysis of a transnational CPD course in digital and data-driven healthcare hosted in Denmark. The course was developed as a blended format combining e-learning, expert presentations, site visits, participatory exercises, and action-plan development. Denmark functions throughout the course as a reference case, not as a model to replicate, but as a shared point of departure for reflection and discussion among participants from different healthcare settings in Asia and Latin and South America.

The paper asks: **How can a transnational CPD format be staged to move participants from shared input to negotiated comparison and towards context-sensitive action in their own healthcare settings?**

To answer this question, we analyse the course through three interrelated design components. First, we examine how blended learning and expert-led input establish a common empirical and conceptual reference point. Second, we analyse how a ranking-based negotiation game structures comparison by making national priorities explicit and discussable across countries. Third, we examine how action plans function as a translation device through which participants attempt to relate course learning to their own institutional settings.

The contribution of the paper is twofold. Empirically, it offers an account of how a transnational CPD course in digital and data-driven healthcare was organised across these three stages. Analytically, it shows that the movement from input, to comparison, to action is uneven: while shared input and negotiated comparison can be staged relatively effectively, translating course learning into concrete short-term action remains difficult. On this basis, the paper contributes design knowledge for transnational CPD in digital and data-driven healthcare by showing how comparison and translation can be structured without reducing contextual differences to best-practice transfer.

2 Study Scenario and Analytical Approach

This paper examines the CPD course, Digital and Data-driven Healthcare, delivered in Denmark from 2022 to 2025 through a collaboration between Danida Fellowship Centre and Aalborg University as part of the Strategic Sector Cooperation (SSC) under the Danish Ministry of Foreign Affairs. The SSC is a development policy initiative, with the overall purpose to promote cooperation between Danish authorities and similar authorities in the countries with which Denmark has a strategic cooperation. The sectors have been selected according to the criterion that Denmark has a leading role within the sectors and will be able to contribute to the development of the sectors in the cooperative countries and, in general, to strengthen professional cooperation with the countries. Other courses under the SSC address environmental aspects, energy, food security, among others. The CPD course, Digital and Data-driven Healthcare, is designed for healthcare-sector professionals working with digitalisation, health data, planning, implementation, and related policy or organisational tasks. Participants are selected through the SSC and typically come from countries in Asia and Latin and South America. Across the course iterations included here, the annual cohort size ranged from 21 to 24 participants.

The course combines virtual preparation, a two-week in-country programme in Denmark, and follow-up activities after participants return to their home country. Denmark functions throughout as a reference case. Danish digital health infrastructures, registries, governance arrangements, and implementation examples are presented as a shared empirical point of departure for discussion. The intention is not that participants should replicate Danish models in their own countries. Rather, the Danish case is used to make central issues in digital and data-driven healthcare discussable in a concrete way and to provide a common reference point against which participants can compare their own experiences, constraints, and priorities.

The course content is organised around two interconnected themes. The first concerns digital health transformation and implementation, including planning and strategy, implementation conditions, and examples of digital solutions such as tele-health and AI-supported decision-making. The second concerns health data and health economics, including the use of data for planning and decision-making, DRG and cost-effectiveness, monitoring and quality development, and the role of registries, clinical quality databases, and electronic health records. Across both themes, issues such as interoperability, classification, coordination, and data use are treated as practical and organisational questions rather than purely technical matters.

Participants represent a heterogeneous group of professional roles spanning health policy, economy and administration (e.g. health ministries, health insurance, social security, disease control management), clinical services (e.g. pharmacist, medical doctors), IT/technical staff, researcher and lectures at a university level, and allied organisational functions. This heterogeneity is analytically important. The course does not assume a shared baseline of professional responsibilities, health system organisation, or digital maturity. Instead, such differences are treated as central to the learning situation itself. The pedagogical challenge is therefore not only to provide relevant content, but also to create formats in which participants can compare how similar issues are prioritised and handled across markedly different healthcare settings.

The empirical material for the present analysis consists of three main sources:

1. Written individual and group action plans produced during the course from 2022 to 2025–the action plan format is described in Sect. 3.3.
2. Written and verbal course evaluations.
3. Facilitator observations and informal follow-up conversations during and after the course.

For the negotiation game introduced in 2024, the analysis also draws on photographs of game outputs and workshop situations. The material is not used to evaluate long-term organisational impact. Rather, it is used to analyse how the course format stages different parts of the learning process and what kinds of opportunities and frictions become visible across them.

Analytically, we focus on three interrelated design components. First, we examine how e-learning, expert presentations, and site visits establish a shared empirical and conceptual reference point. Second, we analyse how the workshop-based ranking negotiation game introduces a different mode of engagement by structuring cross-country comparison and requiring participants to articulate and prioritise national healthcare challenges in a shared format. Third, we examine how action plans function as a translation device through which participants attempt to relate shared input and cross-country comparison to context-sensitive action in their own healthcare settings.

Taken together, these three components form the analytical structure of the paper. They are not treated as separate course activities, but as linked stages in a broader progression: from shared input to negotiated comparison to situated action. The analysis that follows in the results section examines what each stage makes possible, and where the movement from one stage to the next becomes difficult (Table 1).

Table 1. Overview of the course format and analytical focus.

Course phase	Main activities	Pedagogical function	Analytical focus in this paper
Pre-course	E-learning materials, video lectures, readings, short tasks, introductory meetings	Establish a shared reference point and surface participants' own contexts and priorities	Shared input
In-country course in Denmark	Expert presentations, campus sessions, site visits	Provide concrete cases, infrastructures, and examples for reflection and discussion	Shared input
During course workshops	Ranking-based negotiation game and other participatory formats	Make national priorities explicit and discussable across contexts	Negotiated comparison
Return-home / follow-up phase	Individual and group action plans, follow-up meetings	Support translation of course learning into participants' own institutional settings	Situated action

3 Results

This section outlines three progressive, interlinked course components—shared input, negotiated comparison, and situated action—showing what each stage makes possible and where moving from one stage to the next becomes difficult.

3.1 Shared Input: Building a Common Reference Point without Assuming Transfer

The first stage of the course is organised around shared input. This includes e-learning materials, video lectures, campus-based expert presentations, and site visits during the in-country programme in Denmark. Across these formats, the pedagogical aim is to establish a common empirical and conceptual point of departure for participants who enter the course with very different professional backgrounds, roles in healthcare, and national health system conditions.

This common point of departure matters because the course does not assume that participants already share a baseline understanding of digital and data-driven healthcare. Participants work in different parts of the healthcare sector and come from healthcare systems that vary in infrastructure, governance, funding, workforce organisation, and levels of digital maturity. In this context, shared input is needed not to create sameness, but to create a sufficiently concrete basis for later comparison.

Denmark plays a central role in this first stage as a reference case. Through presentations and site visits, participants are introduced to Danish digital health infrastructures, governance arrangements, and implementation practices, including examples related to telehealth, health data, registries, electronic health records, and data use for planning and monitoring. These examples are not presented as universal models to be replicated. Rather, they function as a shared empirical point of reference that makes otherwise abstract issues more tangible and discussable. The Danish case thus serves less as an answer than as an object of interrogation: what conditions make particular digital arrangements possible, what forms of coordination sustain them, and what kinds of organisational and infrastructural work do they depend on?

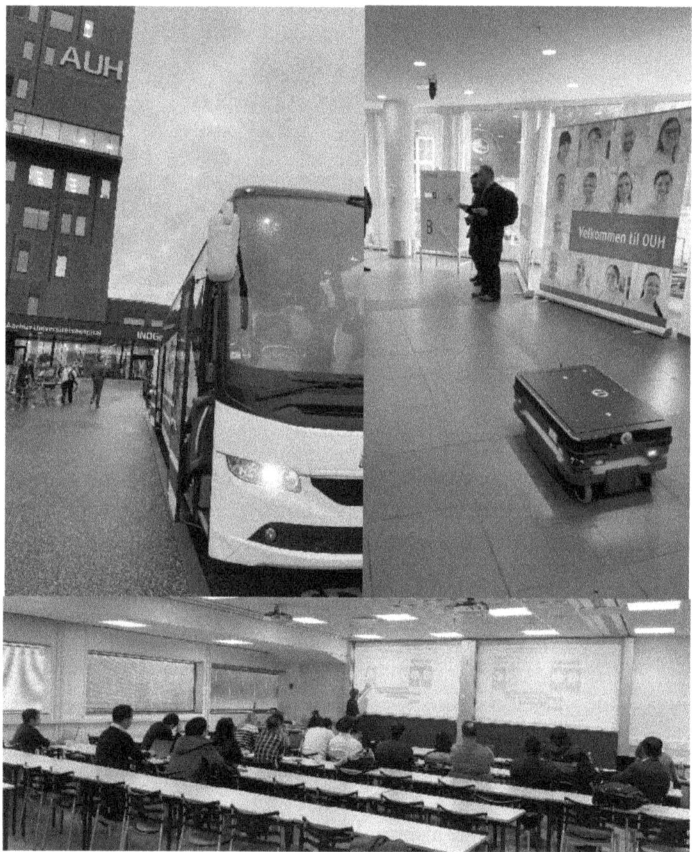

Fig. 1. Photograph from field trips and lectures.

The blended design strengthens this common reference point by distributing input across multiple formats. Before arriving in Denmark, participants engage with e-learning materials, readings, and video lectures that introduce key themes and concepts. This preparatory phase helps surface participants' own interests and contexts before the in-country part of the course begins. During the in-country programme, campus sessions and site visits build on this initial preparation by providing situated exposure to concrete organisational and infrastructural arrangements. Together, these formats create a shared language and a common set of examples that participants can draw on in later course activities.

This first stage also has clear limitations. Shared input can expose participants to relevant examples and provide conceptual orientation, but it does not by itself require participants to position their own priorities in relation to those of others. Participants may find the same presentation or site visit highly relevant, but for different reasons rooted in their own healthcare settings, professional roles, and institutional concerns. These differences remain largely implicit unless the course includes formats that actively require participants to articulate and compare them.

The value of this stage therefore lies in establishing the empirical and conceptual groundwork on which later comparison can be staged. It creates common reference points but not yet negotiated comparison (Fig. 1).

3.2 Negotiated Comparison: Making National Priorities Explicit and Discussable

If the first stage of the course establishes a shared reference point, the second stage introduces a different mode of engagement: negotiated comparison. This shift takes place in the workshop-based participatory formats, most clearly in the ranking-based negotiation game introduced during the course. Whereas expert presentations and site visits provide examples and concepts for reflection, the workshop format requires participants to position their own healthcare realities in relation to a shared set of concerns and, in doing so, to make their priorities visible to others.

The negotiation game was developed as a lightweight comparison format tailored to the course context (cf. Fig. 2). Participants were grouped by country and asked to rank eight predefined healthcare challenges according to their perceived severity in their national context. The challenges represented recurring concerns identified through prior work on healthcare systems and cross-sector collaboration and included shortage of specialists, distance to services, chronic disease management, avoidable readmissions, health information exchange, high costs, variation in quality, and lack of collaboration across professions [17].

The design of the format was deliberately simple. Each group worked with the same set of challenge cards and was asked to produce a single ordered ranking from most to least severe. This constraint was analytically important. In many healthcare settings, the challenges represented on the cards are experienced as tightly interconnected. The ranking task therefore did not merely ask participants to identify relevant issues, but to negotiate how these issues should be prioritised relative to one another.

Within the country groups, the task moved quickly beyond simple sorting. Participants discussed not only which challenges mattered most, but also how specific challenges should be understood in their own context. For some groups, lack of collaboration was primarily discussed as an organisational issue. For others, it was closely connected to infrastructural or data-sharing conditions. Likewise, challenges such as chronic disease management or readmissions were interpreted differently depending on how care pathways, access conditions, and workforce responsibilities were organised nationally. For instance, one country group prioritised shortage of specialists and distance to services near the top of the ranking, while another group placed health information exchange and cross-professional coordination higher, linking them more directly to fragmentation across providers. The shared card set did not remove contextual differences; it made them explicit in a comparable form.

The requirement to arrive at one ranked sequence per country group also mattered. Participants could not simply state parallel views; they had to work towards a collective ordering. In several groups, this appears to have generated discussion around trade-offs between challenges that were initially treated as equally urgent. The no-tie rule therefore functioned as more than a procedural device. It structured the activity as a negotiation of priorities rather than as a general exchange of experiences.

In the subsequent plenary session, the ranked sequences became shared reference points for cross-country discussion. Participants could see that the same challenges recurred across countries, but that they were ranked differently and often linked to different underlying conditions. A particularly clear point of recognition across groups was shortage of specialists. Participants from several countries related this challenge to their own healthcare systems while pointing to different local manifestations, such as uneven geographical distribution, difficulties recruiting to rural areas, or broader pressure on existing services. In this way, the exercise did not only surface differences in prioritisation; it also established certain challenges as recognisable across otherwise heterogeneous settings. Rather than asking participants to speak in general terms about their healthcare systems, the format provided a common set of elements through which national priorities could be articulated, compared, and briefly related to other contexts.

Analytically, the contribution of the negotiation game lies less in demonstrating specific learning outcomes than in how it structures comparison. The format translates heterogeneous experiences into a common set of tangible elements, requires prioritisation under constraint, and produces visible outputs that can circulate in plenary discussion. In this way, it creates a temporary setting in which differences in priorities become explicit and discussable across countries without assuming direct transferability between healthcare systems [17].

The analysis of this part of the course is based on photographs of game outputs and workshop situations, facilitator observations, and participant evaluations. This material does not allow for detailed interaction analysis of the workshop conversations themselves. It does, however, provide sufficient insight into how the format functioned as part of the course design and how it supported negotiated comparison in practice.

Seen in relation to the first stage of the course, the negotiation game marks an important shift. Shared input creates a common reference point, but it leaves participants' own priorities largely implicit. The workshop format, by contrast, requires these priorities to be articulated, ordered, and made visible to others. This does not yet amount to situated action in participants' own settings, but it creates a necessary intermediate step between receiving examples and articulating how one's own context differs from, resembles, or resists those of others.

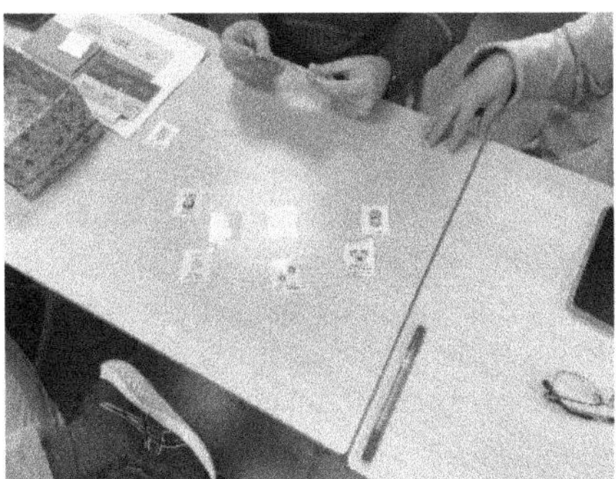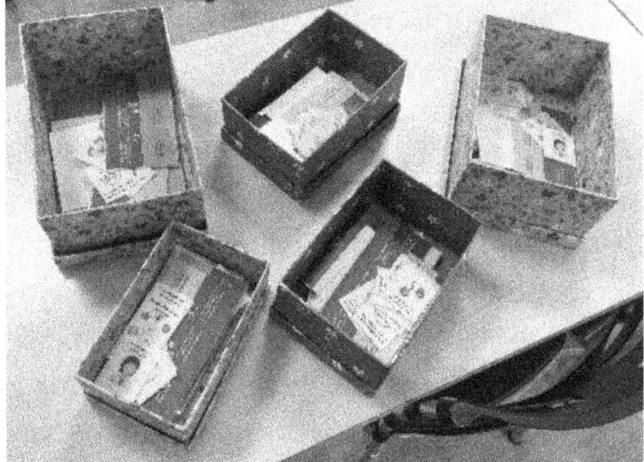

Fig. 2. Photograph from the ranking-based negotiation game.

3.3 Situated Action: Action Plans and the Difficulty of Translation

If the negotiation game structures comparison across countries, the action plans introduce a third mode of engagement: situated action. At this stage, participants are no longer asked primarily to reflect on examples or compare national priorities, but to formulate how course learning might be translated into feasible action in their own healthcare settings. In this sense, the action plans function as a translation device. They connect shared input and negotiated comparison to participants' own organisational realities by requiring them to identify a focal problem, consider relevant stakeholders, and outline possible next steps.

The action-plan format was explicitly designed to support this movement. Rather than ending the course with general reflection, participants were asked to work with a template structured around phases: before the course, during the course, and after the course. Section 1) Before the course starts: the participants formulated expectations to their application of learning and 5 possible and realistic actions upon returning home, including resources to conduct actions) Sect. 2) During the course: participants formulated key learning points to bring home, including five implications for their work responsibilities, organizational priorities, and five adjusted concrete actions to take to use the course learnings at home, including reflections on who can support the implementation of the actions, and how Sect. 3) Three months after the course participants formulated status on the process of implementing the actions in connection with an online follow-up seminar.

This format encouraged participants to connect what they had encountered in the course to their own settings over time. It also invited them to distinguish between broader ambitions and more immediate actions, thereby shifting the focus from inspiration to implementation.

Analytically, the action plans are important because they make visible what happens when course learning is brought back into participants' own contexts. Unlike the first stage of the course, where participants encounter shared input, and unlike the negotiation game, where they compare their settings in a common frame, the action plans require participants to work within the practical constraints of their own institutions. This shift changes the character of the learning process. The question is no longer only what seems important or interesting, but what appears possible, relevant, and actionable given local conditions.

Across the material, the action plans suggest that this stage is also where the progression becomes most difficult. Many participants were able to formulate relevant focal issues and broader ambitions in relation to their own healthcare settings and work context. They identified challenges, articulated concerns, and in some cases drew clearly on course themes such as interoperability, health information exchange, coordination, or data use for planning and improvement. However, when asked to specify concrete short-term actions, the plans often became less precise, unless these concerned dissemination activities such as presentations of course insights for colleagues and management. Long-term intentions were easier to formulate than near-term operational steps.

This difficulty is analytically significant. It suggests that the central challenge in transnational CPD is not only exposure to relevant examples, nor even comparison across settings, but the translation of these into context-sensitive and feasible action. Participants may recognise relevant problems, see parallels with other countries, and identify promising directions, while often struggling to identify realistic actions of precisely what should happen first, by whom, and under which institutional conditions.

From this perspective, the action plans do more than document participants' intended next steps. They also reveal the limits of the course format. While the course appears able to support common reference-making and structured comparison, the translation into concrete action remains fragile and uneven. This does not mean that the action plans fail. Rather, it shows that they surface precisely the friction that a transnational CPD format must contend with: the gap between recognising what matters and identifying what is feasible to do next in a particular socio-technical setting.

This friction also points to a practical design implication. If action plans are to function as a stronger bridge between course learning and local implementation, participants may need more scaffolding in formulating short-term experiments, first steps, or dissemination strategies that are modest enough to be realistic, yet concrete enough to move beyond general aspiration. In that sense, the value of the action plans lies not only in their role as a pedagogical output, but in how they make the difficulty of translation visible.

Seen across the three stages of the course, the action plans complete the progression from shared input to negotiated comparison to situated action. At the same time, they show that this final stage cannot be treated as a straightforward consequence of the preceding ones. Shared examples and cross-country comparison may create orientation and momentum, but they do not automatically generate implementable action. The action plans therefore reveal the most demanding part of the course design: not creating engagement or recognition but supporting participants in turning these into context-sensitive steps within their own healthcare systems.

4   Discussion

The main contribution of the course does not lie in any single activity, but in how the activities are arranged as a progression from shared input to negotiated comparison, to situated action. The three stages do different kinds of work, and the analysis shows that they address different parts of the challenge of transnational professional learning in digital and data-driven healthcare.

A first point concerns the limits of shared input. E-learning, expert presentations, and site visits are important because they establish a common empirical and conceptual reference point across a highly heterogeneous participant group. In a transnational CPD setting, this common ground cannot be taken for granted. At the same time, shared exposure should not be equated with mutual learning. Participants may be introduced to the same examples and infrastructures, but this does not in itself make their own priorities explicit, nor does it ensure that similarities and differences across contexts become discussable.

A second point concerns the role of negotiated comparison. The ranking-based negotiation game matters because it introduces a learning dynamic that expert-led formats do not produce on their own. By requiring participants to prioritise a shared set of healthcare challenges without ties, the format moves the course from exposure to articulation. National priorities do not simply appear; they are produced through a situation in which participants must negotiate meaning, weigh trade-offs, and externalise their ordering in a visible form. Because data-driven change involves many interdependent roles [12, 18] learning health system capacity is partly the capacity to coordinate and translate across these roles. The course format addresses this by assembling a temporary "actorscape" of health sector professionals and by structuring interaction so that participants must surface their assumptions, priorities, and constraints across national as well as professional boundaries. At the same time, the comparison did not only make differences visible. It also established certain challenges as recognisable across otherwise heterogeneous settings. In the plenary discussions, shortage of specialists emerged as a particularly clear point of cross-country recognition, even though participants related it to different local conditions. This is important in digital and data-driven healthcare, where recurrent issues may be widely recognised across settings without carrying identical meanings or implications [12, 18].

The third point concerns translation and the difficulty of situated action. This is where the course progression becomes most demanding. Shared input can create orientation, and negotiated comparison can make priorities explicit and discussable, but neither guarantees that participants can formulate feasible first steps in their own setting. The action plans show that participants were often able to identify relevant concerns, formulate broader ambitions, and connect course themes to their own contexts. However, they also reveal that the movement from comparison to action is not straightforward. Many participants found it easier to articulate what matters than to specify what should happen first in their own setting. This suggests that the central challenge in transnational CPD is not simply a lack of knowledge or inspiration. It is the difficulty of translating shared learning into feasible action under local organisational and institutional constraints [11].

These findings qualify how transnational learning should be understood. If mutual learning is defined too loosely, it risks being reduced to exposure, recognition, or general inspiration. The analysis here suggests a more demanding view: transnational learning becomes meaningful when participants are able to move from shared examples to comparison of priorities, and further towards context-sensitive action. This also points to an important design implication for CPD formats. If action is the most fragile stage in the progression, then it is not enough to provide participants with examples and opportunities for discussion. Greater attention must also be given to the scaffolding of translation, including support for identifying modest first steps, concrete experiments, and contextually feasible forms of dissemination or implementation.

Seen from a learning health system perspective, this progression is particularly relevant. Learning health systems depend not only on data infrastructures and technological capabilities, but also on professionals' capacity to interpret, coordinate, and act across multiple organisational and disciplinary boundaries [6, 13]. The course examined here suggests that such capacity cannot be built through expert-driven teaching alone. It requires learning situations in which professionals are exposed to concrete examples, compelled to compare how recurring concerns are prioritised across contexts, and supported in relating these insights to their own setting.

The contribution of this paper should therefore be understood as design knowledge rather than evidence of downstream impact. The course does not demonstrate that participants implemented change after returning home, nor that the negotiation game or action plans produced measurable organisational outcomes. What it does show is how a transnational CPD format can be staged to support different parts of a learning process that are often collapsed into one another: common reference-making, structured comparison, and attempted translation into action. By analysing where this progression holds and where it becomes difficult, the paper contributes a more precise understanding of what transnational professional learning in digital and data-driven healthcare may require in practice.

4.1 Design Implications for Transnational CPD

Three design implications follow from the analysis. First, shared input should be organised around reference cases rather than models for replication. The value of a case such as Denmark lies in creating a common empirical point of departure, not in presenting a template to be copied. Second, transnational CPD formats benefit from inserting a structured comparison stage before asking participants to formulate local action. The ranking-based negotiation game was useful here because it made national priorities explicit and discussable in a shared frame. Third, the transition from comparison to action requires more scaffolding than the course currently provided. Future formats may therefore benefit from requiring participants to define a modest short-term experiment, a small stakeholder map, and one or two concrete indicators of progress, in order to support translation from broad ambition to feasible first steps.

5 Conclusion

This paper has analysed a transnational CPD course in digital and data-driven healthcare through a progression from shared input, to negotiated comparison, to situated action. Rather than treating transnational learning as a matter of expert-led inspiration or best-practice transfer, the course was staged to support a more structured movement in which participants first encountered a common reference case, then compared national priorities through a negotiation format, and finally attempted to translate these insights into action in their own healthcare settings.

The analysis shows that these stages do different kinds of work. Shared input established a common empirical and conceptual point of departure, while the negotiation game made differences in national priorities explicit and discussable across contexts. The action plans, in turn, revealed that translation into situated action was the most difficult part of the progression. Participants were often able to identify relevant concerns and longer-term ambitions, but less able to specify concrete short-term steps.

The paper contributes design knowledge for transnational CPD in digital and data-driven healthcare by showing that mutual learning does not emerge from exposure alone. It depends on how learning formats are staged to support comparison and translation without erasing contextual differences. For digital health and learning health system ambitions alike, the challenge is therefore not only to share examples across countries, but to structure the movement from shared input towards context-sensitive action in practice.

References

1. Monaghesh, E., Hajizadeh, A.: The role of telehealth during COVID-19 outbreak: a systematic review based on current evidence. BMC Public Health. **20**(1), 1193 (2020). https://doi.org/10.1186/s12889-020-09301-4
2. Shaver, J.: The state of telehealth before and after the COVID-19 Pandemic. Prim. Care. **49**(4), 517–530 (2022). https://doi.org/10.1016/j.pop.2022.04.002
3. World Bank: Digital-in-Health: Unlocking the Value for Everyone. World Bank, Washington, DC (2023)
4. Friedman, C.P., Wong, A.K., Blumenthal, D.: Achieving a nationwide learning health system. Sci. Transl. Med. **2**(57), 29 (2010). https://doi.org/10.1126/scitranslmed.3001456
5. Coiera, E.: The forgetting health system. Learn. Health Syst. **1**(4), e10023 (2017). https://doi.org/10.1002/lrh2.10023
6. Steel, P.A.D., Wardi, G., Harrington, R.A., Longhurst, C.A.: Learning health system strategies in the AI era. npj Health Syst. **2**(1), 21 (2025). https://doi.org/10.1038/s44401-025-00029-0
7. Topol, E.: The Topol Review–Preparing the Healthcare Workforce to Deliver the Digital Future. NHS. Health Education England (2019)
8. do Nascimento, I.J.B., et al.: Barriers and facilitators to utilizing digital health technologies by healthcare professionals. NPJ Digit. Med. **6**(1), 161 (2023). https://doi.org/10.1038/s41746-023-00899-4
9. Car, J., et al.: The digital health competencies in medical education framework: an international consensus statement based on a Delphi study. JAMA Netw. Open. **8**(1), e2453131 (2025). https://doi.org/10.1001/jamanetworkopen.2024.53131
10. Thye, J., et al.: What are inter-professional eHealth competencies? In: German Medical Data Sciences: a Learning Healthcare System, pp. 201–205. IOS Press (2018) https://ebooks.iospress.nl/doi/10.3233/978-1-61499-896-9-201
11. Knudsen, C., Villumsen, S., Krejberg, L., Nøhr, C.G.: The last mile problem and beyond in HIT – the role of context-sensitive digital Integrators. In: Digital Professionalism in Health and Care: Developing the Workforce, Building the Future, Ed., European Federation for Medical Informatics (EFMI) and IOS Press, pp. 97–101 (2022). https://doi.org/10.3233/SHTI220915
12. Bertelsen, P.S., Bossen, C.: Data professionals in healthcare: who they are and what they do? Health Inf. Manag. J. **00**(0), 1–13 (2025). https://doi.org/10.1177/18333583251393395
13. Bertelsen, P.S., Bossen, C., Knudsen, C., Pedersen, A.M.: Data work and practices in healthcare: a scoping review. Int. J. Med. Inform. **184**, 105348 (2024). https://doi.org/10.1016/j.ijmedinf.2024.105348

14. United Nations (UN): The Age of Digital Interdependence: Report of the UN Secretary-General's High-Level Panel on Digital Cooperation. UN, New York (2019)
15. World Health Organization (WHO): Global Strategy on Digital Health 2020–2025, 1st edn. World Health Organization, Geneva (2021)
16. Mehl, G., et al.: WHO SMART guidelines: optimising country-level use of guideline recommendations in the digital age. Lancet Digit. Health. **3**(4), e213–e216 (2021). https://doi.org/10.1016/S2589-7500(21)00038-8
17. Pedersen, S., Dorland, J.: Staging situated negotiation games for (re)designing local healthcare facilities and services. Des. Health. **9**(1), 94–120 (2025). https://doi.org/10.1080/24735132.2025.2454731
18. Bossen, C., Bertelsen, P.S.: Digital health care and data work: who are the data professionals? Health Inf. Manag. J. **53**(3), 243–251 (2023). https://doi.org/10.1177/18333583231183083

Medical Students' Experiences of Digital Collaborative Learning in eHealth Training

Paula Veikkolainen[1]([✉]) [iD], Erika Jarva[2] [iD], Timo Tuovinen[1,3] [iD], Petri Kulmala[4,5] [iD], Tiina Salmijärvi[4] [iD], Jonna Juntunen[2] [iD], Annukka Tuomikoski[5] [iD], Jarmo Reponen[1] [iD], and Merja Männistö[6] [iD]

[1] FinnTelemedicum, Research Unit of Health Sciences and Technology, Faculty of Medicine, University of Oulu, Oulu, Finland
paula.veikkolainen@oulu.fi
[2] Research Unit of Health Sciences and Technology, Faculty of Medicine, University of Oulu, Oulu, Finland
[3] Medical Reasearch Center Oulu, University of Oulu and Oulu University Hospital, The Wellbeing Services County of North Ostrobothnia, Oulu, Finland
[4] Education Development and Service Unit, Faculty of Medicine, University of Oulu, Oulu, Finland
[5] North Ostrobothnia Wellbeing Services County, Oulu University Hospital, Oulu, Finland
[6] School of Health and Social Studies, Jamk University of Applied Sciences, Jyväskylä, Finland

Abstract. There are growing global demands for digital health competencies in undergraduate medical education. At the same time, digital learning environments are increasingly used to support collaborative learning, yet the implementation of eHealth education in medical curricula remains challenging. This paper presents an example of integrating nationally agreed eHealth competence themes into undergraduate medical training through a digital, collaborative learning event. The intervention was an annual eHealth seminar day (2021–2025) for fifth-year medical students at the University of Oulu, including expert lectures and small-group work on assigned competence themes. Students' perceptions of collaborative learning were collected using a previously validated questionnaire and analysed descriptively. A total of 410 students participated across five cohorts. Perceptions of group atmosphere, active participation, peer support, and students' confidence in their own study skills in supporting collaborative learning were strongest, whereas students' own motivation, course materials, and teacher feedback received lower endorsement. Perceptions remained largely stable, with a temporary decline in 2023 - particularly related to teacher input and the digital learning environment - followed by at least partial recovery. Integrating collaborative learning into a digital environment appears to be a feasible and effective approach for delivering eHealth education to medical students. However, improvements in teacher support, learning materials, and motivation-promoting strategies are warranted. Ongoing evaluation and refinement of teaching models and tools are essential to match the rapidly evolving healthcare landscape.

Keywords: Medical education · eHealth · Digital health · Collaborative learning · Digital learning

M. Särestöniemi et al. (Eds.): NCDHWS 2026, CCIS 3009, pp. 423–431, 2026.
https://doi.org/10.1007/978-3-032-28812-7_29

1 Introduction

The application of digital health and use of eHealth tools has rapidly expanded worldwide, which in turn requires that future healthcare professionals possess adequate digital health competencies [1]. This creates a corresponding demand for integrating these competencies into basic medical education. Recent consensus work proposes a global competency framework spanning professionalism in digital health, health information systems, and health data science signalling broad agreement that such skills also belong in undergraduate medical training [2]. Students likewise consider incorporating digital health topics in to basic medical education important [3–5]. Despite this momentum, integrating eHealth into medical programs remains challenging, with barriers including overloaded curricula, variation in faculty readiness, and inconsistent institutional strategies and guidelines [6, 7].

The use of digital learning environments has been present in use of medical education for at least couple of decades [8, 9]. The COVID-19 pandemic forced a rapid shift toward remote teaching strategies, accelerating the adoption of digital learning tools [10, 11]. Evidence suggests that students learn equally well through digital formats as they do in face-to-face settings [12]. A combination of digital and face-to-face learning, often referred to as blended learning, appears to yield better learning outcomes compared to traditional classroom methods [13]. Research also shows that the use of digital learning tools in medical education is associated with higher student satisfaction [14]. Limitations of digital learning include challenges related to social interaction, increased responsibility placed on students, and the need for adequate support [15].

Collaborative learning is an approach in which students jointly construct understanding and knowledge through interaction [16]. It is considered to build competencies, such as teamwork and problem-solving, that are highly valued in the 21st century [17]. Research demonstrates that collaborative learning can be effectively implemented in digital environments with healthcare students, and that well-designed online collaborative settings can successfully foster their competence development [18–20].

In Finland, there has been a growing effort to incorporate digitalisation into the education and training of healthcare professionals. The national MEDigi project (2018–2021) aimed to harmonise, modernise, and digitalise medical education by integrating digital tools into undergraduate medicine and dentistry teaching [21]. The project's key objectives included defining medical core competences, producing electronic learning materials, developing digital examination and assessment methods, and improving the digital pedagogy of teaching staff. Another aim was to train students in the use of eHealth tools. Over the course of the project, 12 thematic eHealth competence areas were defined for the first time in national level in Finland [22]. The ongoing digital transformation of healthcare highlights the need for a systematic approach to professional training [23].

In this paper, we present preliminary results on medical students' perceptions of collaborative learning in a digital environment in the context of healthcare digitalisation and eHealth education, based on the MEDigi recommendations of thematic eHealth competence areas between 2021 and 2025. Drawing on students' experiences, the survey aims to support the iterative and long-term development of medical education, including the refinement of learning contents, teaching methods, and the dynamic use of student feedback.

2   Materials and Methods

A multi-year repeated cross-sectional observational design was used. Survey data were gathered from separate cohorts of fifth-year medical students at the University of Oulu who attended a one-day (7.5 h) eHealth seminar over five consecutive years (2021–2025). The educational event was compulsory for students and part of the fifth-year general practice course. The aim of the intervention was to provide essential knowledge of digital health and its applications from the perspective of healthcare professionals. The event was delivered entirely online. Although the seminar day involved also nursing students in most years, curriculum-related factors prevented their participation in all iterations. Therefore, this study focuses exclusively on medical students.

The first half (3.5 h) of the education event consisted of online expert lectures delivered via Zoom, providing an overview of digital health concepts, the role of digital tools in clinical practice and current eHealth services. During the second half (4 h), students were placed in Zoom breakout rooms and divided into small (interdisciplinary) groups of 2–4 students. The grouping approach differed across years; in 2022, 2023 and 2025 the groups were interdisciplinary and included nursing students, whereas in 2021 and 2024 they did not. Each small group was assigned a specific eHealth theme, and each breakout room had a facilitator to support the group work. Although the overall structure of the event remained consistent across years, minor updates were made annually to the lecture content, group work materials, and teaching personnel.

In the Moodle environment, information on various eHealth services and products was collected and organized into 12 thematic areas based on the competence areas defined in the MEDigi project. Each theme included curated materials such as videos, links to reports, and references to relevant websites. Students worked in small groups to familiarize themselves with the assigned theme and produced a short presentation, which served as their method for teaching the core concepts of the theme to their peers at the end of the day. The event was evaluated as pass or fail.

The theoretical framework for collaborative learning in digital learning environment, applicable to both healthcare students and social and healthcare educators, has been described in earlier doctoral research [24].

Data on medical students' perceptions of collaborative learning were collected using a previously validated instrument with a 5-point Likert scale (from fully disagree to fully agree) [19]. The instrument consists of three sub-dimensions: 1) promoting collaborative group work (six items: S6–S11), 2) the teacher's role in the collaborative learning environment (four items: S2–S5), and 3) the student's own role in collaborative learning (three items: S1, S12, and S13). Responses were collected using web-based survey tool (Webropol). Students were invited to complete the questionnaire after the day's program in Moodle and via email. Participation in the study were voluntary, students were informed about the purpose of the study, and all responses were collected anonymously. No incentives were provided, and the anonymous design ensured that participation could not lead to any adverse consequences, such as influencing the students' evaluations. The response window remained open for one week after events.

Responses were dichotomized into 'agree' (fully or somewhat agree) and 'disagree' (neither agree nor disagree, somewhat disagree, or disagree) to reflect whether students endorsed each statement at a practically meaningful level. Analyses were limited to descriptive summaries; no further statistical testing was performed.

3   Preliminary Results

In total, 410 medical students participated in the study across the five data-collection years (2021: n = 106, 2022: n = 64, 2023: n = 55, 2024: n = 99, 2025: n = 86).

Table 1. Percentages of students agreeing with statements related to their perceptions of collaborative learning during the one-day eHealth education event. Data represent pooled responses from 2021–2025, with percentages calculated as n (students agreeing) / n (total number of students).

Statement		Students who agreed with the statement (%)
S13	My own study skills, such as good interaction skills, are an important prerequisite for successful collaborative learning.	90,5
S9	My fellow students support my learning.	88,8
S8	The members of the group are active and participate equally in the work.	86,3
S7	The group has a positive atmosphere that encourages and motivates us to work together.	86,3
S3	The actions of the teachers and tutors during the course support collaborative learning.	75,9
S11	The interaction in the group is fluent and the discussions are profound.	75,9
S6	Our group has a clear shared goal.	75,6
S1	Formatting of the learning task required collaborative learning.	73,7
S10	The group members have adequate prior knowledge of the course themes, enabling us to address the content in a versatile manner.	73,2
S5	The digital learning environment enables flexible group work.	71,5
S12	My own motivation is an important prerequisite for the success of collaborative learning.	67,3
S2	The course material offers ingredients for versatile group discussion.	67,1
S4	Feedback from the teacher and the tutors promotes my learning.	62,7

Table 1 presents the percentages of students who agreed with statements concerning their perceptions of collaborative learning. Perceptions of group atmosphere, active participation, and the role of fellow students (Table 1; S7–S9) were strong, with agreement levels exceeding 85%. Students also expressed particularly strong confidence (over 90%) in their own study skills as a foundation for successful collaborative learning (Table 1; S13). In contrast, lower agreement was observed for statements addressing students' own motivation for collaborative learning, the motivating role of course materials, and the contribution of teachers' and tutors' feedback, all of which were endorsed by fewer than 70% of respondents (Table 1; S12, S2, and S4).

Figure 1 shows that collaboration and student self-efficacy remained consistently strong from 2021 to 2025. This is reflected in a sustained positive group atmosphere, experiences of equal participation in group work, and the perceived positive role of other students (Fig. 1; S7–S9), as well as the continued emphasis students placed on their own learning skills in collaborative contexts (Fig. 1; S13). However, perceptions of the role of fellow students (Fig. 1; S9) display a modest downward trend over the period. Student agreement across multiple statements shows a clear dip in 2023, followed by at least partial recovery in 2024–2025. Teachers' input and the digital learning environment were the most volatile dimensions, declining sharply in 2023 but also demonstrating the strongest rebound in the subsequent years, although levels remained below those observed in 2021 (Fig. 1; S3-S5).

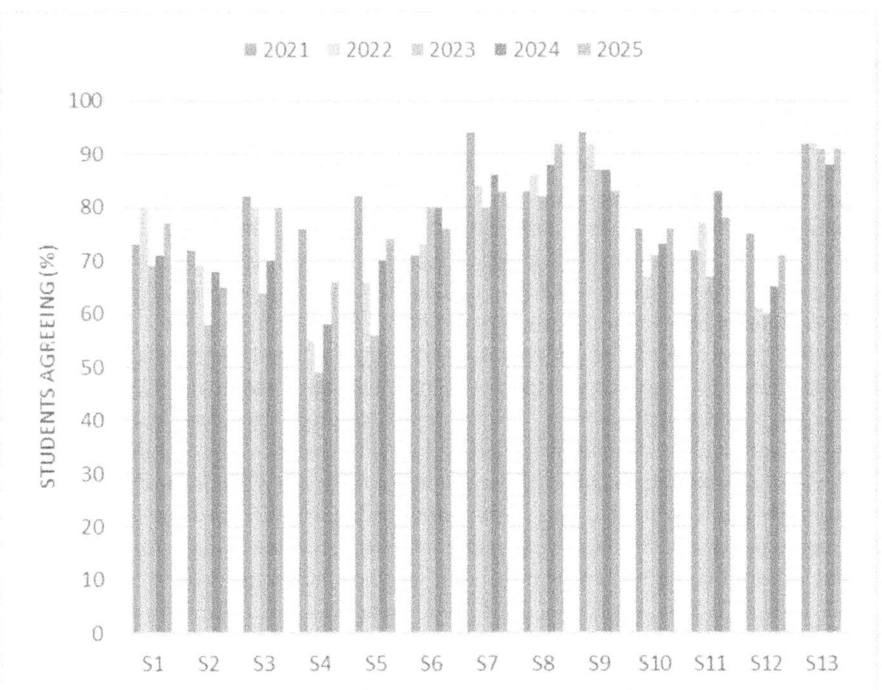

Fig. 1. Percentage of students agreeing with survey statements S1–S13 across survey years 2021–2025. S1–S13 correspond to survey statements listed in Table 1.

4 Discussion

To our knowledge, this is the first study to examine the provision of eHealth education for medical students aligned with nationally agreed competence areas [22] in a digital learning environment, with a specific focus on collaborative learning elements. Earlier research has addressed collaborative learning in digital contexts with medical students, but with different educational settings and aims. For example, a study published in 2011 applied collaborative learning in anatomy teaching using virtual reality [25], rather than integrating broader digital health competencies into medical training through a focused educational intervention.

It seems collaborative learning has been more extensively studied other health science education fields [19, 20, 26]. In the study by Männistö et al., nursing students participating in digital group learning reported higher satisfaction with aspects related to promoting collaborative work than those in control groups, while the teacher's role in the collaborative learning environment was evaluated less positively in the digital context [19]. The findings of our study with medical students are mostly consistent with these observations: high levels of agreement were observed for statements related to promoting collaborative group work (Table 1; S7–S9), whereas teacher feedback and support were rated lowest (Table 1; S4). This suggests that while digital environments may effectively support peer interaction and group processes, the pedagogical role of teachers and tutors in such settings may require further development.

Furthermore, our findings suggest that students' perceptions of their own learning skills play a key role in successful collaborative learning (Table 1: S13), consistent with prior research indicating that interaction among learners with diverse knowledge bases and perspectives enhances their communication and critical thinking skills [27]. In fully online collaborative environments, students' capacity for self-regulation and active engagement may be particularly important, as responsibility for learning is often shifted more strongly to the learner [28]. In addition to pedagogical design, emerging educational technologies can further support collaborative learning [29, 30]. For example, previous studies suggest that generative artificial intelligence can play a significant role in motivating students, enhancing collaborative writing processes, and fostering a positive collaborative learning atmosphere [31].

Although perceptions of collaborative learning remained largely stable across the five-year period, a notable dip in students' agreement was observed in 2023 (Fig. 1). This fluctuation suggests that students' collaborative learning experiences may be sensitive to contextual or implementation-related factors. For instance, the decline observed in 2023 may be partly attributable to the gradual lifting of COVID-19-related isolation measures, as the accumulated stress from the preceding period of strict restrictions could have contributed to more negative perceptions of fully online classes. Importantly, this decline does not appear to correspond with whether the groups were interdisciplinary (2022, 2023, 2025) or not (2021, 2024), indicating that other elements beyond group composition may have contributed. Further research is therefore needed to explore the underlying factors driving this temporary decrease and to identify conditions that support more consistent learning experiences.

5   Conclusions

Our results indicate that integrating collaborative learning with a digital learning environment offers a feasible and effective approach for delivering eHealth education within the medical curriculum. Students consistently reported positive experiences related to group dynamics, peer interaction, and the role of their own learning skills in supporting collaboration. In contrast, lower levels of agreement for items concerning teacher and tutor feedback, course materials, and students' motivation suggest that the pedagogical role of instructors, the clarity and design of materials, and strategies to sustain learner motivation require further development.

Given the rapidly evolving healthcare landscape, continuous refinement of teaching approaches and tools for digital health is essential. Systematic collection of student feedback and iterative course development will be important for maintaining both relevance and quality. Further research examining different models and practices for learning, investigating the factors that influence longitudinal trends in students' perceptions, and assessing the impact of digital approaches on learning outcomes would deepen understanding of how eHealth education can be most effectively integrated into undergraduate medical training.

Acknowledgments. The MEDigi project 2018-2021 and its implementation was supported by Finnish Ministry of Education and Culture (MEDigi OKM/270/523/2017). This work was supported by the University of Oulu and the Research Council of Finland, Profi6 336449.

Disclosure of Interests The employer of PV, PK, TT, TS and JR received support for salaries from the MEDigi project funded by Finnish Ministry of Education and Culture (MEDigi OKM/270/523/2017). The other authors declare no competing interests relevant to the content of this article.

References

1. Global Strategy on Digital Health 2020–2025. World Health Organization, Geneva (2021). https://www.who.int/publications/i/item/9789240020924
2. Car, J. et al.: The digital health competencies in medical education framework: an international consensus statement based on a Delphi study. JAMA Netw. Open. **8**, e2453131–e2453131 (2025). https://doi.org/10.1001/jamanetworkopen.2024.53131
3. Poncette, A.S., Glauert, D.L., Mosch, L., Braune, K., Balzer, F., Back, D.A.: Undergraduate medical competencies in digital health and curricular module development: mixed methods study. J. Med. Internet Res. **22** (2020). https://doi.org/10.2196/22161
4. Veikkolainen, P. et al.: eHealth competence building for future doctors and nurses – attitudes and capabilities. Int. J. Med. Inform. **169**, 104912 (2023). https://doi.org/10.1016/j.ijmedinf.2022.104912
5. Veikkolainen, P. et al.: The evolution of medical student competencies and attitudes in digital health between 2016 and 2022: comparative cross-sectional study. JMIR Med. Educ. **11**, e67423–e67423 (2025). https://doi.org/10.2196/67423
6. Vossen, K., Rethans, J.J., van Kuijk, S.M.J., van der Vleuten, C.P., Kubben, P.L.: Understanding medical students' attitudes toward learning eHealth: questionnaire study. JMIR Med. Educ. **6**, e17030 (2020). https://doi.org/10.2196/17030

7. Tumuhimbise, W. et al.: Opportunities and Challenges of Integrating Digital Health into Medical Education Curricula: a Scoping Review., https://www.researchsquare.com/article/rs-6254999/v1 (2025). https://doi.org/10.21203/rs.3.rs-6254999/v1

8. Ellaway, R., Masters, K.: AMEE guide 32: e-learning in medical education part 1: learning, teaching and assessment. Med. Teach. **30**, 455–473 (2008). https://doi.org/10.1080/01421590802108331

9. Ogundiya, O., Rahman, T.J., Valnarov-Boulter, I., Young, T.M.: Looking Back on digital medical education over the last 25 years and looking to the future: narrative review. J. Med. Internet Res. **26**, e60312 (2024). https://doi.org/10.2196/60312

10. Haleem, A., Javaid, M., Qadri, M.A., Suman, R.: Understanding the role of digital technologies in education: a review. Sustain. Oper. Comput. **3**, 275–285 (2022). https://doi.org/10.1016/j.susoc.2022.05.004

11. MacNeill, H., Masters, K., Nemethy, K., Correia, R.: Online learning in health professions education. Part 1: teaching and learning in online environments: AMEE guide no. 161. Med. Teach. **46**, 4–17 (2024). https://doi.org/10.1080/0142159X.2023.2197135

12. Pei, L., Wu, H.: Does online learning work better than offline learning in undergraduate medical education? A systematic review and meta-analysis. Med. Educ. Online. **24**, 1666538 (2019). https://doi.org/10.1080/10872981.2019.1666538

13. Vallée, A., Blacher, J., Cariou, A., Sorbets, E.: Blended learning compared to traditional learning in medical education: systematic review and meta-analysis. J. Med. Internet Res. **22**, e1f6504 (2020). https://doi.org/10.2196/16504

14. McGee, R.G., Wark, S., Mwangi, F., Drovandi, A., Alele, F., Malau-Aduli, B.S.: The Achieve Collaboration: Digital learning of clinical skills and its impact on medical students' academic performance: a systematic review. BMC Med. Educ. **24**, 1477 (2024). https://doi.org/10.1186/s12909-024-06471-2

15. Pramila-Savukoski, S. et al.: The influence of digital learning on health sciences students' competence development– a qualitative study. Nurse Educ. Today. **120**, 105635 (2023). https://doi.org/10.1016/j.nedt.2022.105635

16. Laal, M., Laal, M.: Collaborative learning: what is it? Procedia. Soc. Behav. Sci. **31**, 491–495 (2012). https://doi.org/10.1016/j.sbspro.2011.12.092

17. Shengqiang, L., Srikhao's, S., Nankhantee, A.: Combining inquiry-based learning and collaborative learning: a new model for improving students' teamwork and problem-solving skills. JoEED. **12**, 13–38 (2025). https://doi.org/10.22555/joeed.v12i1.1296

18. Luk, P., Tsang, J., Tsoi, H.-S., Chan, K., Chen, J.: Collaborative Online Learning in Undergraduate Medical Education: a Scoping Review., https://www.researchsquare.com/article/rs-28397/v2 (2020). https://doi.org/10.21203/rs.3.rs-28397/v2

19. Männistö, M. et al.: Effects of a digital educational intervention on collaborative learning in nursing education: a quasi-experimental study. Nord. J. Nurs. Res. **39**, 191–200 (2019). https://doi.org/10.1177/2057158519861041

20. Männistö, M., Mikkonen, K., Kuivila, H., Virtanen, M., Kyngäs, H., Kääriäinen, M.: Digital collaborative learning in nursing education: a systematic review. Scand. Caring Sci. **34**, 280–292 (2020). https://doi.org/10.1111/scs.12743

21. Levy, A., Reponen, J.: Digital Transformation of Medical Education. MEDigi Project Report. University of Oulu (2021) https://urn.fi/URN:ISBN:9789526232454

22. Tuovinen, T. et al.: Sähköisten terveyspalveluiden opetus lääketieteessä [Education of eHealth in Medicine]. Duodecim. **137**, 1807–1813 (2021) http://hdl.handle.net/10138/349511

23. Kautto, M., Koskela, T., Kulmala, P., Tuovinen, T., Reponen, J.: Digi- ja etälääketieteen osaaminen – tietoa, taitoa ja soveltavaa osaamista. Duodecim. **140**, 1984–9 (2024). https://www.duodecimlehti.fi/duo18552

24. Männistö, M.: Hoitotyön opiskelijoiden yhteisöllinen oppiminen ja sosiaali- ja terveysalan opettajien osaaminen digitaalisessa oppimisympäristössä [Collaborative learning of nursing students and social and health care educators' competence in a digital learning environment] (2020). https://urn.fi/URN:ISBN:9789526225081
25. Huang, H.-M.: A collaborative virtual learning system for medical education. In: The 3rd International Conference on Data Mining and Intelligent Information Technology Applications, pp. 127–130 (2011)
26. Pramila-Savukoski, S. et al.: Competence development in collaborative hybrid learning among health sciences students: a quasi-experimental mixed-method study. Comput. Assist. Learn. **39**, 1919–1938 (2023). https://doi.org/10.1111/jcal.12859
27. Irzawati, I.: The pros and cons of integrating Collaborative learning into lesson plan Desing. PRO. **4**, 1–11 (2023). https://doi.org/10.29303/prospek.v4i1.325
28. Sharma, K., Nguyen, A., Hong, Y.: Self-regulation and shared regulation in collaborative learning in adaptive digital learning environments: a systematic review of empirical studies. Br. J. Educ. Technol. **55**, 1398–1436 (2024). https://doi.org/10.1111/bjet.13459
29. Kuikka, P., Veikkolainen, P., Salmijärvi, T., Tuovinen, T., Kulmala, P., Reponen, J.: Initial experiences of electronic medical record simulation environment in eHealth education course for medical students in Finland. In: Särestöniemi, M., Keikhosrokiani, P., Singh, D., Harjula, E., Tiulpin, A., Jansson, M., Isomursu, M., Van Gils, M., Saarakkala, S., Reponen, J. (eds.) Digital Health and Wireless Solutions, pp. 169–180. Springer Nature, Switzerland, Cham (2024). https://doi.org/10.1007/978-3-031-59080-1_12
30. Borycki, Elizabeth M., Kushniruk Andre, W.: Educational electronic health Records at the University of Victoria: challenges, recommendations and lessons learned. In: Studies in Health Technology and Informatics. IOS Press (2019). https://doi.org/10.3233/SHTI190141
31. Gong, R., Jiang, R., Guo, C., Hu, W., Li, Y.: Roles emerging during the knowledge construction process in collaborative learning: does a generative AI-support chatbot matter? In: Proceedings of the 2024 16th International Conference on Education Technology and Computers, pp. 8–16. ACM, Porto Vlaams-Brabant Portugal (2024). https://doi.org/10.1145/3702163.3702165

Digital Competence of Filipino Nurses Working in Finland: A Cross-Sectional Study

Erika Jarva[1]([✉]) [iD], Floro Cubelo[2,3] [iD], and Elina Laukka[2,4] [iD]

[1] Faculty of Medicine, Research Unit of Health Sciences and Technology, University of Oulu, P.O. BOX 8000, 90014 Oulu, Finland
erika.jarva@oulu.fi
[2] School of Wellbeing and Culture, Oulu University of Applied Sciences, Oulu, Finland
[3] International Management and Affairs, The Filipino Nurses Association in the Nordic Region, Oulu, Finland
[4] Department of Public Health, Faculty of Medicine, University of Helsinki, P.O. BOX 00020, 00014 Helsinki, Finland

Abstract. The evolution of digital health services demands new types of competencies from nurses. Digital competence of nurses has been extensively discussed in research, particularly in relation to aging populations. However, other potentially vulnerable groups, such as foreign nurses, also require attention.

A cross-sectional survey was conducted to assess the digital competence of Filipino nurses working in Finland. The goal was to provide information on the current state of digital competence, potential skill gaps and associated factors to support the development of training and competence development methods.

According to the respondents' (n = 90) self-evaluation, ethical competence related to digital solutions was evaluated as the highest competence area (M = 3.55, SD = 0.63). Competence in utilizing and evaluating digital solutions received the lowest score in self-evaluation (M = 3.24, SD = 0.65). Work experience in healthcare and social welfare was associated with attitude towards using digital solutions at work. Respondents with master's degree evaluated their competence levels significantly lower compared to lower educational levels. Females evaluated human-centred remote counselling competence and ethical competence related to digital solutions higher compared to males.

Filipino nurses' self-evaluated digital competence reached high scores across the competence domains. However, individuals with higher education evaluated their competences significantly lower. This potentially indicates a lack of understanding of the contents of digital competence across the lower educated respondents as previous research has established a connection between higher digital competence and higher education. It is essential that Filipino nurses receive additional training on understanding what digital competence entails and increase their competence to utilize and evaluate digital solutions in the workplace.

Keywords: Digital competence · Foreign · Nurses · Survey · Telemedicine

© The Author(s) 2026
M. Särestöniemi et al. (Eds.): NCDHWS 2026, CCIS 3009, pp. 432–445, 2026.
https://doi.org/10.1007/978-3-032-28812-7_30

1 Introduction

The role of digital services and solutions has grown significantly in social and health-care, especially during and after the COVID-19 pandemic [1–3]. The importance of digital solutions is further emphasized by their potential cost-effectiveness during times of tight resources [4]. Digital services and solutions refer to the utilization of various information and communication technology solutions in social and healthcare products, services, and processes [5]. According to meta-analyses, services provided through digitalization generally produce equally effective services as those provided face-to-face [4]. Additionally, they often appear to be a more cost-effective option [1, 4, 6]. In the social and healthcare digitalization and information management strategy for 2023–2035, the development of digital competence and ensuring sufficient digitalization skills for both citizens and professionals are recognized as one of the cornerstones of successful digitalization [7]. In terms of citizens' digital competence and use of digital services, segmentation thinking has been utilized [8, 9], but this thinking model has been used less for social and healthcare professionals. For example, in citizens' digital competence, those with immigrant backgrounds have been identified as a vulnerable group in terms of digital competence [10], but research on the digital competence of this target group among social and healthcare professionals is lacking.

The proliferation of digital services and solutions in social and healthcare has transformed the service, technology, clinical, and substantive competencies, as well as the ethical skills of social and healthcare professionals. For example, technological competence requires mastery of information and communication technology, while clinical and substantive competencies emphasize digital skills to provide quality care. Additionally, professionals' attitudes, courage, and readiness for change are crucial in the adoption and development of digital services [11]. Digital competence, or digital skills, of professionals includes knowledge, skills, capabilities, and attitudes related to remote guidance, information technology management, identification, utilization, and evaluation of digital solutions and services, recognition of ethical perspectives, and attitudes towards the digitalization of work tasks and environments [12]. The promotion of professionals' digital competence is significantly influenced by psychosocial and organizational factors, such as changing healthcare practices, support from the organization and colleagues, regular training, and previous use of technology [13]. The future of social and healthcare services emphasizes the importance of digital service channels, and their development plays a central role in significantly increasing digital customer interactions. The use of digital services improves operational efficiency and offers opportunities to promote customer well-being and manage everyday matters. The shift towards a more digital service model affects the competency requirements of social and healthcare professionals, emphasizing interdisciplinary collaboration, remote communication, and the management of new technological solutions as part of customer work [14].

Research on digital competence has been conducted relatively extensively in various wellbeing services countries in Finland, but not specifically for nurses with immigrant backgrounds. Internationally, this research is also scarce although several countries are recruiting foreign nurses. According to some estimates, Finland will need a net immigration of 44,000 people with the current age and gender structure of migration to stabilize the size of birth and working-age cohorts [14] and maintain Finland's status as a welfare state. Finland also faces a significant shortage of social and healthcare resources, making nurses with immigrant backgrounds crucial for securing social and healthcare services. To address this shortage, Finland has been actively recruiting internationally educated nurses (IENs) from the Philippines [15].

Finland is one of the most digitalized countries in the world [16], and the basics of digitalization are introduced to residents from primary school onwards. Nurses with immigrant backgrounds may be in a very different position regarding their digital competence, even though basic skills in digitalization and informatics have been implemented more into higher education institutions since 2015 [17]. Language-related challenges can also affect nurses' work, for example, in documentation [18]. To provide adequate and needs-based training and support to nurses and nursing students with immigrant backgrounds, it is necessary to assess their digital competence levels and identify aspects that are associated with their digital competence. Adequate training can also ensure safe and effective care.

The study consists of a cross-sectional survey aimed at assessing the digital competence of Filipino nurses working in Finland. The goal is to provide information on the current state of digital competence and skill gaps to support the development of training and competence development methods. The research questions are:

1. What is the self-assessed digital competence of Filipino nurses?
2. What factors are associated with the digital competence of Filipino nurses?

2 Materials and Methods

2.1 Population

The data for the study was collected from the registry of Filipino nurses under the Filipino Nurses Association in the Nordic Region, which included 206 members. Registry members were also instructed to forward the survey to individuals who are not members of the organization. A survey was sent to the nurses in the network through one author. The response period for the survey was between June 1, 2025, and October 15, 2025.

The data was collected using the email list of the non-profit organization for Filipino nurses who had listed themselves in the organization's data registry under the Webropol survey platform. Reminders have been systematically disseminated on a weekly basis, preceding the initiation of the online survey.

Filipino nurses have been selected as the target group for this study because Finland has been actively recruiting internationally educated nurses from outside the European Union/European Economic Area (EU/EEA), with a particular focus on nurses from the Philippines [19]. However, the digital competencies have not been explored, despite their status as a requisite component within the Finnish healthcare system.

2.2 Data Collection

Validated instruments measuring digital competence (DigiHealthCom) and factors influencing digital competence (DigiComInf) [12] were used for data collection. The DigiHealthCom instrument consisted of five dimensions: human-centred remote counselling competence (16 items), digital solutions as part of work (9 items), information and communication technology (ICT) competence (5 items), competence in utilizing and evaluating digital solutions (8 items) and ethical competence related to digital solutions (4 items). DigiComInf consists of three dimensions (15 items): support from management (6 items), organizational practices as part of digital competence development (4 items) and colleagues' adoption and influence (5 items). According to Jarva et al. [12], the psychometric properties of the instruments demonstrated high reliability and validity, with Cronbach's alpha coefficients ranging between 0.91–0.97 for DigiHealthCom and 0.74–0.88 for DigiComInf.

Background questions were used to gather information on respondents' age, gender, previous degrees and education level, length of residence in Finland, work experience in social/health services, continuing education related to digitalization, experience working with digital services, and methods preferred to develop digital competence.

Digital competence and its influencing factors were assessed using a 4-point Likert scale (1 = Strongly disagree, 2 = Somewhat disagree, 3 = Somewhat agree, 4 = Strongly agree). In the beginning of the survey, the respondent could choose whether to answer to the survey in Filipino, English or Finnish as the instruments have been validated in all three languages.

2.3 Analysis

The data of this cross-sectional study was analyzed using statistical methods with IBM SPSS Statistics 29 for Windows. Statements and composite variables from the instruments were examined using descriptive statistics such as measures of central tendency and dispersion, as well as percentage and frequency distributions. DigiHealthCom and DigiComInf factors were transformed as sum-variables and dependence between the background variables were analysed by using One-way ANOVA, Chi square and Mann-Whitney U tests. The DigiHealthCom sum-variables were converted as dichotomous to divide the sample into lower (1–2.49) and higher (2.5–4) competence categories. There were no missing values in the data.

2.4 Ethical Considerations

The study adhered to the guidelines for responsible conduct of research issued by the Finnish National Board on Research Integrity [20]. In addition, the ethical principles outlined in the Declaration of Helsinki [21] for medical research involving human subjects were followed. According to the Finnish National Board on Research Integrity [20], an application for ethical approval was not required, as the study did not involve minors and posed no direct or indirect psychological or physical harm to the participants [22].

The research data was collected from a network of Filipino nurses, which did not have the administrative structures required to grant a formal research permit. Participation in the study was voluntary, and by responding to the survey, participants gave their informed consent to take part in the research. Responses were provided in a pseudonymized format, meaning that individual respondents could not be identified from their answers.

3 Results

3.1 Respondent Characteristics

A total of 90 Filipino nurses answered to the survey (Table 1), yielding a response rate of 43,7%. Majority of the respondents were female (72,2%) with a college/bachelor's degree from a University of Applied Sciences as the highest degree (47,8%). The respondents' age range was from 28 to 57 years (mean 37 years) and the median length of residence in Finland was 3 years (IQR 3 years) and the median experience in healthcare and social services was 4 years (IQR 9 years). Over half of the respondents (51,1%) use digital remote working tools daily and have participated in training organized by the workplace to develop digital competence (53,3%). One third of the respondents (32,2%) have not participated in any developmental activities related to digital solutions.

Table 1. Characteristics of the respondents.

Characteristics	Respondents (n = 90)
Gender	
Female	65 (72,2%)
Male	21 (23,3%)
Rather not say	4 (4,4%)
Age	
Mean	37
Min - Max	28–57
SD	4.3
Education level (highest degree)	
Vocational qualification	13 (14,4%)
College degree / Bachelor's degree (University of Applied Sciences)	43 (47,8%)
Bachelor's degree (University)	31 (34,4%)
Master's degree (University of Applied Sciences or University)	3 (3,3%)
Length of residence in Finland (in years)	
Median	3
IQR	3
Work experience in social/health services (in years)	
Median	4
IQR	9
Use of working hours in clinical work with digital remote working tools	
Daily	46 (51,1%)
Weekly	5 (5,6%)
Monthly	3 (3,3%)

(continued)

Table 1. (*continued*)

Characteristics	Respondents (n = 90)
Rarely	10 (11,1%)
None	26 (28,9%)
Experience working with digital services	
I have participated in the development of digital solutions (e.g., digital care pathways, digital services)	21 (23,3%)
I have participated in training organized by my workplace to develop my digital competence	48 (53,3%)
I have developed my digital competence independently (e.g., online courses/lectures, not organized by my workplace)	29 (32,2%)
Worked as a trainer (related to digital competence or digitalization in the social and health care sector)	5 (5,6%)
I have not participated in any of the above	29 (32,2%)

3.2 Filipino Nurses' Digital Competence and Factors Associated with Digital Competence

The mean value of Filipino nurses' digital competence only slightly varied across the DigiHealthCom and DigiComInf domains (Table 2). Ethical competence related to digital solutions was evaluated as the highest among the respondents (mean 3.55, SD 0.63). Competence in utilizing and evaluating digital solutions received the lowest score (mean 3.24, SD 0.65). In DigiComInf, all domains had nearly the same mean values, ranging from 3.16 (SD 0.79) in support from management to 3.18 (SD 0.72) in colleagues' adoption and influence.

Table 2. Filipino nurses' self-evaluated digital competence and aspects associated with digital competence.

DigiHealthCom dimension	M	SD
Human-centred remote counselling competence (Counselling)	3.26	0.63
Digital solutions as part of work (Attitude)	3.31	0.65
ICT competence (ICT)	3.42	0.63
Competence in utilizing and evaluating digital solutions (Evaluation)	3.24	0.65
Ethical competence related to digital solutions (Ethics)	3.55	0.63
DigiComInf dimension	**M**	**SD**
Support from management (Management)	3.16	0.79
Organizational practices (Organization)	3.17	0.78
Colleagues' adoption and influence (Collegiality)	3.18	0.72

(*continued*)

Table 2. (*continued*)

DigiHealthCom dimension	M	SD
M = Mean, SD = Standard Deviation		

When analysing the background factors and the aspects associated with digital competence, highest education, managerial, organizational and collegial factors were found to be statistically significantly associated with self-evaluated digital competence (Table 3). In addition, work experience in healthcare and social welfare was associated with attitude towards using digital solutions at work.

Table 3. Factors associated with digital competence domains.

	Counselling (low = 7, high = 83)		Attitude (low = 8, high = 82)		ICT (low = 5, high = 85)		Evaluation (low = 7, high = 83)		Ethics (low = 4, high = 86)	
	$F/X^2/Z$	p	$F/X^2/Z$	p	$F/X^2/Z$	p	$F/X^2/Z$	p	$F/X^2/Z$	p
Age[a]	2.672	0.106	0.114	0.737	0.251	0.618	0.012	0.913	0.351	0.555
Gender[b]	4.430	0.074	3.148	0.202	3.645	0.196	4.194	0.109	5.309	0.068
Highest education[b]	11.578	**0.015**	11.166	**0.017**	13.203	**0.006**	11.578	**0.015**	15.227	**0.002**
Work experience[c]	−1.783	0.075	−2.216	**0.027**	−1.568	0.117	−0.831	0.406	−1.713	0.087
Years in Finland[c]	−1.398	0.162	−1.359	0.174	−1.044	0.296	−1.801	0.072	−0.807	0.420
Use of remote digital tools[b]	3.624	0.385	3.323	0.442	2.427	0.625	1.327	0.869	1.742	0.846
Management[c]	−3.274	**.001**	−4.324	**<.001**	−3.686	**<.001**	−3.900	**<.001**	−3.244	**.001**
Organization[c]	−3.515	**<.001**	−4.265	**<.001**	−3.758	**<.001**	−3.985	**<.001**	−3.305	**<.001**
Collegiality[c]	−3.963	**<.001**	−4.244	**<.001**	−3.797	**<.001**	−4.032	**<.001**	−3.350	**<.001**

Note. Statistically significant (p < 0.05) mean differences are marked in bold

[a]One-way ANOVA F test
[b]Chi-square and Fisher exact test (X^2)
[c]Mann-Whitney U test (Z)

Respondents with a master's degree evaluated their competence as statistically significantly lower compared to lower educational levels across all digital competence domains (Tables 4 and 5). When considering the evaluation of the managerial, organizational and collegial factors, respondents who perceived lower support from management, organizational practices and colleagues, evaluated their digital competence statistically significantly lower across all domains. In addition, females evaluated their competence in remote counselling and ethics statistically significantly higher compared to males and individual who didn't want to disclose their gender.

Table 4. Analysis of variance: counselling, attitude and ICT.

Measure	Counselling			Attitude			ICT		
	M	SD	p	M	SD	p	M	SD	p
Work experience			.911			.264			.474
<10 years	3.26	0.71		3.25	0.73		3.38	0.72	
≥10 years	3.27	0.49		3.41	0.48		3.48	0.45	
Gender			.003			.464			.147
Female	3.40	0.52		3.35	0.52		3.49	0.49	
Male	2.91	0.84		3.16	0.97		3.18	0.94	
Rather not say	2.85	0.33		3.44	0.45		3.50	0.60	
Highest education			<.001			<.001			<.001
Vocational qualification	3.48	0.44		3.46	0.49		3.56	0.48	
College degree	3.25	0.57		3.29	0.60		3.39	0.56	
Bachelor's degree	3.34	0.54		3.41	0.51		3.53	0.49	
Master's degree	1.70	1.22		1.85	1.47		1.93	1.61	
DigiComInf - Management			<.001			<.001			<.001
Low	2.41	0.74		2.55	0.98		2.60	0.91	
High	3.42	0.47		3.45	0.45		3.57	0.43	
DigiComInf – Organization			<.001			<.001			<.001
Low	2.45	0.73		2.46	0.86		2.61	0.89	
High	3.42	0.47		3.48	0.44		3.58	0.42	
DigiComInf - Collegiality			<.001			<.001			<.001
Low	2.34	0.79		2.33	0.87		2.48	0.92	
High	3.40	0.48		3.46	0.45		3.56	0.43	

Table 5. Analysis of variance: evaluation and ethics.

Measure	Evaluation			Ethics		
	M	SD	p	M	SD	p
Work experience			.863			.895

(continued)

Table 5. (*continued*)

Measure	Evaluation			Ethics		
	M	SD	*p*	M	SD	*p*
<10 years	3.23	0.73		3.56	0.70	
≥10 years	3.26	0.48		3.54	0.50	
Gender			.125			.027
Female	3.33	0.55		3.64	0.48	
Male	3.00	0.86		3.23	0.94	
Rather not say	3.12	0.42		3.81	0.37	
Highest education			<.001			<.001
Vocational qualification	3.50	0.46		3.78	0.36	
College degree	3.25	0.53		3.50	0.58	
Bachelor's degree	3.26	0.61		3.70	0.43	
Master's degree	1.83	1.44		1.75	1.29	
DigiComInf - Management			<.001			<.001
Low	2.29	0.82		2.91	1.08	
High	3.42	0.42		3.67	0.43	
DigiComInf - Organization			<.001			<.001
Low	2.38	0.87		2.88	1.03	
High	3.41	0.42		3.69	0.41	
DigiComInf - Collegiality			<.001			<.001
Low	2.17	0.84		2.77	1.10	
High	3.41	0.41		3.67	0.42	

4   Discussion

This paper aims to provide insights into the current state of digital competence, potential skill gaps and associated factors to support the development of continuous education, training and other competence-building methods for Filipino nurses working in Finland. Our findings revealed that ethical competence related to digital solutions was rated highest among respondents, whereas competence in utilizing and evaluating digital solutions received the lowest scores in self-assessment. However, all competence areas were evaluated strikingly high compared to earlier research.

Compared to an earlier study by Jarva et al. [23] conducted with nurses working in Finland, the results of this study suggest that Filippino nurses' overall digital competence would be comparable to high competence profile. However, the responses of Filipino nurses differ from those of nursing staff more generally. Filipino nurses evaluated their ethical competence as the strongest area, which bridges similar results to Finnish nurses according to Kinnunen et al. [24]. In other studies, nurses have typically assessed ICT competence as the strongest digital competence domain [23, 25, 26]. In addition, Filipino nurses rated their human-centered remote counselling competence at a high level, while aspects within this domain, such as work in the digital healthcare environment and digital patient counselling, have been previously evaluated as the weakest among nursing and other healthcare professionals in Finland [23, 24]. Notably, approximately 50% of the respondents in this study reported daily use of digital remote tools which might explain the higher competence evaluation in digital patient counselling.

Similarities between the results from this study and a recent international digital competence survey to healthcare professionals (majority associate and registered nurses) [25] can be identified in the competence evaluation in the utilisation and evaluation of digital solutions domain. The results from both studies reveal that nurses' competence to recognize the potential of digital solutions in patient care has been widely experienced as insufficient. Cultural differences in the use of digital services may partly explain these findings, as previous studies have shown that culture strongly shapes access, adoption and user engagement in digital health services [27, 28].

Overall, Filipino nurses appear to be more satisfied with support from management, organizational practices, and the adoption and influence of colleagues compared to nurses in Finland in general [23]. Additionally, among Filipino nurses, management support, organizational practices, and colleagues' adoption and influence were systematically significant predictors across all domains of digital competence. In contrast, among nurses in general, colleagues tend to be prioritized as the primary influencing factor, whereas the roles of management and organizational structures are typically evaluated as less influential [25, 26]. One potential explanation for these differences may be cultural factors, as previous research has shown that cultural norms strongly influence how digital health support, leadership, and collegial structures are perceived and utilized in healthcare settings [27]. The findings of the study were not entirely unanticipated, considering the cultural conception of Filipino nurses as exemplifying qualities such as compassion, care, reliability, and a sense of professional ethics [29].

While further efforts are required in Finland and other countries, nursing pro-grams are designed to incorporate components on the use of digital services [17, 30]. Our findings support previous understanding that the ability to utilize and critically evaluate digital solutions should be emphasized more strongly within nursing education. Furthermore, comprehensive continuous training on the use of digital solutions in healthcare should also be provided to nurses already working in health and social care services to ensure continuous competence development [17].

In the future, Filipino nurses' digital competence could be explored through qualitative methods such as interviews to gain a deeper understanding of their experiences and development of digital competence, especially from the perspective of understanding the scope and breadth of digital competence. Furthermore, research should also focus on the digital competence and related needs of both Filipino, and other immigrant nurses as well as international nursing students to improve educational practices and build sustainable and inclusive digital competence training.

4.1 Study Strenghts and Limitations

A relatively high response rate was achieved as 43.7% (99/206) of the survey receivers answered the questionnaire. The study used validated instruments, which have been previously used in both national [23, 26] and international settings [25]. However, self-evaluated competence presents subjectivity which may result in either overestimation or underestimation of competence or differing interpretations of the items due to cultural viewpoints. In addition, the study may include self-selection bias as individuals more interested in the topic might have been more prone to respond. Moreover, only three respondents in this study held a master's degree and therefore, the influence of higher education degree in this population cannot be generalized according to the results of this study and the topic needs more investigation to address the needs of healthcare workers with an immigrant background.

Filipino nurses in Finland exhibit a distinctive migratory pattern. A significant proportion of these nurses are recruited as nursing assistants within the framework of practical nursing apprenticeship programs. Subsequently, they elect to pursue the registered nurse pathway. Therefore, within this context, the term "nurse" encompasses nursing assistants, licensed practical nurses, and registered nurses. Due to the heterogeneity of the group and the similarity of their migratory patterns [15], it was deemed appropriate to categorize the nurses as a single group to obtain a comprehensive overview of their digital competencies within the Finnish context. Therefore, it is imperative to exercise caution when generalizing the results of this study to other healthcare settings. Further research is necessary to comprehend the actual and in-depth experiences of Filipino nurses regarding orientation, education, and training to enhance digital competencies.

5 Conclusions

The recruitment of foreign nurses will continue in Finland to address the rising care needs of the aging population. An essential competency that must be evaluated is digital competence and its alignment with the host country.

It is essential that Filipino nurses receive additional training on basic knowledge of healthcare digitalization and the know-how of utilizing and evaluating digital solutions in the workplace, as this competence is a fundamental component of their daily work tasks.

Nurse leaders, work communities and peer workers should prioritize enhancing their readiness to assist newly recruited nurses with an immigrant background in acclimatizing to a workplace where digital technology is integral to their duties and responsibilities. This readiness should ensure that ethical principles and organizational guidelines are adhered to, in accordance with established protocols.

Acknowledgments. We would like to thank all the study participants for answering the survey.

Disclosure of Interests. None.

References

1. Härkönen, H., Lakoma, S., Verho, A., Torkki, P., Leskelä, R.L., Pennanen, P., et al.: Impact of digital services on healthcare and social welfare: an umbrella review. Int. J. Nurs. Stud. **152**, 104692 (2024). https://doi.org/10.1016/j.ijnurstu.2024.104692
2. Ndayishimiye, C., Lopes, H., Middleton, J.: A systematic scoping review of digital health technologies during COVID-19: a new normal in primary health care delivery. Health Technol. (Berl). **13**(2), 273–284 (2023). https://doi.org/10.1007/s12553-023-00725-7
3. Rosenlund, M., Kinnunen, U.M., Saranto, K.: The use of digital health services among patients and citizens living at home: scoping review. J. Med. Internet Res. **25**, e44711 (2023). https://doi.org/10.2196/44711
4. Laukka, E., Jansson, M., Suonnansalo, P., Ojanperä, R., Härkönen, H., Lakoma, S., et al.: Impact of interactive digital health services on outcomes in non-communicable diseases: an umbrella review and evidence synthesis from 17 meta-analyses. Int. J. Nurs. Stud. **147**, 105277 (2026). https://doi.org/10.1016/j.ijnurstu.2025.105277
5. Chidambaram, S., Jain, B., Jain, U., Mwavu, R., Baru, R., Thomas, B., et al.: An introduction to digital determinants of health. PLOS Digit Health. **3**(1), e0000346 (2024). https://doi.org/10.1371/journal.pdig.0000346
6. Laukka, E., Härkönen, H., Lakoma, S., Jansson, M., Torkki, P.: Outcomes and economic effects of digital health services: an umbrella review. Value Health **27**(12) (2024)
7. Ministry of Social Affairs and Health. Strategy for digitalization and information management in healthcare and social welfare. Helsinki: Ministry of Social Affairs and Health; 2024. Publications of the Ministry of Social Affairs and Health; 2024:1. Available from: https://urn.fi/URN:ISBN:978-952-00-5404-5
8. Rantanen, T., Juujärvi, S., Silvennoinen, P., Järveläinen, E.: Haavoittuvassa asemassa olevien ryhmien digitaalinen syrjäytyminen sosiaali- ja terveysalan osaamisen haasteena. Ammattikasvatuksen Aikakauskirja. **25**(3), 50–69 (2023)
9. Virtanen, L., Kaihlanen, A., Kouvonen, A., Safarov, N., Laukka, E., Valkonen, P. et al.: Hyvinvointiyhteiskunnan digitaaliset palvelut yhdenvertaisiksi–9 kriittistä toimenpidettä haavoittuvassa asemassa olevien huomioimiseksi. Helsinki: Valtioneuvosto; 2022. Päätöksen tueksi; 1/2022. Available from: https://urn.fi/URN:ISBN:978-952-343-811-8
10. Ghorbanian Zolbin, M., Kujala, S., Huvila, I.: Experiences and expectations of immigrant and nonimmigrant older adults regarding eHealth services: qualitative interview study. J. Med. Internet Res. **27**, e64249 (2025). https://doi.org/10.2196/64249
11. Pennanen, P., Jansson, M., Torkki, P., Harjumaa, M., Pajari, I., Laukka, E. et al.: Digitaalisten palvelujen vaikutukset sosiaali- ja terveydenhuollossa. Helsinki: Valtioneuvosto; 2023. Valtioneuvoston selvitys- ja tutkimustoiminnan julkaisusarja 52 (2023). [in Finnish]. Available from: https://julkaisut.valtioneuvosto.fi/handle/10024/165147
12. Jarva, E., Oikarinen, A., Andersson, J., Tomietto, M., Kääriäinen, M., Mikkonen, K.: Healthcare professionals' digital health competence and its core factors: development and psychometric testing of two instruments. Int. J. Med. Inform. **171**, 104995 (2023). https://doi.org/10.1016/j.ijmedinf.2023.104995
13. Konttila, J., Siira, H., Kyngäs, H., Lahtinen, M., Elo, S., Kääriäinen, M., et al.: Healthcare professionals' competence in digitalisation: a systematic review. J. Clin. Nurs. **28**(5–6), 745–761 (2019). https://doi.org/10.1111/jocn.14710
14. Ministry of Social Affairs and Health. Competence required for the integration of healthcare and social welfare. Helsinki: Ministry of Social Affairs and Health; 2024. Reports and Memorandums of the Ministry of Social Affairs and Health; 2024:2. Available from: https://urn.fi/URN:ISBN:978-952-00-5412-0

15. Cubelo, F.: Building pathways for Filipino internationally educated nurses' mobility to the Nordic region: recruit, integrate, retain and sustain. Kuopio: University of Eastern Finland (2025). Available from: https://urn.fi/URN:ISBN:978-952-61-5601-9
16. Government of Finland. Government report: Digital Compass. Helsinki: Publications of the Finnish Government (2022). Available from: https://urn.fi/URN:ISBN:978-952-383-609-9
17. Kaihlanen, A.M., Gluschkoff, K., Kinnunen, U.M., Saranto, K., Ahonen, O., Heponiemi, T.: Nursing informatics competences of Finnish registered nurses after national educational initiatives: a cross-sectional study. Nurse Educ. Today **106**, 105060 (2021). https://doi.org/10.1016/j.nedt.2021.105060
18. Joensuu, R., Suleiman, K., Koskenranta, M., Kuivila, H., Oikarinen, A., Juntunen, J., et al.: Factors associated with the integration of culturally and linguistically diverse nurses into healthcare organizations: a systematic review of qualitative studies. J. Nurs. Manag. (2024). https://doi.org/10.1155/2024/5887450
19. Cubelo, F., Turunen, H., Jokiniemi, K.: Recruit, integrate, and retain: internationally educated nurses' mobility to the Nordic region: a two-round policy Delphi study. Nurs. Outlook **72**(6), 102299 (2024). https://doi.org/10.1016/j.outlook.2024.102299
20. Finnish National Board on Research Integrity TENK. The Finnish Code of Conduct for Research Integrity and procedures for handling alleged violations of research integrity in Finland. Helsinki: TENK; 2023. Publications of TENK; 4/2023. Available from: https://tenk.fi
21. World Medical Association. Declaration of Helsinki: ethical principles for medical research involving human subjects. 2013. Available from: https://www.wma.net/policies-post/wma-declaration-of-helsinki/
22. Medical Research Act (488/1999). Finland. Available from: https://finlex.fi
23. Jarva, E., Oikarinen, A., Andersson, J., Pramila-Savukoski, S., Hammarén, M., Mikkonen, K.: Healthcare professionals' digital health competence profiles and associated factors: a cross-sectional study. J. Adv. Nurs. **80**(8), 3226–3252 (2024). https://doi.org/10.1111/jan.16096
24. Kinnunen, U.M., Kuusisto, A., Koponen, S., Ahonen, O., Kaihlanen, A.M., Hassinen, T., et al.: Nurses' informatics competency assessment of health information system usage: a cross-sectional survey. Comput. Inform. Nurs. **41**(11), 869–876 (2023). https://doi.org/10.1097/CIN.0000000000001026
25. Mikkonen, K., Tomietto, M., Lee, J.J., Ye, F., Mandysova, P., Pekara, J. et al.: Digital health competence among healthcare professionals: a cross-sectional cluster analysis across 19 countries and regions. Int. J. Nurs. Stud., 105348 (2026). https://doi.org/10.1016/j.ijnurstu.2026.105348
26. Ylönen, M., Forsman, P., Karvo, T., Jarva, E., Antikainen, T., Kulmala, P., et al.: Social services and healthcare personnel's digital competence profiles: a Finnish cross-sectional study. Int. J. Med. Inform. **193**, 105658 (2025). https://doi.org/10.1016/j.ijmedinf.2024.105658
27. Nittas, V., Daniore, P., Chavez, S.J., Wray, T.B.: Challenges in implementing cultural adaptations of digital health interventions. Commun. Med. **4**, 7 (2024). https://doi.org/10.1038/s43856-023-00426-2
28. Zhou, S., Shen, M., Tao, X., Han, S.: Cultural adaptation of digital healthcare tools: a cross-sectional survey of caregivers and patients. Glob Health Res. Policy. **10**, 36 (2025). https://doi.org/10.1186/s41256-025-00439-5
29. Salinda, M.T.: Development of a cross-cultural competence healthcare model for Filipino nurses. Asian J. Res. Nurs. Health. **8**(1), 165–175 (2025). https://doi.org/10.9734/ajrnh/2025/v8i1193
30. Finnish Nurses Association. Finnish Nurses Association digital social and health services strategy. Helsinki: Finnish Nurses Association; 2021. Available from: https://sairaanhoitajat.fi

Exploring Digital Health Concepts
Through Hands-On Education
in Biomedical Engineering

Christian Schuss[1(✉)] (iD), Atte Koskela[1], Anuradha Athukorala[1],
Tapio Seppänen[2] (iD), and Tapio Fabritius[1] (iD)

[1] Optoelectronics and Measurement Techniques (OPEM) Research Group, University
of Oulu, 90014 Oulu, Finland
`christian.schuss@oulu.fi`
[2] Center for Machine Vision and Signal Analysis (CMVS) Research Group,
University of Oulu, 90014 Oulu, Finland

Abstract. This paper presents insights and experiences from *Wireless Measurements Project* (course code 521168S), a course delivered at the University of Oulu, Finland. As a compulsory element of the newly established master's programme in Biomedical Engineering within the Faculty of Information Technology and Electrical Engineering (ITEE), the course introduces students to practical wireless measurement techniques through a hands-on, project-based methodology. At the beginning of the course, students receive an Internet of Medical Things (IoMT) starter kit comprising an ESP8266 microcontroller, an analog heart-rate sensor, and basic electronic components. Using this kit as a foundation, they design and implement their own IoMT prototypes, addressing themes such as physiological monitoring, wireless data transmission, embedded signal processing, and cloud-based health applications. In this paper, we describe the pedagogical design of the course, present representative student projects, and examine the challenges and opportunities of integrating wireless biomedical measurements into engineering education.

Keywords: Internet of Medical Things (IoMT) · Wireless Measurements · Engineering Education

1   Introduction

Digital health technologies have expanded rapidly in recent years, driven by advances in connectivity, sensing, wireless communication, and data analytics. Despite fluctuations in funding, innovation in digital health remains strong, with new tools for diagnosis, treatment, and remote monitoring entering an increasingly mature global marketplace. Within this evolving landscape, the Internet of Medical Things (IoMT) has emerged as a key enabler of remote and continuous healthcare delivery. Recent literature highlights the rapid expansion of IoMT

M. Särestöniemi et al. (Eds.): NCDHWS 2026, CCIS 3009, pp. 446–461, 2026.
https://doi.org/10.1007/978-3-032-28812-7_31

technologies, supported by improvements in embedded sensing, wireless communication, and the growing demand for remote healthcare solutions [1–3]. This sustained growth underscores the need for biomedical engineers who understand wireless sensing, real-time embedded systems, and data-driven health technologies, as these competencies form the foundation of modern digital health solutions.

Despite the rapid growth of digital health technologies, biomedical engineering (BME) education continues to face challenges in preparing students for practical work with wireless sensing and embedded systems. Recent work has demonstrated that structured, hands-on device activities can substantially enhance student learning and confidence, underscoring the limitations of purely lecture-based instruction [4]. At the same time, embedded-systems education in BME programmes often suffers from large disparities in students' prior experience, making it difficult to ensure consistent skill development across diverse cohorts [5]. These issues are particularly pronounced in internationally diverse programmes, where students arrive with varying backgrounds in electronics, programming, and data analysis. As a result, many students struggle to engage with more advanced IoMT project work, especially when they have limited exposure to laboratory environments or lack confidence in using measurement equipment. Together, these findings highlight the need for inclusive, flexible, and practice-oriented learning approaches that better support students in acquiring the foundational skills required for modern digital health engineering.

To address these challenges, this paper examines a project-based course designed to introduce biomedical engineering students to practical wireless measurement concepts within the broader IoMT landscape. The study outlines the pedagogical rationale, describes the multimodal learning ecosystem supporting the course, and presents representative student projects that illustrate learning outcomes and common challenges. Through this work, we contribute insights into scalable and adaptable approaches for integrating hands-on IoMT education into biomedical engineering curricula.

Similar observations have been made in embedded-systems education, where heterogeneous student preparation complicates skill development and highlights the need for practice-oriented instructional approaches [5]. The pedagogical design of the course is further supported by evidence showing that project-based learning effectively enhances engagement and practical skill acquisition in eHealth and biomedical engineering domains [6]. Likewise, experiential and transdisciplinary approaches have been shown to improve students' ability to apply theoretical concepts to authentic engineering tasks [8]. Finally, hands-on design experiences are known to strengthen student self-efficacy, autonomy, and confidence when working with real-world biomedical technologies [9]. Together, these insights reinforce the value of a practice-oriented, iterative, and inclusive learning environment for supporting heterogeneous student cohorts.

A key element of the course design is the provision of an IoMT starter kit to every student, consisting of a low-cost microcontroller, an analog heart-rate sensor, and a set of basic electronic components. This ensures that all participants begin with a common foundation for exploring wireless biomedical measurement, regardless of their prior technical background [4,5]. Based on their chosen project ideas, students can request and integrate additional materials, allowing them to tailor their prototypes to specific application needs. This structure mirrors real-world IoMT development workflows, where engineers iteratively expand system capabilities in response to design requirements [7]. By working directly with hardware, students learn to acquire, process, and transmit physiological signals while gaining practical insight into the constraints, trade-offs, and design decisions that shape modern digital health solutions. The modularity of the kits supports experimentation and progressive refinement, enabling students to advance from basic signal acquisition to more sophisticated applications at their own pace. Such hands-on, project-based engagement has been shown to enhance technical competence, foster creativity, and strengthen students' confidence in applying engineering concepts to authentic biomedical challenges [6,8,9].

In addition to the physical IoMT starter kits, the course integrates a suite of virtual and AI (artificial intelligence)-enhanced learning environments that support flexible, inclusive, and self-paced study. Moodle serves as the central hub, providing structured access to course materials, simulation tools, and interactive tutorials. Cloud-based and browser-based simulation platforms enable students to prototype and test embedded systems without requiring immediate access to hardware, reducing barriers for learners who are new to electronics or who study remotely. The value of such virtual laboratory environments in engineering education is well documented, with systematic reviews highlighting their role in improving accessibility, supporting experimentation, and preparing students for hands-on work [10–12]. AI tools, including Microsoft Copilot, further assist students by offering guidance, explanations, and examples during programming and system design tasks, reflecting broader findings on the pedagogical potential of large language models in higher education [13]. Complementing these resources, the virtual Super FabLab Oulu provides an immersive environment in which students can explore laboratory equipment, safety protocols, and standard workflows before engaging with the physical facilities. Together, these digital tools create a rich, multimodal ecosystem that enhances accessibility, supports diverse learning preferences, and strengthens students' readiness for hands-on biomedical engineering work.

This paper presents the design, implementation, and evaluation of a student-driven course that integrates IoMT starter kits, virtual laboratory environments, and AI-enhanced learning tools to support hands-on biomedical engineering education. We describe the pedagogical rationale behind the course structure, outline the multimodal learning ecosystem that enables flexible participation, and illustrate how students engage with the complete IoMT workflow from sensor acquisition to wireless data transmission. In addition, we report observations on student learning experiences and highlight the benefits and challenges associated with combining physical prototyping, simulation platforms, and virtual laboratory exploration. By sharing these insights, the paper contributes a scalable and transferable model for teaching practical digital health competencies in higher education.

2   Course Design and Pedagogical Framework

2.1   Educational Context and Course Design

The course is offered in the first year of the Biomedical Engineering master's programme at the University of Oulu. Because many international students enter the programme after completing their bachelor's studies at universities around the world, the cohort brings a diverse range of prior knowledge in electronics, programming, and mathematical foundations. In contrast, most students have limited prior exposure to healthcare systems, clinical workflows, or user requirements in medical contexts. As a result, the course places emphasis on identifying intended use cases, clarifying user needs, and understanding basic principles of safety and reliability when designing measurement solutions.

Although the course does not include formal clinical placements, students are encouraged to select project topics inspired by real-world healthcare challenges, such as fall detection, posture monitoring, and remote rehabilitation. Informal discussions with healthcare professionals have occasionally informed project themes, but structured interdisciplinary collaboration with medical or nursing students was not implemented during the analysed course iterations. Such collaboration is a promising direction for future development, as interdisciplinary engagement could strengthen students' ability to design feasible and context-aware IoMT solutions.

Peppi, the University of Oulu's official information system for curriculum and course management, defines the following learning outcomes (LOs) for this course: After completing the course, the student (i) are able to understand and solve practical challenges associated with wireless measurement solutions, (ii) are able to apply relevant standards when designing such systems, and (iii) are able to set up wireless measurement architectures for specific target applications (*e.g.*, industrial, environmental, traffic, home, or healthcare contexts). These LOs provide the foundation for the pedagogical approach described in Sect. 2.3.

The course is also connected to the broader aims of the SUSA project (Digital Europe Programme), which develops a shared European framework for digital health education. SUSA identifies core competencies in areas such as medical IoT, data analytics, cybersecurity, and digital infrastructures. Several of the course's learning outcomes intersect with these SUSA learning objectives, particularly those related to medical IoT (LO11), wireless communication and interoperability (LO13), data handling and visualisation (LO4 and LO5), and basic security considerations (LO15 and LO16). This alignment highlights how the course contributes to wider European efforts to strengthen digital health competencies.

Students may work individually, in pairs, or in small groups depending on their schedules, interests, and project scope. The course can be completed as either a 5 ECTS or 10 ECTS module, corresponding to different levels of independent project work.

2.2 Pedagogical Approach and Rationale

At the heart of the learning experience is an emphasis on the full end-to-end chain of wireless measurements, taking students from raw sensor voltages to processed data visualised on a smartphone. A central motivation for the course design was to provide students with a clear understanding of how IoMT systems operate across the entire workflow, from sensor level signal acquisition to data processing, wireless transmission, and application level visualisation. This approach aligns with recent analyses of the IoMT landscape, which emphasise the importance of understanding full pipeline architectures and the practical challenges associated with real world deployment [7]. By engaging with this complete pipeline, students gain a holistic perspective on how modern digital health solutions are engineered and deployed. Prior work further demonstrates that hands-on, device centred activities can significantly enhance student confidence and competence in biomedical engineering contexts [4].

This approach is grounded in project based learning and hands-on experimentation, enabling students to actively engage with real measurement challenges rather than only theoretical concepts. The course design follows principles of constructive alignment, ensuring that learning activities, project tasks, and assessment criteria consistently support the intended learning outcomes. More concretely, constructive alignment is implemented by explicitly linking learning outcomes to both practice oriented activities and the final assessment. For instance, the outcome of being able to configure microcontrollers and acquire physiological signals is introduced through guided starter kit exercises and supported by browser based simulations, and it is assessed through the successful operation of the student's prototype.

Likewise, the outcome of constructing a wireless data pipeline is addressed through short demonstrations and self paced experimentation with Message Queuing Telemetry Transport (MQTT) or Hypertext Transfer Protocol (HTTP) communication, and subsequently evaluated via the functionality and reliability of the implemented transmission link. Higher level outcomes, such as analysing physiological data or justifying design decisions, are reinforced through reflective writing and peer discussions and evaluated in the final project report, where students must explain their signal processing methods, measurement choices, and system limitations. This alignment ensures that students encounter each learning outcome through multiple, mutually reinforcing modalities.

The use of IoMT starter kits further motivates students by providing accessible, tangible tools that allow them to prototype and test their own biomedical measurement solutions in a realistic and application oriented context.

2.3 Course Structure and Implementation

Students can engage with the course through a multi-modal structure, attending sessions either in person or remotely via Microsoft Teams. All sessions are recorded and made available for asynchronous viewing, allowing students to follow the course at their own pace. The primary learning environment is Moodle, where students can access all course materials, including supplementary tutorials designed to familiarise them with AI tools such as Microsoft Copilot, browser-based simulation platforms like TinkerCad and Wokwi, and both basic and advanced electronics. The main course webpage also features an AI-enhanced AR/VR-based 360-degree digital learning environment, as shown in Fig. 1, where students can navigate the space and interact with virtual instruments such as oscilloscopes and function generators (see Fig. 2). This approach reflects prior work on remote and hybrid laboratory instruction [14].

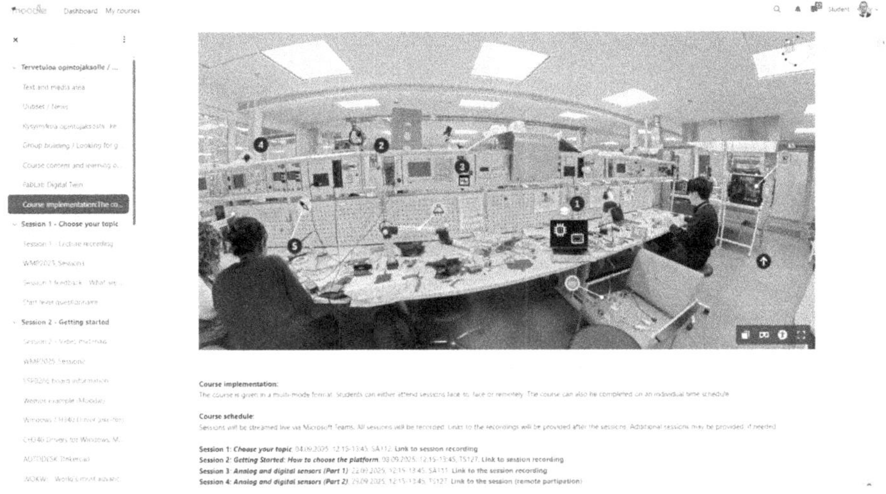

Fig. 1. Screenshot of the virtual FabLab environment integrated into the course's Moodle workspace.

For example, if soldering is required or a circuit needs to be debugged using a digital multimeter or oscilloscope, students can virtually visit the Super FabLab Oulu and familiarise themselves with the available equipment and working practices. This virtual environment allows them to explore tools, become familiar with laboratory workflows and essential safety protocols, and gain confidence before engaging with the physical facilities on campus. It also supports students who may have limited prior experience with electronics by providing a low-threshold, self-paced introduction to the laboratory setting. In this way, the virtual FabLab acts as a bridge between conceptual understanding and hands-on technical competence.

2.4 IoMT Starter Kit and Technical Components

Figure 3 illustrates the core architecture of an IoMT system as implemented in the course. The system begins with an analog photoplethysmography (PPG) heart-rate sensor that acquires real-time physiological data from the user. These

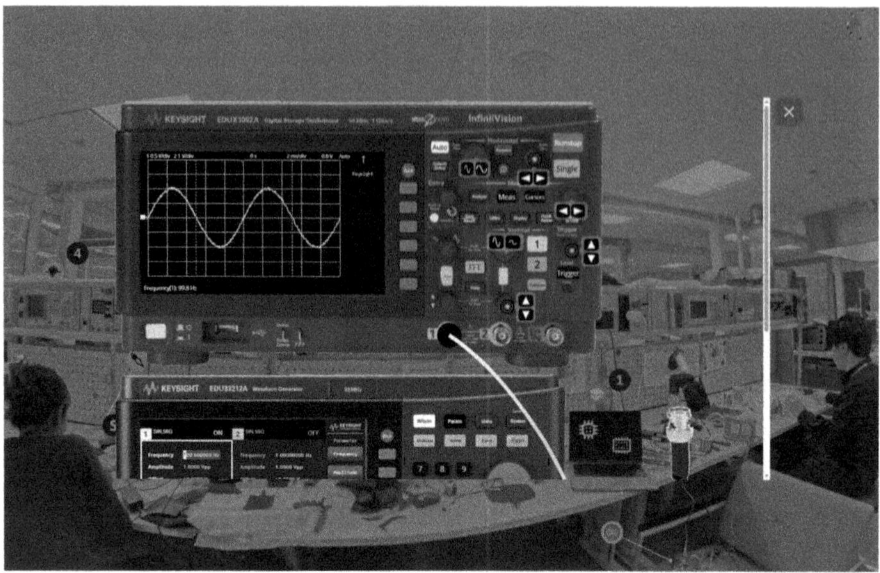

Fig. 2. Screenshot of the virtual FabLab in Moodle, showing interaction with VR/AR tools like a virtual oscilloscope.

signals are processed by a microcontroller unit (MCU), which serves as the central middleware component responsible for signal conditioning, data conversion, data formatting, and wireless transmission. The resulting data is then sent to external endpoints such as cloud platforms or mobile devices, where it can be stored, visualised, or further analysed. In parallel, the MCU may also control actuators that respond to sensor input, enabling closed-loop interaction. This modular architecture reflects the typical structure of modern IoMT systems and provides students with a conceptual and practical framework for designing and implementing wireless biomedical applications.

Each starter kit includes a solderless breadboard, a MCU (*i.e..*, ESP8266 or Wemos D1 Mini), jumper wires, a USB cable, an analog PPG-based heart-rate sensor, and an LED with an appropriate current-limiting resistor. All components are housed in a compact box to support easy transport and organisation. The kit enables students to construct and test complete IoMT systems, covering signal acquisition, preprocessing, wireless data transmission, and visualisation on external devices. Working directly with physical hardware gives students practical experience in circuit design, sensor integration, and embedded programming. The low-cost and reusable nature of the kit supports iterative prototyping and encourages experimentation, making it suitable for both classroom-based and remote learning contexts. Figure 4 shows the contents of the starter kit provided to students.

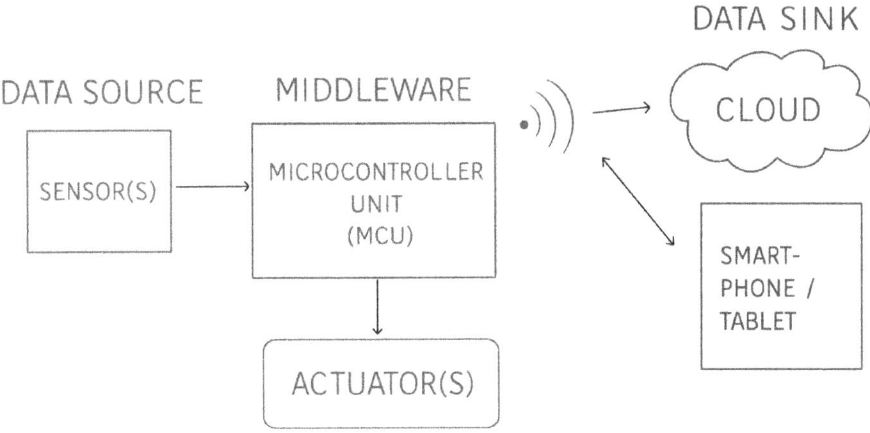

Fig. 3. Block diagram illustrating the core architecture of an IoMT system.

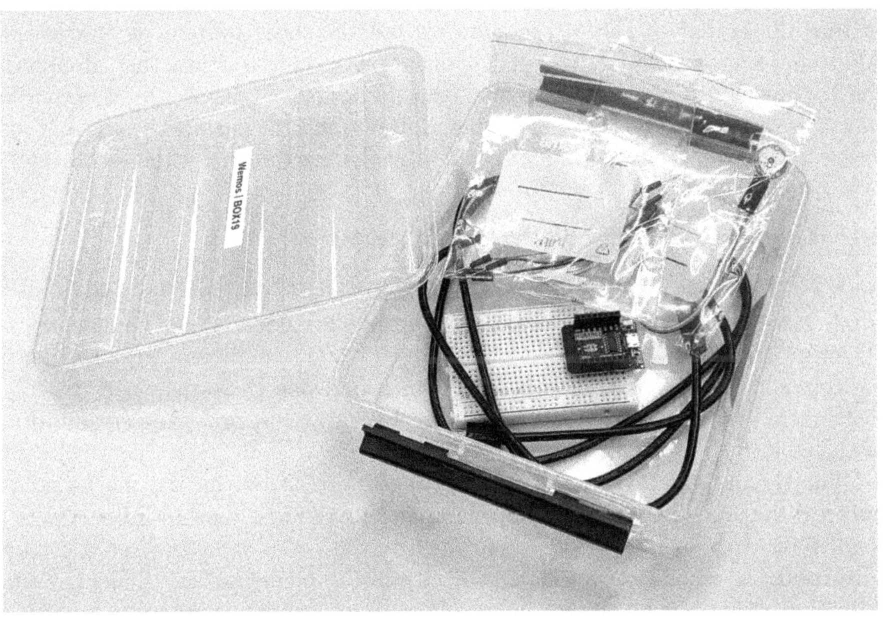

Fig. 4. IoMT starter kit used in the course, containing a breadboard, microcontroller module, jumper wires, sensor, and electronic components.

2.5   Student Support and Learning Environment

To complement the physical IoMT starter kit, the course integrates a set of virtual tools and simulation platforms that enable flexible, accessible, and low-risk experimentation. Moodle serves as the central learning environment, providing structured access to instructional materials, programming exercises, and interactive tutorials. The Wokwi simulator allows students to prototype embedded systems directly in the browser, offering real-time visualisation of circuit behaviour and microcontroller code execution without requiring immediate access to hardware. This reduces barriers for students who are new to electronics or who participate remotely. In addition, AI-assisted tools such as Microsoft Copilot support learners during programming and debugging tasks by offering contextual explanations, examples, and guidance. Together, these virtual resources create a multimodal learning ecosystem that reinforces conceptual understanding, supports self-paced study, and prepares students for more advanced hands-on work with physical IoMT devices.

3   Student Projects and Learning Outcomes

The project component forms the core of the course, enabling students to apply theoretical concepts to authentic engineering tasks and gain hands-on experience with wireless measurement systems. Building on the conceptual IoMT architecture illustrated in Fig. 3, students extend the basic system by integrating additional sensors, electronics, and application-specific features that align with the particular use-case scenarios they aim to address. This section presents an overview of the project themes, highlights representative student work, and discusses the learning outcomes and challenges observed during implementation.

3.1   Overview of Student Project Themes

Across the two academic years (*i.e.*, 2024 and 2025) analysed in this study, a total of 35 student projects were completed by 52 students. The flexible course structure allows students to work individually or in small groups, resulting in 17 individual projects, 17 two-person teams, and one three-person team. This distribution reflects the diverse schedules, backgrounds, and project ambitions of the cohort.

The thematic analysis of all project reports followed the six-phase process outlined by Braun and Clarke [15]. All reports were first read in full to develop familiarity with their content, after which initial codes were generated to capture recurring technical decisions, project aims, implementation challenges, and reflections described by the students. These codes were then reviewed and iteratively refined, with related codes grouped into preliminary themes. The themes were compared against the full dataset to ensure they accurately reflected patterned meaning across projects. Although the analysis was conducted inductively, several themes naturally aligned with the functional elements of the IoMT architecture presented in Fig. 3, reflecting how students themselves conceptualised and structured their systems. Throughout the process, analytic decisions were revisited to enhance the coherence and trustworthiness of the findings.

Drawing on this analysis, six major themes were identified, representing common IoMT application domains and technical approaches found across the 35 student projects. These themes provide a structured foundation for analysing project strategies and learning outcomes across the full set of prototypes. It is important to note that a single project could contribute to more than one theme, as IoMT prototypes often integrate multiple system components and technical approaches; themes therefore reflect recurring patterns rather than mutually exclusive categories.

- **Physiological monitoring** (12 projects): heart rate, SpO_2, respiration, stress estimation, and peripheral perfusion.
- **Posture and movement analysis** (8 projects): fall detection, tilt monitoring, slouching alerts, and ergonomic assessment.
- **Wearable health devices** (4 projects): multi-sensor wearable prototypes and compact form-factor systems.
- **Wireless data transmission pipelines** (4 projects): MQTT, HTTP, Bluetooth Low Energy (BLE), and custom local-server communication.
- **Cloud-based dashboards and IoT health applications** (21 projects): real-time visualisation, remote monitoring, medication reminders, and cloud-integrated health tools using platforms such as ThingSpeak, Firebase, Azure IoT Hub, Blynk, and Arduino IoT Cloud.
- **Embedded signal processing** (11 projects): filtering, peak detection, Fast Fourier Transformation (FFT) analysis, feature extraction, and lightweight machine-learning models.

3.2   Representative Project Examples

One representative project focused on developing a fall-detection system using an ESP32 microcontroller and an MPU6050 6-axis inertial measurement unit (IMU). The student designed a compact prototype, shown in Fig. 5, which continuously measures tri-axial acceleration and processes the data in real time. To evaluate system behaviour, the student implemented a live visualisation and binary classification interface, with example outputs illustrated in Fig. 6. These screenshots demonstrate how the system distinguishes between normal movements and abrupt acceleration patterns indicative of a fall, highlighting the student's integration of embedded sensing, signal processing, and user-facing feedback.

While this student concentrated primarily on the software aspects of reliable fall detection, other groups evaluated their prototypes more extensively in practical scenarios. As shown on the left side of Fig. 7, one pair of students explored fall detection using an ESP8266 mounted on a bicycle, whereas the team on the right side of Fig. 7 investigated the same use-case with a wrist-worn ESP8266-MPU6050 prototype. In their implementation, a detected fall triggered an

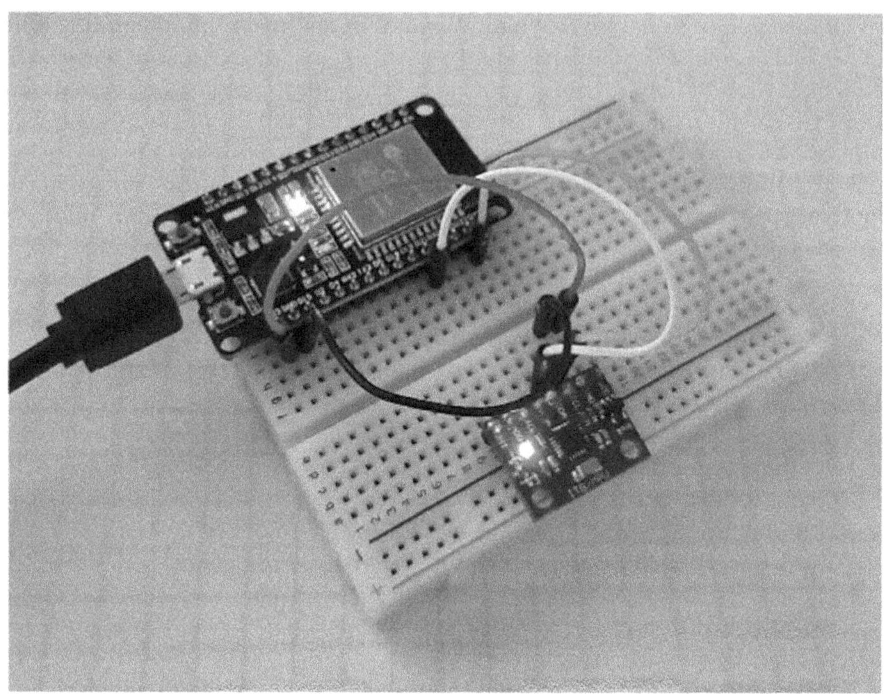

Fig. 5. ESP32-MPU6050 prototype used for fall-detection measurements.

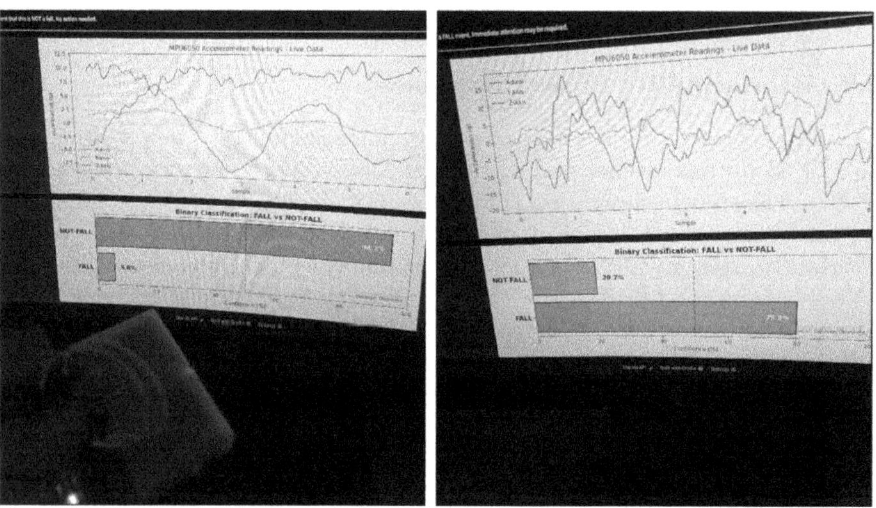

Fig. 6. Live accelerometer data and binary fall-detection output from the prototype.

automated SMS alert to a designated caregiver, as illustrated in Fig. 8. Beyond fall detection, the MPU6050 IMU also supported additional application scenarios, including a neck-posture monitoring system demonstrated in Fig. 9.

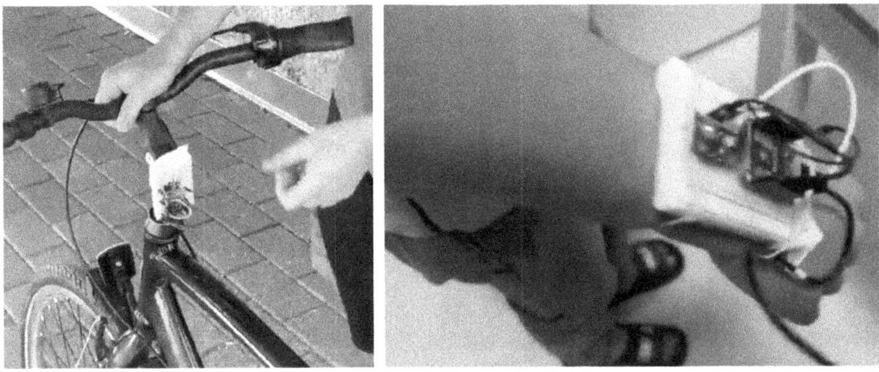

Fig. 7. Two student implementations of fall-detection prototypes: bicycle-mounted ESP8266-based system (left) and wrist-worn ESP8266-MPU6050 version (right).

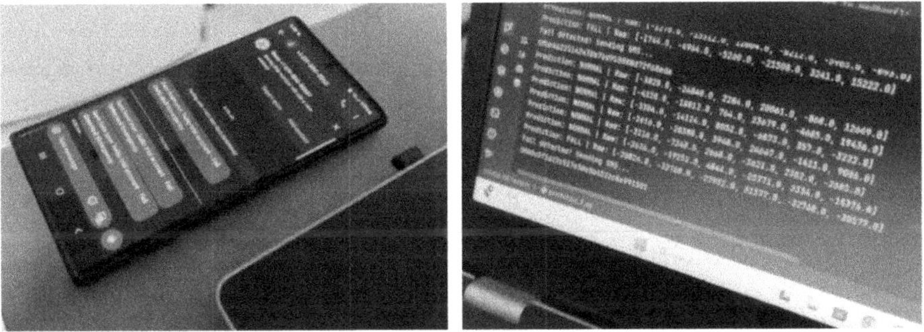

Fig. 8. Demonstration of the wrist-worn fall-detection prototype triggering an automated SMS alert after a detected fall event.

Other notable projects include:

- Cloud-connected heart-rate monitoring systems, where students implemented analog PPG acquisition, signal preprocessing, and wireless transmission to cloud platforms such as ThingSpeak or Azure IoT Hub.
- Wearable stress-monitoring prototypes, combining heart-rate variability estimation with simple machine-learning models running on the microcontroller.
- Home-based rehabilitation tools, where students designed simple exercise-tracking systems with real-time feedback delivered via mobile applications.

These examples illustrate the breadth of possible applications and highlight the creativity and autonomy fostered by the project-based approach.

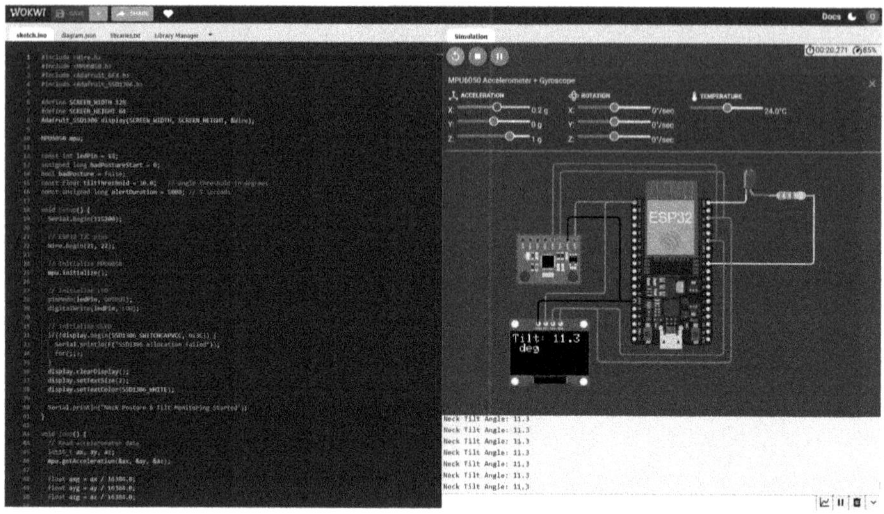

Fig. 9. Wokwi-based simulation of a neck-posture monitoring system using an ESP32 microcontroller, MPU6050 sensor, OLED display, and LED alert.

3.3 Technical and Pedagogical Challenges

While the open-ended nature of the projects supports exploration and innovation, it also introduces several challenges. Students often encounter difficulties related to:

- heterogeneous prior experience, particularly in electronics, programming, and signal processing,
- debugging embedded systems, including issues with wiring, sensor calibration, and timing,
- wireless connectivity, such as unstable Wi-Fi connections or protocol-level errors,
- signal quality, especially when working with low-cost analog sensors in non-ideal conditions,
- time management, as iterative prototyping can require substantial effort.

To address these challenges, the course integrates simulation tools, AI-assisted programming support, and virtual laboratory environments that allow students to experiment safely and at their own pace. These resources help reduce frustration, promote self-directed learning, and ensure that students with varying backgrounds can progress effectively.

3.4 Learning Outcomes and Skill Development

Across the cohort, students demonstrate significant growth in both technical and transversal competencies. Key learning outcomes include:

- embedded programming skills, including microcontroller configuration, interrupt handling, and data processing;
- circuit design and sensor integration, with hands-on experience in building and testing functional prototypes;
- wireless communication, covering Wi-Fi protocols, data formatting, and cloud integration;
- data analysis and visualisation, enabling students to interpret physiological signals and present results meaningfully;
- problem-solving and troubleshooting, developed through iterative experimentation and debugging;
- teamwork and project management, particularly for students working in pairs or small groups.

By the end of the course, students gain a holistic understanding of how modern IoMT systems are engineered, from sensor-level acquisition to application-level deployment. This practical experience strengthens their readiness for advanced coursework, research projects, and professional roles in digital health and biomedical engineering.

4 Discussion and Conclusion

The project outcomes presented in Sect. 3 illustrate how a lightweight starter kit, combined with an open-ended assignment structure, enables students to explore a wide range of IoMT use-case scenarios. Despite the diversity of topics, including fall detection, posture monitoring, newborn-health applications, hand-hygiene monitoring, and home-based rehabilitation tools, the projects shared several common characteristics. Students demonstrated an ability to integrate microcontrollers, inertial sensors, and electronics into functional prototypes, and to reason about sensor behaviour, noise, and threshold-based decision logic. The examples also highlight how quickly students progress from basic data acquisition to more advanced features such as real-time dashboards, automated notifications, and user-centred interaction concepts.

At the same time, the projects reveal typical challenges encountered in early-stage IoMT development. Many students focused heavily on software logic or signal processing while spending less time on enclosure design, long-term usability, or robustness in real-world conditions. Hardware limitations, short project timelines, and varying levels of prior experience also influenced the depth of each prototype. Nevertheless, the hands-on approach proved effective in helping students understand the constraints and opportunities of embedded health-monitoring systems.

In addition to functioning as a course implementation, the integrated combination of IoMT starter kits, virtual laboratory environments, browser-based simulations, and AI-assisted programming tools can also be viewed as a multimodal educational platform for practical learning in IoT, wireless communication, and cloud-connected health applications. This platform-oriented perspective highlights the reusability and extensibility of the environment beyond the specific course setting, and aligns the work with comparable educational toolkits discussed in the literature.

Overall, the course demonstrates that even modest hardware platforms can support meaningful learning experiences in IoMT design. By combining a conceptual architecture with a practical starter kit, students were able to create personalised solutions that addressed real or imagined health-related needs. Future iterations of the course may expand the sensor set, introduce optional cloud-integration modules, or incorporate lightweight machine-learning components to support more advanced analytics. Taken together, the results show that project-based learning remains a powerful method for engaging students in the multidisciplinary landscape of digital health technologies.

Acknowledgments. We thank our students at the University of Oulu for their effort in their course projects. This work has been supported by the SUSA project, funded by the European Union's Digital Europe Programme (DEP) under grant agreement No 101190010.

Disclosure of Interests. The authors declare no competing interests.

AI Use and Tools. Artificial intelligence tools were used for language editing during the preparation of this manuscript. All content was reviewed and approved by the authors.

References

1. El-Saleh, A.A., Sheikh, A.M., Albreem, M.A.M., Honnurvali, M.S.: The Internet of Medical Things (IoMT): opportunities and challenges. Wirel. Netw. **31**, 327–344 (2024)
2. Huang, C., Wang, J., Wang, S., Zhang, Y.: Internet of medical things: a systematic review. Neurocomputing **557**, 126719 (2023)
3. El-deep, S.E., Abohany, A.A., Sallam, K.M., El-Mageed, A.A.A.: A comprehensive survey on impact of applying various technologies on the internet of medical things. Artif. Intell. Rev. **58**(3), 86 (2025)
4. Pennes, A., et al.: A hands-on medical mechatronics exercise to pump up student learnings. Biomed. Eng. Educ. (2023)
5. Caffarena, G., Raya, R., Urendes, E., Otero, A., Mennard, D.: Teaching embedded systems in biomedical engineering degrees: a case study. In: 2021 IEEE Mysore Sub Section International Conference (MysuruCon), pp. 1–7. IEEE (2021)
6. Young, J., Spichkova, M., Simic, M.: Project-based learning within eHealth, bio-engineering and biomedical engineering application areas. Procedia Comput. Sci. **192**, 4952–4961 (2021)
7. Alturki, B., et al.: IoMT landscape: navigating current challenges and pioneering future research trends. Discov. Appl. Sci. **7**, 26 (2024)
8. Montesinos, L., Salinas-Navarro, D.E., Santos-Diaz, A.: Transdisciplinary experiential learning in biomedical engineering education for healthcare systems improvement. BMC Med. Educ. **23**, 207 (2023)
9. Higbee, S., Harrell, D., Chase, A., Miller, S.: A study of biomedical engineering student self-efficacy toward design throughout an undergraduate BME curriculum. Biomed. Eng. Educ. **5**(1), 15–36 (2025)

10. Wahyudi, M.N.A., Budiyanto, C.W., Widiastuti, I., Hatta, P., bin Bakar, M.S.: Understanding virtual laboratories in engineering education: a systematic literature review. Int. J. Pedagogy Teach. Educ. **7**(2), 102–118 (2024)
11. Potkonjak, V., et al.: Virtual laboratories for education in science, technology, and engineering: a review. Comput. Educ. **95**, 309–327 (2016)
12. Balamuralithara, B., Woods, P.: Virtual laboratories in engineering education: the simulation lab and remote lab. IEEE Trans. Learn. Technol. **2**(4), 273–287 (2009)
13. Kasneci, E., et al.: ChatGPT for good? On opportunities and challenges of large language models for education. Learn. Instruct. **90**, 101678 (2023)
14. Schuss, C., Maanselkä, A., Kaikkonen, M., Fabritius, T.: Teaching instrumentation and measurement in local and remote laboratories. In: 2022 IEEE International Instrumentation and Measurement Technology Conference (I2MTC), pp. 1–6. IEEE (2022)
15. Braun, V., Clarke, V.: Using thematic analysis in psychology. Qual. Res. Psychol. **3**(2), 77–101 (2006)

A Phenomenographic Research of Physiotherapy Teachers' Perceptions of Digitalization

Hilkka Korpi[1,2,3]($\boxtimes$) , Mari Harjunen[2,4], and Tuulikki Sjögren[2]

[1] Oulu University of Applied Sciences, Welfare and Culture, Yliopistonkatu 9, 90570 Oulu, Finland
hilkka.korpi@oamk.fi

[2] Faculty of Sports and Health, University of Jyväskylä, University of Jyväskylä, PL 35, 40014 Jyväskylä, Finland

[3] Faculty of Medicine, University of Helsinki, University of Helsinki, PL 63, 00014 Helsinki, Finland

[4] South Kymenlaakso Vocational Collage, Kymenlaaksonkatu 29, 48100 Kotka, Finland

Abstract. This study examines physiotherapy teachers' perceptions of digitalization at a time when digital tools are reshaping higher education and professional practice. As digital technologies influence teaching methods, competency needs, and professional expectations, teachers play a pivotal role in integrating these tools into learning environments. However, little is known about how physiotherapy educators perceive digitalization in their daily work. The aim of the study was to describe physiotherapy teachers' perceptions on their digital skills for developing teaching. A qualitative phenomenographic approach was used in this study. Data consisted of three group interviews with seven physiotherapy educators from two Finnish universities of applied sciences. Interview themes focused on teacher competence, continuing education, and digital proficiency. All participants were women, with an average age of 54.5 years and an average of 19.5 years of teaching experience. The analysis produced four hierarchical categories of conceptions: challenging digitalization, limited digitalization, existing digitalization, and enabling digitalization. These were shaped by three cross-cutting themes: devices and applications, student activity, and teachers' own competence. At the lower levels of the hierarchy, digitalization was perceived as unreliable, resource intensive, and sometimes detrimental to student engagement. At the higher levels, it was viewed as an integrated part of everyday work, offering new pedagogical opportunities, increasing motivation, and enabling innovative approaches such as VR, simulation-based learning, and data-driven tools. The findings illustrate a developmental shift from technology related challenges toward pedagogical and professional opportunities enabled by digitalization. This underscores the need for institutional support, equitable access to digital tools, and continuous professional development. When supported with adequate resources and thoughtful pedagogical design, digitalization holds strong potential to enhance physiotherapy education.

Keywords: Physiotherapy education · Teachers' perceptions · Digital competence · Educational technology · Phenomenography

M. Särestöniemi et al. (Eds.): NCDHWS 2026, CCIS 3009, pp. 462–477, 2026.
https://doi.org/10.1007/978-3-032-28812-7_32

1 Introduction

Digitalization is transforming society on multiple levels, reshaping how individuals work, communicate, learn, and share knowledge [1]. These changes strongly influence professional competence requirements and educational structures across sectors. In higher education, teachers increasingly operate in virtual learning environments, and digitalization - through online teaching and the reusability of digital learning materials-enables instruction for larger groups and more flexible delivery formats [2, 3].

The competence of health and rehabilitation educators plays a critical role in students' professional development in a rapidly changing world. Mikkonen et al. [4] found that the core skills of health science teachers include teaching-related knowledge, skills, and attitudes, with teachers generally assessing their competence highly. Factors influencing competence included academic qualification, teaching position, healthcare experience, research activity, age, and organizational context. A qualitative metasynthesis by Korpi et al. [5] identified six key competence domains essential for educators' continuous development: self-development, supervision, interaction, research, subject-specific expertise, networking, and multicultural competence.

The core of physiotherapy teachers' professional competence is grounded in the essential areas of physiotherapists' work. According to Finnish Physiotherapists [6], physiotherapy is built on the promotion of health, movement, mobility, and functional capacity. Central methods include guidance and counselling, therapeutic exercise, manual and physical therapy, and assistive technology services. Core competence areas include assessment, counselling, therapy, ethical and societal competence, technology competence, and accessibility-related expertise.

Digitalization and advanced technology are highlighted as a major future direction in physiotherapy. Digital tools, applications, and smart technologies support self-monitoring, self-care, diagnostic insight, and individually tailored health solutions. Digital rehabilitation, based on client-reported outcomes, increases the importance of physiotherapists' skills in motivation, guidance, and the use of emerging technologies. These developments strongly shape physiotherapy education, requiring teachers to be proficient in digital tools and capable of guiding students in their use [6]. Educational institutions also need adequate technological resources to support this shift.

As digitalization advances, teachers increasingly integrate digital tools into education, creating a need for innovative pedagogical approaches [2, 7]. Digital learning environments support flexible, time- and place-independent instruction [8], though rapid technological development challenges teachers to maintain sufficient digital competence and support students through ongoing changes [9]. Kullaslahti et al. [10] identified four competence areas required in online teaching: professional, pedagogical, technical, and personal, emphasizing the integration of strong pedagogical and digital knowledge. In their scoping review, Sormunen et al. [11] examined digital learning interventions in higher education, including health sciences education, and concluded that the effective use of digital technologies depends on deliberate pedagogical design, educators' digital pedagogical competence, and empirically demonstrated effectiveness.

In physiotherapy education, digital learning designs, such as blended and distance learning, have shown comparable or even improved effectiveness relative to traditional classroom teaching [12, 13]. Narratively summarized results indicate positive effects of flipped classrooms, interactive apps, and student-generated videos on learning outcomes, though more high-quality trials are needed. Digital learning has been found to enhance practical skills, knowledge acquisition, and reflective thinking [12]. Systematic review and meta-analysis indicate a wide range of digital technologies, including interactive websites, multimodal online environments, simulation videos, and educational games, are used to support the development of practical skills and theoretical knowledge in physiotherapy education [13].

As physiotherapy graduates are expected to practice as independent, autonomous professionals [14], understanding how educators perceive digitalization is essential for aligning educational practices with evolving professional demands. Despite this, physiotherapy education has been critiqued for insufficient grounding in theoretical learning perspectives and for being under-researched compared to other health professions [15, 16].

This study is part of the TerOpe - Competent Teachers Together! project, which aimed to develop and reform health sciences teacher education and continuing education in the social, health, and rehabilitation fields in Finland. The project (2017–2019) was funded by the Ministry of Education and Culture and involved several Finnish universities, including Oulu, Tampere, Jyväskylä, Turku, Eastern Finland, Åbo Akademi and Tampere University of Applied Sciences [17].

The purpose of this study was to investigate physiotherapy teachers' perceptions of digitalization as a work tool and how these perceptions differ. The aim of the study was to describe physiotherapy teachers' perceptions on their digital skills for developing teaching. The results of the study can be used to develop and update physiotherapy education and continuing education to meet future needs. Research Question: What are physiotherapy teachers' perceptions of digitalization as a work tool?

2 Materials and Methods

The data consisted of three group interviews carried out in two Universities of Applied Sciences with a total of seven physiotherapy teachers. The semi-structured interviews were conducted in Finnish. At the beginning of the interview, the participants were given the interview themes, which were associated with social and health care educator competences, continuing education, and integration of digital technology into teaching. Group interviews were considered appropriate because shared discussions can help participants recall experiences and support one another's reflections [18]. The interviews were conducted using a method in which the interviewer had the opportunity to ask the participants to clarify or justify their answers. The questions asked by the interviewer were semi-structured and the following conversation was reciprocal between the interviewer and the interviewees The interviews were conducted by three interviewers from the broader Finnish national project who were not authors of this article. The verbatim transcription was carried out by an individual not affiliated with the project. All three interviewers were experienced health science educators and researchers; two held doctoral degrees and one was a doctoral candidate. The size of the interview material of physiotherapy educators was 86 A4 sheets of transcribed interview material written in

Times New Roman font 12 with 1.5-line spacing. The Ethics Committee of the University of Jyväskylä ensured the appropriateness of our interviews in its statement on November 29, 2017.

Among the interviewed educators, five taught bachelor's-level physiotherapy students enrolled in universities of applied sciences, whereas two were responsible for instruction in master's and doctoral physiotherapy programs at a research university. The mean age of the physiotherapy educators was 54.5 years (range 35–64). On average, they had 19.5 years (range 3–33) of professional teaching experience.

The interview material was analyzed using a phenomenographic research approach. Phenomenography investigates the qualitatively different ways individuals understand or experience a phenomenon, as well as the structural relationships between these conceptions [19–21]. It was chosen for this study because it enables exploration of variation in teachers' conceptions related to thinking, learning, and teaching [20, 22], with a focus on collective, not individual, understandings [23].

Data analysis followed the iterative steps typical of phenomenography. The transcripts were read multiple times to identify expressions related to the research question on physiotherapy teachers' perceptions of digitalization as a working tool [24]. A total of 72 meaning units were highlighted, coded, and in some cases divided further to avoid loss of contextual meaning [23, 25]. To facilitate the analysis, meaning units were assembled into a "pool of meaning" [24], where they were compared, sorted, and grouped based on similarities and differences. Context was repeatedly checked to ensure interpretive accuracy [26].

Through this inductive process, four preliminary descriptive categories were developed to represent distinct ways in which teachers perceived digitalization as a work tool [26]. Categories were refined according to phenomenographic criteria: they must be qualitatively distinct, logically related, and limited in number [24, 27].

The final stage involved identifying structural relationships across the categories and determining critical aspects that appeared in all of them. These aspects formed the themes that traverse the categories [28]. The resulting outcome space represents a hierarchical structure of physiotherapy teachers' conceptions of digitalization, where broader and more complex ways of understanding build upon narrower ones.

3 Results

The phenomenographic analysis resulted in a category system consisting of four hierarchically structured categories of physiotherapy teachers' perceptions of digitalization as a work tool. Digitalization as a work tool was seen as challenging (I), limited (II), existing (III), and enabling (IV). The hierarchy is visible in the category system, with physiotherapy teachers' perceptions of digitalization as a work tool becoming more diverse and deeper from the lowest category of challenging (I) to the highest category of enabling (IV). Differences between the categories were formed through the following themes: devices and applications, student activity, and the teacher's own competence. The descriptive categories and themes together constitute the outcome space (Table 1), in which the hierarchical structure of the categories is visible.

Table 1. Physiotherapy teachers' perceptions of digitalization as a working tool.

Themes	Challenging digitalization (I)	Limited digitalization (II)	Existing digitalization (III)	Enabling digitalization (IV)
Devices and applications	Does not always meet the needs	Does not always provide a solution	An everyday phenomenon	Versatile pedagogy
Student activity	Discourages participation	Insufficient resources	Need for skills in working life	Motivating learning tool
Teacher´s own competence	Technology proficiency is lacking	Limited resources	Continuous need for training	Workmate of tomorrow

3.1 Challenging Digitalization (Descriptive Category I)

The first descriptive category that emerged from the analysis was challenging digitalization. This category illustrates the kinds of difficulties that digitalization creates when used as a teacher's working tool.

According to the participants, one major challenge is that digital devices and systems do not always function as expected. This was seen as particularly problematic in teaching situations where some students are present in the classroom and others participate online—so-called hybrid teaching. The teachers described difficulties in simultaneously managing the needs of students attending remotely and on site, while also trying to control the digital tools required for instruction.

Then, for example, when guiding students using digital tools, yes, that has certainly caused a lot of grey hair. The devices don't work, and then there may be a situation where some students are sitting here and others are online, and you're supposed to manage the remote participants and talk with the hybrid teaching and those who are physically present, like a kind of split personality, and then still control the technology itself. It's quite challenging.

The continuously advancing digital environment was also perceived as having a potentially passivating effect on students. Teachers felt that when materials are readily available in digital form, students do not necessarily engage in active note-taking. Physiotherapy teachers expressed concern that students might not effectively process or internalize digital material and that this could negatively affect learning.

It also gives me the feeling that when they don't make any kind of notes - I have always been absolutely sure that young people today, when they don't write but just sit there, where are their brains then? I don't know. But I am completely sure that they do not absorb the material as well, because they cannot be so different from what we used to be.

Teachers also reported that their own digital competence posed challenges. The rapid development of technology requires continuous familiarization, but they felt that time and resources for this were insufficient. Limited digital skills made it difficult to fully focus on teaching content, as managing the technological aspects required considerable attention during lessons.

I notice that I cannot concentrate on the content as well if I'm giving a webinar about something. If I have to manage the technology - people dropping out of the session and then bringing them back, giving permissions to do this or that, getting their presentations onto the screen and so on...

3.2   Limited Digitalization (Descriptive Category II)

The second descriptive category identified in the analysis was limited digitalization. This category describes perceptions of the limitations of digitalization as a working tool for physiotherapy teachers. As in the first category, digitalization was viewed as challenging, but here it was specifically perceived as limited in its usefulness.

A central issue highlighted in the interviews was the limited capacity of digital devices, particularly within physiotherapy education. The participants felt that digital tools alone are insufficient for teaching the analytical and hands-on skills required in physiotherapy practice. The teachers emphasized that not all competencies can be learned in a digital environment, even though digital tools can serve as a valuable supplement. Additionally, online teaching platforms were perceived as restricting discussion during teaching situations.

In our field, devices provide certain results, but for example when observing someone's movement, you still need to be able to analyze the numbers and understand what they actually mean. It's not enough to just look at the figures; you must interpret what they mean for the person themselves. That's where the challenge lies - many tools give results, but the actual analysis is missing

Because the online environment, in a way, prevents free discussion, and then...

The limitations of digitalization were considered especially relevant for distance and blended learning students. Teachers noted that students do not have access at home to the same equipment that is available in on-campus teaching. As a result, the advantages of digitalization are not equally accessible to all learners.

But we really do not have the kind of equipment or devices that would truly support learning, because the same devices should be available to every student - for example, if we provide remote teaching at home: 3D equipment and all that.

Teachers also recognized limitations in terms of time and resources needed to familiarize themselves with digital tools. They felt a continuous need to stay updated with new technologies, yet lacked sufficient time to do so. They acknowledged that designing and implementing high-quality online courses is time-consuming, while time resources remain inadequate. Additional training opportunities existed, but teachers felt they did not have the resources to attend them. Some participants also believed that hybrid teaching would ideally require two teachers. While technology was seen to offer opportunities, its optimal use was limited by the teachers' own skill level.

It requires quite a lot of familiarization and time from us as well.

There should be more of it, and we should practise it. New things keep coming all the time - last autumn we had those short trainings, and...

3.3 Existing Digitalization (Descriptive Category III)

The third descriptive category identified in the analysis was existing digitalization, which illustrates physiotherapy teachers' perceptions of digitalization as an established and present phenomenon in their everyday work. In this category, digitalization expands from being challenging and limited to being a normal, integrated part of professional practice. The physiotherapy teachers emphasized that digitalization is not merely a future development but a current reality, and an essential part of their work in both teaching and student guidance.

It is not only the future - it is already part of everyday life.

The use of various online teaching platforms was seen as providing the necessary basis for hybrid teaching, and new technologies were described as part of daily instructional practice. Participants explained that tools such as Skype meetings were routinely used in student supervision, making them a normal component of everyday interactions. In teaching, physiotherapy educators reported utilizing walking robots, wrist-worn devices, artificial intelligence, and virtual reality, technologies that are also increasingly present in rehabilitation settings, including forms of gamification. These digital tools are likewise part of the working environments students will encounter in their future professions.

Digitalization was thus perceived not only as a tool for teaching and learning but also as content within physiotherapy education and professional practice. Because digital technologies are constantly present and continually evolving, teachers felt that they face an ongoing need for further training to keep pace with developments.

It will be part of the future, and it is already part of the present - we already have walking robots, wrist devices, artificial intelligence, virtual reality, augmented reality, and these are used in teaching and in rehabilitation directly with clients. Things are being gamified, so digitalization is part of our work.

3.4 Enabling Digitalization (Descriptive Category IV)

The fourth descriptive category that emerged from the analysis was enabling digitalization. This category describes how physiotherapy teachers perceived digitalization as a tool that expands possibilities in their work. In this category, perceptions of digitalization broaden further, encompassing the earlier categories of challenge, limitation, and existing presence.

Digitalization was seen as bringing new opportunities to teachers' work. Various digital devices and applications were perceived to enable more diverse forms of learning. Participants felt that digitalization increases versatility, supports new ways of working, and introduces new pedagogical approaches into teaching.

It certainly diversifies basic teaching and brings new ways of working and new kinds of pedagogy.

Digital technology was also viewed as supportive and motivating for students. For example, the use of virtual reality in teaching was described as providing new sparks for learning. Teachers felt that digital tools can help bring practical experiences closer to students, such as through VR headsets or three-dimensional simulations. Online platforms for examinations, such as EXAM halls or digital exams, as well as online information retrieval, were seen as time-saving and beneficial for students. Hybrid teaching was perceived as enabling studies from anywhere in the world.

What I've often noticed in clinical work as well as in teaching is that it motivates students differently, because for them certain things - like virtual reality are still new to some extent. It creates completely new stimuli and helps ignite that spark.

Participants also viewed digital technology as a future colleague. They believed that technology will offer new opportunities to better understand human body functions. Digitalization was thought to have the potential to replace some older teaching methods. Teachers described how emerging analytical technologies can provide data on the body's movements and positions, and how artificial intelligence may increasingly generate direct insights relevant to rehabilitation.

I do believe that technology may even replace certain things. There are different analytical technologies that tell us about our bodies, movements, and postures, and we can get that data without making the interpretations ourselves. Artificial intelligence may directly provide information like: you have this type of rupture,' and then suggest how rehabilitation should proceed. So, I believe it will be our coworker in the future.

3.5 Relationships Between the Categories

The analysis resulted in four hierarchical categories (Table 1) describing physiotherapy teachers' perceptions of digitalization as a working tool: challenging digitalization (I), limited digitalization (II), existing digitalization (III), and enabling digitalization (IV). Differences between the categories were shaped by three overarching themes that cut across all four categories: devices and applications, student activity, and the teacher's own competence.

Variation within these themes created the hierarchical structure among the categories, such that the understanding of physiotherapy teachers' perceptions of digitalization expands progressively from Category I to Category IV (Fig. 1).

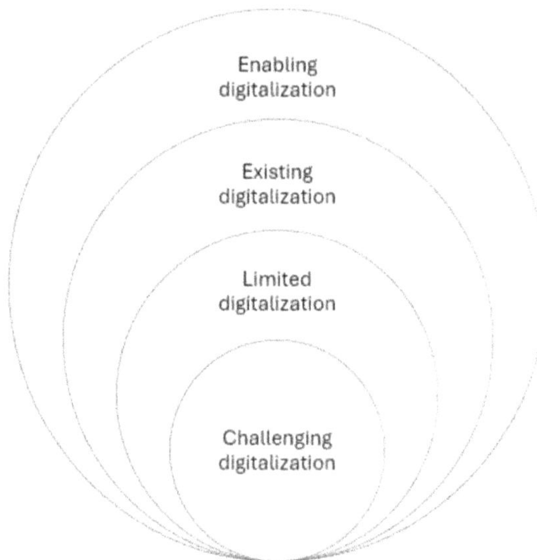

Fig. 1. Hierarchical depiction of physiotherapy teachers' perceptions of digitalization as a working tool

3.6 Devices and Applications

Physiotherapy teachers' perceptions of devices and applications expanded from seeing them as insufficient to enabling diverse pedagogical practices. In the narrowest sense, in Category I (challenging digitalization), devices and applications were seen as not meeting the needs of teaching. In Category II (limited digitalization), teachers' views broadened to recognize that devices and applications do not always provide a solution. In Category III (existing digitalization), teachers' views deepened as devices and applications were seen as part of the everyday working tools of a physiotherapy teacher. Finally, in Category IV (enabling digitalization), the role of devices and applications expanded further, as they were perceived to enable versatile and multifaceted pedagogy.

3.7 Student Activity

Physiotherapy teachers' perceptions of student activity expanded from passivity to viewing digitalization as a motivating learning tool. In the narrowest interpretation, within Category I (challenging digitalization), digitalization was seen as causing passivity among students. In Category II (limited digitalization), teachers noted that resources were limited, particularly for blended-learning students who do not have access to the same equipment at home as in classroom environments. In the third category (existing digitalization), digital competence was viewed as a necessary part of students' future professional practice. In the final category (enabling digitalization), digitalization was seen most broadly as a motivating learning tool that offers students new types of learning experiences.

3.8 Teacher's Own Competence

Physiotherapy teachers' perceptions of their own competence expanded from insufficient technological control to seeing digitalization as a future work partner. In the narrowest view, within Category I (challenging digitalization), teachers described their technological skills as inadequate. In Category II (limited digitalization), teachers perceived their resources for developing digital competence as limited. In Category III (existing digitalization), teachers recognized the need for continuous further training to maintain and develop their skills. In the final category (enabling digitalization), digitalization was seen most broadly as a future "colleague" that will increasingly support physiotherapy teachers' work.

4 Discussion

This phenomenographic study explored physiotherapy teachers' perceptions of digitalization as a working tool and identified a hierarchical continuum of conceptions: from challenging and limited, through existing, to enabling digitalization. The three cross-cutting themes: devices and applications, student activity, and teachers' own competence structure how these conceptions expand in scope and complexity. Overall, the outcome space suggests a developmental trajectory from technology-driven constraints to pedagogically meaningful and professionally integrated use of digitalization in physiotherapy education [24, 28].

At the challenge, teachers described technology that is unreliable in hybrid settings, uneven access to equipment (particularly for distance/blended students), and time and resource shortages to keep pace with rapid technological change. These findings echo prior work showing that accelerating technological development in higher education places substantial demands on teachers' digital competence and support structures [2, 9]. They also align with calls to develop digital learning solutions that match authentic workplace needs and pedagogical aims [3, 7].

Moving toward existing, digitalization is perceived as part of daily work, both a tool and content for teaching and supervision, mirroring the profession's trajectory where technology, data, and remote solutions are increasingly embedded in rehabilitation practice [6, 14]. At the enabling end, teachers framed digitalization as a source of new pedagogical possibilities (e.g., VR/AR, simulations, data-informed analysis, gamification), consistent with evidence that well-designed digital learning (e.g., flipped classrooms, interactive apps, student-generated video) can enhance learning outcomes in physiotherapy education [11–13]. The hierarchy thus captures a shift from technology as a problem to be managed toward technology as a partner and amplifier of pedagogy.

Teachers' accounts highlight a capability-context gap: devices may generate numerical data or visualizations, but analytical interpretation and hands-on skill development remain challenging to teach purely digitally. This aligns with critiques that digital initiatives in physiotherapy education have not always been grounded in robust learning theory or sufficiently targeted toward practical skills [15, 16, 29, 30, 32]. In addition, continuous reflection on physiotherapy students' professional development is essential as they acquire new skills [31, 33]. At the same time, the shift toward existing/enabling conceptions reflects how platforms and tools (e.g., VR, motion analysis, 3D visualizations) are becoming everyday resources when institutions invest in infrastructure and support [2.3]. An equity issue also emerged strongly: students' unequal access to equipment at home underscores the need for programme-level strategies (e.g., loan schemes, on-campus access, minimum technology standards) to prevent digitalization from widening learning gaps [7, 9].

Teachers worried that ready-made digital materials may reduce active engagement. These concerns are valid if digital use is content-delivery-oriented. However, the literature suggests that pedagogical design drives learning: blended learning can be as effective or superior to traditional teaching when it leverages active, interactive tasks (e.g., flipped learning, formative quizzes, peer production) [12, 13]. In the enabling conception, teachers report that digital tools motivate students and bring practice "closer" (e.g., via VR, simulations, EXAM/online assessment), consistent with evidence that multimodal and interactive designs support knowledge and reflective thinking and can scaffold aspects of practical skill learning [12, 13]. The implication is to purposefully design for activity (problem-solving, analysis, creation) rather than passive consumption.

The trajectory from insufficient technological control to viewing technology as a future colleague reflects the competence integration described in earlier research: effective digital teaching requires professional (discipline-specific), pedagogical, and technical knowledge, supported by personal attributes such as motivation and self-efficacy [8, 10]. The present findings are also consistent with broader work on health sciences educators' competence [4] and the emphasis on continuous professional development (CPD) and networking [5]. However, teachers reported limited time and resources to upskill and to design high-quality online/hybrid courses, an organizational barrier well documented in higher education digitalization [2, 9].

The study provided new perspectives specifically on physiotherapy teachers' perceptions of digitalization as a work tool. The results of the study can be used to develop the work of physiotherapy teachers, especially in higher education, but also for teachers working at other educational levels, in terms of digitalization. As this study was nearing completion, schools transitioned to online teaching due to the coronavirus. As teaching moved online, the importance of teachers' digital skills became even more emphasized. Therefore, it is essential to enhance teachers' digital competence to enable them to design effective digital pedagogy and support students in their digital learning [32].

Currently, in addition to the technologization of education, developments related to artificial intelligence pose significant challenges to teaching, placing new demands on teachers' pedagogical competence, digital literacy, and the ethical foundations of education.

4.1 Methodological Reflections and Limitations

Phenomenography aims to describe the qualitatively different ways in which a collective experiences a phenomenon, represented in an outcome space consisting of logically related categories [24, 28, 35]. In this study, established phenomenographic procedures were followed, including iterative reading of the transcripts, identification and coding of meaning units, construction of a "pool of meaning," refinement of descriptive categories, and interpretation of structural relations among them. Despite these strengths, several methodological limitations require consideration. The sample size was small (n = 7), drawn from two Universities of Applied Sciences and research university, and all participants were women. Although small samples are common in phenomenography, and variation rather than quantity is the key criterion, this may nonetheless limit the transferability of the findings. Trigwell [22] suggests that an optimal phenomenographic sample comprises 15–20 participants, but several scholars [35, 36] argue that the decisive factor is whether the sample sufficiently represents variation within the phenomenon, rather than the number of participants. In this study, the participants formed a heterogeneous group in terms of age (35–64 years) and teaching experience (3–33 years), and the resulting variation in conceptions indicates that the data were sufficiently rich for phenomenographic analysis.

The reliability of phenomenographic research is strengthened when the analytic process is transparently described, allowing another researcher to follow the steps of the analysis [27, 37]. In this study, trustworthiness was enhanced by repeatedly returning to the original transcripts to ensure that the descriptive categories accurately represented the data. Clear articulation of the differences between and within categories is also essential for reliability [27] and this study presented these distinctions systematically, ensuring that no categories overlapped. A common challenge in phenomenographic analysis is incomplete categorization or insufficiently defined final categories [27]. To mitigate this, the analytical process and the resulting outcome space were described in detail, and the final categories were carefully defined based on the data.

Trustworthiness was further supported by the inclusion of verbatim interview excerpts, enabling readers to evaluate the interpretations in relation to the original data [27, 37]. However, the use of pre-transcribed interview material collected in an earlier project may have constrained the researcher's access to contextual nuances, and the group interview format may have influenced responses through peer interaction. The researchers of this study are experienced experts in physiotherapy, and they have also formal teacher qualifications and a strong research background. (HK, MH, TS). Researcher triangulation during the various stages of phenomenographic analysis occurred within three researchers.

Finally, the credibility of this study is also linked to the researcher's ethical conduct. Following the Finnish Advisory Board on Research Integrity [38] the study adhered to principles of good scientific practice, including honesty, accuracy, and diligence throughout the research process [39]. An AI-assisted tool (Microsoft Copilot) was used to support language clarity and proofreading. All content and interpretations remain the author's own.

4.2 Practical Implications

The findings of this study highlight several practical implications for physiotherapy education. To fully realize the pedagogical benefits of digitalization, institutions need to invest in reliable hybrid learning environments and provide adequate technical and instructional support so that teachers can focus on teaching rather than troubleshooting. Ensuring equity of access is crucial, especially for blended and distance learners; this may require systematic solutions such as equipment-loan schemes, minimum technology standards, or extended on-campus access to digital tools. Furthermore, high-quality online and hybrid teaching requires time for careful planning, design, and continuous professional development, and institutions should acknowledge this by allocating sufficient resources and opportunities for teacher training. Digitalization also offers valuable opportunities to enrich learning through simulation, VR/AR technologies, motion-analysis tools and other innovations that can complement—rather than replace—hands-on physiotherapy instruction. Team-teaching or support-staff models may help manage the demands of hybrid teaching environments. Finally, digital competence should be integrated into physiotherapy curricula not only as a tool for delivery but also as essential content, including data literacy, ethical use of technology, and understanding the role of AI and analytics in future rehabilitation practice.

4.3 Future Research

Future research should examine how the rapid development of digitalization and artificial intelligence can be effectively integrated into physiotherapy education. As digital learning environments continue to evolve, AI-based tools are expected to influence both the content and the processes of teaching and learning. Consequently, future studies should investigate how AI can support students' clinical reasoning, practical skill development, and reflective learning. In addition, attention should be given to how the use of AI reshapes assessment practices, introduces new ethical considerations, and alters the professional competencies required of physiotherapists. A deeper understanding of these dynamics will be essential to ensure that physiotherapy education remains aligned with emerging technological possibilities while upholding high pedagogical and professional standards. Ultimately, future research should clarify how AI can serve as an enabling tool that enhances students learning in physiotherapy education.

5 Conclusion

Physiotherapy educators' digital competence greatly influences students' professional development. The findings portray a developmental shift in physiotherapy teachers' perceptions from digitalization as a source of difficulty to a pedagogically enabling partner that is both tool and content in education. Realizing the benefits requires systemic support for teachers, equitable access for students, and deliberate pedagogical design. Aligning these elements advances programs toward preparing graduates for autonomous, digitally competent practice consistent with professional expectations.

Acknowledgements. Acknowledgements. The reported research is part of the TerOpe project funded by the Ministry of Education and Culture in Finland. We would like to acknowledge the Ministry for providing us the opportunity to research and extend knowledge of teacher competence. We would also like to express our appreciation to the research assistants who participated in data collection during this research.

Disclosure of Interests. The authors have no competing interests to declare that are relevant to the content of this article.

References

1. Virtanen, L., Kaihlanen, A.-M., Kainiemi, E., Saukkonen, P., Valtokari, M., Väre, A., Nurmi-Koikkalainen, P., Heponiemi, T.: Realisation of the goals of digitalisation in disability work: analysis of work environment and professionals' educational background. Finnish J. eHealth eWelfare **16**(4), 415–439 (2024). https://doi.org/10.23996/fjhw.141124
2. Töytäri, A.: Näkökulmia ammattikorkeakouluopettajan oppimiseen ja osaamishaasteisiin. Doctoral dissertation. University of Jyväskylä (2019)
3. Visio 2030. Visio 2030 reports. Available from: https://minedu.fi/documents/1410845/120 21888/Visiotyo%CC%88ryhmien+yhteinen
4. Mikkonen, K., et al.: Competence areas of health science teachers: a systematic review. Nurse Educ. Today **70**, 77–86 (2018)
5. Korpi, H., Sjögren, T., Mikkonen, K., Piirainen, A., Ojala, T., Koskinen, C., Koskinen, M., Salminen, L., Koivula, M., Lähteenmäki, M.-L., Saaranen, T., Sormunen, M., Koskimäki, M., Kääriäinen, M.: A systematic review and metasynthesis of qualitative studies on the competencies of health and rehabilitation science educators. Nursing Educ. Res. Practice **10**(2), 42–51 (2020). https://nerp.lsmuni.lt/a-systematic-review-and-metasynthesis-of-qualitative-studies-onthe-competencies-of-health-and-rehabilitation-science-educators/
6. Finnish Physiotherapists. Fysioterapeutin ydinosaaminen. 2016. Available from: https://www.suomenfysioterapeutit.com/ydinosaaminen/FysioterapeutinYdnosaaminen.pdf
7. Brauer, S.: Digital open badge-driven learning: Competence-based professional development for vocational teachers. Doctoral dissertation. University of Lapland (2019)
8. Kullaslahti, J.: Ammattikoulun verkko-opettajan kompetenssi ja kehittyminen. Doctoral dissertation. University of Tampere (2011)
9. Paavilainen, S., Rantanen, M., Torikka, S.: Opiskelijat verkkoympäristössä. In: Määttä, J., Pohjanmäki, T., Timonen, P. (eds.), Kohti digikampusta. Humanistinen ammattikorkeakoulu; pp. 89–95 (2016)
10. Kullaslahti, J., Karento, H., Töytäri, A.: Opettajien digipedagoginen osaaminen FUAS-liittouman ammattikorkeakouluissa (2015) (HAMKin e-julkaisuja 35/2015). https://www.theseus.fi/bitstream/handle/10024/103253/fuas_opettajien_digipedagoginen_osaaminen_2015_ekirja.pdf
11. Sormunen, M., et al.: Digital learning interventions in higher education: a scoping review. Comput. Inform. Nurs. **38**(12), 613–624 (2020)
12. Mącznik, A.K., Ribeiro, D.C., Baxter, G.D.: Online technology use in physiotherapy teaching and learning: a systematic review of effectiveness and users' perceptions. BMC Med. Educ. **15**, 160 (2015). https://doi.org/10.1186/s12909-015-0429-8
13. Ødegaard, N.B., Myhaug, H.T., Dahl-Michelsen, T., Røe, Y.: Digital learning designs in physiotherapy education: a systematic review and meta-analysis. BMC Med. Educ. **21**, 48 (2021). https://doi.org/10.1186/s12909-020-02483-w
14. World Confederation for Physical Therapy. World physiotherapy. 2020. Available from: https://www.wcpt.org/node
15. Unge, J., Lundh, P., Gummesson, C., Amnér, G.: Learning spaces for health sciences: the role of e-learning in physiotherapy and occupational therapy education. Phys. Therapy Rev. **23**(1), 50–60 (2018). https://doi.org/10.1080/10833196.2018.144742
16. Veneri, D.: The role and effectiveness of computer-assisted learning in physical therapy education: a systematic review. Physiother. Theory Pract. **27**(4), 287–298 (2011). https://doi.org/10.3109/09593985.2010.493192
17. Mikkonen, K., Koivula, M., Sjögren, T., Korpi, H., Koskinen, C., Koskinen, M., Kuivila, H.-M., Lähteenmäki, M.-L., Koskimäki, H., Mäki-Hakola, H., Wallin, O., Saaranen, T.,

Sormunen, M., Kokkonen, K.-M., Kiikeri, J., Salminen, L., Ryhtä, I., Elonen, I., Kääriäinen, M.: TerOpe-kärkihanke: Sosiaali-, terveys- ja kuntoutusalan opettajien osaaminen ja kehittäminen. Juvenes Print (2019)
18. Eskola, J., Suoranta, J.: Johdatus laadulliseen tutkimukseen. Jyväskylä. Vastapaino (2008)
19. Marton, F.: Phenomenography: describing conceptions of the world around us. Instr. Sci. **10**(2), 177–200 (1981)
20. Marton, F.: Qualitative research in education: Focus and methods. In: Sherman, R.R., Webb, R.B. (eds.) Qualitative research in education, pp. 140–162. Taylor & Francis (2005)
21. Marton, F., Pong, Y.Y.: On the unit of description in phenomenography. High. Educ. Res. Dev. **24**, 335–348 (2005)
22. Trigwell, K.: A phenomenographic interview on phenomenography. In: Bowden, J.A., Walsh, E. (eds.) Phenomenography, pp. 62–82. RMIT University Press (2000)
23. Åkerlind, G., Bowden, J., Green, P.: Learning to do phenomenography: a reflective discussion. In: Bowden, J., Green, P. (eds.) Doing developmental phenomenography, pp. 74–100. RMIT University Press (2005)
24. Marton, F., Booth, S.: Learning and awareness. Lawrence Erlbaum Associates (1997)
25. Bowden, J.A.: The nature of phenomenographic research. In: Bowden, J.A., Walsh, E. (eds.) Phenomenography, pp. 11–31. RMIT University Press (2000)
26. Åkerlind, G.S.: Variation and commonality in phenomenographic research methods. High. Educ. Res. Dev. **31**(1), 115–127 (2012)
27. Huusko, M., Paloniemi, S.: Fenomenografia laadullisena tutkimussuuntauksena kasvatustieteissä. Kasvatus. **37**(2), 162–173 (2006)
28. Åkerlind, G.S.: Academic growth and development: how do university academics experience it? High. Educ. **50**(1), 1–32 (2005). https://doi.org/10.1007/s10734-004-6345-1
29. Korpi, H., Piirainen, A., Peltokallio, L.: Practical work in physiotherapy students' professional development. Reflective Pract. **18**(6), 821–836 (2017). https://doi.org/10.1080/14623943.2017.1361920
30. Kurunsaari, M., Tynjälä, P., Piirainen, A.: Stories of professional development in physiotherapy education. Physiother. Theory Pract. **38**(11), 1742–1755 (2022). https://doi.org/10.1080/09593985.2021.1888341
31. Korpi, H., Peltokallio, L., Piirainen, A.: Problem-based learning in professional studies from the physiotherapy students' perspective. Interdisciplinary J. Probl. Based Learning **13**(1), Article 4 (2019). https://doi.org/10.7771/1541-5015.1732
32. Røe, Y., Torbjørnsen, A.C.V., Admiraal, W.: Educators' digital competence in physiotherapy and health professions education: insights from qualitative interviews. Digital Health. **10**, 1 (2024). https://doi.org/10.1177/20552076241297044
33. Makkonen, K., Korpi, H., Sjögren, T.: Clinical reasoning competence of Finnish physiotherapy students: a cross-sectional study. Europ. J. Physiotherapy. **28**(1), 39–50 (2026). https://doi.org/10.1080/21679169.2025.2469104
34. Paakkari, L.: Widening horizons: a phenomenographic study of student teachers' conceptions of health education and its teaching and learning. Doctoral dissertation. University of Jyväskylä (2012)
35. Collier-Reed, B., Ingerman, Å.: Phenomenography: from critical aspects to knowledge claim. In: Tight, M., Huisman, J. (eds.) International Perspectives on Higher Education Research, Vol. 9. Emerald, pp. 243–260 (2013)
36. Åkerlind, G.S.: Growing and developing as a university researcher. High. Educ. **55**, 241–254 (2008)
37. Laitila, M., Pietilä, A.-M., Nikkonen, M.: Fenomenografinen lähestymistapa hoitotieteellisessä tutkimuksessa. Hoitotiede **24**(4), 258–270 (2012)

38. Tutkimuseettinen neuvottelukunta. Hyvä tieteellinen käytäntö ja sen loukkausepäilyjen käsitteleminen Suomessa 2023 (2023). Available from: https://tenk.fi/fi/ohjeet-ja-aineistot/htk-ohje
39. Tuomi, J., Sarajärvi, A.: Laadullinen tutkimus ja sisällönanalyysi. Tammi (2013)

SurgiVerse-6G: AI Surgical Intelligence for Education

Ricardo Zugaib Abdalla[1], Paulo Sergio Rufino Henrique[2,3]([✉]),
Wagner de Oliveira[4], Marco Antonio[4], Graça Bressan[4],
Pavlos I. Lazaridis[2], and Ramjee Prasad[3]

[1] Clinical Hospital of the Faculty of Medicine, University of São Paulo (FMUSP),
São Paulo, Brazil
`abdalla@hc.fm.usp.br`
[2] University of Huddersfield, Huddersfield, UK
`p.lazaridis@hud.ac.uk`
[3] CTIF Global Capsule, Paris, France
`{paulo,prasad.ramjee}@ctifglobalcapsule.org`
[4] University of São Paulo (USP),São Paulo, Brazil
`{wagner.de.oliveira,marco.sousa,graca.bressan}@usp.br`
`https://ctifglobalcapsule.org/`

Abstract. The launch of 6G around 2030 is expected to enable a hyperconnected society by uniting physical environments with the metaverse, in accordance with the United Nations Sustainable Development Goals (SDGs) and Japan Society 5.0 vision. This paper studies remote surgical training and support, both with and without robotic systems, and addresses the challenges presented by Brazil's extensive geography and regional inequalities. These limitations restrict access to specialised care and training in public hospitals and remote areas such as the Amazon, where shortages of medical specialists contribute to preventable mortality. This study draws on the experience of the Laboratory for Teaching, Research, and Innovation in Surgery (LEPIC) at the Hospital das Clínicas in São Paulo, where medical students are trained in advanced technologies, including robotics and telesurgery in simulated operating rooms. It also incorporates insights from ongoing projects on remote medical assistance in the Amazon, supported by 5G and Digital Health applications. The proposed framework, termed SurgiVerse 6G, is designed for high-impact and time-critical clinical scenarios, including obstetric emergencies, orthopaedic fractures, and laparoscopic surgical procedures. It leverages Terahertz communications, AI, and video-based ML to generate privacy-preserving semantic clinical and educational data. Supported by ultra-low-latency wireless infrastructure, AI-driven augmented reality, and UHD video transmission, the framework merges multimodal data to enable coordinated decision-making and distributed collaboration. This analysis presents a conceptual and architectural framework to improve clinical results and expand access to high-quality care and training in underserved zones.

M. Särestöniemi et al. (Eds.): NCDHWS 2026, CCIS 3009, pp. 478–487, 2026.
https://doi.org/10.1007/978-3-032-28812-7_33

Keywords: 6G · SurgiVerse · Medical Education · Semantic Video Search · Laparoscopy

1   Introduction

1.1   Challenges in Contemporary Surgical Training and Clinical Practice

6G aims to support the needs of a hyperconnected digital society by enabling seamless integration between physical and cyber environments [1]. 6G evolution aligns with the United Nations (UN) Sustainable Development Goals (SDGs) and the Japan Society 5.0 vision [2]. Within this context, 6G is expected to enable new forms of interaction through immersive environments, intelligent systems, and real-time data-driven services. This research addresses remote surgical training and remote surgical support, with and without the presence of robotic systems, while contributing to SDG goals (3) good health and well being, (4) quality of education, (9) industry, innovation and infrastructure, and (10) reduction of inequalities.

6G networks will enable terahertz communications and ultra-low latency below one millisecond, supporting real-time interaction in hyperconnected environments. These capabilities are critical for clinical applications that require precision and rapid decision-making, transforming surgical education and support.

Brazil presents a critical case due to its continental geography and diverse economic conditions across states. Providing well-distributed medical specialisation, high-quality training, and emergency surgical care remains a challenge. Many patients die due to the lack of trauma specialists or limited access to affordable and specialised procedures in public hospitals and remote regions such as the Amazon [3]. These challenges are worse in laparoscopy training, where proper learning and supervision are limited in the public health system (SUS) in Brazil, leading to preventable deaths.

This study builds on the experience of the Laboratory for Teaching, Research, and Innovation in Surgery (LEPIC) [4] at the Hospital das Clínicas in São Paulo, where medical students are trained using advanced technologies, including robotics and telesurgery in simulated operating rooms. These environments support minimally invasive surgery training, especially laparoscopy, which depends on visual skills and precision. SurgiVerse 6G builds on this by using artificial intelligence, video data, and telementoring to enable remote surgical training.

The need for remote surgical support is not new. Historical evidence illustrates early forms of remote assistance before the emergence of modern communication systems. During the Brazilian military dictatorship in the1960 s Dr Nagib Cury [5] performed a complex surgery outside his speciality with guidance by telephone. This example highlights the need for real-time expert support and the role of modern communication and artificial intelligence in preventing avoidable deaths.

Further evidence of the importance of remote and autonomous surgical capabilities is found in extreme environments such as space missions. Kirkpatrick et al., including trauma surgeon Dr Kenneth L Mattox, identified significant challenges in managing severe injuries during long-duration spaceflight in their work titled "Severe traumatic injury during long-duration spaceflight Light years beyond ATLS" [6]. The authors emphasise that future missions will require highly trained medical professionals capable of operating under constrained conditions with limited resources. These environments require advanced decision support and autonomy, highlighting the importance of intelligent connected medical platforms.

6G will support these applications through reliable high-speed communication beyond current fifth-generation capabilities, benefiting both space exploration and remote healthcare in underserved regions.

In this context, this paper proposes SurgiVerse 6G, a 6G-enabled surgical intelligence framework designed for remote education and clinical support in time-critical scenarios. The framework integrates Gigahertz and Terahertz wireless systems [7], artificial intelligence (AI), augmented reality (AR), ultra high definition (UHD) video, and video-based machine learning (ML) to enable real-time analysis and interaction. The initial focus is on laparoscopic interventions, extending to obstetric emergencies and trauma cases where rapid decisions and coordinated remote medical support are essential.

SurgiVerse 6G transforms surgical procedures into privacy-preserving and semantically structured clinical and educational data. By integrating multimodal data, the framework supports training and real-time assistance, with a focus on laparoscopy for minimally invasive surgery. It provides a conceptual and architectural approach to extend surgical expertise and improve access to care in underserved regions.

2   SurgiVerse 6G for Medical Education and Surgical Training

SurgiVerse 6G is proposed as an advanced framework for medical education and surgical training, extending established Minimally Invasive Surgery (MISS) training practices into a next generation digital and connected environment enabled by Sixth Generation (6G) wireless systems. The framework builds on core MISS elements such as structured video repositories, simulation based learning, and guided supervision, while introducing intelligent and immersive capabilities for remote surgical education.

At its foundation, SurgiVerse 6G integrates semantic Artificial Intelligence (AI) tagging based on medical corpora, cloud based video databases, Virtual Reality (VR) and Augmented Reality (AR) simulators, gamified learning approaches, and haptic feedback systems. Patient data protection is ensured through anonymization using UTF 8 (Unicode Transformation Format 8 bit) encoding standards, enabling compliance with the General Data Protection Regulation (GDPR) and the Brazilian Lei Geral de Proteção de Dados (LGPD).

The architecture incorporates terahertz communications to support Ultra High Definition (UHD) video and haptic data transmission, enabling immersive and precise interaction. AI and Machine Learning (ML) techniques enable privacy preserving semantic indexing and retrieval of surgical content. AR overlays provide real time telementoring support, enhancing both training and live surgical procedures.

The system processes multimodal inputs, including video, sensor data, and patient telemetry, through edge AI to ensure low-latency decision-making. This extends MISS telemetry into digital twin representations of surgical procedures, enabling real time monitoring, analysis, and feedback. The framework supports both robotic and non-robotic scenarios and enables remote supervision at scale, extending training capabilities from specialised centres such as the Laboratory for Teaching, Research, and Innovation in Surgery (LEPIC) to broader healthcare systems, including the Brazilian Unified Health System.

The educational model focuses on time-critical scenarios, particularly laparoscopic procedures and haemorrhage control, where low-latency communication enables accurate kinesthetic feedback and coordinated team interaction. During procedures, operating rooms are equipped with wireless UHD cameras and sensors that capture surgical activity and patient telemetry in real time. Procedures are recorded, structured, and semantically tagged to create searchable educational assets.

Successful procedures generate summary reports and indexed learning content, while unsuccessful cases are analysed with highlighted errors to support training and continuous improvement. An AI assistant provides real time guidance through audio and visual feedback displayed within the operating environment. The system operates over dedicated 6G network slices [8]using Ultra Reliable Low Latency Communications (URLLC), enabling high data rate transmission and real-time synchronisation between local and remote teams.

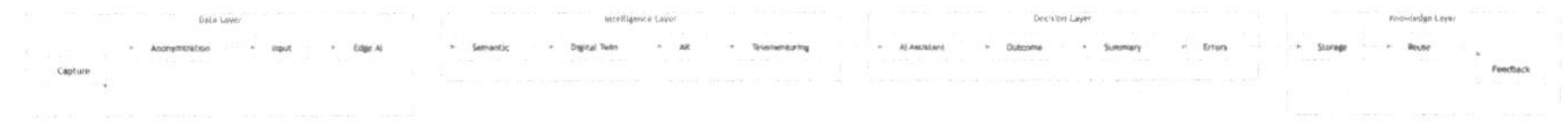

Fig. 1. Workflow of SurgiVerse 6G medical training

Figure 1 presents the horizontal workflow of the SurgiVerse 6G framework for medical training and surgical support. The process begins with data acquisition and anonymisation, followed by multimodal data integration and low-latency edge processing. The framework then applies artificial intelligence for semantic tagging and digital twin generation, enabling augmented reality guidance and remote telementoring. In the next stage, an artificial intelligence assistant supports decision-making during procedures, while outcomes are recorded, summarised, and analysed. Finally, the system stores data in the cloud, enabling knowledge reuse and a continuous feedback loop that enhances training and improves surgical performance over time.

Figure 2 illustrates a 3D conceptual representation of the SurgiVerse 6G AI Surgical Lab, where a surgical procedure is performed in a fully connected and intelligent operating environment. The scene highlights the integration of advanced medical equipment, ultra high definition cameras, and real time wireless communication, represented by visible signal exchanges between devices. The presence of the 6G infrastructure enables seamless data transmission and coordination across the surgical ecosystem. The environment emphasizes the role of artificial intelligence and connectivity in supporting surgical teams, enhancing precision, and enabling real time collaboration within a digitally augmented clinical setting.

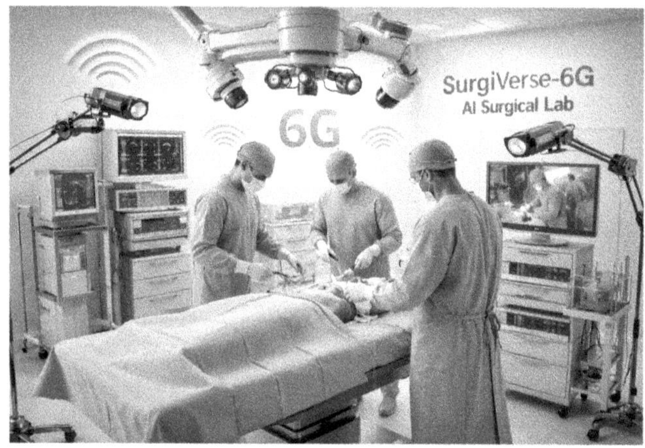

Fig. 2. 3D representation of the SurgiVerse 6G AI Surgical Lab

In summary, SurgiVerse 6G provides a scalable framework that combines advanced communication, artificial intelligence, and immersive technologies to enhance surgical training and support. By enabling real-time guidance and continuous learning, it has strong potential to improve clinical outcomes, particularly in underserved regions.

3   Cross Disciplinary Methodology

The development of **SurgiVerse 6G Framework** follows a cross-disciplinary methodology that draws on telecommunications, artificial intelligence, medical training, and clinical practice. The approach is structured into three progressive phases, ensuring a smooth transition from conceptual development to real-world validation. The methodology leverages Minimally Invasive Surgery (MISS) training frameworks, extended through Sixth Generation devices.

A critical enabler of this methodology is the use of *6G Ultra Reliable Low Latency Communications* (6G-URLLC), which provides ultra-low latency below one millisecond, high data throughput, and enhanced security. These capabilities are essential for supporting time-critical surgical applications, where real-time responsiveness, reliable communication, and secure transmission of sensitive medical data are required. The combination of URLLC with advanced network slicing mechanisms ensures deterministic performance, enabling precise coordination between surgical teams, remote experts, and intelligent systems.

In the first phase, existing MISS prototypes are adapted to 6G simulation environments. This includes the use of three-dimensional organ reconstruction, Natural Language Processing (NLP) based interaction, and structured surgical video datasets derived from the Laboratory for Teaching, Research, and Innovation in Surgery (LEPIC). The objective is to establish a controlled environment in which advanced communication and intelligence capabilities supported by URLLC can be evaluated without clinical risk.

The second phase focuses on experimental validation through pilot deployments in 6G testbeds in collaboration with University of São Paulo (USP) partners. During this stage, the framework is evaluated with a cohort of 100 trainees, including both medical and non-medical participants. Performance is assessed using the *Objective Structured Assessment of Technical Skills* (OSATS), enabling quantitative evaluation of skill acquisition, procedural understanding, and decision-making under simulated and assisted conditions. The high throughput and low latency characteristics of 6G networks are critical to ensure seamless interaction, real-time feedback, and synchronisation across distributed environments.

The third phase extends the framework into real clinical environments through multicenter trials across the *Brazilian Unified Health System* (SUS) and remote regions such as the Amazon. This phase evaluates system performance under operational constraints, including communication latency below one millisecond, secure data exchange, skill transfer effectiveness, and clinical outcomes compared to conventional approaches. Ethical approval is obtained through the Faculty of Medicine, University of São Paulo (FMUSP) Institutional Review

Table 1. Cross Disciplinary Methodology for SurgiVerse 6G

Phase	Timeline	Description
Phase 1	Year 1	Adapt MISS prototypes to 6G simulations using LEPIC data, including 3D organ reconstruction and NLP interaction, supported by URLLC for low latency evaluation.
Phase 2	Years 2–3	Deploy pilot 6G testbeds with USP partners and evaluate 100 trainees using OSATS metrics, leveraging high throughput and real time feedback enabled by 6G.
Phase 3	Year 4	Conduct multicenter trials in SUS and Amazon regions, evaluating latency, security, skill transfer, procedural accuracy, and complication rates under real conditions.

Board (IRB). Key evaluation metrics include procedural accuracy, complication rates, and the ability to capture and integrate data from interconnected medical devices alongside patient physiological signals.

Table 1 outlines the cross disciplinary methodology for SurgiVerse 6G across three phases. The first phase focuses on adapting MISS prototypes into 6G simulation environments using LEPIC data, enabling controlled evaluation of advanced techniques and URLLC. The second phase introduces pilot testbeds with USP partners, where 100 trainees are assessed using OSATS to measure performance and real-time feedback supported by 6G. The third phase extends the framework to clinical settings within SUS and the Amazon, evaluating latency, security, skill transfer, procedural accuracy, and complication rates under real conditions.

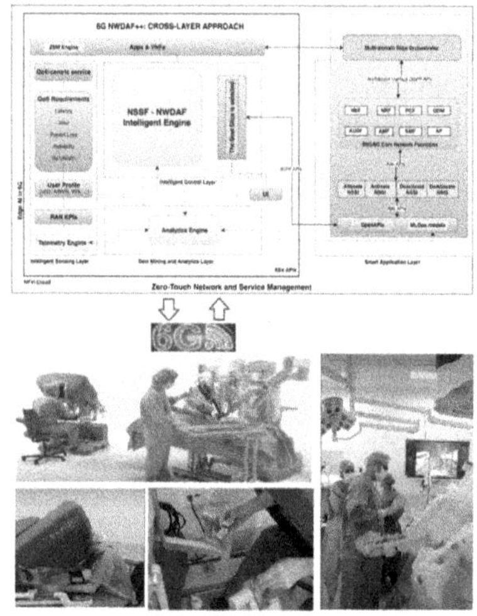

Fig. 3. 6G NWDAF SurgiVerse Framework

Figure 3 illustrates the 6G Network Data Analytics Function (NWDAF) enabled SurgiVerse framework, presenting an integrated architecture that combines communication, artificial intelligence (AI), and network orchestration for real-time surgical applications. At the upper layer, the Sixth Generation (6G) Network Slice Function provides dedicated connectivity, tightly coupled with the Video Semantic AI module and telemetry engine within the Network Slice Selection Function (NSSF). A Network Slice Selector, accessible via Third Generation Partnership Project (3GPP) Application Programming Interfaces (APIs), enables multidomain orchestration through Machine Learning Operations (MLOps) models, including OpenAI models, within a Zero Touch Network and Service Management (ZSM) environment.

At the application layer, Ultra High Definition (UHD) wireless cameras capture and transmit real-time surgical video streams, ensuring seamless data flow across the surgical ecosystem. The NSSF DAF++ (Network Slice Selection Function Decision-Aid Framework Plus) solution is inherently versatile, supporting integration with Internet of Things (IoT) data and cloud services, and enabling specialised network slicing, including FeMBB (enhanced mobile broadband), mMTC (ultra-massive machine-to-machine communication), and eURLLC (extremely reliable low-latency communication).

This work extends the NSSF DAF++ framework to address 6G-specific requirements, including support for Cloud Radio Access Network (C-RAN) Key Performance Indicators (KPIs), integration of MLOps pipelines, and deployment of intelligent agents within the SurgiVerse environment. Operating in the centimetre wave (cmWave) spectrum (100–1000 GHz), the framework enables near-zero latency (microseconds) and ultra-high data rates, critical for real-time medical applications.

As depicted in Fig. 3, 6G networks incorporate native AI capabilities to enhance diagnostic accuracy and automate minimally invasive surgical procedures, while balancing wide-area coverage with high-bandwidth support for robotic operations. The framework transforms surgical processes into structured, privacy-preserving clinical and educational data streams. Through multimodal data integration, it enables advanced video semantics, encompassing understanding, segmentation, and context-aware content generation, facilitating real-time interaction and training for medical professionals.

Finally, the framework supports dynamic evaluation and adaptation of Quality of Service (QoS), Quality of Experience (QoE), and RAN KPIs across heterogeneous services, user profiles, and specialised network segments.

4   Expected Outcomes

SurgiVerse 6G is expected to enhance access to Minimally Invasive Surgery (MISS) training and support through 6G-enabled telementoring, particularly in remote and resource-constrained operating rooms. By leveraging ultra-low latency communication, real-time guidance, and semantically structured surgical knowledge, the framework aims to improve procedural accuracy and decision-making. A key projected outcome is the reduction of preventable mortality, targeting improvements of up to 50 per cent in critical surgical scenarios, in line with MISS performance benchmarks. The framework is designed to be scalable across global low-resource settings and is supported by open-source semantic tools that enable interoperability, broader adoption, and continuous knowledge sharing.

5   Conclusions and Future Work

SurgiVerse 6G presents several challenges related to deploying 6G infrastructure, particularly in underserved regions, as well as to data privacy and secure transmission in terahertz communication environments. Ensuring reliable and compliant handling of sensitive medical data remains a critical requirement.

Future work will focus on integrating the Industrial Internet of Medical Things (IIoMT) to enable predictive analytics based on real-time patient data and surgical performance metrics. In addition, the framework will be extended towards full robotic telesurgery, enabling higher levels of automation and precision, while further validating its effectiveness across diverse clinical environments.

Disclosure of Interests. This study was partially financed by ICESP (Cancer Institute of the State of São Paulo), LEPIC (Laboratory for Teaching, Research and Innovation in Surgery) of the Faculty of Medicine of the University of São Paulo (FMUSP), Brazil, and by the Coordenação de Aperfeiçoamento de Pessoal de Nível Superior - Brasil (CAPEX/PROEX - Doutorando do PPGEE da POLI-USP).

References

1. International Telecommunication Union, "Focus: The 5G era and beyond, ITU Journal on Future and Evolving Technologies, vol. 1(1) (2020). https://www.itu.int/pub/S-ITUJNL-JFETS.V1I1-9-2020. Accessed: 8 Apr 8 2026
2. Cabinet Office of Japan, Society 5.0, Council for Science, Technology and Innovation, Japan. https://www8.cao.go.jp/cstp/english/society5_0/index.html. Accessed 7 Apr 2026
3. De Angelis, M., et al.: Artificial intelligence for surgical video analysis: a comprehensive review. Sensors**23**(2), Art. no. 1047 (2023). https://doi.org/10.3390/s23021047
4. ABC News, Doctor robot perform telesurgery on patient thousands of miles away, ABC News Video. https://abcnews.go.com/Technology/video/doctor-robot-perform-telesurgery-patient-thousands-miles-122914343
5. Jornal da USP, "Cirurgia para correção do peito de sapateiro: uma história de inovação e colaboração. Jornal da USP, 25 Sept. (2023). https://jornal.usp.br/artigos/cirurgia-para-correcao-do-peito-de-sapateiro-uma-historia-de-inovacao-e-colaboracao/. Accessed 31 Jan 2026
6. Kirkpatrick, A.W., et al.: Severe traumatic injury during long duration spaceflight: light years beyond ATLS. World J. Emergency Surgery **3**(4) (2009). https://pubmed.ncbi.nlm.nih.gov/19320976/. Accessed 28 Jan 2026
7. Henrique, P.S.R., Prasad, R.: 6G: The Road to the Future Wireless Technologies 2030. River Publishers, Herning, Denmark (Mar 2021), ISBN: 9788770224390
8. Da Silva, D.C., et al.: NSSF function in 6G networks based on MLOps deployment model. In: Proc. 2024 27th Int. Symp. Wireless Personal Multimedia Communications (WPMC), Greater Noida, India, pp. 1–6 (2024). https://doi.org/10.1109/WPMC63271.2024.10863370. https://ieeexplore.ieee.org/document/10863370

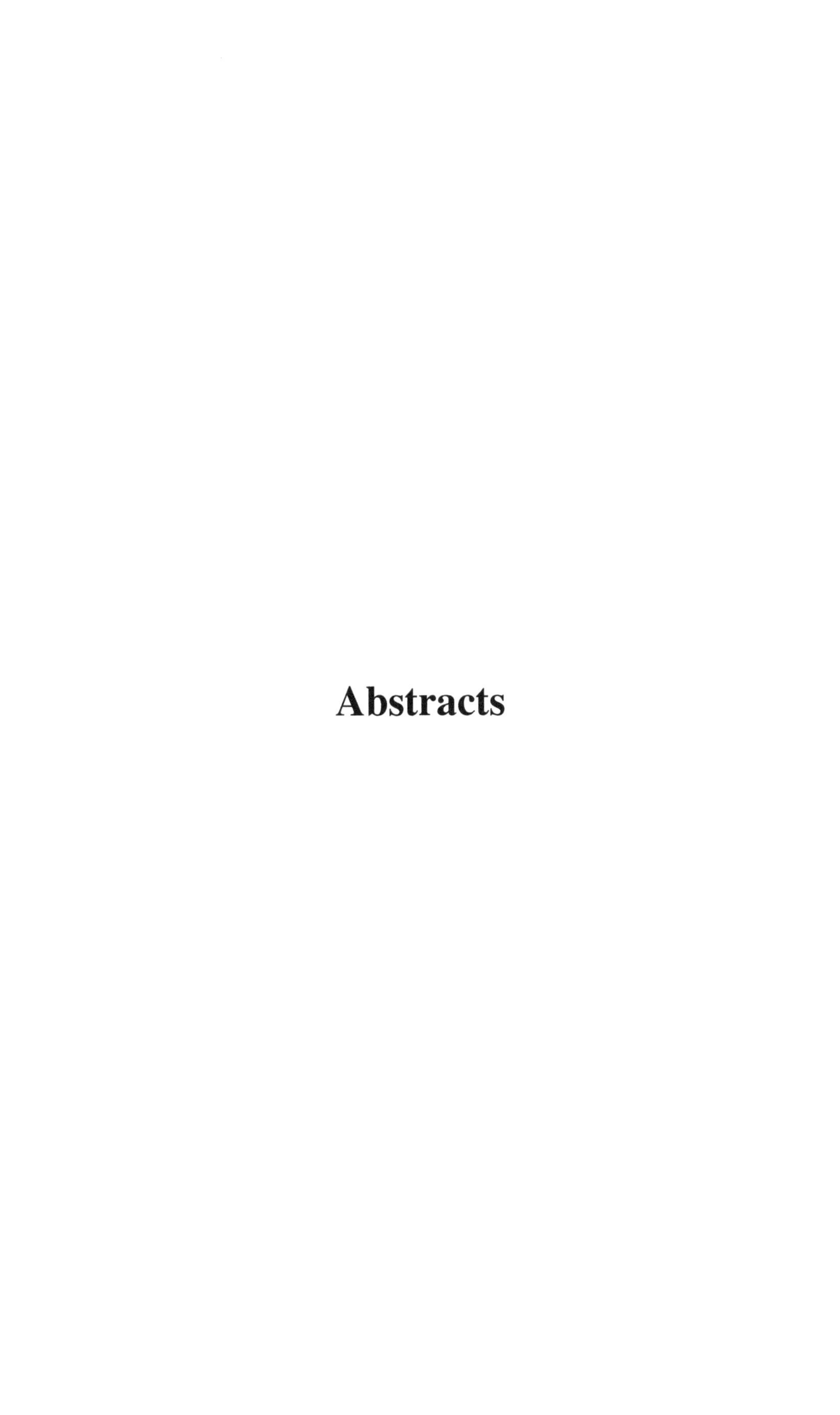

Abstracts

Toward Standardized Quality Evaluation of Synthetic Health Data for the European Health Data Space

Aino-Lotta I. Alahäivälä[1]($\boxtimes$) , Tunc Asuroglu[2] , Juha Pajula[2] ,
Ileana Montoya Perez[3] , Tapio Pahikkala[3] , and Antti Airola[3]

[1] VTT Technical Research Centre of Finland, Microkatu 1, 70211 Kuopio, Finland
`aino.alahaivala@vtt.fi`
[2] VTT Technical Research Centre of Finland, Visiokatu 4, 33720 Tampere, Finland
[3] Department of Computing, University of Turku, 20014 Turku, Finland

Abstract. Research and development in healthcare, including early-stage research, testing, and demonstrational data catalogues, is significantly hindered by strict data use restrictions imposed by regulations such as GDPR and HIPAA. Acquiring high-quality, real-world health data is often expensive and labor-intensive for researchers, data owners, and companies. Synthetic data (SD) has emerged as a complementary approach, aiming to improve data accessibility while addressing privacy and regulatory constraints. Unlike traditional anonymization methods for real-world health data, SD generation enables controlled trade-offs between data quality and privacy, depending on the data type and intended use. However, despite rapid methodological advances, there is no consensus on how SD quality should be evaluated across modalities, purposes of use, and intended use cases. Data privacy is often compromised by the high fidelity or resemblance of the SD, and vice versa; therefore, the selection of metrics and evaluation thresholds should be carefully considered and tailored to the specific purpose of use and use case [1]. Current literature lacks standardized, use-case–aware quality evaluation and reporting, limiting comparability and regulatory interpretability [2]. Typically, health data authorities have no standardized criteria for reporting synthetic data quality within their evaluation frameworks, as their primary focus here is on data anonymization.

We aim to provide a representative guiding approach within the PHASE IV AI (Privacy Compliant Health Data as A Service for AI Development) project [3]. This approach focuses primarily on synthetic tabular health data, expected to be in high demand in the early phases of European Health Data Space (EHDS) implementation, through data-type-dependent quality assessment frameworks applied across representative use cases. Use cases besides tabular are included in an exploratory role to assess the feasibility and limitations of extending quality evaluation principles beyond tabular data, with implications for harmonized reporting under the EHDS.

We will use multiple healthcare datasets covering key data types to evaluate SD generation and quality assessment approaches. The framework development follows a design science research approach, iteratively designing the framework, instantiating it through representative use cases, and empirically evaluating it using

© The Author(s) 2026
M. Särestöniemi et al. (Eds.): NCDHWS 2026, CCIS 3009, pp. 491–492, 2026.
https://doi.org/10.1007/978-3-032-28812-7

established quality metrics. Validation is conducted by applying the framework across use cases, assessing its ability to consistently capture fidelity, utility, and privacy trade-offs and to support transparent, comparable quality reporting. The quality framework will be established and evaluated primarily through tabular electronic health record use cases (e.g., prostate cancer data). Selected medical image use cases (lung cancer and ischemic stroke) are used to explore the transferability and limitations of the proposed quality evaluation dimensions across modalities. The aim is to establish a framework for each use case and data modality that addresses fidelity, utility, and privacy. Widely accepted and well-established metrics will be employed to assess quality across these dimensions [4, 5].

The lack of a gold-standard quality evaluation framework remains a critical barrier, particularly across heterogeneous data types. Given that SD quality assessment is inherently dependent on data type and purpose of use, we propose a harmonized evaluation structure that is immediately applicable to tabular data using standard statistical and privacy metrics. The aim is to provide a foundation that can be incrementally extended to more complex modalities and task-specific metrics as EHDS infrastructure matures. This approach aligns with anticipated early EHDS secondary use needs, while preserving methodological extensibility and supporting development of harmonized SD quality reporting guidelines within the PHASE IV AI project.

Heterogeneity poses challenges for secondary use of synthetic health data under the EHDS, where comparability and auditability are essential. We propose that harmonized quality reporting—built on common evaluation dimensions, while allowing data type- and use case-specific metrics—could address these challenges across EU Member States. Within the EHDS, standardized SD quality documentation could support secondary data use, facilitate cross-border data sharing, and contribute to data protection impact assessments. SD, regardless of modality and strengthened by a robust quality framework, serves as a trusted complementary approach for research and development in a strictly regulated health data environment. In this context, our aim is to establish a starting point for standardized SD quality evaluation, which can be further adapted as a baseline for the EHDS.

Keywords: Synthetic Data · Data Quality Evaluation · Standardized Reporting · European Health Data Space · Secondary Use of Health Data · Regulatory Compliance

References

1. Adams, T., et al.: On the fidelity versus privacy and utility trade-off of synthetic patient data. iScience **28**(5) (2025)
2. Belgodere, B., et al.: Auditing and generating synthetic data with controllable trust trade-offs. IEEE J. Emerg. Sel. Top. Circuits Syst. **14**(4), 773–788 (2024)
3. PHASE IV AI — Privacy Compliant Health Data as a service for AI development. Homepage. https://www.phase4ai-project.eu/. Accessed 22 Jan 2026
4. Hernadez, M., Epelde, G., Alberdi, A., Cilla, R., Rankin, D.: Synthetic tabular data evaluation in the health domain covering resemblance, utility, and privacy dimensions. Methods Inf. Med. **62**(2), E19–E38 (2023)
5. Figueira, A., Vaz. B.: Survey on synthetic data generation, evaluation methods and GANs. Mathematics **10**(15), 2733 (2022)

Cost-Effectiveness of a Metabolomic Risk Score-Based Health Check Combined with a Digital Health Intervention for Cardiometabolic Disease Prevention in Finland

Piia Lavikainen[1]([📧]) [iD], Leena Haikonen-Salo[1] [iD], Aku-Ville Lehtimäki[1] [iD], Kari Jalkanen[1] [iD], Jari Heiskanen[1] [iD], Tiina Laatikainen[2,3] [iD], and Janne Martikainen[1] [iD]

[1] School of Pharmacy, University of Eastern Finland, Kuopio, Finland
`piia.lavikainen@uef.fi`
[2] Institute of Public Health and Clinical Nutrition, University of Eastern Finland, Kuopio, Finland
[3] Wellbeing Services County of North Karelia (Siun Sote), Joensuu, Finland

Abstract. This study used microsimulation modelling to examine the cost-effectiveness of metabolomic risk score-based proactive prevention of cardiometabolic diseases compared with current Finnish practices. Because metabolomics can be derived from a standard blood sample, it enables efficient risk assessment while reducing the time required from healthcare professionals. Metabolomic risk score-based health checks were consistently cost-saving compared with current practices. Among adults aged 50–54, this approach identified cardiometabolic risk more efficiently, saved up to €298 million when combined with enhanced prevention including digital health intervention, and improved quality-adjusted life years in most scenarios, demonstrating strong potential for use in both primary and occupational care.

Keywords: Cost-Effectiveness · Cardiometabolic Disease · Metabolomic Risk Score · Digital Lifestyle Intervention

1 Introduction

Cardiometabolic diseases (CMDs), such as coronary heart disease, stroke, and type 2 diabetes (T2D), are major global health and economic challenges [1, 2]. Healthcare has traditionally been reactive, but growing evidence underscores the importance of proactive prevention, early risk identification, and lifestyle intervention [3, 4]. Predictive metabolomics enables risk assessment from standard blood samples, offering a more efficient approach [5]. This study evaluated the long-term cost-effectiveness of a metabolomic risk score (MRS)-based health check (HC) compared with current practice in Finland's working-age population.

© The Author(s) 2026
M. Särestöniemi et al. (Eds.): NCDHWS 2026, CCIS 3009, pp. 493–495, 2026.
https://doi.org/10.1007/978-3-032-28812-7

2   Materials and Methods

Cost-effectiveness was assessed using an individual-level microsimulation model based on synthetic data from 256,372 Finnish adults aged 50–54 without prior CVD or T2D (see Fig. 1). Three scenarios were assessed: 1) standard HC replaced with MRS-based HC, 2) standard HC replaced with MRS-based HC plus enhanced prevention, and 3) standard HC plus enhanced prevention compared with MRS-based HC plus enhanced prevention. The MRS was derived from nuclear magnetic resonance spectroscopy-based metabolomic biomarkers [6]. Standard HC targeted key risk factors, such as high blood pressure, hyperlipidemia, and smoking, whereas the enhanced prevention arm applied stricter thresholds and included a 12-month interactive web-based digital intervention addressing diet, physical activity, psychological factors, and stress management. Long-term cost-effectiveness was evaluated using literature-based health-state costs and quality-of-life weights to estimate cumulative costs and quality-adjusted life years (QALYs), which were then used to calculate the incremental cost-effectiveness ratios (ICERs) per QALY gained between the study arms.

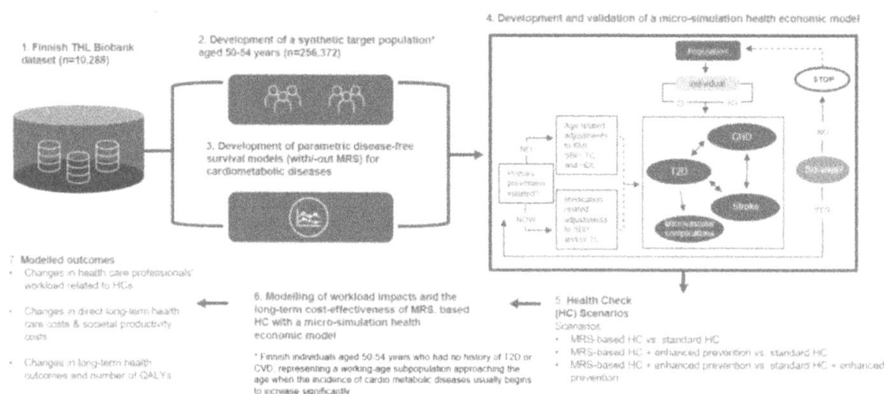

Fig. 1. General workflow of the health economic model development.

3   Results and Discussion

The MRS-based approach was cost-saving in all scenarios. Compared with standard HC, MRS-based HC led to discounted long-term savings of €26 million over the study period. Adding enhanced prevention including digital health intervention to MRS-based HC increased the discounted long-term savings up to €298 million compared with standard HC. In scenarios 1–2, it also improved QALYs, resulting in discounted gains ranging from 2017 to 8550 QALYs. In scenario 3, no QALY gains were observed, and minor losses occurred due to differences in baseline risk stratification.

The findings indicate that MRS-based HC offers a cost-saving alternative for identifying elevated cardiometabolic risk. Savings arise largely from faster, less resource-intensive risk assessment combined with diagnostic performance comparable to existing tools. Early risk detection paired with enhanced preventive measures produced the greatest combined health and economic benefits. Even if current practices were fully optimized MRS-based strategies would still be expected to reduce costs with only small differences in health outcomes.

The evaluation also captures only part of the potential value of MRS testing. The same metabolomic platform provides risk estimates for multiple preventable diseases beyond CVD and T2D, suggesting broader utility for supporting early detection and preventing multimorbidity. This is consistent with its growing use in Finnish occupational healthcare for identifying individuals with elevated risks across several disease categories.

4 Conclusions

Simulations indicate that MRS-based health checks in primary and occupational care are a cost-saving strategy for identifying individuals at risk for cardiometabolic diseases. Enhanced prevention, including digital interventions, may further increase both health benefits and cost savings.

Acknowledgments. The study was financially supported by Nightingale Health Plc.

Disclosure of Interests.   JM is a founding partner of ESiOR Oy. This company was not involved in carrying out this research. PL, LH-S, AVL, KJ, JH, and TL have no competing interests to declare that are relevant to the content of this article.

References

1. OECD. Cardiovascular Disease and Diabetes: Policies for Better Health and Quality of Care. (OECD, 2015). https://doi.org/10.1787/9789264233010-en
2. Institute for Health Metrics and Evaluation (IHME). Global Burden of Disease 2021: Findings from the GBD 2021 Study. (Institute for Health Metrics and Evaluation (IHME), Seattle, WA, 2024)
3. Knowler, W.C., et al.: Diabetes prevention program research group: reduction in the incidence of type 2 diabetes with lifestyle intervention or metformin. N. Engl. J. Med. **346**, 393–403 (2002)
4. Tuomilehto, J., et al.: Finnish diabetes prevention study group: prevention of type 2 diabetes mellitus by changes in lifestyle among subjects with impaired glucose tolerance. N. Engl. J. Med. **344**, 1343–1350 (2001)
5. Buergel, T., et al.: Metabolomic profiles predict individual multidisease outcomes. Nat. Med. **28**, 2309–2320 (2022)
6. Nightingale Health Biobank Collaborative Group, et al.: Metabolomic and genomic prediction of common diseases in 700,217 participants in three national biobanks. Nat. Commun. **15**, 10092 (2024)

A Telemedicine Pathway for Secondary Prevention in Coronary Artery Disease: Real-World Implementation

Outi Haggren[1]([✉]) [iD], Jari Laukkanen[1,5], Anna-Mari Hekkala[3], Sinikka Yli-Mäyry[4], Jaakko Immonen[5], Johanna Keränen[6], Kari Ylitalo[2], and Kari Kaikkonen[2]

[1] School of Medicine, Institute of Clinical Medicine, University of Eastern Finland, Kuopio, Finland
`outi.haggren@fimnet.fi`
[2] Research Unit of Biomedicine and Internal Medicine, Medical Research Center (MRC) Oulu, Oulu University Hospital and University of Oulu, Oulu, Finland
[3] The Finnish Heart Association, Oulu, Finland
[4] Faculty of Medicine and Health Technology, Tampere University, Heart Hospital, Tampere University Hospital, Tampere, Finland
[5] Department of Internal Medicine, Wellbeing Services County of Central Finland, Jyväskylä, Finland
[6] Department of Cardiology, Oulu University Hospital, North Ostrobothnia Wellbeing Services County (Pohde), Oulu, Finland

Abstract. Secondary prevention for coronary artery disease (CAD) remains challenging in routine practice, with suboptimal achievement of guideline-based risk-factor targets and low participation in traditional in-person cardiac rehabilitation programs. This study describes the real-world implementation of an integrated telemedicine pathway embedded in routine care and evaluates its feasibility and effectiveness. The pathway combines remote follow-up, structured eLearning, systematic risk-factor monitoring, and medication optimisation. In a retrospective, longitudinal, registry-based observational cohort of patients undergoing coronary angiography, 1130 patients were diagnosed with CAD, of whom 516 (46%) were referred to the DCP; high enrolment and low dropout indicated strong feasibility. Telemedicine-supported care improved blood pressure, LDL-cholesterol, and smoking cessation, while weight and glycaemic control showed limited improvement, highlighting the need for more intensive digital lifestyle support in these domains.

Keywords: Telemedicine · Remote Healthcare · eRehabilitation · Digital Healthcare Pathways · Secondary Prevention · Chronic Disease Management · Real-World Implementation · Coronary Artery Disease

1 Introduction

Despite robust evidence and guidelines [1], achievement of recommended secondary prevention targets in CAD remains low, and participation in traditional in-person cardiac rehabilitation programs is limited [2]. Barriers include service access, fragmented

© The Author(s) 2026
M. Särestöniemi et al. (Eds.): NCDHWS 2026, CCIS 3009, pp. 496–498, 2026.
https://doi.org/10.1007/978-3-032-28812-7

follow-up, delayed treatment optimisation, and insufficient self-management support. Telemedicine solutions can address these challenges [3], but many digital models are not fully integrated into clinical workflows. To overcome these limitations, the cardiac department at Oulu University Hospital in Finland developed an integrated digital care pathway (DCP) combining telemedicine follow-up, eLearning, remote monitoring, and medication optimization.

2   Materials and Methods/Study Scenario

This retrospective, longitudinal, registry-based observational cohort included patients with newly diagnosed or established CAD undergoing coronary angiography between February 2022 and July 2023. During the study period, 1130 such patients were identified, of whom 516 (46%) with sufficient digital skills were referred to the DCP as part of routine care. A total of 452 patients were enrolled, with follow-up completion rates of 98% at 6 months and 87% at 12 months. The pathway was delivered via a national digital health platform, replacing most in-person visits, and comprised remote follow-up, digital learning, laboratory monitoring, patient-reported outcomes, coordinated care, and an optional rehabilitation programme (TULPPA) (Fig. 1). Routine monitoring was nurse-led, with cardiologist oversight when guideline targets were unmet. Outcomes were assessed against 2021 ESC secondary prevention targets [4].

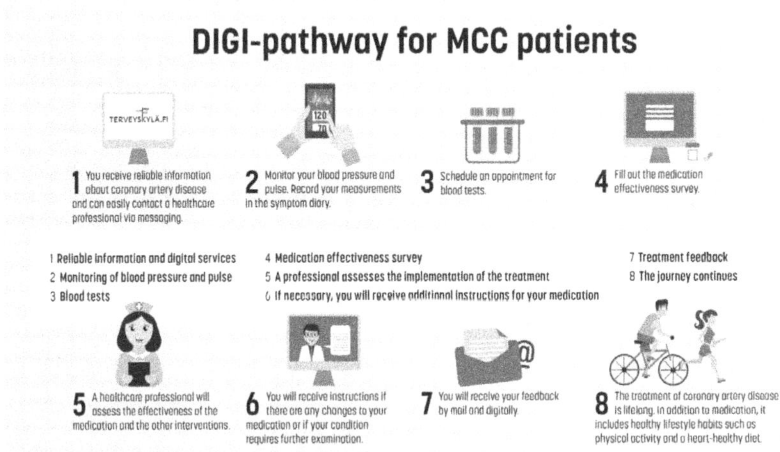

Fig. 1. Key components of the digital care pathway for secondary prevention in coronary artery disease.

3   Results and Discussion

DCP participation was associated with significant improvements in major cardiovascular risk factors. Mean blood pressure decreased markedly, with the proportion achieving <130/80 mmHg increasing from 33% at baseline to 62% at 12 months (p < 0.05).

LDL-cholesterol declined substantially, with attainment of <1.4 mmol/L rising from 11% to 59% (p < 0.05). Smoking prevalence decreased from 22% to 10% (p < 0.05). In contrast, BMI showed no clinically meaningful change (28.7 to 28.4 kg/m^2). Among patients with diabetes, the proportion achieving HbA1c < 53 mmol/mol increased from 63% to 72% (p = 0.07). As this was a real-world observational study without a control group, causality cannot be confirmed. The pathway's effectiveness appears to be driven by structured remote monitoring, eLearning, timely medication titration, and continuity across sectors, consistent with recommendations for comprehensive cardiac rehabilitation [4]. Persistent challenges in weight and glucose control underscore the need for improved digital lifestyle and eRehabilitation components providing nutrition, exercise, and psychosocial support.

4 Conclusions

A telemedicine pathway integrated into routine care was associated with improved control of key risk factors in CAD secondary prevention. While blood pressure, LDL-cholesterol, and smoking improved, persistent challenges in obesity and glycaemic control highlight the need for more advanced digital lifestyle support. Taken together, these findings support the integration of scalable telemedicine and eRehabilitation models into modern CAD secondary prevention.

References

1. Visseren, F.L.J., Mach, F., Smulders, Y.M., Carballo, D., Koskinas, K.C., Bäck, M., et al.: 2021 ESC Guidelines on cardiovascular disease prevention in clinical practice. Eur. Heart J. **42**, 3227–3337 (2021)
2. Kotseva, K., De Backer, G., De Bacquer, D., Rydén, L., Hoes, A., Grobbee, D., et al.: Lifestyle and impact on cardiovascular risk factor control in coronary patients across 27 countries: EUROASPIRE V. Eur. J. Prev. Cardiol. **26**, 824–835 (2019)
3. Shi, W., Green, H., Sikhosana, N., Fernandez, R.: Effectiveness of telehealth cardiac Rehabilitation Programs. J. Cardiopulm. Rehabil. Prev. **44**, 15–25 (2024)
4. Brown, T.M., et al.: Update. Circulation **2024**, 150 (2024)

Decreased Call Volumes and High Satisfaction Observed After Opening the Digital Social and Health Care Center (DSHCC) of Wellbeing Services County of North Karelia – Siun Sote, Finland

Nora Tarvus[1,2](✉) (iD), Mika Kortelainen[3,4], Paulus Torkki[2] (iD), Mikael Ripatti[1], Marjo-Riikka Huppunen-Vänskä[1], and Enni Sanmark[2] (iD)

[1] Wellbeing Services County of North Karelia – Siun sote, Tikkamäentie 16, 80210 Joensuu, Finland
nora.tarvus@gmail.com
[2] Faculty of Medicine, University of Helsinki, Tukholmankatu 8, 00290 Helsinki, Finland
[3] Department of Economics, University of Turku, Rehtorinpellonkatu 3, 20500 Turku, Finland
[4] THL Finnish Institute for Health and Welfare, Mannerheimintie 166, 00280 Helsinki, Finland

Abstract.

Background: Previous research shows that digital services achieve high patient satisfaction [1–6], improve treatment adherence, standardize care needs assessment [7], and provide safety and quality comparable to in-person services [5, 6, 8, 9]. However, evidence from Finnish primary healthcare remains limited [10]. This retrospective study evaluated the centralized Digital Social and Health Care Center (DSHCC) in the Wellbeing services county of North Karelia – Siun sote, describing chat service use and user demographics, reasons for contact, patient and staff satisfaction, resolution rates, and whether predefined targets were met.

Methods: Data on chat volumes, user demographics, and patient satisfaction were extracted from platform provider reports (1 April 2024 – 30 September 2025). Staff satisfaction in the DSHCC and primary care centers was analyzed for the corresponding period. Reasons for contact and repeat visits were assessed using electronic health record statistics, and call volumes to primary care centers and the out-of-hours medical helpline were analyzed using call system data (1 January 2023–30 September 2025).

Results: There were 55 147 chats during the observation period. The chat service was utilized across all municipalities in North Karelia and by all age groups. Calls to primary care centers declined by 22.2% between Q3/2023 and Q3/2025 (131 918 vs 102 665). Most patients of the DSHCC did not recontact for the same issue within 2 days (94.1%) or within 14 days (79.5%). Mean patient satisfaction was 4.4/5, and mean professional satisfaction was 4.0/5. Reasons for contact were diverse. The DSHCC achieved predefined targets.

Conclusions: Digital services may be associated with decreased call volumes

© The Author(s) 2026
M. Särestöniemi et al. (Eds.): NCDHWS 2026, CCIS 3009, pp. 499–500, 2026.
https://doi.org/10.1007/978-3-032-28812-7

alongside high patient and professional satisfaction and effective issue resolution. Similar results might be possible in other wellbeing services counties as well but more data is needed.

Keywords: Telemedicine · Primary Care · Digital Health Transformation

References

1. Härkönen, H., Lakoma, S., Verho, A., et al.: Impact of digital services on healthcare and social welfare: an umbrella review. Int. J. Nurs. Stud. **152**, 104692 (2024)
2. Metsäniemi, P., Sanmark, E.: Mitä tiedämme etävastaanottojen vaikuttavuudesta ja turvallisuudesta? Suom. Lääkäril. **80**, e43465 (2025)
3. Leighton, C., Cooper, A., Porter, A., et al.: Effectiveness and safety of asynchronous telemedicine consultations in general practice: A systematic review. BJGP Open 8(1), BJGPO.2023 (2024)
4. Wec, A., Gleason, K.T., Peereboom, D., et al.: Measurement, drivers, and outcomes of patient-initiated secure messaging use and intensity: A scoping review. JAMIA Open 8(4) (2025)
5. Laukka, E., Jansson, M., Suonnansalo, P., et al.: Effectiveness of interactive digital health services in non-communicable diseases: an umbrella review and evidence synthesis from 26 meta-analyses. Int. J. Nurs. Stud. **174**, 105277 (2026)
6. Ferre, F., Furelau, P., Labaste, F.: Medical-economic and ecological impact of anesthesia teleconsultation: retrospective observational study. JMIR Form. Res. **9**, e70259 (2025)
7. Koskela, T., Kunnamo, I.: Digitaaliset työkalut yleislääkärin tukena. Suom. Lääkäril. **76**(46), 2708–2712 (2021)
8. Dahlberg, A., Jukarainen, S., Kaartinen, T., Orre, P.: Cost minimization analysis of digital-first healthcare pathways in primary care. NPJ Digit. Med. **8**, 546 (2025)
9. Chow, A., et al.: Teledermatology: an evidence map of systematic reviews. Syst. Rev. **13**, 258 (2024)
10. Haaga, T., Herzig, M., Kortelainen, M., et al.: Digitaalisten terveyspalvelujen käyttö, käyttäjät, tuotanto ja vaikuttavuus: esiselvitys. Sosiaali- ja terveysministeriö, Helsinki (2024). ISBN 978-952-00-5665-0

Use of a Gamified Tool for the Promotion of Physical Activity and the Reduction of Obesity in Young Adults

Maria João Trigueiro[✉] (iD), Guilherme Pinto, José Nunes,
Raquel Simões de Almeida (iD), and Vítor Simões-Silva (iD)

LabRP/CIR, E2S, Polytechnic of Porto, Porto, Portugal
mjtrigueiro@ess.ipp.pt

Abstract. Obesity in young adults is a growing public health crisis, frequently associated with sedentary lifestyles consolidated during the transition to higher education. This work describes the development of "OBSCURA: Urban Mystery", a serious game designed to promote physical activity through meaningful gamification and immersive narrative. Unlike traditional fitness apps that rely on extrinsic rewards, this approach utilizes a mystery-driven story where physical effort becomes a "narrative necessity," fostering intrinsic motivation. The methodology utilizes internal smartphone sensors (GPS and accelerometer) to transform real physical effort into in-game progress, eliminating the need for external hardware. Grounded in the ARCS model of motivational design, the tool seeks to ensure long-term engagement by aligning attention, relevance, confidence, and satisfaction with health goals. It is expected that this approach will increase exercise adherence and improve anthropometric indicators such as BMI. Preliminary validation will follow a pilot quasi-experimental design with a single-group pre-post test assessment (n = 30) to evaluate the feasibility, retention rates, and impact on participants' physical activity levels.

Keywords: Obesity · Young Adults · Gamification · mHealth · Physical Activity

1 Introduction

Obesity prevalence has tripled over the last four decades, becoming a critical public health crisis and a primary risk factor for systemic comorbidities [1]. This scenario is particularly alarming in young adults aged 20 to 39, where prevalence rates approach 40% due to sedentary lifestyles and poor dietary habits established during the transition to higher education and professional life [1]. Beyond weight loss, current clinical concerns focus on the decline of functional capacity, reduced cardiorespiratory fitness, and the psychological impact of social stigma and depression, necessitating multidisciplinary interventions that combine structured exercise with health education [1, 2].

To address these challenges, the integration of mobile health (mHealth) and gamification offers a robust strategy by transforming exercise into a personalised and interactive

© The Author(s) 2026
M. Särestöniemi et al. (Eds.): NCDHWS 2026, CCIS 3009, pp. 501–504, 2026.
https://doi.org/10.1007/978-3-032-28812-7

experience [3]. By utilising real-time feedback, progress monitoring, and reward systems, these digital tools enhance intrinsic motivation and mitigate common barriers such as low adherence and lack of social support [3, 4]. Furthermore, digital platforms facilitate the delivery of effective high-intensity protocols, such as HIIT, which are proven to improve cardiorespiratory health and reduce visceral fat, providing a response tailored to the media preferences of contemporary young adults [2, 4].

The objective of this work is the development of an mHealth solution specifically designed to combat sedentary behaviour and promote active lifestyles. By empowering users in the self-management of their physical condition, the proposal uses structured exercise as a primary tool for obesity reduction and improved health-related quality of life. This application aims to provide continuous support, facilitating a sustainable transition from inactivity to a healthy lifestyle while integrating international physical activity recommendations.

2 Materials and Methods

The proposed solution results from a convergence between clinical exercise prescription and advanced gamification techniques, transforming traditional rehabilitation into an immersive and interactive experience [4]. "OBSCURA: Urban Mystery" distances itself from conventional fitness tools by adopting the structure of a serious game based on exploration and mystery. Unlike conventional approaches, the project utilises game mechanics that allow for training personalisation and increased active participation [4]. To mitigate the low retention rates typical of mHealth solutions, OBSCURA employs Meaningful Gamification [5]. According to Nicholson [5], this paradigm focuses on using game design to help users find personal meaning in an activity rather than relying on transient external rewards. Instead of superficial 'pointsification,' OBSCURA integrates the narrative as a core mediator where physical effort becomes a 'narrative necessity' for solving enigmas. This represents a strategic advancement in mitigating the lack of motivation and adherence—critical barriers identified in long-term interventions [3]. The immersion is further strengthened by Keller's ARCS Model [6] which foster sustained intrinsic motivation: Attention: Captured through the mystery aesthetic and evolving urban enigmas. Relevance: Exercise is presented as the essential tool for story progression, tailored to the digital preferences of young adults. Confidence: Built through a system of levels and achievements that allow users to control their own avatar's evolution. Satisfaction: Reinforced by social support dynamics and group missions, which are determining factors for well-being and long-term habit maintenance.

The core of the game rests on a narrative where story progression is intrinsically linked to the user's real physical activity, measured through motion sensors [4]. The user takes on the role of an investigator who needs to solve urban enigmas, with story advancement being tied to their actual physical activity. By walking or performing structured workouts, the user accumulates resources and unlocks clues on a virtual map of their city, transforming physical effort into an immediate narrative reward [3]. The interface uses aesthetic elements of mystery and exploration to increase immersion, ensuring that exercise is no longer perceived as an obligation but rather as an essential component of a playful experience. Gamification is implemented through a system of levels and achievements, where meeting health goals allows for avatar evolution, while social support dynamics enable collaboration in group missions—a determining factor for happiness and well-being.

The target audience consists of young adults, identified as a group at high vulnerability for developing sedentary behaviours and excess weight due to life transitions during this phase. This choice is justified by the need for early intervention before metabolic pathologies become chronic, taking advantage of this population's high digital literacy and familiarity with mobile devices [3]. By directing the tool at this audience, the project seeks to establish solid health habits using an interface adapted to the media preferences of young people.

The tool's effectiveness will be tested through a quasi-experimental single-group pilot study with pre- and post-intervention assessments. A convenience sample of 30 sedentary university students will be recruited to monitor: a) Physical Activity Levels: Measured via smartphone sensors (GPS/accelerometer) and the IPAQ-SF questionnaire. b) Clinical Indicators: Assessment of anthropometric data, specifically BMI, to address obesity reduction goals. c) Engagement and Retention: Tracking active participation and the sustainability of healthy behaviors through the game's social components.

3   Results and Discussion

It is expected that the implementation of this tool will result in a sustained increase in moderate-to-vigorous physical activity levels, a significant reduction in sedentary behaviours, and an improvement in the self-perception of happiness and life satisfaction within the target population. To monitor these results, engagement indicators (retention rates), physical activity levels (exercise minutes via sensors), and psychological well-being indicators will be utilised, employing instruments such as the WHO-5 Well-being Index to measure the impact on mental health.

Current evidence suggests that mHealth interventions are more effective when they incorporate gamification elements, which may have an impact on reducing the low adherence typical of conventional programmes. By using the game as a mediator, the perception of effort is reduced, and exercise begins to be seen as a playful activity, facilitating the sustainability of healthy behaviours. However, long-term effectiveness depends on the tool's ability to keep the user engaged after the initial novelty wears off, with the social component of the "OBSCURA" project being a crucial differentiating factor.

4   Conclusions

The development of gamified digital tools represents a paradigm shift in promoting health among young adults. By aligning physical activity recommendations with the technological preferences of this population, it is possible to create more sustainable interventions. The proposed project aims not only for weight reduction but for the promotion of global metabolic and mental health, demonstrating that technology is an indispensable ally in modern rehabilitation and in the fight against the obesity pandemic.

Disclosure of Interests.   The authors have no competing interests to declare that are relevant to the content of this article.

References

1. Jakicic, J.M., Rogers, R.J., Davis, K.K.: Physical activity and weight management. Nutr. Rev. **83**(S1), 45–56 (2025)
2. Hao, M., Glass, S.C., Reid, K.J., Ross, R.: Comparison of high-intensity interval training of different volumes on visceral fat and cardiometabolic risk in persons with obesity. J. Appl. Physiol. **135**(4), 845–855 (2023)
3. Schwarz, A., Winkens, L.H.H., de Vet, E., Ossendrijver, D., Bouwsema, K., Simons, M.: Design features associated with engagement in mobile health physical activity interventions among youth: systematic review. JMIR Mhealth Uhealth **11**, e40898 (2023)
4. Xu, L., Shi, H., Shen, M., Ni, Y., Zhang, X., Pang, Y., et al.: The effects of mHealth-based gamification interventions on participation in physical activity: systematic review. JMIR mHealth uHealth. **10**(2), e27794 (2022)
5. Nicholson, S.: A user-centered theoretical framework for meaningful gamification. Games+Learning+Society **8**(1), 1–22 (2012)
6. Keller, J.M.: Development and use of the ARCS model of instructional design. J. Instr. Dev. **10**(3), 2–10 (1987)

A Novel Smartphone App Increases Smoking Cessation, Participants' HRQoL and Cost-Effectiveness in LDCT Lung Cancer Screening of Heavy Smokers

Antti Kurtti[1,2]([✉]), Sanna Iivanainen[1,2], and Jussi Koivunen[1,2,3]

[1] University of Oulu, Oulu, Finland
antti.kurtti@oulu.fi
[2] Oulu University Hospital, Oulu, Finland
[3] FICAN North, Oulu, Finland

Keywords: smartphone app · lung cancer screening · smoking cessation · quality of life · cost-effectiveness

1 Introduction

Lung cancer is the main cause of cancer mortality in the Western world and smoking is the most important risk-factor for the disease [1]. Lung cancer screening of heavy smokers with low-dose computed tomography (LDCT) decreases lung cancer mortality while a smoking cessation intervention is highly recommended within screening programs as its efficacy may be enhanced in such a setting, although specific cessation methods are not well established [2–4].

The ubiquity of smartphones means new opportunities for scalable and individualized smoking cessation approaches. However, the effects of lung cancer screening, smoking cessation, and the use of smartphone apps on health-related quality of life (HRQoL) are widely unknown [5, 6]. An analysis of cost-effectiveness is crucial in considering the feasibility and implementation of cancer screening programs [7].

2 Materials and Methods

The study was a randomized controlled trial comparing two different smoking cessation methods in participants undergoing LDCT lung cancer screening. All study participants (n = 201) met the inclusion criteria: aged 50–74 years, heavy smoking history (smoked ≥15 cigarettes per day for ≥25 years or smoked ≥10 cigarettes per day for ≥30 years), an active smoking status, and access to a smartphone. Participants were randomized 1:1 to a yearly LDCT with standard smoking cessation (written material) or the standalone smartphone app–based cessation. Self-reported smoking cessation at three and six months were the primary endpoints of the study. HRQoL, an exploratory study end point,

© The Author(s) 2026

M. Särestöniemi et al. (Eds.): NCDHWS 2026, CCIS 3009, pp. 505–508, 2026.
https://doi.org/10.1007/978-3-032-28812-7

was assessed at baseline and at one year with Quality-of-Life Questionnaire Core 30 (QLQ-C30) and EQ-5D. Cost-effectiveness was analyzed using a Markov model to find the incremental cost-effectiveness ratios (ICER) for screening with smoking cessation application. Costs included the annual smoking cessation intervention, LDCT scans, and estimated diagnostic and treatment costs. Since no predefined willingness-to-pay threshold exists in Finland, a WTP of 50000$ was chosen based on literature.

3   Results

Participants randomized to the smartphone app arm had significantly higher rates of self-reported smoking cessation at three and six months (Table 1). Individuals with frequent use of the app had a higher chance for smoking cessation at three (p < 0.001) and six months (p = 0.003).

We did not detect a significant change in HRQoL between baseline and at one year using QLQ-C30 global health status score or EQ-5D index score, nor with achieving smoking cessation at one year in overall study population. However, improved HRQoL was observed by EQ-5D at one year in the app arm (improved in 17/93, 18% of controls vs 29/93, 31% in app arm). EQ-5D means at one year (Table 1). Furthermore, the app arm reported reduced pain (EQ-5D effect size [ES] 0.049; P = .01; QLQ-C30 ES 0.076; P < .001) and increased mobility (EQ-5D ES 0.031; P = .02) at one year. The number of completed questionnaires in the app was associated with improved HRQoL by EQ-5D (ES 0.073; P = .04; adjusted ES 0.071; P = .04).

The ICER of the screening program in standard-of-care arm was 28116$, and 12535$ in the app arm.

Table 1. Smoking cessation rates at three and six months, between arms of the study. SC = smoking Cessation, mo = month, oR = odds Ratio, CI = confidence Interval, y = year

	SC at 3mo % of group	OR for SC (95% CI)	p-value	SC at 6mo % of group	OR for SC (95% CI)	p-value	EQ-5D at 1y mean (SD)	p-value
App	19.8	3.2 (1.2–7.9)	0.010	18.8	2.8 (1.1–7.1)	0.021	0.8 (0.2)	0.007
Control	7.1			7.1			0.7 (0.2)	

4   Discussion

To our knowledge, our study is the first to report the results of a smartphone app–based smoking cessation in a randomized controlled trial setting among individuals participating in LDCT lung cancer screening and the associated effects on participants' HRQoL. The developed smartphone app improved smoking cessation 3-fold, surpassing the ORs of similar interventions [8]. Functionalities of the app include e.g. weekly questionnaires, and personalized feedback, meant to enhance goal setting, and personal empowerment to support smoking cessation as well as overall management of health. Interestingly, smoking cessation did not translate to altered HRQoL, contrary to what might have been expected. However, the participants in the app arm reported improved HRQoL, which mainly arose from decreased pain and increased mobility. Self-reported smoking cessation is widely used in smoking cessation trials, although, the reliability of the data could be increased with biochemical verification. However, the use of multiple timepoints increases the credibility of our results. Furthermore, in smoking cessation trials, an abstinence of one year is considered as a long-term outcome. The addition of smoking cessation app improved the cost-effectiveness of LDCT lung cancer screening markedly.

As greater extent of app use was associated with cessation success and improved overall HRQoL, this suggests that the app has a direct impact on the observed outcomes. Future efforts to amplify app adherence may further enhance the favorable effects on smoking cessation and HRQoL. Furthermore, the cost-effectiveness analysis indicated that the integration of the developed smoking cessation app lowered the ICER of LDCT lung cancer screening substantially.

5 Conclusions

In conclusion, the study showed that the developed smoking cessation app provides a feasible and effective smoking cessation intervention that is applicable in population-based lung cancer screening programs, with health benefits beyond mere smoking cessation as well as a chance for improving the overall cost-effectiveness of such screening programs.

Acknowledgments. The study was funded by Roche and AstraZeneca.

Disclosure of Interests. The authors have no competing interests to declare that are relevant to the content of this article.

References

1. Tesfaw, L.M., Dessie, Z.G., Mekonnen Fenta, H.: Lung cancer mortality and associated predictors: systematic review using 32 scientific research findings. Front. Oncol. **13** (2023). https://doi.org/10.3389/FONC.2023.1308897
2. de Koning, H.J., van der Aalst, C.M., de Jong, P.A., et al.: Reduced lung-cancer mortality with volume CT screening in a randomized trial. N. Engl. J. Med. **382**, 503–513 (2020). https://doi.org/10.1056/NEJMOA1911793
3. Wood, D.E., Kazerooni, E.A., Aberle, D., et al.: NCCN Guidelines® insights: lung cancer screening, version 1.2022. J. Natl. Compr. Cancer Netw. **20**, 754–764 (2022). https://doi.org/10.6004/JNCCN.2022.0036
4. Brain, K., Carter, B., Lifford, K.J., et al.: Impact of low-dose CT screening on smoking cessation among high-risk participants in the UK Lung cancer screening trial. Thorax **72**, 912–918 (2017). https://doi.org/10.1136/THORAXJNL-2016-209690
5. Taylor, G., et al.: Change in mental health after smoking cessation: systematic review and meta-analysis. BMJ **348** (2014). https://doi.org/10.1136/BMJ.G1151

6. Tomioka, H., Sekiya, R., Nishio, C., et al.: Impact of smoking cessation therapy on health-related quality of life. BMJ Open Respir. Res. **1**, 47 (2014). https://doi.org/10.1136/BMJRESP-2014-000047
7. ten Berge, H., Willems, B., Pan, X., et al.: Cost-effectiveness analysis of a lung cancer screening program in the Netherlands: a simulation based on NELSON and NLST study outcomes. J. Med. Econ. **27**, 1197–1211 (2024). https://doi.org/10.1080/13696998.2024.2404359
8. Sha, L., et al.: Automated digital interventions and smoking cessation: systematic review and meta-analysis relating efficiency to a psychological theory of intervention perspective. J. Med. Internet Res. **24** (2022). https://doi.org/10.2196/38206

Coverage and Utilization of Digital Healthcare Services: A Registry-Based Observational Study

Alexandra Dahlberg[1,2,3]($\boxtimes$) iD, Taavi Kaartinen[1,2,3], Sakari Jukarainen[2,3] iD, and Petja Orre[2,3] iD

[1] Harjun Terveys, Lahti, Finland
alexandra.dahlberg@harjunterveys.fi
[2] Faculty of Medicine, University of Helsinki, Helsinki, Finland
[3] Mehiläinen, Helsinki, Finland

Keywords: Digital Healthcare · Digital Healthcare Pathways · Telemedicine · Health Services Accessibility · Patient Demographics

1 Background

Chat-based digital clinics are increasingly integrated into public primary care systems, offering an additional modality for accessing healthcare services. However, there is limited real-world evidence on how their introduction affects overall service coverage and utilization across care modalities, as well as which population groups use these services. This study evaluated a 24/7 chat-based digital clinic integrated into Harjun terveys, Päijät-Häme, Finland.

2 Methods

The study utilized data from 2,796,975 primary care encounters recorded between 2019 and 2025 to examine patterns of care following the digital clinic's introduction. Outcomes included annual service coverage (proportion of residents with ≥ 1 encounter) and utilization (encounters per 1,000 residents), stratified by modality. Demographics (age, sex), comorbidity (Charlson Comorbidity Index [CCI]), and diagnostic profiles were compared using $\chi 2$ tests and t-tests (two-tailed, $P < .05$).

3 Results

Coverage increased from 36.5% in 2019 to 40.7% in 2025, and utilization rose from 1,211 to 1,567 encounters per 1,000 residents: digital clinic encounters accounted for 29.8% of all primary care encounters in 2025. During 2023–2025, the digital clinics patients were significantly younger than those utilizing only traditional healthcare services (mean age 33.5 vs 52.5 years; $P < .001$) and had fewer comorbid conditions (CCI $\geq$ 1: 11.3% vs

M. Särestöniemi et al. (Eds.): NCDHWS 2026, CCIS 3009, pp. 509–510, 2026.
https://doi.org/10.1007/978-3-032-28812-7

21.0%; $P < .001$). Coverage among adults$\geq$75 years remained near pre-pandemic levels, indicating a potential digital divide. Digital clinic encounters predominantly addressed minor acute conditions, including respiratory infections, general health maintenance or preventive issues, dermatologic conditions, and throat or eye complaints. Among digital physician consultations, common ICD-10 diagnoses included conjunctivitis, acute cystitis, and prescription renewal requests. Following a digital nurse consultation, 18.0% of patients received a same-day physician consultation and 14.0% had a new appointment booked. Excluding pre-scheduled follow-up, 5.2% had another encounter within 48 h, 16.8% within 14 days, and 23.4% within 30 days; most of these follow-ups were in person.

4 Conclusions

Findings indicate that an integrated digital clinic can broaden access and resolve a substantial share of minor acute conditions at the nurse-led level, with nearly half of care pathways terminating already without a digital physician consultation and the remainder efficiently triaged to appropriate follow-up. However, lower uptake among older adults and patients with chronic illnesses highlights the importance of developing targeted approaches to support engagement with digital services in these populations.

Disclosure of Interests. The authors declare the following competing interests: All authors are employed by Harjun terveys and/or Mehiläinen, the healthcare provider responsible for developing and operating the digital clinic evaluated in this study. Some authors hold personal financial interests in Mehiläinen. The study was funded by Mehiläinen, and the leadership of Harjun terveys provided institutional support throughout the research process.

Service Demand Predictive Models
in Well-Being Services Counties
Qualitative Research on Project Team Members' Experiences

Helmi Virtanen[✉]

Oulu University of Applied Sciences, Oulu, Finland
`helmi.virtanen@oamk.fi`

Abstract. Predicting future service demand is vital in healthcare for shaping health policies and ensuring the efficient use of health resources. While Knowledge Management (KM) offers a strategy for evidence-informed decision-making and resource efficiency, its full potential is often hindered by the fragmented nature of healthcare systems. KM must evolve from efficiency practices to effectiveness by fully leveraging existing data. Predictive Models (PMs) have been and are being developed in well-being services counties of Finland to support strategic planning and use of resources by offering nationally comparable information. Literature shows examples of PMs demonstrating high predictive accuracy, yet there is a widespread lack of validation and follow-up on model performance causing a need to determine the models' usefulness. For now, PMs are deployed to aid and assist medical staff locally, but in the future their integration is expected to grow, leading to more standardized and wide-spread use. The purpose of this research is to describe the experiences of project team members who have participated in developing service demand PMs in well-being services counties of Finland through qualitative research. The aim is to produce information that can be utilized in the future development of PMs, possibly improving the development process and/or outcomes. Preliminary results show recurrent themes in developing experiences, especially challenges within utilizing the PMs.

Keywords: Predictive Model · Knowledge Management · Service demand

1 Introduction

Despite enormous resources – an annual average of 10% of GDP worldwide – aimed at improving health, modern healthcare globally is said to be characterized by low quality [1], with costly results [2]. The healthcare sector is not optimized sufficiently and the use of services may be uncontrolled and coordinated by no-one [3, 4]. However, medical facilities are moving towards data-based healthcare together with its benefits [5] and the healthcare sector is being revolutionized by digital transformation with key services such as Artificial Intelligence (AI), Machine Learning (ML) and Big Data Analytics (BDA) [6]. One example is the developing of service demand Predictive Models (PMs) in well-being services counties of Finland, allowing to predict the development of service needs and its impact on costs. PMs serve the counties' long-term strategic planning and the need to allocate resources based on needs [7].

M. Särestöniemi et al. (Eds.): NCDHWS 2026, CCIS 3009, pp. 511–514, 2026.
https://doi.org/10.1007/978-3-032-28812-7

While Knowledge Management (KM) offers a strategy for evidence-informed decision-making and resource efficiency [8, 9], the healthcare system has been described as fragmented and driven by multiple interests, harming the sharing and efficient use of knowledge [10]. Accordingly, the WHO European Pro-gramme of Work emphasizes the critical need for countries to strengthen their health data and information systems to ensure that decisions are data driven and facilitate public health monitoring [11].

Cozzoli et al. [12] state that integrating large amounts of data and exploiting PMs and up-to-date views supports professionals and managers in decision-making processes. PMs are tools that predict future events or trends in populations by analyzing historical data with various algorithms. They are crucial in the healthcare system providing insights for strategic decision-making [13], significantly enhancing resource optimization, enabling accurate disease prevalence predicting and improving the identification of high-risk populations [14]. However, PM development faces challenges such as model performance, validation [13, 15] and data availability [16] in addition to ethical, legal and infrastructural challenges [14] and challenges regarding Big Data and its analysis since it is produced rapidly in huge quantities and varied formats [6, 17, 18].

2   Material and Methods

Qualitative research is a justified approach in this research as it aims to examine the experiences of project team members. The methodological choice is semi-structured interview, in which the interview questions are based on previous knowledge and offer a focused structure for the discussion during the interviews but are not meant to be followed strictly [19]. Here, a qualitative descriptive design is most appropriate as it recognizes the subjective nature of the problem, the different experiences participants have and presents the findings in a way that directly reflects or closely resembles the terminology used in the initial research question [20].

The target group is sampled based on knowledge and experience. Participants consist of project team members who have worked or are working on PM development projects in well-being services counties in Finland. The interviews are conducted with 3–4 wellbeing services counties that have developed PMs.

Once the data collection is complete around February 2026, the data is transcribed and sorted and ready for analysis. In this research we utilize qualitative content analysis which is very utilized in qualitative descriptive research. The analysis is built up inductively from a close reading of the texts rather than searching the text for a predetermined list of content items [21]. Qualitative descriptive research is purely data-derived in that codes are generated from the data through the research [22]. Analysis proceeds by grouping or coding the data and trying to identify similar patterns, phrases, themes, relationships and consequences to gradually form generalisations [23, 24].

3   Results

Preliminary results indicate that there have been multiple and partially similar challenges in the processes of developing PMs among the experiences. Difficulties in setting the goal, exploiting data and fulfilling the goal of utilizing the developed PM seem to be recurring themes. To some extent, challenges in resources or their use have been brought up. On the other hand, interesting and enlightening points have also been made regarding some recognized possibilities within the developing process. Additionally, there are plenty of utilizable and experience-based recommendations to consider in future PM development. A deeper analysis will be conducted during spring 2026 with conclusions and further discussion.

Acknowledgments. This study is not funded.

Disclosure of Interests. The author has no competing interests to declare that are relevant to the content of this article.

References

1. Djulbegovic, B., Hozo, I.: Threshold Decision-making in Clinical Medicine. vol. 189. Springer, Cham (2023). https://doi.org/10.1007/978-3-031-37993-2
2. Warda, E.R.: Does missing trust lead to overuse or underuse of health care services? Am. J. Manag. Care **29**(8) (2023). https://www.proquest.com/scholarly-journals/does-missing-trust-lead-overuse-underuse-health/docview/2852407548/se-2
3. Humphreys, P., et al.: An overview of hospital capacity planning and optimisation. Healthcare **10**(5), 826 (2022)
4. Koivisto, J., Tiirinki, H.: Monialaisen palvelutarpeen tunnistaminen sosiaali-, terveys ja työvoimapalveluissa. Valtioneuvoston selvitys- ja tutkimustoiminnan julkaisusarja **38** (2020)
5. Batko, K., Ślęzak, A.: The use of big data analytics in healthcare. J. Big Data **9**(1), 3 (2022)
6. Babar, M., Qureshi, B., Koubaa, A.: Review on federated learning for digital transformation in healthcare through big data analytics. Futur. Gener. Comput. Syst. **160**, 14–28 (2024)
7. THL. Sote-palvelujen johtaminen. Hyvinvointialueen palvelutarpeen ennakointityökalu
8. El-Jardali, F., et al: Knowledge management tools and mechanisms for evidence-informed decision-making in the WHO European Region: a scoping review. Health Res. Policy Syst. **21**(1) (2023)
9. Karamitri, I., Talias, M.A., Bellali, T.: Knowledge management practices in healthcare settings: a systematic review. Int. J. Health Plann. Manage. **32**(1), 4–18 (2017)
10. Kohn, M. S., Kush, R., Whalen, M., Tobin, M., Dori, D., Koski, G.: The Future of Health and Science: Envisioning an Intelligent HealthScience System. Pharm. Med. **37**(1), 1–6 (2023)
11. WHO: Knowledge management is key to public health planning, new study shows (2023). https://www.who.int/europe/news/item/13-11-2023-knowledge-management-is-key-to-public-health-planning--new-study-shows
12. Cozzoli, N., Salvatore, F.P., Faccilongo, N., Milone, M.: How can big data analytics be used for healthcare organization management? Literary framework and future research from a systematic review. BMC Health Serv. Res. **22**(1), 1–14 (2022)
13. Grøntved, S., Jørgine Kirkeby, M., Paaske Johnsen, S., Mainz, J., Brink Valentin, J., Mohr Jensen, C.: Towards reliable forecasting of healthcare capacity needs: a scoping review and evidence mapping. Int. J. Med. Informatics **189**, 105527 (2024)
14. Nwoke, J.: Healthcare data analytics and predictive modelling: enhancing outcomes in resource allocation, disease prevalence and high-risk populations. Int. J. Health Sci. **7**(7), 1–35 (2024)
15. de Ruijter, U.W., et al.: Prediction models for future high-need high-cost healthcare use: a systematic review. J. Gen. Intern. Med. **37**(7), 1763–1770 (2022). https://doi.org/10.1007/s11606-021-07333-z

16. Tavazzi, E., et al.: Artificial intelligence and statistical methods for stratification and prediction of progression in amyotrophic lateral sclerosis: a systematic review. Artif. Intell. Med. **142**, 102588 (2023). ISSN 0933-3657. https://doi.org/10.1016/j.artmed.2023.102588
17. Baro, E., Degoul, S., Beuscart, R., Chazard, E.: Toward a literature-driven definition of big data in healthcare. Biomed. Res. Int. **2015**, 1–9 (2015). https://doi.org/10.1155/2015/639021
18. Bellini, V., et al.: Machine learning in perioperative medicine: a systematic review. J. Anesth. Analg. Crit. Care **2**(1), 2 (2022). https://doi.org/10.1186/s44158-022-00033-y
19. Kallio, H., Pietilä, A., Johnson, M., Kangasniemi, M.: Systematic methodological review: developing a framework for a qualitative semi-structured interview guide. J. Adv. Nurs. **72**(12), 2954–2965 (2016). https://doi.org/10.1111/jan.13031
20. Bradshaw, C., Atkinson, S., Doody, O.: Employing a qualitative description approach in health care research. Glob. Qual. Nurs. Res. **2017**, 4 (2017)
21. Vears, D.F., Gillam, L.: Inductive content analysis: a guide for beginning qualitative researchers. Focus Health Prof. Educ. **23**(1), 2022 (2022)
22. Lambert, V.A. Lambert, C.E.: Editorial: qualitative descriptive research: an acceptable design. Pac. Rim Int. J. Nurs. Res. **16**(4), 255–256 (2012)
23. Doyle, L., McCabe, C., Keogh, B., Brady, A., McCann, M.: An overview of the qualitative descriptive design within nursing research. J. Res. Nurs. **25**(5), 443–455 (2020). https://doi.org/10.1177/1744987119880234
24. Elo, S., Kajula, O., Tohmola, A., Kääriäinen, M.: Laadullisen sisällönanalyysin vaiheet ja eteneminen. Hoitotiede **34**(4), 215–225 (2022)

Impact of XR-Based Training on Radiation Knowledge and Workflow Performance in Healthcare Professionals

Marja Jaronen[1]([✉]), Karoliina Paalimäki-Paakki[1,2], Adam Graham[1], Tanja Schroderus-Salo[2], Niko Männikkö[2], Tuulikki Keskitalo[3], Milla Immonen[3], and Kristina Mikkonen[1]

[1] University of Oulu, 90570 Oulu, Finland
marja.jaronen2@oulu.fi
[2] Oulu University of Applied Science, 90570 Oulu, Finland
[3] Lapland University of Applied Science, 96300 Rovaniemi, Finland

Keywords: Extended reality (XR) · Radiation safety · Healthcare professionals

1 Background

Extended reality (XR) technologies enable immersive, risk-free training for radiation protection by simulating real-world scenarios. Evidence indicates that XR-based training reduces occupational radiation exposure more effectively than traditional classroom instruction among interventional radiology and cardiology professionals [1, 2] XR offers manipulable environments, instant feedback, and visualisation of exposure consequences, supporting behavioural changes. Integrating XR into radiation safety education may enhance occupational safety and long-term compliance as well as patient safety. Furthermore, XR simulations provide an opportunity to practice workflow and teamwork in high-risk clinical environments [3].

This study investigates the impact of XR training on healthcare professionals' radiation-related knowledge and workflow performance.

2 Materials and Methods

Systematic searches of the CINAHL (EBSCO), ProQuest, PubMed, Scopus and Web of Science databases were conducted in May 2025. Search terms such as "extended reality", "radiation protection" and "competence" using the Boolean operator "AND" across all databases. The review considered studies that included healthcare workers (P), interventions evaluating extended reality (I), traditional safety training (C) and confidence in radiation safety as outcome (O). The systematic review was carried out in accordance with the JBI Reviewers' Manual. The Preferred Reporting Items for Systematic reviews (PRISMA) was utilized. Covidence tool (Covidence org.) was used to handle the scientific data (n = 14 386). After the screening process and quality appraisal, all nine studies

M. Särestöniemi et al. (Eds.): NCDHWS 2026, CCIS 3009, pp. 515–516, 2026.
https://doi.org/10.1007/978-3-032-28812-7

(n = 9) met the inclusion criteria. Due to the broadness of the research topic and the multidisciplinary data collection, all identified articles were included in the systematic review, and the results were presented as a synthesis.

3   Results

Integrating XR into radiation safety training improves healthcare professionals' confidence, reflecting better understanding and knowledge consolidation on radiation safety, while its intuitive and pedagogically relevant design encourages deeper learning. XR enhances both theoretical knowledge and practical skills, such as minimizing scattered radiation through visualization of radiation exposure. Additionally, XR training boosts confidence in teamwork, workflow, and communication, and improves procedural efficiency through feedback, thereby enhancing patient and occupational safety. This effect may be especially evident among less experienced team members, particularly in terms of communication.

4   Conclusion

XR's interactive, immersive nature offers a safe, effective tool for radiation protection education, providing realistic learning environment and instant visual feedback on radiation dose. Additionally, XR is an effective tool to optimize interprofessional workflow, teamwork and communication in a safe immersive environment. Although interventional radiology and cardiology are based on teamwork, XR can be used for education in a single-user or multi-user format. The rapidly evolving nature of XR in healthcare, with new applications and use cases emerging continuously, may limit the timeliness of the findings. As most of the included studies focused on single-user XR, further research is needed specifically on multi-user XR.

Acknowledgments. This study was funded by the European Union (DTRIP4H, No. 101188432).

Disclosure of Interests. The authors have no competing interests to declare that are relevant to the content of this article.

References

1. Khamis, K.K., Bello, A.S., Abdullahi, M.L.: Assessing the impact of virtual reality training on radiation dose reduction among interventional radiology nurses: a multicenter crossover study. J. Radiol. Nurs. **44**(3), 300–305 (2025). https://doi.org/10.1016/j.jradnu.2025.05.005
2. Tortora, M., et al.: Current applications and future perspectives of extended reality in radiology. Radiol. Med. (Torino) **130**(6), 905–920 (2025). https://doi.org/10.1007/s11547-025-02001-2
3. Fugelli, C.G., Hansen, B.S., Ersdal, H., Kurz, M.: Unveiling team needs: a qualitative study of simulation training for endovascular cerebral thrombectomy. BMJ Open Qual. **14**(3), e002981 (2025). https://doi.org/10.1136/bmjoq-2024-002981

Co-Teaching with Machines: Generative Artificial Intelligence in Healthcare Simulation-Based Education

Nicholas Wee Siong Neo[1]([✉]) [iD], Joko Gunawan[1] [iD], Tracy Levett-Jones[2] [iD], Eng Tat Khoo[3] [iD], Wei Ling Chua[1] [iD], and Sok Ying Liaw[1] [iD]

[1] Alice Lee Centre for Nursing Studies, Yong Loo Lin School of Medicine, National University of Singapore, Singapore, Singapore
nicholaswsneo@u.nus.edu
[2] Faculty of Health, University of Technology Sydney, Ultimo, NSW, Australia
[3] Engineering Design and Innovation Centre, College of Design and Engineering, National University of Singapore, Singapore, Singapore

1 Background

Generative artificial intelligence (GenAI) is increasingly used in healthcare simulation-based education to generate rich contexts and support individualized learning experiences. GenAI-simulated conversational agents offer greater interactivity and adaptability due to their exceptional natural language capabilities and contextual awareness, surpassing earlier rule-based systems constrained by pre-scripted branching logic. Despite these advantages, GenAI-enhanced simulation modalities remain in their early stages of development and empirical evaluation. This review aimed to explore the current state of GenAI use in simulation-based healthcare education through a comprehensive examination of GenAI types, applications and reported outcomes.

2 Materials and Methods

A scoping review was conducted utilizing the Joanna Briggs Institute's methodological guidance [1]. Six databases (Medline, CINAHL, Embase, Web of Science, PsycINFO, ERIC) were searched from their inception until 21 February 2025. A limited search for grey literature was also conducted on Proquest Dissertations and Theses Global and Google Scholar. The search strategy utilized the population, context and context framework, searching key terms such as "health personnel", "artificial intelligence", "simulation training" and "education". Simulation-based education activities were defined as activities that comprised of a simulation activity or scenario, with or without debriefing. The initial search yielded 2,355 records. After removing duplicates (n = 674), two independent reviewers screened 1,681 records at the title and abstract level, followed by full-text assessment 186 records. This review mapped study characteristics and GenAI-related features across included studies. Outcome measures were categorized based on the New World Kirpatrick Model, with all included studies reporting learning reactions (Level 1) and outcomes (Level 2). Benefits, limitations, and ethical considerations associated with GenAI use in healthcare simulation were also summarized.

M. Särestöniemi et al. (Eds.): NCDHWS 2026, CCIS 3009, pp. 517–518, 2026.
https://doi.org/10.1007/978-3-032-28812-7

3   Results

We included 28 articles that were published between 2023 and 2025. Included studies were predominantly situated within medicine (n = 14) and nursing (n = 10). An emerging trend towards the adoption of newer GPT-models and the integration of advanced GenAI functionalities via developer interfaces were observed. Several studies also reported on the use of prompt engineering strategies and testing frameworks. Across the simulation phases, GenAI was employed to design and develop simulation activities (n = 7), portray simulated characters (n = 16) and deliver automated feedback (n = 7). Only one study utilized GenAI-produced video backstories as part of pre-briefing, while another study supplemented instructor-led debrief with GenAI. Overall, GenAI-enhanced simulation was perceived as accurate, realistic and feasible (Kirkpatrick Level 1), with early evidence indicating benefits as an adjunct to conventional simulation and in improving knowledge, communication and non-technical skills (Kirkpatrick Level 2). Prior to transitioning to GenAI-enhanced modalities, simulation faculty and researchers should review the benefits and limitations identified in this review. Ethical considerations related to biases, privacy and security, accountability, copyright and equal access should also be considered. Finally, practice recommendations were identified to inform future GenAI-enhanced simulation research and innovations.

4   Conclusion

GenAI-enhanced simulation is increasingly being adopted and is likely to develop in parallel with human-facilitated simulation. Future works should focus on GenAI innovations in under-explored phases of simulation (e.g. pre-briefing, debrief), AI capacity building among simulation educators and hybrid intelligence approaches that integrate human and AI cognition. Further rigorous research is needed to establish best practices.

Acknowledgments. We would like to thank the review team for their dedication, support and expertise which facilitated the production of this interesting and timely work in the area of simulation-based education.

Disclosure of Interests.   The authors have no competing interests to declare that are relevant to the content of this article. This research did not receive any specific grant from any funding agency in the public, commercial or not-for-profit sectors.

Reference

1. Neo, N.W.S., Gunawan, J., Levett-Jones, T., Khoo, E.T., Chua, W.L., Liaw, S.Y.: Generative artificial intelligence in healthcare simulation-based education: a scoping review. Clin. Simul. Nurs. **108**, 101819 (2025). https://doi.org/10.1016/j.ecns.2025.101819

MetaHealth Infra and MetaHealth Infra Development Projects: Building an Immersive Digital Development and Testing Environment for the Health Sector

Mika Paldanius[(✉)] and Outi Kajula

Oulu University of Applied Sciences, Kiviharjuntie 4, 90220 Oulu, Finland
`mika.paldanius@oamk.fi`

Abstract. The MetaHealth Infra and MetaHealth Infra Development projects address the rapidly evolving competence requirements and innovation needs of the social and healthcare sector by establishing a comprehensive digital development and learning environment. The projects focus on the integration of immersive technologies, gamification, and artificial intelligence to support education, research, and business collaboration. The MetaHealth environment is designed to be mobile, scalable, and remotely accessible, enabling realistic simulation, product testing, and skills development across diverse healthcare contexts.

Keywords: Immersion · Gamification · Artificial intelligence

1 Introduction

Digital transformation in healthcare has created new demands for flexible learning environments and innovation infrastructures. Immersive technologies such as Virtual Reality, Augmented Reality, and Mixed Reality are increasingly applied in healthcare education and professional training [1–3]. Research highlights their potential to support experiential learning, observation, embodiment, and learner engagement, while also emphasizing the need for sustainable and accessible deployment models.

2 Project Overview and Objectives

The MetaHealth Infra project aims to develop a digital development and learning environment that supports future skills in healthcare. The environment is mobile, adaptable, and designed for remote access. The MetaHealth Infra Development project expands this foundation by establishing a structured business collaboration model, enabling cooperation between higher education institutions, research and development staff, healthcare professionals, and regional companies.

M. Särestöniemi et al. (Eds.): NCDHWS 2026, CCIS 3009, pp. 519–520, 2026.
https://doi.org/10.1007/978-3-032-28812-7

3 Implementation

Implementation activities include multidisciplinary workshops involving educators, healthcare professionals, and companies. Immersive scenarios are co-created to reflect authentic healthcare situations. The environment supports immersive simulation, gamification, remote access, portability, and collaboration, enabling safe testing and development of digital solutions.

4 Results and Impact

The projects have resulted in a unique digital learning and development environment that enhances innovation capacity and competence development. The MetaHealth collaboration model supports local companies in developing and scaling digital health solutions. The environment improves accessibility, supports low-carbon participation, and ensures sustainability beyond the project lifecycle.

5 Conclusion

The MetaHealth projects demonstrate how immersive and intelligent digital environments can support future healthcare education and innovation needs. The combination of technology, collaboration, and sustainability offers a transferable model for other regions and sectors.

Acknowledgments. This study was funded by the Council of Oulu Region from the European Regional Development Fund (ERDF).

Disclosure of Interests. The authors have no competing interests to declare that are relevant to the content of this article.

References

1. Morgado, L., Beck, D., O'Shea, P.: Bridging the gaps: an updated mapping of the uses of immersive learning environments. Virtual Real. **29**, 134 (2025). https://doi.org/10.1007/s10 055-025-01208-y
2. Ryan, G.V., Callaghan, S., Rafferty, A., Higgins, M.F., Mangina, E., McAuliffe, F.: Learning outcomes of immersive technologies in health care student education: systematic review of the literature. J. Med. Internet Res. **24**(2), e30082 (2022). https://doi.org/10.2196/30082
3. Ricci, S., Penza, V., Neri, F.: Editorial: VR, AR, MR in healthcare: the role of immersive technologies in medical training. Front. Digit. Health **7**, 1669899 (2025). https://doi.org/10.3389/fdgth.2025.1669899

Pioneering the Future of Healthcare: The Development and Implementation of an Interdisciplinary Master's Program in Digital Health in Japan - A Case of Regional University

Kakuya Kitagawa[✉], Yasuko K. Bando, Hiroharu Kawanaka, Yusuke Sugitani, and Hajime Sakuma

Mie University, Tsu-City, Mie 5148507, Japan
kakuya@med.mie-u.ac.jp

Abstract. To address the systemic pressures threatening the sustainability of Japan's healthcare system — including an aging population and chronic personnel shortages — Mie University has developed a novel interdisciplinary educational framework to cultivate "hybrid professionals" at the intersection of clinical practice and information technology. While the Japanese government has prioritized Medical Digital Transformation (DX), a persistent gap remains between IT development and clinical application.

This program bridges that divide by leveraging a regional digital health platform that enables students to engage in real-world projects and clinical implementation. The curriculum aims to produce "Problem-Solving Digital Medical Personnel" proficient in three core competencies: solution design, ethical and regulatory governance, and collaborative implementation.

The pedagogy utilizes a cross-disciplinary approach where medical and engineering students take courses in each other's fields, fostering a shared technical and clinical language. The training model progresses from theoretical foundations to practical On the Project Training (OPT), culminating in Master's theses derived from real-world clinical interventions. The effectiveness of the program is evaluated based on student project outcomes, competency assessments, and feedback from clinical implementation sites.

By integrating academic research with tangible regional needs, the program produces graduates capable of serving as health-tech product managers or clinical digital health coordinators. This practice-oriented model not only strengthens regional healthcare resilience but also provides a scalable blueprint for cultivating the digital talent essential for the future of healthcare.

Keywords: Digital health · Interdisciplinary education · Project-Based Learning

M. Särestöniemi et al. (Eds.): NCDHWS 2026, CCIS 3009, pp. 521–523, 2026.
https://doi.org/10.1007/978-3-032-28812-7

1 Introduction

1.1 Background and Rationale

To address systemic pressures threatening the sustainability of Japan's healthcare system - including an aging population, chronic personnel shortages, and regional disparities - Mie University has developed a novel interdisciplinary educational framework. This program cultivates a new generation of "hybrid professionals" at the intersection of clinical practice and information technology. While the Japanese government has prioritized Medical Digital Transformation (DX) in its '2024 Basic Policy,' a fundamental gap persists between IT developers and clinical practitioners [1, 2]. Successful DX requires more than just technical deployment; it necessitates a deep, mutual understanding of clinical workflows and technological capabilities.

Mie University's program is designed to bridge this communication gap, creating professionals capable of navigating both worlds. The program leverages a mature regional digital health platform [3] that enables students to engage in real-world projects and clinical implementations.

1.2 Program Design and Curriculum

The program aims to develop graduates who possess three core competencies:

Solution Design: Analyzing complex clinical needs to design and propose effective, technology-driven solutions.

Ethical and Regulatory Governance: Mastering the legal and ethical frameworks governing sensitive medical data to ensure secure, compliant implementations.

Collaborative Implementation: Leading the adoption of digital tools by facilitating collaboration among physicians, nurses, and administrators to optimize patient care.

Students from engineering backgrounds undertake medical electives (e.g., Clinical Medicine Overview), while those from medical backgrounds enroll in engineering courses (e.g., Mathematical Statistics & Multivariate Analysis). This cross-disciplinary approach ensures a shared language and foundational knowledge across cohorts.

1.3 Educational Approach and Implementation

The pedagogy systematically guides students from theory to research:

Fundamental Learning: Establishes theoretical foundations in AI, IoT, and data analysis using Problem-Based Learning (PBL) with guest lecturers from industry and clinical practice.

Practical Learning: Centers on On the Project Training (OPT). Students participate in real-world digital health projects and are responsible for specific tasks and project outcomes within multidisciplinary teams.

Research Activities: Students develop their Master's thesis directly from their OPT project outcomes, ensuring academic research contributes to solving tangible clinical problems.

The program effectiveness is evaluated through student project outcomes, competency assessments, and feedback from clinical implementation sites. Graduates earn a

Master of Digital Health. The program maintains a selective annual quota of 10 students to ensure high-quality, supervised OPT placements at Mie University Hospital and regional partner hospitals.

2 Anticipated Impact and Future Directions

2.1 Anticipated Impact

The program is expected to produce a significant return on investment by strengthening regional healthcare resilience through diverse career trajectories:

For IT Professionals: Graduates become health-tech product managers or AI engineers with a distinct competitive advantage rooted in clinical experience.

For Healthcare Professionals: Graduates return to clinics as Digital Health Coordinators or Medical Data Analysts, acting as catalysts for DX adoption.

Beyond individual careers, the program serves as a replicable blueprint for other regions. Its focus on regional networking, industry co-design, and project-based learning offers a scalable model for cultivating digital health talent nationwide.

2.2 Future Directions

The challenges facing Japan's healthcare system require professionals fluent in both medicine and technology. Mie University's Master's program in Digital Health is a practice-oriented response to this need. By immersing students in a proven ecosystem of regional collaboration, the program produces the architects of a digital healthcare future, ensuring that technological advancements translate directly into improved patient outcomes and a more resilient medical system.

Acknowledgments. This program is conducted in collaboration with the Organization for Research Initiative and Promotion, Mie University, as well as Mie University Hospital and its affiliated hospitals.

Disclosure of Interests. The authors have no competing interests to declare that are relevant to the content of this article.

References

1. Japan Cabinet Decision: Policy on Economic and Fiscal Management and Reform (2024). https://www5.cao.go.jp/keizai-shimon/kaigi/cabinet/honebuto/2024/2024_basicpolicies_en.pdf. Accessed 2026 Feb 03
2. Japan Cabinet Secretariat: Grand Design and Action Plan for a New Form of Capitalism (2024). https://www.cas.go.jp/jp/seisaku/atarashii_sihonsyugi/pdf/ap2024en.pdf. Accessed 2026 Feb 03
3. MUDX Initiative Homepage. https://mudx.jp/link. Accessed 2026 Jan 31

Industry-Driven Project-Based Learning in Digital Health Education

Raquel Simões de Almeida[✉] [iD], Vítor Simões-Silva [iD], and Maria João Trigueiro [iD]

LabRP/CIR, ESS, Polytechnic of Porto, Porto, Portugal
afa@ess.ipp.pt

Abstract. Preparing graduates for the fast-evolving field of digital health requires learning models that integrate theory and practice through authentic, interdisciplinary collaboration. This paper presents an industry-driven project-based learning (PBL) approach implemented in the Laboratory of Rehabilitation and Digital Health IV within the Digital Health Bachelor's Degree Program. Students work in diverse teams to design and develop digital health solutions addressing real-world challenges defined by industry mentors. The project integrates knowledge from multiple disciplines (data analysis and visualization, mobile health technologies, gamification, and digital rehabilitation) fostering creativity, teamwork, and problem-solving. The implementation emphasizes agile methods and iterative refinement supported by mentor feedback. Assessment comprises prototype development (60%) and public oral defense (40%), judged on innovation, technical quality, and communication. Results show high student motivation and strong performance, alongside significant engagement from external stakeholders. This case study shows how interdisciplinary, industry-linked PBL enhances practical competence, critical thinking, and innovation capacity, preparing students to meet the demands of the digital health sector.

Keywords: Digital Health · Higher Education · Pedagogy · Industry-Driven Approach · Project Based Learning · Interdisciplinary Learning

1 Introduction

The digital transformation of healthcare is reshaping professional roles and competencies, calling for innovative approaches to higher education. Digital health professionals must navigate complex, interdisciplinary environments that combine healthcare knowledge with data analytics, software development, ethics, design thinking, and patient-centered innovation [1]. Traditional education often remains siloed and content-based, providing limited opportunities for experiential learning and cross-disciplinary collaboration.

Project-based learning (PBL) has demonstrated value in addressing these gaps by promoting authentic, team-oriented, and problem-based experiences [2]. In the field of digital health, PBL provides a platform for integrating diverse perspectives (technical, clinical, and human-centered) while fostering innovation and professional readiness [3].

© The Author(s) 2026

M. Särestöniemi et al. (Eds.): NCDHWS 2026, CCIS 3009, pp. 524–526, 2026.
https://doi.org/10.1007/978-3-032-28812-7

Building on these pedagogical foundations, the Laboratory of Rehabilitation and Digital Health IV (LabRDH IV) was designed to bridge academia and industry through co-creation. This paper reports on the design, implementation, and preliminary outcomes of this educational intervention that took place in Porto, in the north of Portugal.

2 Materials and Methods

The LabRDH IV course was delivered in the second year of the Digital Health Bachelor Degree Program. The course structure was based on four key principles:

- Interdisciplinarity: intentionally diverse teams combined health and technology expertise.
- Authenticity: project themes reflected current industry and healthcare challenges, proposed by external mentors.
- Agility: iterative design and evaluation cycles promoted adaptability and reflection.
- Mentorship: professionals from partner organizations offered guidance and feedback throughout the process.

Students were introduced to agile project management, user research, and evidence-based design before forming teams. Projects incorporated knowledge from other curricular units (Data Analysis and Visualizations, Mobile Health Technologies, Gamification in Health, and Digital Technologies in Rehabilitation). Each team developed a functional prototype addressing a real-world issue (e.g. remote rehabilitation adherence, patient engagement through gamification, wearable health monitoring dashboards). Evaluation covered prototype quality (60%), assessing innovation, functionality, and design and an oral defense (40%) during a public seminar. Assessment criteria prioritized creativity, technical depth, user focus, and communication. Data sources included student grades, mentor feedback, and observation of student engagement.

3 Results and Discussion

Over three editions (2022–2025), the course consistently produced measurable improvements in student engagement and performance. Last academic year, grades ranged from 14.23 to 18.74 (mean = 16.88, SD = 1.39), scale 0 to 20, confirming high achievement across cohorts. Students reported increased confidence in applying digital health concepts, greater appreciation for interdisciplinary collaboration, and enhanced problem-solving autonomy. Several projects advanced beyond the academic context: one mobile application prototype for physical activity monitoring was tested in a clinical setting; another gamified intervention was incorporated into a partner rehabilitation center's innovation agenda. External mentors emphasized the realistic alignment of student outputs with ongoing sector demands.

These outcomes support prior findings that authentic, industry-linked PBL enhances motivation and creativity. Participation in public presentations and peer debates further strengthened professional identity and communication competence. Importantly, the iterative collaboration between academia and the digital health sector produced reciprocal benefits students gained contextual insight, while partners accessed fresh, evidence-informed prototypes for potential development. Departing from traditional passive and theory-heavy models, this active-learning approach replaces rote memorization with industry-aligned co-creation, shifting students from passive recipients to proactive innovators. Nevertheless, challenges included balancing group workload, harmonizing interdisciplinary terminology, and managing project scope within semester constraints. Future iterations will integrate digital collaboration tools and embed early-stage co-design workshops to optimize workflow.

4 Conclusions

The LabRDH IV initiative illustrates how an interdisciplinary and industry-driven project-based model can effectively prepare students for the multifaceted demands of digital health professions. By merging academic instruction with authentic industry challenges, the approach cultivates technical capability, empathy, and innovation, which key attributes for navigating the complexities of digital transformation in healthcare. Institutional investment in such pedagogical formats can strengthen employability pathways, while contributing to the broader digital health ecosystem through relevant, student-generated innovation.

References

1. Fagherazzi, G., Goetzinger, C., Rashid, M.A., Aguayo, G.A., Huiart, L.: Digital health strategies to fight COVID-19 worldwide: challenges, recommendations, and a call for papers. J. Med. Internet Res. **22**(6), e19284 (2020)
2. Naseer, F., Tariq, R., Alshahrani, H.M., et al.: Project based learning framework inte-grating industry collaboration to enhance student future readiness in higher educa-tion. Sci. Rep. **15**, 24985 (2025). https://doi.org/10.1038/s41598-025-10385-4
3. Ferreira, J.C., Elvas, L.B., Correia, R., Mascarenhas, M.: Empowering health professionals with digital skills to improve patient care and daily workflows. Healthcare **13**(3), 329 (2025). https://doi.org/10.3390/healthcare13030329

A User-Centred mHealth Approach to Remote Routine Management and Mental Health Promotion in Higher Education

Vitor Simões-Silva⬥, Maria João Trigueiro⬥, and Raquel Simões da Almeida⬥

CIR, ESS, Polytechnic of Porto, Porto, Portugal

Abstract. The transition to higher education is a critical developmental stage often marked by increased stress, challenges in time management, and vulnerability to mental health problems. Poor organisation of daily routines negatively impacts students' wellbeing and academic performance. Digital health interventions, especially mobile health (mHealth) tools, offer scalable opportunities for self-management and mental health promotion. This study aimed to define the functional and non-functional requirements of an mHealth solution to support routine management, self-regulation, and wellbeing in higher education students. A project-based methodology was implemented in two phases: (1) a systematic analysis of existing mobile applications for routine management; and (2) a qualitative focus group with seven university students using a semi-structured interview guide. Thematic content analysis guided data interpretation. Existing tools were found to be fragmented and mainly focused on scheduling. Three key components emerged: (1) a personalised digital calendar with visual analytics to improve time awareness; (2) a moderated peer-support forum to foster collaborative learning and social support; and (3) a learning module offering brief educational content on daily living skills, stress management, and wellbeing. Gamification elements were highlighted as essential to enhance engagement.

This mHealth proposal fills a gap in remote healthcare by integrating routine management, peer support, and health education into a unified and scalable digital platform.

Keywords: Digital health · mHealth · Remote healthcare · Routine management · Mental health promotion · Self-management

1 Introduction

The transition to higher education represents a major developmental milestone that is frequently associated with increased stress, reduced wellbeing, and heightened vulnerability to mental health problems [1, 2]. University students face significant changes in their daily routines, including increased academic demands, relocation, social network changes, and the need for greater autonomy [3, 4]. Empirical evidence consistently shows that difficulties in time and routine management are among the most common stressors experienced during this period, negatively affecting academic performance, mental health, and participation in daily life [5–7].

© The Author(s) 2026

M. Särestöniemi et al. (Eds.): NCDHWS 2026, CCIS 3009, pp. 527–530, 2026.

https://doi.org/10.1007/978-3-032-28812-7

Epidemiological data indicate that approximately one in three first-year university students presents symptoms of at least one diagnosable mental disorder, most commonly depression or anxiety [1]. Although pharmacological treatments play an important role, adherence remains challenging, often due to side effects and low illness insight [8]. Consequently, non-pharmacological and digital interventions have gained increasing relevance. Internet-based psychological interventions and mobile health (mHealth) applications have been recognised as effective, scalable, and low-cost strategies for mental health promotion and early intervention [9].

A systematic analysis of current market solutions (e.g., iStudiez, Time Tune, For-est) conducted in the initial phase of this study indicates that most existing mHealth apps for students focus narrowly on scheduling and task reminders. These tools offer limited support for holistic routine management, wellbeing, and the psychosocial adaptation required during the transition to higher education.

2 Objective

This study aimed to develop the functional and non-functional requirements for a mobile mHealth solution designed to support routine management, self-regulation, and wellbeing among higher education students, contributing to accessible and scalable remote healthcare delivery.

3 Methods

A project-based research methodology was adopted, comprising two sequential phases. First, a systematic search was conducted in digital repositories (IEEE Xplore, PubMed, Google Scholar) and app stores using the query: ("All Metadata": app) AND ("All Metadata": routines) AND ("All Metadata": students). This analysis focused on routine and time management because, according to the ICF (b1642), these are core mental functions; stabilizing these patterns is a foundational step for mental health promotion. Second, a qualitative focus group was held with seven students (aged 19–22) from various health programmes. Data were collected via a validated semi-structured guide, transcribed, and analyzed through thematic content analysis [10]. Ethical approval was granted by the ESS-P.Porto Ethics Committee (CE0109C/2022).

4 Results

The study identified three core integrated components for the mHealth solution:

- **Personalized Digital Calendar with Visual Analytics**: Allows task categorization by life domains using color coding. Visual feedback through graphs improves time awareness and self-regulation [11].
- **Moderated Peer-Support Forum:** A collaborative space for sharing experiences and peer knowledge. It promotes social connectedness, a critical protective factor during life transitions [12, 13].

- **Digital Learning Module (Digital Academy):** Offers brief educational content (videos and texts) on daily living skills and stress management. Knowledge reinforcement is provided through integrated quizzes [14, 15].

Additionally, gamification emerged as a transversal requirement, using points and rewards to enhance engagement and adherence to the platform [16].

5 Conclusion

This study proposes an integrated mHealth solution that addresses a critical gap in remote healthcare for higher education students. By combining routine management, peer support, and digital health education in a single mobile platform, the proposed tool has the potential to promote self-regulation, autonomy, and mental wellbeing. As a scalable, low-cost, and accessible digital health strategy, this solution contributes to the advancement of remote healthcare models tailored to young adult populations during key life transitions.

Disclosure of Interests. It is now necessary to declare any competing interests or to specifically state that the authors have no competing interests. Please place the statement with a third level heading in 9-point font size beneath the (optional) acknowledgments, for example: The authors have no competing interests to declare that are relevant to the content of this article. Or: Author A has received research grants from Company W. Author B has received a speaker honorarium from Company X and owns stock in Company Y. Author C is a member of committee Z.

References

1. RP Auerbach 2018 WHO world mental health surveys international college student project: prevalence and distribution of mental disorders J. Abnorm. Psychol. 127 7 623 638
2. Padovani, R.C., et al.: Vulnerability and psychological well-being of college student. Rev Bras. Ter. Cogn. **10**(1) 2014
3. Soares, A.B., dos Santos Mello, T.V., Baldez, M.D.O.M.: Vivências acadêmicas em estudantes universitários do Estado do Rio de Janeiro. Interação Em Psicologia **15**(1) (2011)
4. de Oliveira, C.T., Carlotto, R.C., Teixeira, M.A.P., Dias, A.C.G.: Oficinas de Gestão do Tempo com Estudantes Universitários. Psicologia: Ciência e Profissão **36**(1), 224–233 (2016)
5. BF Dear 2019 Examining an internet-delivered intervention for anxiety and depression when delivered as a part of routine care for university students: a phase IV trial J. Affect. Disord. 256 567 577
6. R García-Ros F Pérez-González J Pérez-Blasco LA Natividad 2012 Evaluación del estrés académico en estudiantes de nueva incorporación a la universidad Rev. Latinoam. Psicol. 44 2 143 54
7. S Michelato Yoshiy N Kienen 2018 Time management: a behavior analysis interpretation Psicol Educ. 47 67 77
8. A Semahegn K Torpey A Manu N Assefa G Tesfaye A Ankomah 2020 Psychotropic medication non-adherence and its associated factors among patients with major psychiatric disorders: a systematic review and meta-analysis Syst. Rev. 9 1 17
9. EB Davies R Morriss C Glazebrook 2014 Computer-delivered and web-based interventions to improve depression, anxiety, and psychological well-being of university students: a systematic review and meta-analysis J. Med. Internet Res. 16 5 e3142

10. V Braun V Clarke 2006 Using thematic analysis in psychology Qual. Res. Psychol. 3 2 77 101

11. SA Murray J Davis HD Shuler EC Spencer A Hinton 2022 Time management for STEMM students during the continuing pandemic Trends Biochem. Sci. 47 4 279 283

12. Camarero, C., Rodríguez, J., José, R.S.: An exploratory study of online forums as a collaborative learning tool. Online Inf. Rev. **36**(4), 568–586 (2012)

13. Jovenn, C., Subaramaniam, K., Jalil, A.: The development of a forum mobile application for students. In: 2019 IEEE 9th International Conference on System Engineering and Technology, ICSET 2019 - Proceeding, pp. 90–95 (2019)

14. P Cuijpers 2016 Psychological treatment of depression in college students: a metaanalysis Depression Anxiety 33 5 400 414

15. J Galante 2018 A mindfulness-based intervention to increase resilience to stress in university students (the mindful student study): a pragmatic randomised controlled trial Lancet Public Health 3 2 e72 e81

16. D Johnson S Deterding KA Kuhn A Staneva S Stoyanov L Hides 2016 Gamification for health and wellbeing: a systematic review of the literature Internet Interv. 6 89 106

Author Index